DIABETES: CURRENT PERSPECTIVES

DIABETES: CURRENT PERSPECTIVES

Edited by

D *John Betteridge,* BSc PhD MD FRCP
Consultant Physician UCL Hospital Trust, and
Professor of Endocrinology and Metabolism
University College London
Department of Medicine
Royal Free and University College Medical School
London W1N 8AA
UK

MARTIN DUNITZ

© Martin Dunitz Ltd 2000

First published in the United Kingdom in 2000 by
Martin Dunitz Ltd
The Livery House
7–9 Pratt Street
London NW1 0AE

Tel: +44 (0)207 482 2202
Fax: +44 (0)207 267 0159
E-mail: info@mdunitz.globalnet.co.uk
Website:http://www.dunitz.co.uk

A CIP catalogue record for this book is available
from the British Library

ISBN 1–85317–555–2

Distributed in the United States by:
Blackwell Science Inc.
Commerce Place, 350 Main Street
Malden MA 02148, USA
Tel: 1 800 215 1000

Distributed in Canada by:
Login Brothers Book Company
324 Salteaux Crescent
Winnipeg, Manitoba R3J 3T2
Canada
Tel: 1 204 224 4068

Distributed in Brazil by:
Ernesto Reichmann Distribuidora de Livros, Ltda
Rua Coronel Marques 335
03440–000 São Paulo–SP
Brazil

Composition by Scribe Design, Gillingham, Kent
Printed and bound in Great Britain by
Biddles Ltd, Guildford, Surrey

CONTENTS

List of contributors   vii

Preface   xi

Chapter 1   1
Diabetes: quantifying the burden for patients and health-care systems
Rhys Williams

Chapter 2   13
Genetics of diabetes: unravelling the complexities
Marco Giorgio Baroni, David Leslie, Paolo Pozzilli and Raffaella Buzzetti

Chapter 3   33
Prevention of Type 1 diabetes: what are the possibilities?
Polly Bingley and Nicky Leech

Chapter 4   53
Glucotoxicity: a role for protein kinase C activation?
Douglas Kirk Ways and George King

Chapter 5   67
Advanced glycation end-products: impact on diabetic complications
Alan W Stitt and Helen Vlassara

Chapter 6   93
Insulin resistance: the prime mover in Type 2 diabetes?
Eleuterio Ferrannini

Chapter 7   111
Impaired glucose tolerance and Type 2 diabetes: a role of obesity and leptin?
Asjid Qureshi and Peter Kopelman

Chapter 8   125
Diabetic dyslipidaemia: metabolic and epidemiological aspects
Francine V van Venrooij, Ronald P Stolk, Manuel Castro Cabezas and D Willem Erkelens

Chapter 9   141
Endothelial dysfunction
John Cockcroft and Jonathan Goodfellow

Chapter 10   165
New targets for the prevention and treatment of diabetic nephropathy
Paula Chattington and Mark Cooper

Chapter 11   179
The diabetic foot
Edward B Jude and Andrew JM Boulton

Chapter 12   197
Erectile failure: the complication 'that dare not speak its name'
Julian Shah

Chapter 13   209
Acute coronary syndromes: impact of diabetes on pathophysiology, outcome, and management
Laura Benzaquen and Richard Nesto

Chapter 14   223
Designer insulins: have they revolution-
ized insulin therapy?
David Owens and Anthony Barnett

Chapter 15   267
Insulin sensitizers: a new era in the
management of Type 2 diabetes
John J Nolan

Chapter 16   295
Optimal control of Type 2 diabetes:
current and future prospects
*Robert J Heine, Jeroen JJ de Sonnaville and
Stephan JL Bakker*

Chapter 17   317
Optimum dietary approach in Type 2
diabetes
Joyce Barnett and Abhimanyu Garg

Chapter 18   341
Patient self-empowerment: the route to
improved clinical outcome and patient
satisfaction
John Day

Index   355

List of contributors

Stephan JL Bakker MD
Internist–Diabetologist, Department of
Endocrinology, Academic Hospital Vrije
Universiteit, 1007 MB Amsterdam, The
Netherlands

Anthony Barnett BSc, MD, FRCP
Professor of Medicine, Department of
Medicine, University of Birmingham and
Birmingham Heartlands Hospital,
Birmingham B9 5SS, UK

Joyce Barnett MS, RD/LD
Department of Clinical Nutrition, The
University of Texas Southwestern Medical
Center at Dallas, Dallas, Texas, TX 75235,
USA

Marco Giorgio Baroni MD, PhD
Department of Clinical Science, Division of
Endocrinology, University 'La Sapienza' of
Rome, 00161 Rome, Italy

Laura Benzaquen MD
Cardiovascular Division, Beth Israel
Deaconess Medical Center, Harvard
Medical School, Boston, MA 02215, USA

Polly Bingley MD, FRCP
Senior Lecturer in Diabetic Medicine,
University of Bristol, Diabetes and
Metabolism, Medical School Unit,
Southmead Hospital, Bristol BS10 5NB, UK

Andrew JM Boulton MD, FRCP
Professor of Medicine, M7 Records,
Department of Medicine, Manchester Royal
Infirmary, Manchester M13 9WL, UK

Raffaella Buzzetti MD
Department of Clinical Science, Division of
Endocrinology, University 'La Sapienza' of
Rome, 00161 Rome, Italy

Manuel Castro Cabezas MD, PhD
Department of Internal Medicine,
University Hospital Utrecht, 3584 CX
Utrecht, The Netherlands

Paula Chattington MD, MBChB
Specialist Registrar in Endocrinology,
University Hospital Aintree, Liverpool,
UK

John Cockcroft FRCP
Senior Lecturer in Cardiology, Department
of Cardiology, Wales Heart Research
Institute, and Honorary Consultant
Cardiologist, University of Wales College of
Medicine, Cardiff CF4 4XN, UK

Mark Cooper MD
Associate Professor, Austin and
Repatriation Medical Centre, Repatriation
Campus, University of Melbourne, West
Heidelberg, Victoria 3081, Australia

John Day MD, FRCP
Consultant Physician, The Diabetes Centre,
Department of Medicine, The Ipswich
Hospital NHS Trust, Ipswich, Suffolk IP4
5PD, UK

D Willem Erkelens MD
Professor and Chairman, Department of Internal Medicine, University Hospital Utrecht, 3584 CX Utrecht, The Netherlands

Eleuterio Ferrannini MD
Professor of Internal Medicine, Department of Internal Medicine, University of Pisa School of Medicine, and Chief Metabolism Unit, CNR Institute of Clinical Physiology, 56100 Pisa, Italy, and Adjunct Clinical Professor of Medicine, University of Texas Health Science Center at San Antonio, San Antonio, Texas, USA

Abhimanyu Garg MD
Associate Professor of Internal Medicine, The Center for Human Nutrition, and Associate Program Director, General Clinical Research Center, The University of Texas Southwestern Medical Center at Dallas, Dallas, Texas, TX 75235, USA

Jonathan Goodfellow MD
Senior Lecturer in Cardiology, Department of Cardiology, Wales Heart Research Institute, University of Wales College of Medicine, Cardiff CF4 4XN, and Consultant Cardiologist, Princess of Wales Hospital, Bridgend, Mid Glamorgan CF31 1RQ, UK

Robert J Heine MD, PhD
Professor of Diabetology, Department of Endocrinology, Academic Hospital Vrije Universiteit, 1007 MB Amsterdam, The Netherlands

Edward B Jude MD, MRCP
Clinical Research Fellow, M7 Records, Department of Medicine, Manchester Royal Infirmary, Manchester M13 9WL, UK

George King MD
Senior Investigator and Section Head, Section on Vascular Cell Biology, Joslin Diabetes Center, and Professor of Medicine, Harvard Medical School, Boston, MA 02215, USA

Peter Kopelman MD, FRCP
Professor of Clinical Medicine, St Bartholomew's and the Royal London School of Medicine and Dentistry, London E1 2AD, UK

Nicky Leech MD, MRCP
Clinical Lecturer in Medicine, University of Bristol, Diabetes and Metabolism, Medical School Unit, Southmead Hospital, Bristol BS10 5NB, UK

David Leslie MD, FRCP
Professor, St Bartholomew's and the Royal London School of Medicine and Dentistry, Department of Diabetes and Metabolism, Dominion House, London EC1A 7BE, UK

Richard Nesto MD
Cardiovascular Division, Beth Israel Deaconess Medical Center, Associate Professor of Medicine, Harvard Medical School, Boston, MA 02215, USA

John J Nolan BSc, FRCPI
Consultant Endocrinologist, St James's Hospital, Dublin 8, Ireland

David Owens MD, FRCP, FIBiol.
Professor and Consultant Diabetologist, Diabetes Research Unit, Department of Medicine, Academic Centre, Llandough Hospital, Penarth, South Glamorgan CF64 2XX, UK

Paolo Pozzilli MD
Professor, University of Rome 'Tor Vergata' and Campus Biomedico, Rome, Italy

Asjid Qureshi MB, MRCP
Specialist Registrar, St George's Hospital, Tooting, London SW17 0RE, UK

Julian Shah FRCS
Senior Lecturer, Academic Unit, Institute of Urology and Nephrology, UCL Medical School, London W1P 7PN, and Consultant Urologist to St Peter's Hospital at the Middlesex Hospital and to the Spinal Cord Injuries Unit, Royal National Orthopaedic Hospital, Stanmore, Middlesex, UK

Jeroen JJ de Sonnaville MD, PhD
Internist–Diabetologist, Department of Endocrinology, Academic Hospital Vrije Universiteit, 1007 MB Amsterdam, The Netherlands

Alan W Stitt PhD
Lecturer in Ophthalmology, Department of Ophthalmology, School of Clinical Medicine, The Queen's University of Belfast, The Royal Victoria Hospital, Belfast BT12 6BA, Northern Ireland

Ronald P Stolk MD, PhD
Julius Centre of Patient-Oriented Research, University Hospital Utrecht, 3584 CX Utrecht, The Netherlands

Francine V van Venrooij MD
Department of Internal Medicine, University Hospital Utrecht, 3584 CX Utrecht, The Netherlands

Helen Vlassara MD
Director, Division of Experimental Diabetes and Aging, Department of Geriatrics, Mount Sinai Medical Center, New York, NY 10029, USA

Douglas Kirk Ways MD, PhD
Senior Clinical Research Physician, Lilly Research Laboratories, A Division of Eli Lilly Company, Lilly Corporate Center, Indianapolis, IN 46285, USA

Rhys Williams MA, PhD, FFPHM, FRCP
Professor of Epidemiology and Public Health at the University of Leeds, Nuffield Institute for Health, Leeds LS2 9PL, UK

Preface

The importance of diabetes mellitus as a major cause of mortality and morbidity and its claim on healthcare provision is increasingly recognized not only in developed countries but also in developing countries. The International Diabetes Federation estimates the worldwide prevalence at over 143 million with projections to 300 million by 2025.

It is only relatively recently that major end-point trials, DCCT and UKPDS, have facilitated evidence-based strategies for glycaemic control in diabetic patients, which should reduce mobidity particularly from microvascular complications. The prevention of atherosclerosis-related disease remains a major challenge and the importance of multirisk factor approach is accepted.

This book is designed to highlight important areas in the pathophysiology of diabetes and its complications together with a particular focus on common clinical problems and newer therapies. Moving from epidemiology and genetics to potential mechanisms of tissue damage, in-depth considerations of neuropathy, the diabetic foot, erectile failure and acute coronary syndromes, newer therapies and patient empowerment, this book will provide up-to-date, highly readable reviews of topics of current interest not only to diabetologists and endocrinologists but also general physicians, cardiologists and basic scientists.

I would like to thank the contributors for their enthusiastic support of this project and for their prompt delivery of manuscripts. As always the publishers Martin Dunitz have been highly efficient and helpful, and grateful thanks are due to Alan Burgess and Mike Meakin.

Finally, this book is dedicated to the dogged determination of our patients who despite the shadow of diabetes continue to live life to the full and to the physicians and other members of the team who have the privilege of looking after them.

1

Diabetes: quantifying the burden for patients and health-care systems

Rhys Williams

Life with diabetes – background and terminology

Most health professionals have some insight into what it is like to live with diabetes. The depth of that insight will vary depending on the extent of their contact with patients who have diabetes, the rapport they are able to create and sustain with them and, of course, whether they themselves have diabetes or live with someone who has. It has been said that there are *four* types of diabetes – Types 1 and 2, already recognized, 'type 3 diabetes' – that experienced by the relatives and friends of those affected – and 'type 4 diabetes' – that affecting professionals who specialize in diabetes care. No one who has close contact with diabetes can escape its influence.

The terms 'cost', 'burden' and 'impact' have, in some senses, similar meanings in the context of describing the effects of disease. 'Cost', though usually taken to imply financial consequences, is used more widely than this in the field of health economics. Some of the costs of diabetes may be readily translated into financial terms. Examples of this are the direct costs of diabetes to health care systems or the 'out-of-pocket' costs of diabetes to the individual and family (both of which will be dealt with later). Less easily translated into financial terms are the 'indirect costs' of diabetes to society – the effects, in terms of lost production, of diabetes-related sickness absence from work, disability, premature retirement, or death during an individual's 'economically active' years. Of even greater difficulty in terms of quantification are the 'intangible costs' – those resulting from the anxiety, discomfort, pain, guilt, and other emotions associated with having the disorder or living with someone who has.

The term 'burden' can also be used to describe the effects of a disease on the individual, the family, and on society. It has the useful implication that the effects are reversible. If the burden can be reduced or cast aside completely then the individual, family, or society will be the lighter for it. 'Impact' is perhaps an even better term because this can be positive as well as negative. As will be mentioned below, there are reasons to suppose that, in certain circumstances, having diabetes *might* be of some advantage to the individual and perhaps to the family.

The theme chosen for World Diabetes Day 1999 – the costs of diabetes – is an indication that there is considerable current interest in quantifying the costs, burden or impact of diabetes. This interest is likely to be most productive if the widest possible connotations are placed on these terms – the costs, burden, and impact with regard to individuals, families, and societies; the financial and non-financial costs; the existing and preventable burden; and the positive as well as negative impact.

Living with diabetes – psychosocial effects on the person with diabetes

There are a number of accounts of the personal burden of having diabetes. Wainwright,[1] for example, from the point of view of a person with diabetes, comments on three main areas – psychological, social, and financial. These are summarized in *Table 1.1*. Although Wainwright lists a number of ways in which these psychosocial costs are manifest, it is interesting that fears of the longer term consequences of diabetes – blindness, renal failure, leg ulceration, amputation, and ischaemic heart disease – are not at all emphasized. It is the shorter term consequences, particularly hypoglycaemia, that dominate in his account.

Kangas[2] (like Wainwright, a person with long-standing insulin-dependent diabetes) provides another individual perspective. In this he emphasizes the crucial role of the affected individual in obtaining metabolic control through behavioural change. Health-care professionals, as he says, 'can, at best, only be advisers'. Central to his statement is the concept of 'empowerment' – 'giving people with diabetes the knowledge and other things they need to manage their disease'. The key to empowerment, in his opinion, is education – a notion which is, to a certain extent, borne out by the evidence.

The somewhat conflicting nature of the current evidence on the psychosocial impact of

Area of costs	Details
Psychological	Feeling 'different'
	'Continual and added responsibility for caring for oneself'
	Fear of hypoglycaemia
	Potential for obsessive behaviour
	Concern about long-term complications*
Social	Restricted lifestyle – the result of the need to inject with insulin, take regular meals etc.
	Restricted range of employment
	Potential restrictions on driving
Financial	Costs of additional episodes of health care
	Time away from work to attend these episodes or for sickness absence
	Purchase of insulin, drugs, and blood and urine testing equipment
	Additional costs of diet
	Extra costs of special footwear
	Higher premiums for health and other insurance

* Brief mention only in the original article.

Table 1.1
The costs of having diabetes (adapted from Wainwright[1]).

diabetes on affected children, both as children and when they become adults, has been well summarized by Jacobson *et al*.[3] As they point out, some studies (e.g. Dunn and Turtle[4]), including some of their own,[5,6] have claimed that experiences of low self-worth, distress or alterations in personality are no commoner in young people with diabetes than would be expected. On the other hand, other studies have described adolescents with Type 1 diabetes as more socially isolated,[7] having lower levels of well-being[8] and an increased prevalence of eating disorders[9] compared with people of the same ages without diabetes. In their own study,[3] a 10-year follow-up of children and adolescents with Type 1 diabetes, the most striking findings were the lower perceived individual competence, negative views on physical appearance and on sociability, and lower global self-worth.

A number of explanations are possible for the conflicting results in this area of research. First, it is an area in which the basic instruments of measurement – psychometric scales for the assessment of well-being, self esteem, competence, and so on – are being rapidly developed and refined. It is a complex and methodologically difficult area in which the validity, reliability, and transferability of instruments from population to population need particularly careful attention.[10]

Secondly, several of the studies available in the literature are on comparatively small groups of subjects studied once or on a few occasions only. This is partly a consequence, of course, of the complexity of the measurements required and the limited resources available. Given that variability, both intra-individual and inter-individual, is likely to be considerable, small samples studied in this way will give rise to contrasting results.

Added to the above, there are likely to be cross-cultural differences in the responses of children and adolescents to their own diabetes, and there may be secular changes, with different cohorts of people experiencing different psychosocial consequences of diabetes. Methods of treatment and support change over time, as do public knowledge about diabetes and the attitudes of society towards it. It is likely that individuals' attitudes to their own diabetes will be changed as a result.

A particularly striking example of cross-cultural differences are the findings of Shobhana.[11] She carried out a detailed psychometric study of 150 children and adolescents with diabetes in Madras, India, with comparison groups consisting of 44 of their non-diabetic sibs and 109 non-diabetic children of ages similar to those of the affected subjects. The children affected by diabetes showed significantly *better* psychosocial adjustment than both comparison groups, except for interpersonal relationships, where no differences were found. The diabetic children had significantly *lower* scores on the depression inventory (Children's Depression Inventory) (i.e. they were less depressed).

Although studies from Western populations have failed to show differences (see above), none have reported positive effects of having diabetes. Shobhana's interpretation of these findings was that, at least for the 150 children receiving diabetes care in the Madras Centre, the diagnosis of diabetes had positive effects because of more parental attention and better nutrition, general care, education, and counselling compared with their non-diabetic sibs and peers.

Adults with diabetes have also been studied. Karlson and Agardh,[12] in their study of 200 people (mean age around 35 years) with Type 1 diabetes in Sweden, obtained postal questionnaire data from 155 of them. The essence of their findings was that there were 'modestly elevated' degrees of depression in the 155 diabetic subjects compared with non-diabetic subjects. The instrument used was part of the Symptom Check List SCL-90. Their finding of a lack of association between measures of metabolic control and self-reported burden of illness is perhaps not surprising, as is their finding that self-reported burden of illness was strongly (and positively) related to depression. Their subjects with the lowest HbA_{1c} levels were significantly worried about long-term complications. It is difficult to judge from this whether the intermediate outcome of good metabolic control is, at least in part, causally linked to the concern about complications or whether both are the result of a particular outlook on the disease and life in general. The authors are appropriately cautious about this aspect of their conclusions. Those with poor metabolic control were found to have depressive symptoms related to their difficulties with achieving good control.

Living with diabetes – psychosocial effects on relatives

An interesting and potentially important facet of the psychosocial impact of diabetes is the impact, not on patients themselves, but on their relatives. Gonder-Frederick and colleagues[13] have explored this in relation to the impact of severe hypoglycaemia on the spouses of people with Type 1 diabetes.

The study subjects chosen for their investigation were the spouses of 67 people with Type 1 diabetes who themselves were taking part in a study of behavioural interventions aimed at improving their ability to 'recognize and prevent blood glucose extremes'.[14] Eight of the spouses who were invited to participate refused. Of the remaining 61, 41 had diabetic partners

who had not reported severe hypoglycaemia in the previous year, while 20 were married to partners who had had at least one such episode. In the first of these groups, 16 were wives and 25 were husbands. In the second, seven were wives and 13 were husbands. (It is interesting that the paper includes only married couples and no unmarried partnerships. Given that recruitment took place fairly recently and that the mean age of those who took part was under 40, this is somewhat surprising.)

Some of the results of this study are predictable in that spouses in the second of the above groups (those whose diabetic spouses reported hypoglycaemia) showed significantly more fear of hypoglycaemia, more marital conflict about diabetes management and more sleep disturbance caused by hypoglycaemia than those in the first group. What is noteworthy, however, is that spouses of diabetic subjects who had reported severe hypoglycaemia showed greater fear of the possibility of hypoglycaemic episodes than did their diabetic husband or wives. Also, important from the methodological point of view, all of the group differences that were apparent between the two groups were noted in the diabetes-specific measures. These were the 'Diabetes conflict' subscale of the Dyadic Adjustment Scale (DAS) of Spanier,[15] the 'Behaviour subscale' of the Hypoglycaemia Fear Survey (HFS),[16] the 'Worry subscale' of the HFS, and a three-item sleep disturbance scale developed specifically for the study. None of the generic instruments or subscales identified differences between the two groups of spouses.

Financial costs to the individual and family

Whether the financial costs of diabetes care fall mainly on the state health sector, on health

Income group	Patients attending a government general hospital	Patients attending a private hospital for diabetes
High	0	8.9
Upper middle	0	8.8
Middle	1.0	18.8
Low	3.3	53.5

Table 1.2
Percentages of family incomes spent on diabetes care – patients attending two hospitals in Madras (adapted from reference 17).

insurance companies, or on the individual and the family depends on the particular health-care funding mechanism which applies in that instance. Ironically, where the individual and the family have to pay, 'out-of-pocket', these costs may fall heaviest on those who can least afford it. There is not much published evidence on this for developing countries, but Shobhana et al.,[17] again studying individuals with diabetes treated in Madras, have collected data which strongly suggest that this is the case. They interviewed 174 patients attending a government general hospital and 322 attending an independently financed private hospital for diabetes. Amongst other things, the interviews with these subjects covered the contributions made from their families' incomes to the treatment of their diabetes. *Table 1.2* presents the most important finding from this study – that the proportion of each family's income which was devoted to the care of their diabetic member was significantly higher in the 'low-income' families than it was in the other groups. The irony is further compounded by the fact that, in the government hospital group, although most of the subjects did not contribute to their treatment out of their own family's income, the few that did were found in the poorer income groups.

In the USA, Songer et al.[18] have investigated patterns of financial outlay on diabetes care in the families of children with diabetes (identified through the Allagheny County IDDM Register) compared with families with children of the same age without diabetes. As would be expected, families with the lowest household incomes were those which were least likely to have health insurance cover. Even for those who had insurance cover, many (10%) had no reimbursement for insulin or syringes or for blood testing strips (30%). The amount of their income that families with diabetic children devoted to health was 56% higher than for families with no child with diabetes. Again, as in the Madras study, the family financial burden inflicted by diabetes was highest in the low-income families.

Kangas[19] has made an interesting observation on the personal costs of the disease and its relationship to the proportion of the burden taken up by the state. He has calculated that the time spent by each person in Finland with Type 1 diabetes in managing his or her condition (blood testing, injecting with insulin, attending for follow-up care, etc.) can be costed at US$2,500 per person per year. The implication from his findings is that the motivated, empowered person with diabetes contributes a substantial amount of his or her own resources to diabetes management, even when, because of the state-funding health-care system, they do not contribute 'out-of-pocket' expenses. This is a fact that is frequently not recognized in economic studies of diabetes.

Diabetes and the health-care sector

A clutch of recent papers from the group working in Cardiff, UK[20–24] has added considerably to our understanding of the burden of diabetes on the acute health-care sector. Their estimates are likely to be more precise than those previously published from the UK because they have been able to overcome some of the known deficiencies of routine hospital data in the UK[25] by linking a number of local databases. These were the hospital in patient and out patient databases for all hospitals in their district and a primary care database constructed during a district-wide audit of diabetes care. Thus, they were able to overcome the problem of known under-recording of the diagnosis of diabetes in a substantial number of hospital episodes.[25] After having ascertained all

relevant hospital admissions using these databases, they were able to report that 45% of them would have remained unrecognized as being for people with diabetes if they had relied on the hospital information system alone.

Their exclusive concentration on acute sector activity was determined by the availability of validated data, but this is not a major drawback since hospital costs are, by far, the largest single element in direct health-care costs[26] and the acute sector bears the main brunt. Their findings are summarized in *Tables 1.3a* and *1.3b*. The relative risk estimates shown in *Table 1.3a* are not adjusted for age (though age-specific data are reported in the paper[20] from which they are taken). *Table 1.3b* shows, for selected age groups, the numbers of admissions and numbers of bed days in one year (1994/95) for people with and without diabetes. Also shown are their estimates for the mean cost of each stay, using nationally available cost weightings[27,28] associated with the relevant diagnosis-related groups (DRGs) within the case mix of each age group's admissions.

Table 1.3a

Main findings of Currie et al.[20–24] on acute health sector usage by people with diabetes compared with people without diabetes: relative risks of admission to hospital.

Reason for admission (ICD* 9 codes)	Relative risk†	95% confidence interval
Coronary heart disease (401–428)	11.8	11.4–12.3
Cerebrovascular disease (434–438)	11.8	10.8–12.8
Neuropathy and peripheral vascular disease (354–447)	15.6	13.6–17.9
Eye complications (362–366)	10.4	9.3–11.7
Renal disease (581–586)	14.7	12.6–17.3

* ICD = International Classification of Diseases.
† Relative risk calculated with reference to non-diabetic population of the district.

Table 1.3b
Main findings of Currie et al.[20–24] on acute health sector usage by people with diabetes compared with people without diabetes: excess use and costs of hospital in-patient facilities (selected age groups; 1994/95).

Age group (years)	No. of admissions		No. of bed days		Mean LOS (days)		Mean cost (£)	
	Diab	Non-diab	Diab	Non-diab	Diab	Non-diab	Diab	Non-diab
10–14	57	2,697	230	4,442	4.0	1.6	1,065	894
40–44	194	4,682	727	12,293	3.7	2.6	1,163	1,074
60–64	753	5,375	9,261	27,450	12.3	5.1	1,520	1,336
80–84	746	5,992	22,487	144,362	30.1	24.1	1,707	1,557

Most work on the direct costs of diabetes to the health-care sector has been carried out in the USA. Songer[29] has summarized the estimates made in that country from 1969 to 1992. These studies, with the addition of the more recently published American Diabetes Association (ADA) study,[30] are summarized in *Fig. 1.1*. This figure also contains estimates of indirect costs (see below) set beside those for direct costs in the same years.

The direct health-care cost estimates increase markedly from the US$1 billion reported in 1969 to the US$44.1 billion reported by the ADA in 1997. Inflation and an increased prevalence of clinically diagnosed diabetes over this time period might, quite reasonably, be postulated as two contributory factors to this increase. Recent work by Songer and Ettaro[31] has shown that, when these estimates are corrected for the effects of inflation and

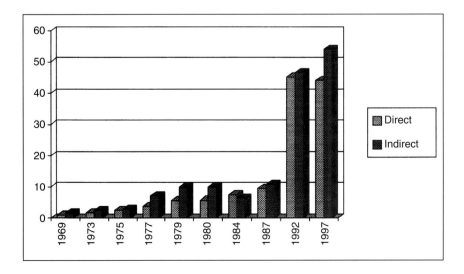

Fig. 1.1
Estimates of direct and indirect costs (US$ billions) as summarized by Songer[29] with the addition of the most recently published estimate from the American Diabetes Association[30].

increased prevalence, there is little 'real' rise for 1969 to 1987. Thereafter, the estimates fluctuate (partly because of differences in methodology), but the general trend is upwards, though not as dramatically as the impression given by the uncorrected estimates.

One of the problems in drawing together health economic data from a number of research studies is the difficulty of comparing costs, prices, or charges from one country to another. The most common method for doing this is the conversion of local currencies to a common currency and the most commonly chosen is US dollars. Although convenient, this ignores the fact that the true value, in terms of its buying power, of a US dollar is likely to be different in the countries being compared and at the times being compared, even within the same country. The cost of labour, the cost of raw materials, and the cultural value placed on different goods and services are likely to be different in different places and at different times.

One novel method of avoiding these problems is to express the monetary results of economic studies in a common unit derived from a product which is available almost everywhere and is manufactured in the country within which it is purchased. The so-called 'standard hamburger' has been advocated as such a product. Items sold by the large and ubiquitous fast food chains are manufactured to a common standard in each country in which that particular fast food chain operates. As a matter of company policy, these items are manufactured in the country within which they are sold and from raw materials derived from that country. (There is the occasional exception, for example, that prompted by the BSE (bovine spongiform encephalopathy) 'scare' when 'hamburgers' (actually 'beefburgers') manufactured in the UK were made from imported, not home-grown beef.) However

potentially useful this ploy may be, being able to convert estimates into 'standard hamburger' units does rely on having information about the costs of this product in all countries and at all of the times being compared. This information is not in the public domain, though it can be obtained from companies if required!

An alternative, and simpler, method is to calculate the ratio of the average cost of the care of a person with diabetes divided by the average cost of care of a person without diabetes. As long as these two estimates have been made by the same methods, in the same locality and at the same time, this ratio has validity, has intuitive meaning, and is independent of currency, inflation, and differences in the buying power of 'health dollars' in different places. 'Crude' ratios can be calculated easily from published studies, though age, sex, and ethnic-group-specific ratios are preferable where the availability of data permit.

If this calculation is carried out for the ADA study mentioned above[30] and for a study (one of the few) from a developing country (Tanzania),[32] the results, as shown in *Table 1.4*, are very different. In the USA, the average annual health expenditure on a person with diabetes is 3.8 times that on a person without diabetes. In Tanzania, according to Chale *et al.*,[32] this same ratio is 143.5 for a person treated with insulin and 51.5 for a person treated with oral hypoglycaemic agents. These differences require explanation.

Part of the reason for these large differences is that, although the estimated per capita expenditure on people with diabetes in the Tanzanian study is much lower that that in the US study, the amount spent per head on the health care of the general population is *very much* lower. Also, the estimates from the Tanzania study are of diabetes care in a 'centre of excellence' in Dar es Salaam and, therefore, likely to be much higher than the average cost

Table 1.4
Comparison of average, annual, per person direct health-care costs of diabetes in USA[30] and Tanzania[32].

Country (type of diabetes)	Mean cost (for those with diabetes) (US$)	Mean cost (for those without diabetes) (US$)	Difference (US$)	Ratio
USA (all diabetes)	10,071	2,699	7,372	3.8
Tanzania (insulin-treated diabetes)	287	2	285	143.5
Tanzania (diabetes treated with oral hypoglycaemics)	103	2	101	51.5

of care for people with diabetes being treated elsewhere in the country. This fact, despite the realistically low prevalence (0.2%) assumed for diabetes in Tanzania, means that the extrapolated estimates for the cost of diabetes care in the whole country are probably higher, perhaps much higher, than reality. Nevertheless, this ratio of costs of care, in the presence of diabetes versus without diabetes, deserves to be used and its validity and explanatory value explored.

The indirect costs of diabetes to society

The valuation of lost production, due to sickness absence from work, disability, premature retirement, and premature mortality, is a contentious economic issue. The 'human capital approach'[33] equates the value of lost production with the salary or wage which society would have paid for that work to be done. As can be seen from *Fig. 1.1*, estimates of the indirect cost of diabetes using this approach have suggested that they are at least as great as the direct health-care costs. This is also largely true for studies carried out in countries other than the USA.

While most researchers agree that indirect costs should be estimated, exactly how this should be done is what gives rise to the contention. The details of the debate, essentially between the human capital approach and the 'friction-cost approach',[34] are beyond the scope of this chapter. However, the essence of the argument is that the human capital approach does not apply, except in the case of full employment. When there is unemployment, work does not remain undone when an individual is ill, is disabled, or dies prematurely. To a greater or lesser extent, unemployed or underemployed people are recruited or retrained to make up for this deficiency. The result of this on estimates of indirect costs is that human capital approach estimates are likely to be overestimates. Those based on the friction-cost approach are very much lower.[34]

Nevertheless, despite the likelihood that previous estimates of indirect costs may need to be adjusted downwards, the burden on society resulting from diabetes is significant. All available epidemiological prophecies suggest that this burden is set to increase in all regions of the world.

References

1. Wainwright B. A patient's view of the costs of having diabetes. *IDF (International Diabetes Federation) Bulletin* 1995; **40**: 26–27.
2. Kangas T. In: Gruber W, Leese B, Songer T, Williams R, eds. *The Economics of Diabetes and Diabetes Care*, Brussels and Geneva: International Diabetes Federation (IDF) and World Health Organization (WHO), 1997.
3. Jacobson AM, Hauser ST, Willett JB *et al.* Psychological adjustment to IDDM: 10-year follow-up of an onset cohort of child and adolescent patients. *Diabetes Care* 1997; **20**: 811–818.
4. Dunn SM, Turtle JR. The myth of the diabetic personality. *Diabetes Care* 1984; **4**: 640–646.
5. Jacobson AM, Hauser ST, Noam G, Powers S. The influences of chronic illness and ego development on self-esteem among adolescent diabetic and psychiatric patients. *Youth Adolescence* 1984; **13**: 489–507.
6. Jacobson AM, Hauser ST, Wertlieb D *et al.* Psychological adjustment of children with recently diagnosed diabetes mellitus. *Diabetes Care* 1986; **9**: 323–329.
7. Lloyd CE, Robinson N, Andrews B *et al.* Are the social relationships of young insulin-dependent diabetic patients affected by their condition? *Diabetic Medicine* 1993; **10**: 481–485.
8. Tebbi C, Bromberg C, Sills I *et al.* Vocational adjustment and general well-being of young adults with IDDM. *Diabetes Care* 1990; **13**: 98–103.
9. Rodin GM, Daneman D. Eating disorders and IDDM: a problematic association. *Diabetes Care* 1992; **15**: 1402–1411.
10. Greenhalgh J, Georgiou A, Long AF *et al. Measuring the health outcomes of diabetes care.*

Outcomes Measurement Reviews No. 4. Leeds: Nuffield Institute for Health, UK Health Outcomes Clearing House, 1997.
11. Shobhana R. Psychosocial aspects of diabetes mellitus: experience of depression, behaviour patters, life stress, family attitudes in children with Insulin Dependent Diabetes Mellitus. Doctoral thesis. Madras, India: The Tamil Nadu Dr MGR Medical University, 1997.
12. Karlson B, Agardh C-D. Burden of illness, metabolic control, and complications in relation to depressive symptoms in IDDM patients. *Diabetic Medicine* 1997; **14**: 1066–1072.
13. Gonder-Frederick L, Cox D, Kovatchev B *et al.* The psychosocial impact of severe hypoglycaemic episodes on spouses of patients with IDDM. *Diabetes Care* 1997; **20**: 1543–1546.
14. Cox DJ, Gonder-Frederick LA, Polonsky W *et al.* A multi-center evaluation of Blood Glucose Awareness Training-II. *Diabetes Care* 1995; **18**: 523–528.
15. Carey MP, Spector IP, Lantingua LJ, Krauss DJ. Reliability of the Dyadic Adjustment Scale. *Psychological Assessment* 1993; **5**: 238–240.
16. Irvine A. The fear of hypoglycaemia scale. In: Bradley C, ed. *Handbook of Psychology and Diabetes*. Chur, Switzerland: Harwood Academic, 1994: 133–155.
17. Shobhana R, Rama Rao P, Lavanya A *et al. Cost of diabetes in a developing country. A study from southern India. Diabetes Research and Clinical Practice.* Presented at 'Economic Aspects of Diabetes – The Next Steps' Conference and Workshop, Barcelona, Spain, 6–8 September 1998.
18. Songer TJ, LaPorte RE, Lave JR *et al.* Health insurance and the financial impact of IDDM in families with a child with IDDM. *Diabetes Care* 1997; **20**: 577–584.
19. Kangas T. In: *The Finndiab Report. Health Care of People with Diabetes in Finland.* Research Report No. 58. Helsinki, Finland: Stakes National Research and Development Centre for Welfare and Health, 1995.
20. Currie CJ, Williams DRR, Peters JR. Patterns of in- and out-patient activity for diabetes: a district survey. *Diabetic Medicine* 1996; **13**: 273–280.
21. Currie CJ, Kraus D, Morgan CLl *et al.* NHS acute sector expenditure for diabetes: the

present, future and excess cost of care. *Diabetic Medicine* 1997; **14**: 686–692.

22. Currie CJ, Morgan CL, Peters JR. Patterns and costs of hospital care for coronary heart disease related and not related to diabetes. *Heart* 1997; **78**: 544–549.

23. Currie CJ, Peters JR. Estimation of unascertained diabetes prevalence: different effects on calculation of complication rates and resource utilization. *Diabetic Medicine* 1997; **14**: 477–481.

24. Currie CJ, Morgan CLl, Peters JR. The epidemiology and cost of inpatient care for peripheral vascular disease, infection, neuropathy, and ulceration in diabetes. *Diabetes Care* 1998; **21**: 42–48.

25. Williams DRR, Fuller JH, Stevens L. Validity of routinely collected hospital admissions data on diabetes. *Diabetic Medicine* 1989; **6**: 320–324.

26. Laing W, Williams DRR. *Diabetes: a model for health care management.* Office of Health Economics. No 92 in a series of papers on current health problems. London: OHE, 1989.

27. Bardsley M, Coles J, Jenkins L, eds. *DRGs and Health Care. The Management of Casemix.* London: King Edwards Hospital Fund for London, 1987.

28. Söderland N, Milne R, Gray A, Raftery J. Differences in hospital casemix, and the relationship between casemix and hospital costs. *J Pub Health Med* 1995; **17**: 25–32.

29. Songer TJ. The economics of diabetes care: USA. In: Alberti KGMM, Zimmet P, DeFronzo RA, eds, *International Textbook of Diabetes Mellitus*, Vol 2. Chichester: John Wiley & Sons, 1997: 1762–1772.

30. American Diabetes Association. Economic consequences of diabetes mellitus in the US in 1997. *Diabetes Care* 1998; **21**: 296–309.

31. Songer TJ, Ettaro L (and the Economics of Diabetes Project Panel). *Studies on the Costs of Diabetes.* Report prepared for the Division of Diabetes Translation, Centres for Disease Control and Prevention, Atlanta, GA, 1998.

32. Chale S, Swai ABM, Mujinja PGM, McLarty DG. Must diabetes be a fatal disease in Africa? Study of costs of treatment. *Br Med J* 1992; **304**: 1215–1218.

33. Rice DP. *Estimating the costs of illness.* Health Economic Series, PHS Publ. No. 947–6. Washington: Government Printing Office, 1966.

34. Koopmanschap MA, Rutten FFH, van Ineveld BM, van Roijen L. The friction cost method for measuring indirect cost of disease. *J Health Econ* 1995; **14**: 171–189.

2

Genetics of diabetes: unravelling the complexities

Marco Giorgio Baroni, David Leslie, Paolo Pozzilli and Raffaella Buzzetti

Diabetes mellitus has many different causes. The major two types of diabetes, Type 1 or insulin-dependent diabetes (IDDM) and Type 2 or non-insulin dependent diabetes (NIDDM), are thought to be due to the interaction of genetic and environmental factors. This chapter outlines many of the developments obtained in recent studies on the genetic heterogeneity of Type 1 and Type 2 diabetes.

Approaches to genetic analysis

There are a several research designs used for genetic analysis, each with varying powers to detect linkage disequilibrium between a particular marker and a disease state, and each with different assumptions about the mode of inheritance of the disease. These include population association studies, family or pedigree linkage analysis, and studies in affected sib-pairs. Each of these methods has advantages and disadvantages.

In population association studies, the usual approach is to compare the allelic frequencies and genotype distributions of a candidate gene between affected individuals and carefully chosen controls. A deviation from expected allelic frequencies indicates association between the candidate gene and the disease. Heterogeneity of a disease limits the power of an association study when phenotypically similar individuals with varying constellations of genetic defects are included. Association studies are useful for identifying a single common mutation present in the majority of the patients studied. Thus, a negative result cannot be used as grounds to reject a role for a given gene in disease susceptibility. For minor genes, extremely large numbers of patients and controls (500–1,000 for each group) are probably necessary to identify a significant disease association. Association studies, in an adequately large sample, are therefore suitable to define whether a candidate gene may or may not play a role (major or minor) in the aetiology of a disease.

Linkage analysis in pedigrees is one of the most powerful methods for genetic analysis, in particular for single-gene disorders. The demonstration that a disease co-segregates in families with alleles at a marker locus provides convincing evidence that a major locus contributes to the disease susceptibility. Linkage analysis can be used to study either candidate gene markers or a set of anonymous chromosomal markers, covering the whole genome. Two major requirements are necessary for linkage analysis: first, the mode of transmission of the disease has to be determined, since it requires that assumptions are made about the frequencies and dominance relationships of alleles at the locus. Secondly, families with at least three generations are necessary, in order to determine unequivocally the allele phase in heterozygous parents, otherwise alleles in the offspring would be scored as recombinant or non-recombinant according to the arrangement chosen. In more complex disorders, in which more than one gene interacts to cause the disease, linkage analysis is difficult to perform. In Type 2 diabetes, for example, heterogeneity could be present between pedigrees and within pedigrees, the mode of transmission is unknown, the late age of onset means parents are rarely both affected, and bilinear transmission (inheritance of different disease-related genes from the parents) cannot be excluded.

Linkage analysis has been applied to the analysis of two siblings, both affected by diabetes, as they are likely to have inherited the same susceptibility genes from their parents.[1] Affected sib-pair (ASP) analysis is based on comparison of the observed and expected distribution of the number of shared identical alleles by descent at a marker locus, with significant excess of alleles shared taken as evidence for linkage. Two genes are identical by descent if one is a copy of the other or if they are both copies of the same ancestral gene. The great advantage of sib-pair analysis is that no assumption need be made regarding the mode of inheritance of the disease, and ascertainment bias is not important, as the 'unaffected' siblings are not considered in the analysis. In order to obtain identity-by-descent between two affected siblings, if parents are not available, it is necessary to use extremely polymorphic markers. Usually, highly polymorphic anonymous markers, of which only the chromosomal location is known, are studied in large sets of affected sib-pairs in order to identify the chromosome regions linked to the disease under study (the so called 'genome-wide search'). Within families, we can now determine whether, and if so, what markers are co-inherited with a disease, and whether a marker is transmitted in linkage with that disease. If data suggest linkage, then we can conclude that there is at least one susceptibility gene in the defined region. Nevertheless, the potential of bilinear inheritance and genetic heterogeneity may also be relevant to ASP analysis. Using the ASP method, two research groups have reported some positive evidence of linkage to at least 20 non-HLA loci as well as the major HLA locus for Type 1 diabetes.[2,3] Moreover, a series of interesting, but not definitive, observations have been obtained in 'adult-onset' Type 2 diabetes.[4]

Although ASP linkage studies are robust, a very large number of affected sib-pairs would be needed to map diabetes-predisposing loci which are not associated with a strong excess genetic risk. Moreover, as shown by Kruglyak and Lander,[5] a large number of false linkages may occur by chance in a genome scan. Therefore, it has been suggested[5] that one uses a classification for putative genetic markers based on the number of times one would expect to see positive evidence of linkage at random in a complete genome screening. Four standard levels have been proposed: (1) suggestive; statistical evidence expected to occur one time at random in a genome scan ($p < 0.0007$ or maximum lod score, MLS, = 2.2); (2) significant ($p < 0.00002$ or MLS = 3.6), statistical evidence expected to occur 0.05 times in a genome scan; (3) highly significant, statistical evidence expected to occur 0.001 times in a genome scan ($p < 0.0000003$ or MLS = 5.4); and (4) confirmed linkage, significant linkage from one or a combination of initial studies that has been confirmed in a further data set with a $p = 0.01$. The above standards are very difficult to achieve in practice. Therefore, once a disease gene is localized to a 10–20 cM (centiMorgan) region by linkage, linkage disequilibrium mapping can be used to locate more accurately the position of the gene. Linkage disequilibrium mapping or allelic association can be seen when two loci are so closely positioned that meiotic recombination between the loci is rare.[6]

Genetic susceptibility to Type 1 diabetes

Type 1 diabetes is a typical multifactorial disease caused by a combination of genetic and environmental factors.[7] As regards the genetic component, segregation analysis indicates that Type 1 diabetes cannot be classified according to the genetic model of recessive, dominant, or intermediate inheritance. There are three major differences with respect to Mendelian genetic diseases: (1) more than one gene is involved, therefore the disease is multigenetic rather than monogenic; (2) the genes responsible for the disease are not rare variants or mutations, but are polymorphic genes; these genes show different allelic variants, each with a frequency greater than 1% in the general population and differing in some functional characteristics; and (3) Type 1 diabetes is caused by the interaction between different genetic and different environmental factors. In the next section we present evidence for the genetic susceptibility to Type 1 diabetes and discuss the regions or genes so far identified as responsible for that susceptibility.

Type 1 diabetes and HLA-genes

The association of Type 1 diabetes with HLA antigens has been known for many years;[8] indeed, 90–95% of Caucasian Type 1 diabetic patients, compared with 45–55% of control populations, possess the HLA DR3 or DR4, or both antigens.[8] Subsequently, the importance of HLA–DQ in the genetic susceptibility to diabetes was established. Susceptibility or protection for diabetes is determined by either single genetically determined amino acid substitutions or by the entire class II haplotype.

In 1987, Todd and collaborators[9] observed a significant correlation between amino acid 57 of the DQ beta chain and susceptibility or resistance to the disease. The great majority of neutral haplotypes and haplotypes negatively associated with the disease possess an aspartic acid in position 57 (asp 57), whereas the positively associated haplotypes posses neutral-charge amino acids (alanine, valine, serine). Subsequently, a comparative analysis of the different nucleotide sequences of the HLA–DQA locus showed that all alleles with an arginine in position 52 (arg 52) are associated with the disease.[10] On the basis of this observation, we and others[11,12] suggested that the presence in *cis* or in *trans* of the DQB non-asp 57 allele and DQA 52 allele (DQ alpha/beta-susceptible heterodimer) determined whether an HLA allele would be a marker of susceptibility to Type 1 diabetes. A molecular basis for HLA–DQ association with Type 1 diabetes has recently been proposed,[13] where HLA–DQ genes bias the immunological repertoire towards autoimmune specificities, creating an autoimmune-prone individual, followed by amplification and triggering events that promote subsequent immune activation.

The importance of the entire class II haplotype has recently been stressed[14] since DRB1, DQA and DQB1 have been found to correlate with diabetes differently according to the population studied. Haplotype analysis shows that among the different combinations of DRB1–DQA1–DQB1, a single dose of protective allele (DRB1*0403 or DQB1*0301) is sufficient to confer protection from Type 1 diabetes, whereas susceptibility is due to a

Table 2.1
Loci other than HLA (IDDM1) so far identified as being associated with Type 1 diabetes.

IDDM locus	Chromosome	Candidate genes for the locus	MLS results	Association studies	References
IDDM3	15q26	unknown	2.5	NT	32
			1.6	NT	54
			0.2	NT	55
IDDM4	11q13	ICE,	1.2	NT	2
		CD3, ZMF1, RT6	2.6	NT	3
			0.2	NT	58
			3.9	NT	55
IDDM5	6q25	TNDM, SOD2	1.5	NT	2
			4.5	NT	55
			1.7	NT	59
IDDM6	18q	unknown	1.1	NT	2
			1.6	Significant	60
IDDM7	2q31	IL-1 family,	1.3	Significant	61
		HOXD cluster	1.3	NT	58
			0.4	Not significant	55
IDDM8	6q25–q27	MnSOD2	1.2	NT	2
			2.8	NT	54
			3.6	NT	55
			2.5	Significant	59
IDDM9	3q21–q25	unknown	1.9	NT	2
IDDM10	10p11–q11	unknown	1.3	NT	2
			2.4	Significant	62
IDDM11	14q24–q31	unknown	3.8	NT	63
IDDM12	2q33	CTLA-4, CD28	3.2	Significant	45
			0.6	Significant	51
IDDM13	2q34	IGFBP2, IGFBP5	3.3	NT	53
IDDM15	6q	unknown	6.2	Significant	64
Glucokinase	7q	glucokinase	0.8	Significant	52

CD3, ZMF1, RT6: see text on IDDM4. ICE: Interleukin-converting enzyme. MnSOD2: Mn-superoxide dismutase.
HOXD: homeobox gene CTLA-4. CD28: see text on IDDM12. IGFBP2, IGFBP5: insulin growth factor binding protein.
NT = not tested. MLS = maximum lod score for linkage analysis.

combination of susceptibility alleles, at both DRB1 and DQB1 loci (DRB1*0405, DQB1 *0302, or DQB1*0201).[14,15]

Type 1 diabetes and non-HLA genes

Comparison of disease concordance between HLA-identical siblings (15–20%) and monozygotic twins (35–45%) indicates that genetic loci other than the HLA locus may be involved in the genetic transmission of Type 1 diabetes. We now describe the loci other than HLA (IDDM1) so far identified by linkage and/or linkage disequilibrium. A number has been assigned to each of these loci associated with Type 1 diabetes, but apart from IDDM1, which is most strongly linked to diabetes, the numbers do not represent a hierarchy of importance (*Table 2.1*).

IDDM2

The chromosome region encoding the insulin gene in locus 11p15.5 confers susceptibility to Type 1 diabetes.[16,17] This locus is a 20 kb (kilobase) region and includes the structural genes for tyrosine hydroxylase, IGF2, HRAS1, and insulin. Further studies have restricted the region of susceptibility to a 4.1 kb region containing a cluster of highly associated polymorphisms,[18,19] one or more of which could be responsible for the genetic susceptibility. Bennett *et al.*, by 'cross-match' haplotype analysis, mapped the IDDM2 within the VNTR at 5' of the insulin gene.[20] The polymorphism results from a variable number of tandemly repeated 14 bp oligonucleotides (VNTRs) located at nucleotide 363 from the transcriptional start site. The different types of VNTR are grouped into three classes according to their lengths as measured by standard Southern blotting techniques: class I with an average of 570 bp (base pairs); class II with an average of 1,200 bp;

and class III with an average of 2,220 bp.[18] Homozygosity for short class I VNTR confers a two- to five-fold increase in Type 1 diabetes risk,[21] while class III VNTR alleles are dominantly protective.[21,22] Some studies *in vivo* demonstrate that class III VNTR are associated with lower INS transcription in the pancreas,[21,23,24] compared with class I VNTRs. These results suggest transcriptional effects of VNTR, although it is difficult to explain how lower INS mRNA levels could confer a protection.

To find a plausible mechanism for the dominant protection of class III alleles, the expression of insulin in human thymus, a critical site for induction to self-proteins, was analysed.[24–27] Insulin mRNA expression was detected in all thymus tissues examined.[24,25] Furthermore, it was demonstrated that allelic variations at VNTR loci correlate with differential INS mRNA expression in the thymus, where, in contrast to the pancreas, class III VNTRs are associated with higher levels of INS expression.[25,28] These authors suggested that higher levels of insulin expression in the thymus may promote a deletion of insulin-specific-T lymphocytes, a crucial mechanism for inducing self-tolerance during development. The Type 1 diabetes-associated susceptibility with or without resistance may derive from the VNTR influence on INS transcription in the thymus. These observations represent the first proposed mechanistic link between genetic effect of IDDM2 and insulin as a causative antigen in Type 1 diabetes.

However, the mechanism exerted by INS VNTR alleles to induce different INS transcription remains unknown. One possibility is that a different number of repeats could affect the binding of a nuclear protein important for insulin gene transcription: alternatively, a variety of metabolic activity linked to different VNTR lengths can be associated with hyperactive β-cells being more vulnerable to cellular, antibody, and cytokine-mediated destruction.

In an analysis of diabetic UK multiplex families, the λ value (ratio of the frequency of a disease in siblings relative to the general population) for IDDM2 (the INS locus) was 1.29.[20] Therefore, IDDM2 may contribute 10% of the genetic effect that causes familial clustering of the disease.[20] It appears that IDDM1 and IDDM2 contribute to disease by acting epistatically, i.e. in an additive manner, and together reflect a multiple gene cause for Type 1 diabetes.[29]

HLA and INS regions together explain only a proportion of the familial clustering, suggesting that other susceptibility factors, either genetic, environmental, or both, must exist. The number of susceptibility genes is probably even higher in human Type 1 diabetes than in the NOD mouse,[30,31] due to ethnic and genetic heterogeneity of the disease.

IDDM3

The first evidence of disease linkage with the IDDM3 locus was reported by Field et al., in chromosome region 15q26.[32] A summary of the results of genetic studies on IDDM3 appear in Table 2.1. Interestingly, evidence for linkage of Type 1 diabetes to IDDM3 was contained principally in the subset of families at low risk, as judged by HLA region susceptibility-gene-sharing (HLA DR sharing less than 50% in affected siblings), compared with the high HLA risk families. This finding suggests that IDDM3 falls in the category of genes that act independently on disease predisposition, perhaps playing a greater role in those families where HLA genes are less influential.[32]

IDDM4

IDDM4 is located near the locus FGF3 on chromosome 11q13 and has been reported by different groups (Table 2.1). In humans, several potential candidate genes have been mapped near FGF3. These genes include MDU1, which

encodes a cell-surface protein involved in the regulation of intracellular calcium,[33] and ZFM1, which encodes a putative nuclear protein.[34] Both are expressed in the pancreas. The RT6 gene, encoding a T-cell membrane protein, has been mapped to the same genetic region.[35] Defective expression of this protein has been reported in the BB rat and NOD mouse,[36,37] although this defect is not linked to diabetes development in the BB rat.[37] Interleukin-converting enzyme (ICE) and CD3 are candidate genes for diabetes susceptibility and CD3 maps to the chromosomic locus 11q23. CD3 represents one of the most important membrane complexes involved in the delivery of signals to the T-cell during antigen presentation and is required for T-cell activation.

Studies using a two-locus MLS analysis have shown how IDDM4, 70 cM distant from the INS gene on chromosome 11, could have a joint effect with IDDM1 in an epistatic model.[29] The contribution of such loci to the development of Type 1 diabetes may involve different biological pathways, and these findings suggest the existence of several forms of the disease with different genetic loci.

IDDM5

Linkage analysis performed in Type 1 diabetes multiplex families has suggested that two separate regions on human chromosome 6q are linked to the disease (IDDM5 and IDDM8). The first evidence of linkage for the ESR (IDDM5) marker locus was reported by Davies et al. after a whole genome screening (Table 2.1).[2]

ESR on chromosome 6q maps close to the SOD2 gene encoding for Mn-superoxide dismutase (MnSOD). There is further evidence supporting a role of free oxygen radicals in the immune-mediated β-cell destruction.[38] A limited repertoire of radical scavengers,[39,40] such as MnSOD, could render β-cells more susceptible to free-radical injury. An RFLP of the SOD2 gene has been described to be associated to Type 1 diabetes.[41,42] Structurally polymorphic MnSOD proteins with reduced activity have been also reported,[43] and such variants might increase predisposition to Type 1 diabetes.

IDDM6, IDDM7, IDDM8, IDDM9, IDDM10, IDDM11 and IDDM15

All these loci remain putative, and confirmatory results are needed. See *Table 2.1* for summary of results and possible candidate genes for these loci.

IDDM12

An interesting new locus, IDDM12 on chromosome 2q33, has been identified by our group to be linked to and associated with Type 1 diabetes in different European populations.[44,45] The chromosome region 2q33 is a region of synteny to Idd5, a susceptibility gene located on chromosome 1 in NOD mouse, and contains two autoimmune disease candidate genes, CTLA-4 (cytotoxic T lymphocyte-associated protein 4) and CD28, encoding for T-cell receptors involved in controlling T-cell proliferation.[46-48] CTLA-4 encodes a T-cell receptor that mediates T-cell apoptosis and is a vital negative regulator of T-cell activation;[49] thus it is a strong candidate gene for T-cell-mediated autoimmune diseases. Co-stimulation of CD28 by B7 leads to T-cell proliferation and production of IL-2. Alteration of the delicate balance between CD28 and CTLA-4, which both interact with B7, could lead to autoimmune diseases by preventing apoptosis or down-regulation of activated self-reactive T-lymphocytes.[64]

We performed multipoint linkage studies of the chromsome 2q33 CTLA-4/CD28 region in Italian multiplex families. Maximal evidence of linkage ($p = 0.00006$) was obtained in the D2S72-CTLA-4-D2S116 region, which includes an (AT)n microsatellite in the 3'

untranslated region of the CTLA-4 gene. Since CTLA-4 is a strong candidate susceptibility locus for Type 1 diabetes, we analysed a point mutation of CTLA-4. This is an A–G transition at position 49, encoding a Thr/Ala substitution in the leader peptide located 5.3 kb 5' of the microsatellite locus. The G allele was studied in Italian and in Spanish families. The combined data sets showed that the G allele was preferentially transmitted to the affected siblings ($p = 0.0001$). In collaboration with Todd, we extended our early observations evaluating UK, Sardinian and USA data sets without finding any significant evidence for transmission disequilibrium at this locus, although a trend was observed in the USA families. By combining all data sets from different populations, the G allele was preferentially transmitted ($n = 818$ affected families, $p = 0.002$). Further support for the positive association with IDDM12 was obtained from a large population of Belgian Type 1 diabetic patients.[45] In addition, supporting evidence comes from a case-control study where CTLA-4 was found to be associated with susceptibility to Graves disease, another organ-specific autoimmune disease.[45] More recently, a case-control study in a German population[50] and a large family study performed in multiple ethnic groups[51] confirmed our results.

Overall, these data indicate that the G allele is associated with Type 1 diabetes, at least in certain populations. One possibility for the lack of association in the large UK data set is that the G allele at position 49 is not in as tight a disequilibrium with the predisposing allele of the aetiological mutation as it is in the Mediterranean populations. Another possibility could be that the IDDM12 aetiological mutation may have either an extremely high or low frequency in the UK population, so that its effect cannot be detected by genetic studies. Even though CTLA-4 is the most likely candidate gene for IDDM12, the aetiological mutation has not yet been found. The exon 1 A/G substitution is not expected to affect the function of the CTLA-4 molecule. The CTLA-4 microsatellite $(AT)_n$ repeat itself is a better candidate because it could affect RNA stability, but mapping and identification of the IDDM12 aetiological mutation will require detailed physical mapping of the region, characterization of multiple polymorphisms by DNA sequencing, and analysis of the transmission of multilocus haplotypes in affected families.

The glucokinase gene

Some evidence of linkage to Type 1 diabetes has been reported on chromosome 7p in 186 multiplex families from the USA and the UK using five microsatellites (D7S531, D7S678, GCK, D7S502, and D7S672).[52] Among these markers, the most interesting one was glucokinase (GCK), as it appeared to be the only one to show a significant linkage in all tested families. The authors investigated the closest candidate gene, glucokinase, and a positive association was reported with allele 4 of GCK3. The same authors went on to analyse another data set to reconfirm these data; whereas a significant linkage was found ($p <$ 0.025), the association with the GCK3 allele 4 did not reach statistical significance in the second data set.[52] By single-strand conformational polymorphism, all 12 exons of the GCK gene in 27 diabetic probands were evaluated for evidence of possible variants.[53] None of the several variants previously observed was significantly increased on the chromosome bearing the GCK allele 4. Therefore more studies with different data sets are required. Nevertheless, the study of the GCK gene raises two main points: (1) a gene (not a locus) of susceptibility to Type 1 diabetes has been identified, which, if confirmed, could be added to IDDM1 and IDDM2 to improve the prediction of Type

1 diabetes; and (2) the GCK gene posseses a metabolic, and probably not an immune, function and therefore it is of particular interest that a gene, in addition to IDDM2, involved in controlling a metabolic pathway may be associated with Type 1 diabetes.

IDDM13

Chromosome 2 encodes for three susceptibility loci (IDDM7, IDDM12, and HOXD8). A fourth locus has recently been identified by Morahan et al.[53] By mulitpoint analysis, a peak was reached at 2q34 20 cM, distal to CTLA-4; this was designated IDDM13. However, at this stage it is unclear whether IDDM13 represents a distinct gene effect from IDDM7 and IDDM12, and evidence for linkage requires independent confirmation. Morahan et al.[53] suggested that the genes contained in the IDDM13 region may control an early event in islet cell autoimmunity such as islet cell antibody (ICA) production. They also found that IDDM13 confers susceptibility to islet autoimmunity, notably in females. By testing many structural genes, only IGFBP2 and IGFBP5 were found to be relevant flanking markers.

The linkage analysis showed that the contribution of this gene to the relative risk of developing Type 1 diabetes was as great as that of other non-HLA susceptibility loci. Why IDDM13 was not detected in other studies remains unclear; it probably reflects differences in linkage between different data sets. Such differences could be due to the variations in environment and genetic background between populations.

Type 1 diabetes and non-HLA genes: final comments

In a recent study, we have analysed 265 Caucasian families with Type 1 diabetes for the following loci: IDDM3, IDDM4, IDDM5,

IDDM7 and IDDM8; and we reported evidence of linkage for three loci: IDDM4, IDDM5, and IDDM8, which met the standard for confirmed linkage.[54,55] However, linkage for IDDM3 and IDDM7 was not confirmed.[54] Furthermore, two very recent studies produced contradictory results.[56,57] In the first, Mein *et al.*[56] confirmed their own data (Davies) on affected sib-pairs, whilst the second, by Concannon *et al.*[57], confirmed only the HLA region of all the IDDM genes previously reported. The discrepancy between these two studies is sobering. Why are we unable to replicate linkages in additional data sets? Several explanations could be called upon: the linkages could be spurious, and there could be no disease genes in those regions; alternatively, the linkage could be real, and the problem is our ability to identify disease genes. Mapping complex disease genes is a serious challenge because: (1) heterogeneity of the disease – a considerable number of genes may be involved, each of which may contribute to only a fraction of the total familial aggregation; (2) the frequency of relevant genetic mutations may vary between different populations, as for example in the most common genetic mutation ($\Delta508$) in cystic fibrosis; (3) a range of factors, genetic and environmental, unique to a particular population will influence the detection of genetic linkage and linkage disequilibrium in that population; and (4) current linkage analysis methods, at best, give unambiguous results only for HLA, yet other genes must exist.

In conclusion, the studies performed so far have demonstrated that the major susceptibility locus for Type 1 diabetes resides within the major histocompatibility complex on chromosome 6p21 (DR/DQ). There are seven additional loci for which there is evidence for linkage and association to justify fine mapping: IDDM2, IDDM4, IDDM5, IDDM6, IDDM8, and IDDM12. Seven other loci remain to be replicated: IDDM7, IDDM9, IDDM11, IDDM13, IDDM15, and GCK (*Table 2.3*). Only for two of the confirmed loci, IDDM1 and IDDM2, has the gene involved in the disease been characterized. In the case of IDDM1, the DR/DQ locus is the gene responsible,[8,14] probably in conjunction with other loci. In the case of IDDM2, a repeated sequence at the 5' of the insulin gene which could possibly affect the regulation of insulin secretion has been identified as a susceptibility marker of the disease.[20] In the other cases, the presence of some susceptibility genes can be envisaged. The identification of these additional genes, their products, and the relationship of the gene products to disease susceptibility represents the goal of genetic research in the coming years.

Type 2 diabetes

Type 2 diabetes is strongly inherited, as evidenced by the high concordance in identical twins,[65,66] and by the strong familial aggregation. A first-degree relative of a diabetic sibling has a lifetime risk of around 40%, a risk that doubles if both parents are affected.[67] The hypothesis that there is a strong genetic susceptibility to Type 2 diabetes is supported by the wide variation in prevalence among different ethnic groups and the different disease incidence within populations exposed to identical environmental factors.[68]

Despite such a strong genetic component, a single gene defect is highly unlikely to explain most cases of Type 2 diabetes. Several lines of evidence indicate that genetic heterogeneity exists within the Type 2 phenotype. First, the risks for disease in the first-degree relatives and in monozygotic twins are around 40 and 90%, respectively,[69] not in the expected proportion for a single gene defect. Secondly, more than 60 genetic syndromes are associated with glucose intolerance.[70] Finally, even within maturity onset diabetes of the young (MODY, see below), which shows autosomal dominant inheritance, several genes have been identified in different families and populations.[71]

It is therefore clear that Type 2 diabetes is a heterogeneous disorder, in which most cases appear to be of polygenic inheritance. In fact, formal segregation analysis has confirmed the complex mode of inheritance of Type 2 diabetes. Cook et al.[72] observed that the prevalence of diabetes was higher in sibs with two affected parents (75% of sibs affected) than in sibs with only one parent affected (38%) and sibs with neither parent affected (23%), and concluded that this pattern is compatible with a polygenic inheritance. Rich[69] fitted different models to explore the mode of inheritance of NIDDM, comparing the theoretical relative risks to different family members with those observed, and again found that the best fit was a single locus with polygenes or a few multiplicative loci with polygenes.

Single genes identified and possible functional interaction

Candidate genes: application to the study of monogenic and polygenic Type 2 diabetes

The physiology of Type 2 diabetes has provided some evidences of possible gene defects (Fig. 2.1); insulin resistance is a trademark for Type 2 diabetes, and an enormous body of work demonstrates consistently that insulin resistance is primary in the development of Type 2 diabetes.[73] Studies of patients with Type 2 diabetes have demonstrated a primary defect in insulin-mediated glucose uptake into muscle.[73] Insulin sensitivity is reduced by 50% on average, corresponding to a proportional reduction in glycogen synthesis and storage.[73] Furthermore, the offspring of two diabetic parents are insulin resistant many years before

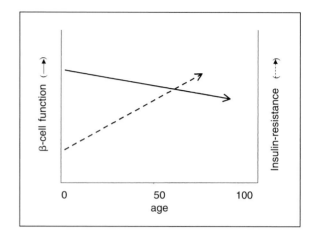

Fig. 2.1

Increasing insulin resistance combines with declining β-cell function to produce Type 2 diabetes mellitus. When insulin resistance is severe, only a small fall in insulin secretion is required to induce overt diabetes.

the disease develops.[74] Individuals with Type 2 diabetes also show various forms of pancreatic β-cell dysfunction.[75] There is progressive failure in insulin secretion as glucose levels rise, by unmasking either a primary defect in insulin secretion, pancreatic exhaustion, or glucose toxicity, or a combination of these defects. Prospective studies of individuals with glucose intolerance have shown a decrease in insulin levels after glucose challenge (secretory defect), and this altered response is a predictor of the development of the disease.[76]

Obesity, finally, has a role in the aetiology of Type 2 diabetes; in epidemiology studies, obesity alone increases the risk of Type 2 diabetes twofold.[77] Obesity, in particular visceral obesity, appears to exert its effects by reducing insulin sensitivity, possibly as the result of the high level of circulating free fatty acids (FFAs) produced by the adipose tissue.[78]

Although it is clear that obesity affects the susceptibility to Type 2 diabetes, the interaction between these two disorders is unclear. Obesity may define a subset of Type 2 diabetic patients with severe insulin resistance and relatively mild β-cell dysfunction, or it may act equally in all susceptible subjects to increase the penetrance of the genetic loci.

Our knowledge of the pathophysiology of Type 2 diabetes has led to the identification of several candidate genes for the disease. Whilst extensive analyses have been performed on many of these candidate genes, most studies have been negative. At present, only a few genes have been identified, with a possible role in the aetiology of Type 2 diabetes (*Table 2.2*). One of these genes, confirmed in several studies, is the insulin-receptor substrate-1 (IRS-1) gene.

The IRS-1 protein is a cytoplasmic molecule expressed in most insulin-sensitive tissue, which has been demonstrated to play a pivotal role in modulating cellular effects of insulin.[79,80] After binding of insulin to its receptor, the intrinsic tyrosine kinase activity of the receptor of the β-subunit is activated and catalyses the phosphorylation of specific tyrosine residues on the IRS-1 protein. Thereafter, phosphorylated IRS-1 binds with high affinity to several cellular signal proteins, thus functioning as a multisite 'docking' protein, linking the receptor kinase to the variety of cell functions regulated by insulin.[81,82] Genetic analysis of the IRS-1 gene has revealed several base-pair changes that result in amino acid substitutions.[83–85] The most common amino acid change is a glycine to arginine substitution at codon 972 (G972R), which has an overall frequency of ~6% in the general population.[86] This mutation has been reported to impair significantly IRS-1 function in experimental models,[87] and clinical studies have shown that this genetic variant is associated with reduced insulin sensitivity.[88] In our study of the IRS-1 gene,[89] we have found that

Table 2.2
Candidate genes for Type 2 diabetes.

Candidate genes for insulin action
Insulin receptor substrate-1 (IRS-1)
Tumour necrosis factor-α (TNF-α)
Peroxisome proliferator activated receptor γ (PPAR-γ)
Glycogen synthase
Leptin
Leptin receptor
Intestinal fatty acid binding protein (FABP2)

the Gly972Arg mutation in the IRS-1 gene is a significant predictor of insulin resistance syndrome and that this effect is independent of obesity. The fact that the diabetics have a lower prevalence of this mutation than do subjects with insulin resistance syndrome indicates that this gene needs the interaction with some other gene(s) to determine the clinical expression of Type 2 diabetes.

Other interesting genes are the glycogen synthetase gene, the tumour necrosis factor-α (TNF-α) gene, and the peroxisome proliferator activated receptor-γ (PPAR-γ) gene.

Glycogen synthetase plays a key role in glycogen synthesis, and the gene is associated with diabetes in a few populations.[90] The TNF-α protein has been shown to modulate gene expression in adipocytes and is implicated in the development of insulin resistance and obesity. TNF-α modulates insulin action through an effect on the insulin signalling pathway, by inhibiting insulin-receptor and IRS-1 phosphorylation.[91] A mutation in the promoter region of this gene in position −308 has been shown to determine increased expression of the TNF-α gene. Association studies of this variant have shown that it is increased in obese patients with visceral adiposity and insulin resistance, but not in diabetes.[92,93] It could therefore influence the genetics of a subtype of patient, who may or may not develop diabetes if other gene(s) are present.

The PPAR-γ gene is a nuclear hormone receptor that is considered potentially important in the activation or differentiation of fat cells.[94] One of the factors controlling fat-cell differentiation is the activation of genes involved in glucose and lipid metabolism. Genetic analysis of PPAR-γ has not been successful, with only a few polymorphisms found in diabetics and obese subjects.[95,96]

The study of the genetics of Type 2 diabetes with onset before the age of 25 years, commonly known as maturity onset diabetes of the young or MODY, has been extremely successful. MODY is unique in that most families show autosomal dominant inheritance, and these subjects are not obese and have a predominant defect in insulin secretion. Linkage analysis of one candidate gene, the glucokinase gene, in this subtype of diabetes showed a very strong linkage with this gene locus, called MODY2.[97] Further studies of the gene sequence have revealed that glucokinase mutations account for almost 50% of MODY in France and in England. These mutations are relatively rare in other populations, where other genes are at play.[98] Several mutations (around 80 identified so far) have been found throughout the gene and appear to alter the glucose set point for insulin secretion. Glucokinase phosphorylates glucose in β-cells and hepatocytes. Expression studies have shown that the enzymatic activity of the mutant proteins is impaired, with a decreased affinity for glucose.[99] Impairment of mutant glucokinase activity results in decreased glycolytic flux in β-cells.[100] This defect translates *in vivo* as a glucose-sensing defect, leading

to an increased threshold for glucose-stimulated insulin secretion.[101] Comparisons of insulin secretion rates in the presence of glucose demonstrate that mutant glucokinase carriers present with a 60% reduction in insulin secretion. Furthermore, decreased accumulation of hepatic glycogen and increased hepatic gluconeogenesis after a meal were observed in glucokinase-deficient patients.[102] Because most glucose is taken up by the liver after a meal to be converted to glycogen, a reduction in glycogen synthesis will exacerbate postprandial hyperglycaemia. Also, suppression of hepatic glucose production contributes to maintain normoglycaemia. Therefore, the observed increased gluconeogenesis in glucokinase-deficient patients is another factor contributing to postprandial hyperglycaemia. These results suggest that abnormalities of liver glucose metabolism play an important part, in addition to defective β-cell function, in the pathogenesis of hyperglycaemia in MODY2 patients.

This gene represents a clear example of the power of linkage analysis of a candidate gene in a single-gene disorder, and also the importance of classification of patients for the analysis.

Type 2 diabetes genes identified by genome-wide searches

As mentioned above, when the candidate gene approach is not successful, an alternative method is to search throughout the whole genome for loci in linkage with the disease. With this method, several other genes for MODY have been found (*Table 2.3*), and a few loci potentially involved in the aetiology of Type 2 diabetes have been reported. It should be pointed out that the primary defect in MODY is an altered insulin secretion, and it was not a surprise therefore that all the genes identified as responsible for MODY were

Table 2.3
MODY genes.

	MODY1	MODY2	MODY3	MODY4	MODYX
Genetic locus	20q	7p	12q	13q	unknown
Gene	HNF4α	glucokinase*	HNF1α*	IPF-1	heterogeneous?
Distribution (% of MODY families)	rare	10–65%	20–75%	rare	10%
Age at diagnosis	>12 years	childhood	post-pubertal	30 years	>25 years
Primary defect	pancreas	pancreas	pancreas/kidney	pancreas	insulin resistance?
Severity of diabetes	severe	mild	severe	mild?	mild
Complications	frequent	rare	frequent	unknown	unknown

* Different in different populations.

implicated in the regulation of insulin secretion.

In MODY, three genes, together with MODY2, have been identified: MODY1, mapped to chromosome 20 in a single large family, has now been identified as the hepatocyte nuclear transcription factor 4α (HNF4α).[103] Mutation at this steroid/thyroid hormone receptor causes a severe form of diabetes with all the complications of Type 2 diabetes. It probably acts by regulating a downstream transcription factor 1α (HNF1α) (see below). The hepatocyte nuclear transcription factor 1α (HNF1α)[104] is responsible for a large proportion of MODY in different populations. This transcription factor, as is HNF4α, is involved in tissue-specific regulation of liver genes, but it is also present in pancreatic islets. More than 50 mutations in the HNF1α gene have been reported so far. An insulin secretory defect, in the absence of insulin-resistance, has been observed in patients carrying the mutations in this gene.[105] Recently, the MODY4 gene has been found in large kindred, where a mutation in exon 1 of the insulin promoter factor (IPF-1) has been found to co-

segregate with the disease.[106] This gene regulates pancreatic development and the expression of various β-cell genes including insulin. The phenotype of heterozygous carriers of a mutated IPF-1 gene varies from impaired glucose tolerance to overt diabetes. One child homozygous for the mutations was born with pancreatic agensis.[107] Finally, a few families with clinical characteristics of MODY do not show mutation at any of the genes described, and the search for other genes is still on-going. As shown in Table 2.3, different clinical characteristics, distribution, and age at diagnosis, are associated with each MODY gene.

Genome-wide searches in families with 'adult-onset' Type 2 diabetes are in progress, and a few loci have been identified. Hanis et al.[108] initially reported linkage to a marker in chromosome 2q (called NIDDM1) in Mexican Americans from Starr County, Texas. This result has not been repeated by other groups. One other study[109] reported a second locus in the MODY3 region in a small subgroup of Bosnian Finnish families that showed the lowest quintile of insulin secretion. Several other studies have reported linkage to different chromosome regions, but no gene has been identified so far.[4]

Type 2 diabetes genes: final comments

Thus far no single gene or locus has been unequivocally confirmed for Type 2 diabetes. A handful of candidate genes, namely IRS-1, glycogen synthase, and leptin receptor, have been found to be associated with the disease in subtypes of Type 2 diabetic patients. Confirmatory genome-wide searches are not concluded. The same question applies to Type 2 as Type 1 diabetes: why are we unable to find the genes? The same answers apply: heterogeneity, stratification, and genetic–environmental interaction. What can be done to find the genes? The use of association studies rather than linkage analysis has been advocated;[110] another approach is to study populations that originate from a small number of founders, and are small and isolated. Presumably the disease loci are few and linkage disequilibrium extends over longer distances. Pima Indians provide an example. It is possible that the Type 2 diabetes phenotype is the end-point of several minor changes in different genes. Finding intermediate phenotypes (for example, subjects with early insulin resistance or β-cell dysfunction) that may be more related to gene action may help us to identify the genes.

Prediction by genetic studies: what is the future?

The induction of immune changes in early childhood and their continuous presence in the prediabetic period suggest that these changes might predict Type 1 diabetes. Numerous studies have demonstrated the value of ICA as a predictor of Type 1 diabetes.[111] Disease risk is most strongly related to the number of autoantibody markers present, so that estimates of prediction are greatly improved by considering combinations of antibodies.[112–114] Why should antibody combinations be of any value as predictors? Presumably, they reflect a spreading of the immune response to include more than one antigenic determinant, with an associated increase in the risk of progression to Type 1 diabetes. Spreading of this immune response may be, in part, genetically determined; thus, identification of genes associated with susceptibility to Type 1 diabetes could be valuable for disease prediction in conjunction with antibody screening. For example, it is well known that non-diabetic relatives with ICA are unlikely to develop diabetes if they have the HLA allele DQB1*0602.[115] The potential value of genetic screening may be reflected in the different positive predictive values for autoantibodies detected in identical twins (100%) as compared with siblings (41%) of Type 1 diabetes patients.

We now know that Type 2 diabetes exists in several subtypes: at least 1–5% of all diabetics are MODY, and another subtype includes those with late autoimmune diabetes of the adult, or LADA. A further subset of early onset Type 2 diabetes is now recognized, termed MODYX. This subset shows autosomal dominant inheritance, but clinically presents with insulin resistance rather than defective insulin secretion. They do not show linkage to known MODY genes. The MODYX subtype is still to be determined. Other subtypes of Type 2 diabetes may soon be recognized, and it is needed to go back to the clinical definition of the disease, since the study of an heterogeneous population is bound to give negative results. Once we are able to classify all patients according to their Type 2 diabetes subtype, all the genetic studies will gain greater power to detect true linkage.

As regards MODY, it is already possible to predict in family members whether they are at risk of developing the disease; soon, with the new DNA chip technology,[116] early prediction will become easily available in clinical practice.

References

1. Risch N. Linkage strategies for genetically complex traits. I. Multilocus models. *Am J Hum Genet* 1990a; **46**: 222–228.
   Linkage strategies for genetically complex traits. II. The power of affected relative pairs. *Am J Hum Genet* 1990b; **46**: 229–234.
   Linkage strategies for genetically complex traits. III. The effect of marker polymorphism on analysis of affected relative pairs. *Am J Hum Genet* 1990c; **46**: 242–248.

2. Davies JL, Kawaguchi Y, Bennett ST *et al*. A genome wide search for human type 1 diabetes susceptibility genes. *Nature* 1994; **371**: 130–136.

3. Hashimoto L, Habita C, Beressi JP *et al*. Genetic mapping of a susceptibility locus for insulin-dependent diabetes mellitus on chromosome 11q. *Nature* 1994; **371**: 161–164.

4. American Diabetes Association Meeting. *Diabetes* 1998; **47**: A170–A171.

5. Kruglyak L, Lander ES. High-resolution genetic mapping of complex traits. *Am J Hum Genet* 1995; **56**(5): 1212–1223.

6. Jorole LB. Linkage disequilibrium mapping as a gene-mapping tool. *Am J Hum Genet* 1995; **56**: 11–14.

7. Atkinson MA, Maclaren NK. The pathogenesis of insulin-dependent diabetes mellitus. *N Engl J Med* 1994; **331**(21): 1428–1436.

8. Wolf E, Spencer KM, Cudword AG. The genetic susceptibility to type 1 (insulin dependent) diabetes analysis of the HLA-DR association. *Diabetologia* 1983; **24**: 224–230.

9. Todd JA, Bell JI, McDevitt HO. HLA-DQ beta gene contributes to susceptibility and resistance to insulin dependent diabetes mellitus. *Nature* 1987; **329** (614D): 599–604.

10. Khalil I, D'Auriol L, Gobet M *et al*. A combination of HLA-DQ beta Asp 57 negative and HLA-DQ alpha Arg 52 confers susceptibility to insulin dependent mellitus. *J Clin Invest* 1990; **85**: 1315–1319.

11. Khalil I, Deschamps I, Lepage V *et al*. Dose effect of *cis* and *trans* encoded HLA-DQ alpha-beta heterodimers in IDDM susceptibility. *Diabetes* 1992; **42**: 378–384.

12. Buzzetti R, Nisticò L, Osborn JF *et al*. HLA DQA1 and HLA DQB1 gene polymorphisms in type 1 diabetic patients from central Italy and their use for risk prediction. *Diabetes* 1993; **42**: 1173–1178.

13. Nepom GT, Kwok WW. Molecular basis for HLA-DQ associations with IDDM. *Diabetes* 1998; **47**: 1177–1184.

14. Cucca F, Lampis R, Frau F *et al*. The distribution of DR4 haplotypes in Sardinia suggests a primary association type 1 diabetes with DRB1 and DQB1 loci. *Hum Immunol* 1995; **43**(4): 301–343.

15. She JX, Bui MM, Tian XH *et al*. Additive susceptibility to insulin-dependent diabetes conferred by HLA-DQB1 and insulin genes. *Autoimmunity* 1994; **18**(3): 195–203.

16. Bell GI, Horita S, Karam JH. A polymorphic locus of the human insulin gene is associated with insulin-dependent diabetes mellitus. *Diabetes* 1984; **33**: 176–183.

17. Julier C, Hyer RN, Davies J *et al*. Insulin-IGF2 region on chromosome 11p encodes a gene implicated in HLA-DR4-dependent diabetes susceptibility. *Nature* 1991; **354**: 155–159.

18. Lucassen AM, Julier C, Beressi JP *et al*. Susceptibility to insulin-dependent diabetes mellitus maps to a 4.1 kb segment of DNA spanning the insulin gene and associated VNTR. *Nature Genet* 1993; **4**: 305–310.

19. Owerbach DE, Gabbay KH. Localitation of a type 1 diabetes susceptibility locus to the variable tandem repeat region flanking the insulin gene. *Diabetes* 1993; **42**: 1708–1714.

20. Bennett ST, Lucassen AM, Gough SC *et al*. Susceptibility to human type 1 diabetes at IDDM2 is determined by tandem repeat variation at the insulin gene minisatellite locus. *Nature Genet* 1995; **9**: 284–292.

21. Pugliese A, Awdeh ZL, Alper CA *et al*. The paternally inherited insulin gene B allele (1,428 Fokl site) confers protection from insulin dependent diabetes in families. *J Autoimmun* 1994; **7**: 689–694.

22. Pugliese A, Zeller M, Fernandez Jr. A *et al*. The insulin gene is transcribed in the human thymus

and transcription levels correlate with allelic variation at the INS VNTR-IDDM2 susceptibility locus for type 1 diabetes. *Nature Genet* 1997; **15**: 293–296.

23. Undlien DE, Bennett ST, Todd JA *et al.* Insulin gene region-encoded susceptibility to IDDM maps upstream of the insulin gene. *Diabetes* 1995; **44**: 620–625.

24. Vafiadis P, Bennett ST, Colle E *et al.* Imprinted and genotype-specific expression of genes at the IDDM2 locus in pancreas and leucocytes. *J Autoimmun* 1996; **9**: 397–403.

25. Matsumoto C, Awata T, Iwamoto Y *et al.* Lack of association of the insulin gene region with type 1 (insulin dependent) diabetes mellitus in Japanese subjects. *Diabetologia* 1994; **37**: 210–213.

26. Saoudi A, Seddon B, Heath V *et al.* The physiological role of regulatory T cells in the prevention of autoimmunity- the function of the thymus in the generation of the regulatory T cell subset. *Immunol Rev* 1996; **149**: 195–216.

27. Randsell F, Fowllkes BJ. Clonal deletion versus clonal anergy: The role of the thymus in inducing self tolerance. *Science* 1990; **248**: 1342–1348.

28. Vafiadis P, Bennett ST, Todd JA *et al.* Insulin expression in human thymus is modulated by INS VNTR alleles at the IDDM2 locus. *Nature Genet* 1997; **15**: 289–292.

29. Cordell HJ, Todd JA, Bennett ST *et al.* Two-Locus Maximum Lod Score Analysis of a Multifactorial Trait: Joint Consideration of IDDM2 and IDDM4 with IDDM1 in type 1 diabetes. *Am J Hum Genet* 1995; **57**: 920–934.

30. Todd JA, Aitman TJ, Cornall RJ *et al.* Genetic analysis of autoimmune type 1 diabetes mellitus in mice. *Nature* 1991; **351**: 542–546.

31. Ghosh S, Palmer SM, Rodrigues NR *et al.* Polygenic control of autoimmune diabetes in non obese diabetic mice. *Nature Genet* 1993; **4**: 404–409.

32. Field LL, Tobias R, Magnus T. A locus chromosome 15q26 (IDDM3) produces susceptibility to insulin-dependent diabetes mellitus. *Nature Genet* 1994; **8**: 189–194.

33. Quackenbush E, Clabby M, Gottesdiener KM *et al.* Molecular cloning of complementary DNAs encoding the heavy chain of the human 4F2 cell–surface antigen: a type II membrane glycoprotein involved in normal and neoplastic cell growth. *Proc Natl Acad Sci USA* 1987; **84**: 6526–6530.

34. Toda T, Iida A, Miwa T *et al.* Isolation and characterization of a novel gene encoding nuclear protein at a locus (D11S636) tightly linked to multiple endocrine neoplasia type 1 (MEN1). *Hum Molec Genet* 1994; **3**: 465–470.

35. Koch F, Haag F, Kashar A, Thiele HG. Primary structure of rat RT6.2, a nonglycosylated phosphatidylinositol-linked surface marker of post-thymic T cells. *Proc Natl Acad Sci USA* 1990; **87**: 964–967.

36. Greiner DL, Mordes JP, Handler ES *et al.* Depletion of RT6.1 T lymphocytes induces diabetes in resistant Biobreeding/Worcester (BB/W) rats. *J Exp Med* 1987; **166**: 461–469.

37. Prochazka M, Gaskin HR, Leiter EH *et al.* Chromosomal localization, DNA polymorphism, and expression of RT-6, the mouse homologue of rat T-lymphocyte differentiation marker RT6. *Immunogenetics* 1991; **33**: 152–156.

38. Mandrup-Poulsen T, Helqvist S, Wogensen LD *et al.* Cytokines and free radicals as a factor molecules in the destruction of the pancreatic β-cell. *Curr Topics Microbiol Immunol* 1990; **164**: 169–193.

39. Malaisse WJ, Malaisse-Lagae F, Sener A, Pipeleers DG. Determinants of the selective toxicity of alloxan to the pancreatic B-cell. *Proc Natl Acad Sci USA* 1982; **79**: 927–930.

40. Asayama K, Kooy NW, Burr IM. Effects of vitamin E deficiency on insulin secretory reserve and free radical scavenging systems in islets. *J Lab Clin Med* 1986; **107b**: 459–464.

41. Pociot F, Lorenzen T, Nerup J. A manganese superoxide dismutase (SOD2) gene polymorphism in insulin-dependent diabetes mellitus. *Disease Markers* 1993; **11**: 267–274.

42. Pociot F, Johannesen J, Nerup J. *J Autoimmunity*: in press.

43. Borgstahl GEO, Parge HE, Hickey MJ *et al.* The structure of human mitochondrial manganese superoxide dismutase reveals a novel tetrameric interface of two 4-helix bundles. *Cell* 1992; **71**: 107–118.

44. Buzzetti R, Nisticò L, Pozzilli P *et al.* The CTLA-4 microsatellite identifies a new region on chromosome 2 linked to IDDM. *Diabetologia* 1995; **38**(1): A29, n: 105.

45. Nisticò L, Buzzetti R, Pritchard LE *et al*. The CTLA-4 gene region of chromosome 2q33 is linked to, and associated with type 1 diabetes. *Hum Molec Genet* 1996; **5**: 1075–1080.

46. Robey E, Alison JP. T cell activation: integration of signals from the antigen receptor and costimulatory molecules. *Immunol Today* 1995; **16**: 306–309.

47. Buonavista N, Balzano C, Pontarotti P *et al*. Molecular linkage of the human CTLA-4 and CD28 Ig superfamily genes in yeast artificial chromosome. *Genomics* 1992; **13**: 856.

48. Harper K, Balzano C, Rouvier E *et al*. CTLA-4 and CD28 activated lymphocyte molecules are closely related in both mouse and human as to sequence, message expression, gene structure and chromosomal location. *J Immunol* 1991; **147**: 1037–1044.

49. Noel PJ, Boise LH, Thompson CB. Regulation of T cell activation by CD-28 and CTLA-4. *Adv Exp Med Biol* 1996; **406**: 209–217.

50. Donner H, Rau H, Walfish PG *et al*. CTLA-4 alanine-17 confers genetic susceptibility to Grave's disease and to type 1 diabetes mellitus. *J Clin Endocrinol Metab* 1997; **82**: 143–146.

51. Marron MP, Raffel LJ, Garchon HJ *et al*. IDDM is associated with CTLA-4 polymorphism in multiple ethnic groups. *Hum Molec Genet* 1997; **6**: 1275–1282.

52. Rowe RE, Wapelhorst B, Bell GL *et al*. Linkage and association between insulin-dependent diabetes mellitus (IDDM) susceptibility and markers near the glucokinase gene on chromosome 7. *Nature Genet* 1995; **10**: 240–242.

53. Morahan G, Huang D, Tait BD *et al*. Markers on distal chromosome 2q linked to insulin dependent diabetes mellitus. *Science* 1996; **272**: 1811–1813.

54. Luo DF, Bui MM, Muir A *et al*. Affected sib-pair mapping of a novel susceptibility gene to insulin-dependent diabetes mellitus (IDDM8) on chromosome 6q25-q27. *Am J Hum Genet* 1995; **57**: 911–919.

55. Luo DF, Buzzetti R, Rotter JI *et al*. Confirmation of three susceptibility genes to insulin-dependent diabetes mellitus: IDDM4, IDDM5, and IDDM8. *Hum Mol Genet* 1996; **5**: 693–698.

56. Mein CA *et al*. A search for Type 1 diabetes susceptibility genes in families from the United Kingdom. *Nature Gen* 1998; **19**: 297–300.

57. Concannon P, Gogolin-Ewens KJ, Hinds DA *et al*. A second-generation screen of the human genome for susceptibility to insulin-dependent diabetes mellitus. *Nature Gen* 1998; **19**: 292–296.

58. Owerbach D, Gabbay KH. The HOXD8 locus (2q31) is linked to type 1 diabetes – interaction with chromosome 6 and 11 disease susceptibility genes. *Diabetes* 1995; **44**: 132–136.

59. Davies JL, Cucca F, Zeinat A *et al*. Saturation multipoint linkage mapping of chromosome 6q in type 1 diabetes. *Hum Molec Genet* 1996; **5**: 1071–1074.

60. Merriman T, Twells R, Merriman M *et al*. Evidence by allelic association-dependent methods for a type 1 polygene (IDDM) on chromosome 18q21. *Hum Molec Genet* 1997; **6**: 1003–1010.

61. Copeman JB, Cucca F, Hearne CM *et al*. Linkage disequilibrium mapping of a type 1 diabetes susceptibility gene (IDDM7) to chromosome 2q31–q33. *Nature Genet* 1995; **9**: 80–85.

62. Read P, Cucca F, Jenkins S *et al*. Evidence for a type 1 diabetes susceptibility locus (IDDM10) on human chromosome 10q11–q11. *Hum Molec Genet* 1997; **6**: 1011–1016.

63. Field LL, Tobias R, Thomson G, Plon S. Susceptibility to insulin-dependent diabetes mellitus maps to a locus (IDDM11) on human chromosome 14q24.3–q31. *Genomics* 1996; **33**: 1–8.

64. Delepine M, Pociot F, Habita C *et al*. Evidence of a non-MHC susceptibility locus in type 1 diabetes linked to HLA on chromosome 6. *Am J Hum Genet* 1997; **60**: 174–187.

65. Barnett AH, Eff C, Leslie RDG, Pyke DA. Diabetes in identical twins: a study of 200 pairs. *Diabetologia* 1981; **20**: 87–93.

66. Newman B, Selby JV, King MC *et al*. Concordance for type 2 (non-insulin-dependent) diabetes mellitus in male twins. *Diabetologia* 1987; **30**: 763–768.

67. Rewers M, Hamman RF. Risk factors for non-insulin dependent diabetes. In: National Diabetes Data Group, eds. *Diabetes in America*. 2nd edn. Bethesda, MD: NIH/NIDDK, 1995, 179–220.

68. Mather HM, Keen H. The Southall Diabetes Survey: prevalence of diabetes in Asian and Europeans. *Br Med J* 1985; **291**: 1081–1084.

69. Rich SS. Mapping genes in diabetes: genetic epidemiological perspective. *Diabetes* 1990; **39**: 1315–1319.

70. Vadheim CM, Rotter JI. Genetics of diabetes. In: Alberti KGMM, De Fronzo RA, Keen H, Zimmet P, eds. *International Textbook of Diabetes Mellitus*. Chichester: J Wiley, 1992; 31–98.

71. Froguel P. Glucokinase and MODY: from the gene to the disease. *Diabetic Med* 1996; **13**: S96–S97.

72. Cook JTE, Shield DC, Page RCL *et al.* Segregation analysis of NIDDM Caucasian families. *Diabetologia* 1994; **37**: 1231–1240.

73. De Fronzo RA, Bonadonna R, Ferrannini E. Pathogenesis of NIDDM. *Diabetes Care* 1992; **15**: 318–368.

74. Warram JH, Martin BC, Krowelski AS. Slow glucose removal rate and hypeinsulinaemia preced the development of type II diabetes in the offspring of diabetic parents. *Ann Intern Med* 1990; **113**: 909–991.

75. Polonsky KS, Sturis J, Bell GI. Non-insulin dependent diabetes mellitus. A genetically programmed failure of the beta cell to compensate for insulin resistance. *N Engl J Med* 1997; **334**: 777–783.

76. Charles MA, Fontbonne A, Eschwege E. Risk factors of type 2 diabetes in Caucasian population. *Diabetologia* 1998; **31**: 479A.

77. Kenny SJ, Aubert RE, Geiss LS. Prevalence and incidence of non-insulin dependent diabetes. In: National Diabetes Data Group, eds. *Diabetes in America*, 2nd edn. Bethesda, MD: NIH/NIDDK, 1995, 47–68.

78. Boden G. Role of fatty acids in the pathogenesis of insulin resistance and NIDDM. *Diabetes* 1997; **45**: 3–10.

79. Kahn CR. Insulin action, diabetogenes and the cause of type II diabetes. *Diabetes* 1994; **43**: 1066–1084.

80. Sun XJ, Rothemberg P, Khan CR *et al.* Structure of the insulin receptor substrate IRS-1 defines a unique signal transduction protein. *Nature* 1991; **352**: 73–77.

81. Meyers MG, White MF. The new elements of insulin signalling. Insulin receptor substrate-1 and proteins with SH2 domains. *Diabetes* 1993; **42**: 643–650.

82. Kanai F, Ito K, Todaka M *et al.* Insulin-stimu-lated GLUT4 translocation is relevant to the phosphorilation of IRS-1 and the activity of PI-3 kinase. *Biochem Biophys Res Comm* 1993; **195**: 762–768.

83. Almind K, Bjorbaek C, Vestergaard H *et al.* Aminoacid polymorphisms of insulin receptor substrate-1 in non-insulin-dependent diabetes mellitus. *Lancet* 1993; **342**: 828–832.

84. Laakso M, Malkki M, Kekalainen P *et al.* Insulin receptor substrate-1 variants in non-insulin-dependent diabetes. *J Clin Invest* 1994; **94**: 1141–1146.

85. Imai Y, Fusco A, Suzuki Y *et al.* Variant sequences of insulin receptor substrate-1 in non-insulin-dependent-diabetes mellitus. *J Clin Endocrinol Metab* 1994; **79**: 1655–1658.

86. Hitman GA, Hawrami K, McCarthy MI *et al.* Insulin receptor substrate-1 gene mutations in NIDDM: implications for the study of polygenic disease. *Diabetologia* 1995; **38**: 481–486.

87. Almind K, Inoue G, Pedersen O, Kahn CR. A common aminoacid polymorphism in insulin receptor substrate-1 causes impaired insulin signalling. *J Clin Invest* 1996; **97**: 2569–2575.

88. Clausen JO, Hansen T, Bjorbaek C *et al.* Insulin resistance: interactions between obesity and a common variant of insulin receptor substrate-1. *Lancet* 1995; **346**: 397–402.

89. Baroni MG, Arca M, D'Andrea MP *et al.* A common mutation in the insulin receptor substrate 1 (IRS-1) is a genetic marker for the insulin resistance syndrome in patients with coronary artery disease. *Diabetes* 1998; **47(1)**: A173.

90. Groop LC, Kankuri M, Schalin Jantti C *et al.* Association between polymorphism of the glycogen synthase gene and NIDDM. *N Engl J Med* 1993; **328**: 10–14.

91. Hotamisligil GS, Spiegelman BM. Tumor necrosis factor alpha: a key component of the obesity–diabetes link. *Diabetes* 1994; **43**: 1271–1278.

92. Fernandez-Real JM, Gutierrez C, Ricart W *et al.* The TNF-α gene Nco I polymorphisms influences the relationship among insulin resistance, percent body fat, and increased serum leptin levels. *Diabetes* 1997; **46**: 1468–1471.

93. Hamman A, Mantzoros C, Vidal-Puig A, Flier J. Genetic variability in the TNF-α promoter is not associated with type 2 diabetes mellitus. *Biochem Biophys Res Comm* 1995; **211(3):** 833–839.

94. Tontonoz P, Hu E, Spiegelman BM. Stimulation of adypogenesis in fibroblasts by PPAR gamma 2, a lipid-activated transcription factor. *Cell* 1994; **79:** 1147–1156.

95. Meirhaeghe A, Fajas L, Helbeque N *et al.* A genetic polymorphism of the PPAR gamma gene influences plasma leptin levels in obese humans. *Hum Molec Genet* 1998; **7:** 435–440.

96. Yen CJ, Beamer BA, Negri C *et al.* Molecular scanning of the human peroxisome proliferator-activated receptor gamma (hPPAR gamma) gene in diabetic Caucasians: identification of Pro12Ala PPAR gamma 2 missense mutation. *Biochen Biophys Res Comm* 1997; **241:** 270–274.

97. Froguel P, Zouali H, Vionnet N *et al.* Familial hyperglycaemia due to mutations in glucokinase: definition of subtype of diabetes mellitus. *N Engl J Med* 1993; **328:** 697–702.

98. Elbein SC, Hoffman MD, Chiu K *et al.* Linkage analysis of the glucokinase locus in familial type 2 diabetes mellitus. *Diabetologia* 1993; **37:** 1412–1445.

99. Gidh-Jain M, Takeda J, Xu LZ *et al.* Glucokinase mutations associated with non-insulin dependent diabetes have decreased enzymatic activity: implications for structure/function relationships. *Proc Natl Acad Sci USA* 1993; **90:** 1932–1936.

100. Sturis J, Kurkland IJ, Byrne MM *et al.* Compensation in pancreatic β-cell function in subjects with glucokinase mutations. *Diabetes* 1994; **43:** 718–723.

101. Vehlo G, Froguel P, Clement K *et al.* Primary pancreatic β-cell secretory defect caused by mutations in the glucokinase gene in kindreds of MODY. *Lancet* 1992; **340:** 444–448.

102. Velho G, Petersen KF, Perseghin G *et al.* Impaired hepatic glycogen synthesis in glucokinase-deficient subjects. *Diabetes Care* 1996; **17:** 1015–1021.

103. Yamagata K, Furuta H, Oda N *et al.* Mutations in the hepatocyte nuclear factor 4α gene in maturity onset diabetes of the young (MODY1). *Nature* 1996; **384:** 458–460.

104. Yamagata K, Oda N, Kaisaki PJ *et al.* Mutations in the hepatocyte nuclear factor 1α gene in maturity onset diabetes of the young (MODY3). *Nature* 1996; **384:** 455–458.

105. Byrne MM, Sturis J, Clement K *et al.* Insulin secretory abnormalities in subjects with hyperglycaemia due to glucokinase mutations. *J Clin Invest* 1994; **93:** 1120–1130.

106. Stoffers DA, Ferrer J, Clarke WL, Habener JF. Early-onset type 2 diabetes (MODY4) linked to IPF1. *Nature Genet* 1997; **371:** 138–139.

107. Stoffers DA, Zinkin NT, Stanojevic V *et al.* Pancreatic agenesis attributable to a single nucleotide deletion in the human IPF1 gene coding sequence. *Nature Genet* 1997; **15:** 106–110.

108. Hanis CL, Boerwinkle E, Chakraborty R *et al.* A genome-wide search for human non-insulin dependent diabetes genes reveals major susceptibility locus on chromosome 2. *Nature Genet* 1996; **13:** 161–166.

109. Mahtani MM, Widen E, Lehto M *et al.* Mapping a gene for type 2 diabetes associated with an insulin secretion defect by a genome scan in Finnish families. *Nature Genet* 1996; **14:** 90–94.

110. Risch N, Merikangas K. The future of genetic studies of complex human diseases. *Science* 1996; **273:** 1516–1517.

111. Bingley PJ, Bonifacio E, Williams AJK *et al.* Prediction of IDDM in the general population. Strategies based on combinations of autoantibody markers. *Diabetes* 1997; **46:** 1701–1710.

112. Verge CF, Gianani R, Kawasaki E *et al.* Prediction of type 1 diabetes in first-degree relatives using a combination of insulin, GAD and ICA512bdc/IA-2 autoantibodies. *Diabetes* 1996; **45:** 926–933.

113. Seissler I, Morgenthaler NG, Achenbach P *et al.* Combined screening for autoantibodies to IA-2 and antibodies to glutamic acid decarboxylase in first-degree relatives of patients with IDDM. *Diabetologia* 1996; **39:** 1351–1356.

114. Dittler J, Seidel D, Schenker M, Ziegler AG. GADIA-2 combi determination as first-line screening for improved prediction of type 1 diabetes in relatives. *Diabetes* 1998; **47:** 592–597.

115. Pugliese A, Gianani R, Moromisato R *et al.* HLA-DQB1*0602 is associated with dominant protection from diabetes even among islet cell antibody first-degree relatives of patients with IDDM. *Diabetes* 1995; **44**: 608–613.

116. Southern EM. DNA chips: analysing sequence by hybridization to oligonucleotides on a large scale. *Trends Genet* 1996; **12**: 110–115.

3

Prevention of Type 1 diabetes: what are the possibilities?

Polly Bingley and Nicky Leech

Introduction

The discovery of islet cell antibodies (ICAs) in 1974, and the observation that they could be detected prior to the onset of clinical disease, gave rise to the possibility that Type 1 diabetes could be prevented rather than controlled.[1] Twenty-five years later, major advances in our understanding of the pathogenesis of the disease, and the development of strategies to assess risk of Type 1 diabetes in unaffected individuals, have brought us closer to the goal of a safe and effective intervention, though much work remains to be done before this target is reached.

In this chapter we first provide an overview of current understanding of the pathogenesis of Type 1 diabetes, and discuss the points at which intervention might be targeted. We then summarize the approaches to diabetes prevention which have been taken or are currently undergoing large clinical trials, and finally we outline prospects for the future. Recent advances in our understanding of autoimmunity have provided novel and more disease-specific approaches to immunotherapy. We review continuing research towards development of immunointerventions for use in humans, and speculate on the realistic possibilities for prevention of Type 1 diabetes.

The pathogenesis of Type 1 diabetes

Type 1 diabetes is the result of T cell-mediated autoimmune destruction of pancreatic islets.[2]

The first appearance of pancreatic autoantibodies in the serum can occur many years before the development of clinical disease,[3] and loss of pancreatic insulin responses can be demonstrated several years prior to clinical hyperglycaemia. Histological studies of pancreata of people who have died at the time of diagnosis suggest that 90% of the islets have been destroyed at the onset of clinical disease.[4] Primate studies confirm that the onset of hyperglycaemia does not occur until only 10–20% of β-cells remain.[5] Current understanding of the pathogenesis of the disease remains incomplete, but does allow potential targets for intervention to be identified. *Fig. 3.1* summarizes the immunological events leading up to the destructive insulitis. Several models have been proposed for the mechanism by which a primary environmental insult may initiate the cascade resulting in insulitis. Direct damage to the β-cell may result in β-cell antigens becoming abnormally displayed on their surface and presented to the T cells.[6] Activated T cells respond by proliferating and secreting cytokines such as interferon gamma (IFN-γ) and tumour necrosis factor alpha (TNF-α), which encourage the cellular response and activate cytotoxic CD8+ T cells, resulting in T cell attack on the β-cell and destructive insulitis. The activated CD4+ T cells also regulate B cells in the production of autoantibodies to islet autoantigens, although these antibodies appear not to play a direct role in β-cell destruction. Alternatively,

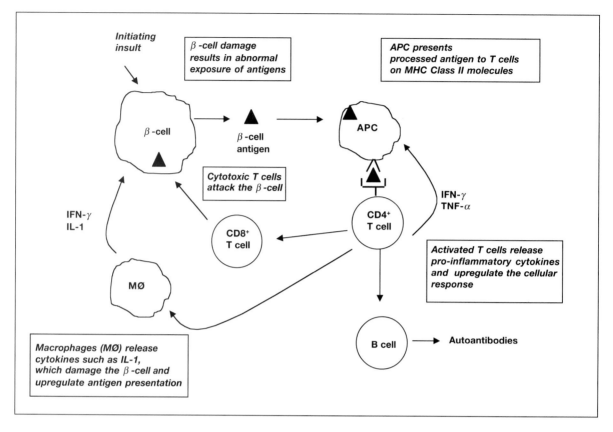

Fig. 3.1
Pathogenesis of pancreatic β-cell destruction.

molecular mimicry may explain the initiating event. There is close-sequence homology between fragments derived from putative pancreatic autoantigens such as glutamate decarboxylase (GAD65) and insulin, and viral proteins, in particular coxsackie, mycobacterium heat-shock protein, and cytomegalovirus.[7] It has been proposed that exposure to such viruses in early life results in a T cell response against these peptides as part of a normal immune response. The homology between the viral peptides and the pancreatic peptides means, however, that the T cells are inappropriately reactive against pancreatic proteins and could initiate the immune cascade resulting in insulitis and diabetes.

Potential targets for intervention therefore include the initiating event, the antigen presenting cell (APC)–T cell interaction, inhibition of T cell proliferation, or protection against the effect of the cytokines. Further details of such approaches will be given below.

Genetic susceptibility

Studies of concordance for Type 1 diabetes in monozygotic twins indicate that the genetic contribution is between 20–60%,[8–10] and 25–50% of genetic susceptibility is accounted for by the major histocompatibility complex (MHC), which codes for the HLA molecules involved in antigen presentation and recognition.[11] Ninety per cent of Caucasians with Type 1 diabetes have either HLA DR3 or DR4 haplotypes, and the combination of DR3 and DR4 carries the greatest risk.[12–13] Possession of the DR2/DQB1*0602 haplotype provides dominant protection against diabetes even in the presence of HLA DR3 or DR4.[14] Genome mapping has identified at least 11 other gene regions contributing to disease susceptibility.[15] Of these, the insulin gene region on chromosome 11 (IDDM2) is most closely associated with disease.[15,16]

Early environmental events

Non-genetic factors account for the remainder of susceptibility. The rising incidence of Type 1 diabetes in a genetically stable population suggests an additional environmental influence.[17] Prospective studies in offspring and siblings of patients with Type 1 diabetes have shown that stable islet autoantibodies appear early in infancy in children at high risk of subsequently developing diabetes.[18] It therefore appears that the initial event precipitating pancreatic autoimmunity in genetically predisposed individuals probably occurs *in utero* or during the neonatal period.

The role of immunoregulation

ICAs are present in 5–10 times the number of children who would be expected to develop Type 1 diabetes.[19,20] It has been thought, therefore, that many more people had evidence of pancreatic autoimmunity than would ever develop clinical diabetes. Long-term follow-up has revealed, however, that most first-degree relatives with high levels of ICAs are likely to eventually develop diabetes.[21] The rate of progression to disease varies from months to over 20 years. There is evidence that age at diagnosis is influenced by genetic susceptibility.[22,23] Immunological mechanisms influencing the rate of progression of pancreatic autoimmunity are still not fully understood, but there is preliminary evidence to suggest that production of cytokines, particularly IL-4, may be important.[24]

Prevention strategies

Our increased understanding of the disease process leading up to insulin-dependent diabetes has suggested a number of points at which it might be possible to intervene to prevent disease, and strategies can be categorized according to the stage of the disease process at which intervention takes place. *Primary* interventions would be applied before the initiation of the autoimmune disease process, *secondary* interventions given to individuals with evidence of ongoing islet autoimmunity in order to slow or stop the destructive process, and *tertiary* interventions used after the clinical onset of diabetes with the aim of preserving residual β-cell function.

Primary intervention

Anti-islet autoimmunity appears to be initiated in intra-uterine or neonatal life, and it is during this period that primary interventions will need to be applied.[18] Depending on the safety profile of an intervention, it could be applied to all newborns or given on the basis of screening for genetic susceptibility. Current strategies for genetic screening are, however, associated with relatively low sensitivity and specificity. Used in the general population, the highest risk combination of genetic markers (HLA-DQA1*0301-DQB1*0302/DQA1*0501-DQB1*0201) would identify some 40% of children destined to develop diabetes before the age of 15 years but it is present in 3% of the background population.[25] At present the only realistic strategy is the avoidance of putative environmental factors triggering the autoimmune process, although some of the novel immunointerventions described in the second half of this chapter, for example those interfering with primary antigen presentation and the interaction between the APC and T lymphocyte, may also fall into this category.

Diet and viral infection, particularly intrauterine enteroviral infection, currently represent the leading candidates for environmental factors triggering the immune response. The hypothesis that early exposure to cow's milk or cow's milk products may have a causative role in Type 1 diabetes is based on animal studies, and on epidemiological and immunological data. While a considerable body of evidence has been presented to the effect that cow's milk may have a role to play, this issue remains controversial.[26-28] The hypothesis is currently being tested in a Finnish randomized placebo-controlled trial of cow's milk avoidance in genetically susceptible infants during the first 6 months of life.[29] Serological and epidemiological studies in newly diagnosed patients have shown associations between enteroviruses, particularly coxsackievirus B (CBV), and Type 1 diabetes.[30] Coxsackievirus and viral RNA sequences have been isolated from the pancreas or serum of patients with newly diagnosed Type 1 diabetes.[31-33] Further studies have suggested that viral infection encountered *in utero* may play a causal role, even when diabetes develops much later in life. This was first demonstrated with congenital rubella, but more recently investigators in Sweden and Finland have found evidence of a higher frequency of maternal enterovirus infection in pregnancy among the mothers of children who subsequently developed diabetes than among controls.[34-37] There is considerable evidence therefore to suggest that viral infection encountered early in life may be a factor in later development of Type 1 diabetes. The mechanism may involve persistent infection, which is more readily established when the immune system is immature, or potential immunological cross-reactivity or 'molecular mimicry' resulting from sequence homologies between viral and host islet antigens.[7] While existing studies have yielded conflicting results, and causality remains unproven, identification of viruses with a role in the aetiology of Type 1 diabetes would give rise to the possibility that immunization against relevant viruses might prevent at least a proportion of cases.[38]

Secondary and tertiary prevention strategies

Recent advances in our ability to identify those at greatest risk of developing Type 1 diabetes have given rise to the possibility of immune intervention to delay or prevent the clinical onset of diabetes, and clinical trials have been started in family members at risk. Risk assessment is based on combined analysis of the four major islet autoantibody markers: antibodies to glutamate decarboxylase (GAD), protein tyrosine phosphatase IA-2, insulin and ICAs. Combinations of these antibodies can identify family members with around 80% risk of diabetes within 10 years, with a sensitivity of 80–90%.[39-41] It seems probable that this approach will also be valuable in general population screening to identify children at high risk of developing IDDM but who have no family history of the disease.[42] Trials can be broadly divided according to the approach

Table 3.1
Approaches taken in randomized clinical intevention trials in Type 1 diabetes.

Agent	Type of prevention	Mechanism	References
Azathioprine	tertiary	non-specific immunosuppression of primary T cell responses	(Harrison *et al.* 1985)[122]
Cyclosporin A	tertiary	Semi-specific immunosuppresion, blocking CD4 activation	(Feutren *et al.* 1986; Canadian–European Randomized Control Trial Group, 1988)[44,45]
Nicotinamide	tertiary and secondary	protection of β-cell against cytokine-mediated cytotoxicity	(Elliot *et al.* 1996; Pozzilli *et al.* 1996; Lampeter *et al.* 1998; Moore *et al.* 1997)[63,65,67,123]
Parenteral insulin	secondary	immunomodulation	(Fuchtensbusch *et al.* 1998; DPT-1 Study Group, 1994)[55,56]
Oral insulin	secondary	immunomodulation	(DPT-1 StudyGroup, 1994)[56]
Bacille Calmette–Guérin Vaccination (BCG)	tertiary	immunomodulation	(Pozzilli and the IMDIAB group, 1997)[70]

used: immunosuppression – generalized or specific – or immunomodulation – attempting to correct or influence a disordered or inappropriate immune response. Early trials have been reviewed elsewhere.[43] Agents which have been, or are currently, under investigation in large randomized controlled human trials are listed in *Table 3.1*.

Cyclosporin A

The controlled trials of cyclosporin A were particularly important, since they showed that treatment with this agent from the time of diagnosis could increase the rate of non-insulin-requiring remission, albeit temporarily.

It was therefore demonstrated that the course of the autoimmune disease process could be altered to achieve a clinically significant effect.[44,45] The Canadian–European trial also found that this effect was concentrated in the patients with shorter duration of symptoms, less weight loss, higher C-peptide secretion, and absence of ketoacidosis at diagnosis. The rate of non-insulin-requiring remission was also higher at both 6 and 12 months in adults than in children.[44] These observations suggest that, as would be predicted from its mode of action, the drug is more effective if given earlier in the disease process and less effective in the more rapid destructive process that occurs in children. Cyclosporin toxicity is, however, generally considered to preclude its use in secondary prevention, though a small pilot study has suggested that it could delay the onset of disease in individuals at very high risk of developing Type 1 diabetes.[46]

Insulin

Subcutaneous insulin reduces the incidence of diabetes in the BB rat and NOD mouse models of Type 1 diabetes.[47,48] Intensive insulin treatment (including 2 weeks of intravenous treatment given via an artificial pancreas) given to patients at the time of diagnosis was associated with lower glycated haemoglobin levels and higher stimulated c-peptide after 12 months than in controls.[49] Proposed mechanisms are immune modulation, tolerance induction, or β-cell rest, whereby reduced insulin secretion causes less antigen expression, rendering the cells less susceptible to immune attack.[50] Both oral and intraperitoneal insulin have been shown to be effective in preventing diabetes in the non-obese diabetic mouse (NOD) mouse[51] and subcutaneous administration of the insulin beta chain is also as effective as injection of the whole molecule.[52] In addition, in the NOD mouse, insulin therapy has been found to increase T cell production of IL-4, a cytokine associated with protection against diabetes.[53] Such data suggest that although β-cell rest may have some effect, the main mechanism of insulin treatment in this context is likely to be immunomodulatory.

A pilot trial of pre-emptive parenteral insulin treatment, given to seven subjects predicted to have a more than 90% risk of developing diabetes within 3 years, produced promising results,[54] and a more recent randomized controlled pilot study from Germany found that parenteral insulin delayed the manifestation of clinical diabetes by 2–3 years.[55] A large multicentre study of subcutaneous insulin with

annual 5-day admission for intravenous insulin infusion is underway in the USA – the Diabetes Prevention Trial-1 (DPT-1).[56] This open randomized controlled study is aiming to recruit 340 first- and second-degree relatives of children with Type 1 diabetes with an ICA ≥10 JDF units and impairment of first-phase insulin secretion who have an estimated risk of more than 50% of developing diabetes within 5 years.

Nicotinamide

Nicotinamide (nicotinic acid amide or niacin-amide) is a water-soluble group B vitamin. Its effect in prevention of toxin-induced models of diabetes has been known for more than 50 years.[57,58] It is also effective in preventing spontaneous diabetes in the NOD mouse and inhibits transplant allograft insulitis, another animal model of immune β-cell damage, as well as preserving residual β-cells in partially pancreatectomized rats and promoting the growth of cultured human islet cells. It appears to act in the final stage of β-cell damage, preventing the cytotoxic effects of cytokines. As outlined in the introduction, current evidence suggests that Type 1 diabetes is a cytokine-mediated, Th-cell and macrophage-dependent disease (*Fig. 3.1*), and that free radicals (NO, $O_2 \cdot -$ and OH-) are intracellular mediators of cell death.[59] These may cause direct damage to intranuclear DNA, resulting in strand breaks. Nicotinamide prevents IL-1-induced islet cell nitric oxide (NO) production by inhibiting the expression of inducible nitric oxide synthase in β-cells.[60] There are two proposed major mechanisms for its action: (1) it acts as a free radical scavenger to reduce DNA damage; and (2) it restores the islet cell content of NAD towards normal by partial inhibition of the DNA repair enzyme poly ADP-ribose polymerase (PARP), a major route of NAD metabolism, and by elevating intracellular NAD.[59,61,62]

The low toxicity and lack of side-effects associated with this agent made it an attractive drug for human trials. Studies in patients with newly diagnosed Type 1 diabetes have yielded variable results, but meta-analysis has suggested that nicotinamide treatment is associated with some preservation of residual β-cell function.[63] In a pilot study of its ability to prevent Type 1 diabetes in first-degree relatives, four out of eight historical controls developed diabetes within 1 year, compared to none of nine receiving nicotinamide. By 2 years, seven of eight in the untreated group and none of six on nicotinamide had developed diabetes.[64] A large population-based trial has subsequently been undertaken in schoolchildren in New Zealand, using randomization by school. In total, 33,658 children aged 5–8 years were offered ICA testing, of whom 20,195 were tested. Of these, 185 children met the criteria for nicotinamide treatment (ICA ≥20 JDF or ICA 10 JDF units and low first-phase insulin response), and 173 received this treatment. The incidence of diabetes over a mean follow-up of 7.1 years in the treated children was 7.1/100,000/year (95% confidence interval (CI) 3.1–14.1), compared with 16.1/100,000/year (95% CI 12.4–20.5) in children from the control schools ($p = 0.008$).[65]

On the strength of these preliminary studies, two large multicentre randomized placebo-controlled trials were initiated. The European Nicotinamide Diabetes Intervention Trial (ENDIT) is the largest randomized placebo-controlled diabetes intervention trial to date. It has screened 40,000 first-degree relatives from 23 countries and recruited those with ICA ≥20 JDF units and a non-diabetic OGTT. Such individuals have an estimated 40% risk of diabetes within 5 years.[66] The recruitment target of 528 individuals was reached in December 1997 and, when recruitment closed in May 1998, a total of 552 individuals had been randomized to 5 years treatment with nicotinamide or placebo. The end-point of the study is diabetes as defined by WHO criteria, and the trial will be unblinded in 2003. ENDIT was designed to have 90% power to detect a 35–40% treatment effect. A smaller German trial, Deutsche Nicotinamide Intervention Study (DENIS), was set up around the same time, with power to demonstrate an 80% treatment effect in children at high risk of rapid progression to diabetes (30% in 3 years). The trial was terminated when the second interim analysis had failed to detect a reduction in the cumulative incidence of diabetes at 3 years from 30 to 3%. Fifty-five children were recruited and, by the end of the trial, seven in the treated group and six on placebo had developed diabetes.[67] The authors concluded 'these data do not exclude the possibility of a less strong but clinically meaningful risk reduction in this cohort or a major clinical effect of nicotinamide in individuals with less risk of progression to IDDM'. These issues should be resolved by ENDIT.

Bacillus Calmette–Guérin (BCG)

Bacillus Calmette–Guérin (BCG) vaccination induces regulatory T cells, and a single injection can decrease the rate of development of diabetes in the NOD mouse.[68] BCG represents an attractive intervention strategy with few side-effects, and its historical widespread use in immunization programmes enables us to feel confident that it is associated with low toxicity. It is, therefore, not surprising that it has already been used in human diabetes prevention trials. A pilot study in 17 diabetic patients showed prolonged remission in 65% of BCG-treated patients when administered at the time of diagnosis, versus 7% of controls.[69] It has been tested in one arm of IMDIAB, a large multicentre trial addressing the role of nicotinamide in tertiary diabetes prevention. Patients with newly diagnosed Type 1 diabetes were randomized to nicotinamide and BCG vaccination or nicotinamide alone. No independent protective effect of BCG could be detected.[70]

Epidemiological studies of BCG vaccination and Type 1 diabetes have also failed to establish any protective effect of BCG. In Sweden, uptake of BCG vaccination of newborn children born before 1975 was almost universal, and following a change in vaccination policy in that year, BCG vaccination was subsequently given to less than 2% of children. There was, however, no change in the cumulative incidence of Type 1 diabetes between the birth cohorts 2 years before and after that time.[71] A case control study of Type 1 diabetes patients in Montreal also failed to show an independent protective effect of previous BCG vaccination.[72] It therefore seems that this immunointervention strategy will not be useful in humans, despite promising results from animal studies.

Future directions

Towards the development of a specific immunotherapy

Although Type 1 diabetes may be modified by general immunosuppressive agents, this approach appears only to control or delay the disease process rather than to cure it, and the generalized immunosuppression and side-effects are a high price to pay for short-term remission. There therefore remains a need for therapy which is long lasting, non-toxic, and targets a specific point in the immune system where dysregulation has occurred. To understand the rationale behind the ongoing attempts to design such a therapy, it is first necessary to review our current understanding of the concepts behind the immunological events resulting in autoimmunity.

Concepts in natural immune tolerance and autoimmunity

There is a fine balance between establishing immunity to exogenous antigens, and autoimmunity. T cells play a pivotal role in the initiation and control of our immune responses and our ability to distinguish self from non-self. When a part of this complex regulatory system fails, autoimmunity may result. The mechanisms involved in normal immune tolerance can be divided into central or thymic tolerance and peripheral tolerance.

Establishing the T cell repertoire: role of the thymus

The initial education of T cells to distinguish self from non-self occurs in the thymus during the neonatal period. Recent studies have demonstrated that T cells with high affinity for self-antigens are selectively destroyed in the thymus,[73] and by this process about 95% of T cell precursors are deleted.[74]

The importance of thymic selection in the development of Type 1 diabetes was initially indicated by studies demonstrating that neonatal thymectomy resulted in autoimmune organ destruction.[75] Thymectomy performed before or after the neonatal period did not have this effect, demonstrating the importance of precise timing of thymic elimination of self-reactive T cells. Further work in the NOD mouse has demonstrated that a defect in HLA Class II expression in the thymus results in failure to delete autoreactive T cells and allows their release into the peripheral circulation.[76,77] This is one way in which autoimmunity may develop.

It has been shown, using both GAD65 and proinsulin, that expression or injection of these antigens in the thymus of the NOD mouse during the neonatal period results in the abolition of T cell reactivity against these antigens and protection against the development of diabetes.[78–80] Such studies establish a role for these antigens in the development of the T cell repertoire.

Regulation of T cell reactivity in the peripheral circulation

Elimination of autoreactive T cells in the thymus is not complete and there are further self-protective mechanisms against autoimmunity acting on peripheral T cells. The T cell responses to a particular antigen can be regulated by three mechanisms. The cell may be rendered temporarily unable to proliferate or respond to antigen (*anergy*). The T cell may be deleted (*apopotosis*), or the cytokine production of the cell may be altered, resulting in modulation of its behaviour (*suppression*) (*Fig. 3.2*).

Immunoregulation: the Th1/Th2 paradigm

T cells are activated as the result of interaction of a cell surface antigen-specific receptor with a peptide fragment of the specific antigen presented to them by an antigen-presenting cell. Activation of the T cell results in proliferation

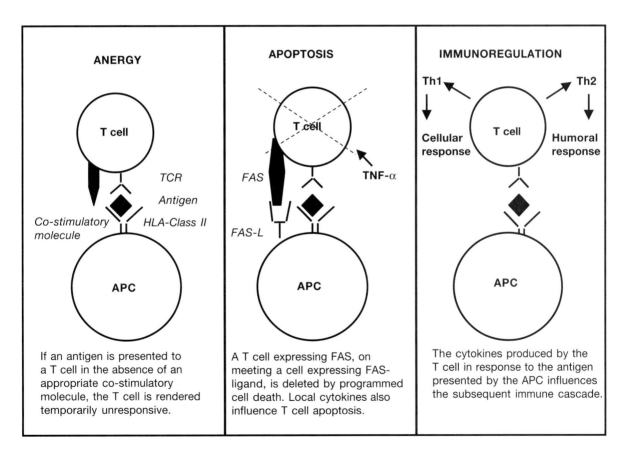

Fig. 3.2
Mechanisms of peripheral tolerance.

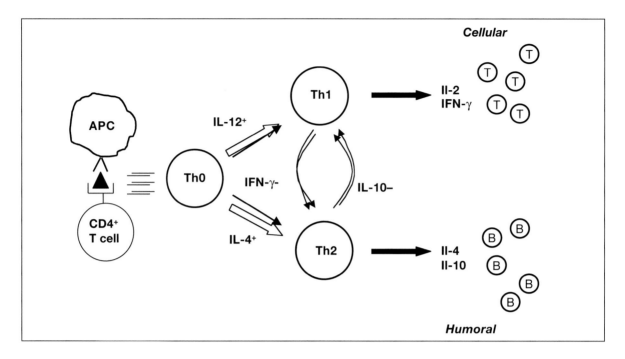

Fig. 3.3
Differentiation of CD4+ T cell subsets according to their cytokine profile.

and cytokine production. The cytokines produced influence the nature of the subsequent immune response. In 1986, Mossman described two distinct CD4+ T cell phenotypes, their types being dependent upon their cytokine production (*Fig. 3.3*). Th1 cells produced IFN-γ and IL-2, and generated a cell-mediated response, while Th2 cells produced IL-4 and IL-10, and promoted humoral responses.[81] Although this polarization of the cytokine response was initially described in mouse T cell clones, similar patterns of response occur in human T cells.

In the NOD mouse, T cells infiltrating the insulitic lesion have been found to produce large amounts of Th1-type cytokines, IL-2 and IFN-γ, whereas T cells producing Th2-type cytokines, IL-4, IL-5, and IL-10, are associated with a non-destructive peri-insulitis.[82,83] The situation in human Type 1 diabetes is less clear. Post-mortem pancreata from patients with newly diagnosed Type 1 diabetes have revealed large amounts of IFN-γ producing infiltrating T cells.[84] *In vitro* studies of human peripheral blood lymphocytes have suggested a bias towards increased concentrations of Th1-type cytokine production[85,86] and a deficit of Th2-type cytokines, associated with the development of Type 1 diabetes.[24]

New approaches to immunointervention

Modification of peripheral tolerance has the greater potential as an immunointervention strategy since it may be effective in children and adults in whom thymic selection has already occurred.

Breaking the Class II–peptide interaction: anti-CD3/CD4 monoclonal antibodies

Disruption of the central interaction, the APC–peptide–T cell trimolecular complex seems a logical approach to preventing progression of autoimmunity. Monoclonal antibodies (MoAbs) have been raised against the T cell CD3 and CD4 receptors. Treatment with either anti-CD3 or anti-CD4 MoAb has prevented the onset of IDDM in the NOD mouse.[87–91] The use of anti-CD3 (OKT3) in human Type 1 diabetes is precluded by the serious side-effects that result from its generalized T cell stimulatory properties.[92] One small trial combining anti-CD4 MoAb with prednisolone in newly diagnosed diabetic children resulted in a transient improvement in three out of five children.[93] Anti-CD4 immunotherapy has undergone more extensive trials in severe rheumatoid arthritis, but, although clinical benefit and significant immunomodulation have been shown,[94] side-effects are common. Anti-CD3 and anti-CD4 monoclonal antibodies are therefore insufficiently specific to be a viable form of immunointervention for Type 1 diabetes.

Diphethia toxin interleukin-2 recombinant fusion protein (DAB486 IL-2)

DAB486 IL-2 represents an elegant development in the development of a more specific immunosuppressant agent. IL-2 molecules are tagged to a cytotoxic agent, in this case a diptheria-toxin-related protein. When T cells are activated, they express IL-2 receptors on their surface. Tagged IL-2 would home to these receptors, and thereby selectively destroy the activated T cells. DAB486 IL-2 has undergone clinical pilot studies in newly diagnosed Type 1 diabetics,[95] but unfortunately the high rate of side-effects precludes its general use.

Changing the Th1/Th2 cytokine balance

Much attention has focused on developing strategies attempting to tip the balance towards a Th2-like cytokine response, which could protect against the development of diabetes. The problem has been approached using (a) cytokines, cytokine antagonists, or monoclonal antibodies against cytokines or their receptors; and (b) antigen-derived peptides which skew the cytokine response.

A number of animal studies have been performed to assess the feasibility of upregulating suppressor (Th2) cytokine production. IL-10 injection in NOD mice has been shown to decrease insulitis and IDDM.[96] IL-4 administration also inhibited the rate of development of IDDM but not insulitis.[97] Increasing IL-4 within the islet resulted in a non-destructive insulitis in NOD mice. Although such results are encouraging, systemic administration of IL-4 in humans can be associated with severe side-effects.

The Th1/Th2 paradigm is, however, an oversimplification. IL-10 administration has been shown to increase rates of diabetes development in the NOD mouse, and IL-4 can augment the development of another T cell-mediated autoimmune disease, experimental uveitis.[98] It therefore appears that the effect of cytokines on immune deviation are more complicated than was originally anticipated, and may be dependent upon factors such as timing of administration, dose, and method of administration.

Inhibition of Th1 responses

Since the administration of Th2 cytokines is problematical, the possibility of blocking the Th1 response has been considered. IL-12 is a Th1-promoting cytokine which accelerates the development of insulitis and diabetes in the NOD mouse.[99] Anti-IL-12 MoAb has been shown to be effective in preventing experimental allergic encephalitis (EAE), the spontaneous animal model of multiple sclerosis,[100] and experimental colitis.[101] Human clinical trials have been undertaken using this approach with anti-TNF-α MoAb in the treatment of established rheumatoid arthritis.[102] Anti-TNF-α appeared to be safe and well tolerated, but there were major limitations in its efficacy, due to the immune response mounted against the antibody itself. Modifications to the antibody to overcome this neutralizing effect by the recipient immune system appear to have improved its efficacy.[103]

Immune deviation by antigenic tolerance

Antigen-specific modification of the immune response was explored as far back as 1911, when HG Wells demonstrated that guinea pigs could be made refractory to anaphylactic reactions to dietary proteins by feeding of peptides derived from the proteins.[104] T cell anergy,[105] immunomodulation of cytokine production,[106] and induction of apoptosis[107] have all been proposed as mechanisms involved in antigen-specific tolerance. The efficacy and mechanisms of tolerance induction are dependent upon the route of administration, the dose

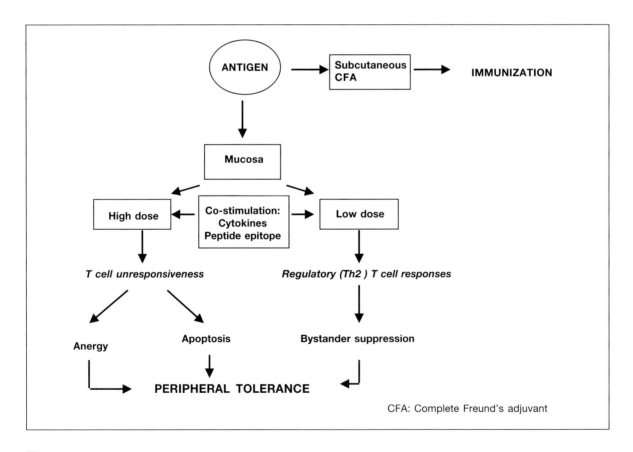

Fig. 3.4
Mechanisms of antigen-induced peripheral tolerance.

of antigen used, whether the whole protein or peptides derived from it are given, and the use of adjuvant. The influence of these factors is summarized in *Fig. 3.4*.

Can an appropriate antigen be identified for human immunointervention?

A drawback to antigen-specific immunotherapy is the identification of an appropriate antigen. Candidate primary antigens for T cells in Type 1 diabetes have predominantly been identified through the study of disease-associated auto-antibodies. The list of candidate antigens is, however, extensive, and it is possible that several antigens can initiate T cell reactivity against the pancreatic islet. Furthermore, although there is some evidence to suggest that T and B cells recognize similar self-proteins in Type 1 diabetes,[108,109] reports from the first Immunology Diabetes Society (IDS) Workshop indicate that the reproducibility and disease specificity of antigen-specific T cell reactivity studies is poor. It is possible, however, that identification of the primary antigen is not essential for effective antigenic tolerance. Early studies of the use of myelin basic protein (MBP) in the prevention of experimentally induced EAE demonstrated a phenomenon now referred to as *bystander suppression*. The administration of oral ovalbumin had no effect on MBP-induced encephalitis in the Lewis rat, but if animals were fed oral ovalbumin and then immunized with subcutaneous ovalbumin following subcutaneous immunization with MBP, the development of encephalitis was suppressed.[106] It could be demonstrated that suppression of the MBP-specific response was mediated by the ovalbumin-specific T cells which migrated to the draining lymph node and produced TGF-β on re-encountering ovalbumin. This TGF-β inhibits the MBP-specific response in the lymph node. The phenomenon of bystander suppression means

that it may be possible to induce tolerance by the induction of a regulatory T cell response, and by directing the T cell to the pancreas, where it can influence the T cells involved in the ongoing autoimmune process.

In the NOD mouse, tolerance (and prevention) of diabetes has been achieved by a variety of routes,[51,52,79,110–112] and with a number of antigens, including insulin,[48,51,52] GAD65,[78,79,112–114] proinsulin,[80] and peptides derived from the heat-shock protein 65.[115] The diabetes-protective effect of oral insulin could be transferred to naïve recipients by the transfer of CD4+ T cells. These experiments provide evidence for the induction of regulatory T cells.[116,117] More recently, several studies have demonstrated the induction of Th2-like T cells.[52,53,112] The mechanism of insulin-induced tolerance therefore appears to be due to a shift from Th1 to Th2 T cell responses.

Antigen-specific imunotherapy in clinical trials

In order to assess the efficacy of antigen-specific immunotherapy in human trials, it is useful to look to the results in other autoimmune diseases. Pilot studies of oral MBP therapy in patients with relapsing and remitting multiple sclerosis (MS) have shown some clinical improvement in a subset of patients carrying a particular MHC, HLA-DR2.[118] In a larger trial of in 515 patients, however, oral MBP therapy resulted in no improvement in disability scores. Pilot studies of oral collagen in patients with rheumatoid arthritis also looked promising, but a larger double-blind placebo-controlled trial failed to show any difference between the placebo and treated groups.[119] No deleterious effects were observed in either trial.

Although these initial results of human oral tolerization studies have so far been disappointing, there is no prior information with regard to dose, route of administration and duration of administration of such therapies. Many manipulations of the treatment principles are likely to be required before successful immunointervention is achieved. Trials of antigen-specific immunotherapy are, however, in progress in Type 1 diabetes. DPT-1 has included an arm of oral insulin therapy in first-degree relatives with intermediate risk (26–59%) of developing Type 1 diabetes over 5 years.[56] Pancreatic β-cell function will be included as a surrogate end-point as well as the clinical end-point of diabetes. Human double-blind placebo-controlled trials of nasal insulin are also underway in Australia in high-risk prediabetic individuals.[120]

Conclusions

Large multicentre diabetes intervention trials such as ENDIT and DPT-1 have demonstrated the feasibility of identifying high-risk first-degree relatives for diabetes intervention. The next few years will provide answers as to whether current strategies such as insulin or nicotinamide are useful agents for prevention. Although such trials are useful for initial study of new therapeutic agents, they intervene at a late stage in the immune process and are therefore less likely to result in long-term remission. Screening strategies and intervention must ultimately be applicable in the general population, where 90% of new cases of Type 1 diabetes occur. Interventions will have to be of sufficiently low toxicity to be applied earlier in the disease process and be relatively easy to administer. We do not currently have sufficient knowledge about the aetiology of Type 1 diabetes to consider population-wide primary prevention. Further work is needed on the earliest stages of the immune process, and the complex interactions with environmental

agents. The role of *in utero* viral infection, and the possibility of vaccination against candidate enteroviruses, may be worth exploring further, but it currently seems naïve to think that any single environmental trigger is responsible for the disease.

The accumulating evidence for the role of Th1/Th2 cytokine balance in progression to diabetes provides a key to the development of immunomodulatory prevention strategies and much-needed immunological surrogate markers of successful intervention. Our current understanding of the role of regulatory T cells and 'bystander suppression' offers hope that antigen-specific therapies can be designed without necessarily identifying the primary antigen involved in the pathogenic process. The considerable success in preventing diabetes in the NOD mouse using antigen-specific therapies from a range of pancreatic antigens provides encouragement for the development of such strategies in humans, though the comparison should not be pushed too far.[121] Much work is required with regard to dose of antigen, route of administration, and modification of the antigen before such therapies are ready for large clinical trials in humans.

Identification of potential agents for intervention is only one step in the process towards prevention of disease. The basic science must be complemented by rigorous clinical evaluation of efficacy, and of the best way to introduce treatments into clinical practice. Laboratory, clinical, and epidemiological researchers all have key roles to play in research towards the prevention of Type 1 diabetes. We have emphasized the limitations of our current knowledge and the distance we have to go to achieve prevention of Type 1 diabetes, but we must remember how far we have already come. We conclude that there are grounds for considerable optimism!

References

1. Gorsuch AN, Lister J, Dean BM *et al*. Evidence for a long prediabetic period in type I (insulin-dependent) diabetes mellitus. *Lancet* 1981; **2**: 1363–1365.

2. Bottazzo G, Dean B, McNally J *et al*. *In situ* characterization of autoimmune phenomena in diabetic expression of HLA molecules in the pancreas in diabetic insulitis. *N Engl J Med* 1985; **313**: 353–360.

3. Eisenbarth GS. Type 1 diabetes: a chronic autoimmune disease. *N Engl J Med* 1986; **314**: 1360–1368.

4. Foulis AK, Stewart JA. The pancreas in recent-onset type 1 (insulin-dependent) diabetes mellitus: Insulin content of islets, insulitis and associated changes in the exocrine acinar tissue. *Diabetologia* 1984; **26**: 456–461.

5. McCulloch DK, Koerker DJ, Kahn SE *et al*. Correlations of *in vivo* β-cell function tests with β-cell mass and pancreatic insulin content in streptozocin-administered baboons. *Diabetes* 1991; **40**: 673–679.

6. Bottazzo GF. Death of a beta cell: Homicide or suicide? *Diabetic Med* 1986; **3**: 119–130.

7. Atkinson MA, Bowman MA, Campbell L *et al*. Cellular immunity to a determinant common to glutamate decarboxylase and coxsackie virus in insulin-dependent diabetes. *J Clin Invest* 1994; **94**: 2125–2129.

8. Kaprio J, Tuomilehto J, Koskenvuo M *et al*. Concordance for type 1 (insulin-dependent) and type 2 (non-insulin-dependent) diabetes mellitus in a population-based cohort of twins in Finland. *Diabetologia* 1992; **35**: 1060–1067.

9. Kyvik KO, Green A, Beck-Nielsen H. Concordance rates of insulin dependent diabetes mellitus: a population based study of young Danish twins. *Br Med J* 1995; **311**: 913–917.

10. Tattersall RB, Pyke DA. Diabetes in identical twins. *Lancet* 1972; **2**: 1120–1125.

11. Davies JL, Kawaguchi Y, Bennett ST *et al*. A genome-wide search for human type 1 diabetes susceptibility genes. *Nature* 1994; **371**: 130–136.

12. Bertrams J, Baur MP. Insulin dependent diabetes mellitus. In: Albert ED, Mayr WR, eds. *Histocompatibility Testing 1984*. Berlin: Springer-Verlag, 1984: 348–358.

13. Wolf E, Spencer KM, Cudworth AG. The genetic susceptibility to type 1 (insulin-dependent) diabetes: analysis of the HLA-DR association. *Diabetologia* 1983; **24**: 224–230.

14. Thomson G, Robinson WP, Kuhner MK *et al*. Genetic heterogeneity, modes of inheritance, and risk estimates for a joint study of Caucasians with insulin-dependent diabetes mellitus. *Am J Hum Genet* 1988; **43**: 799–816.

15. Todd JA. Genetic analysis of Type 1 diabetes using whole genome approaches. *Proc Natl Acad Sci USA* 1995; **92**: 8560–8565.

16. Bennett ST, Wilson AJ, Cucca F *et al*. IDDM2–VNTR-encoded susceptibility to type-1 diabetes: dominant protection and parental transmission of alleles of the insulin gene-linked microsatellite locus. *J Autoimmun* 1996; **9**: 415–421.

17. Gardner SG, Bingley PJ, Sawtell PA *et al*. Rising incidence of insulin dependent diabetes in children aged under 5 years in the Oxford region: time trend analysis. *Br Med J* 1997; **315**: 713–717.

18. Ziegler AG, Hummel M, Schenker M, Bonifacio E. Autoantibody appearance and risk for the development of childhood diabetes in offspring of parents with type 1 diabetes: The 2 year analysis of the German BABYDIAB study. *Diabetes* 1999; **48**: 460–468.

19. Bingley PJ, Bonifacio E, Shattock M *et al*. Can islet cell antibodies predict IDDM in the general population? *Diabetes Care* 1993; **16**: 45–50.

20. Rowe RE, Leech NJ, Nepom GT, McCulloch DK. High genetic risk for IDDM in the Pacific Northwest: First report from the Washington State Diabetes Prediction Study. *Diabetes* 1994; **43**: 87–94.

21. Bingley PJ, Gardner SG, Williams AJK *et al*. Longterm follow-up of family members with ICA≥20 JDF units: will they all develop diabetes? (abstr). *Diabetologia* 1998; **41**(**Suppl 1**): A:87.

22. Tait BD, Harrison LC, Drummond BP *et al*. HLA antigens and age at diagnosis of insulin-dependent diabetes mellitus. *Hum Immunol* 1995; **42**: 116–122.

23. Van der Auwera B, Schuit F, Lyaruu I *et al*, and Belgium Diabetes Registry. Genetic

susceptibility for insulin-dependent diabetes in Caucasians revisited: the importance of diabetes registries in disclosing interactions between HLA-DQ-and insulin gene-linked risk. *J Clin Endocrinol Metab* 1995; **80**: 2567–2573.

24. Wilson SB, Kent SC, Patton KT *et al.* Extreme Th1 bias of invariant Vα24JαQ T cells in type 1 diabetes. *Nature* 1998; **39**: 1177–1181.

25. Ronningen KS, Spurkland A, Iwe T *et al.* Distribution of HLA-DRB1, -DQA1 and -DQB1 alleles and DQA1-DQB1 genotypes among Norwegian patients with insulin-dependent diabetes mellitus. *Tissue Antigens* 1991; **37**: 105–111.

26. Ellis TM, Atkinson MA. Early infant diets and insulin-dependent diabetes. *Lancet* 1996; **347**: 1464–1465.

27. Harrison LC. Cow's milk and IDDM. *Lancet* 1996; **348**: 905–906.

28. Scott FW, Norris JM, Kolb H. Milk and Type 1 diabetes: examining the evidence and broadening the focus. *Diabetes Care* 1996; **19**: 379–383.

29. Åkerblom HK, Paganus A, Teramo K *et al.* Primary prevention of type 1 diabetes by nutritional intervention. Description of a pilot study. *Autoimmunity* 1993; **15(Suppl 1)**: 58.

30. Barrett-Connor E. Is insulin-dependent diabetes mellitus caused by coxsackie B infection? A review of the epidemiologic evidence. *Rev Infect Dis* 1985; **7**: 207–215.

31. Clements GB, Galbraith DN, Taylor KW. Coxsackie B virus infection and onset of childhood diabetes. *Lancet* 1995; **346**: 221–223.

32. Gladisch R, Hofmann W, Waldherr R. Myocarditis and insulitis in Coxsackie virus infection. *Z Kardiol* 1976; **65**: 873–881.

33. Yoon J, Austin M, Onodera T, Notkins AL. Virus-induced diabetes mellitus: isolation of a virus from the pancreas of a child with diabetic ketoacidosis. *N Engl J Med* 1979; **300**: 1173–1179.

34. Ginsberg-Fellner F, Witt ME, Fedun B *et al.* Diabetes and autoimmunity in patients with the congenital rubella syndrome. *Rev Infect Dis* 1985; **7(Suppl 1)**: S170–176.

35. Dahlquist G, Frisk G, Ivarsson SA *et al.* Indications that maternal Coxsackie B virus infection during pregnancy is a risk factor for childhood-onset IDDM. *Diabetologia* 1995; **38**: 1371–1373.

36. Dahlquist G, Ivarsson S, Lindberg B, Forsgren M. Maternal enteroviral infection during pregnancy as a risk factor for childhood IDDM. *Diabetes* 1995; **44**: 408–413.

37. Hyoty H, Hiltunen M, Knip M *et al.* A prospective study of the role of coxsackie B and other enterovirus infections in the pathogenesis of IDDM. *Diabetes* 1995; **44**: 652–657.

38. Graves PM, Norris JM, Pallansch MA *et al.* The role of enteroviral infections in the development of IDDM. Limitations of current approaches. *Diabetes* 1997; **46**: 161–168.

39. Bingley PJ, Christie MR, Bonifacio E *et al.* Combined analysis of autoantibodies improves prediction of IDDM in Islet Cell Antibody-positive relatives. *Diabetes* 1994; **43**: 1304–1310.

40. Christie MR, Roll U, Payton MA *et al.* Validity of screening for individuals at risk for type 1 diabetes by combined analysis of antibodies to recombinant proteins. *Diabetes Care* 1997; **20**: 965–970.

41. Verge CF, Stenger D, Bonifacio E *et al.* Combined use of autoantibodies (IA-2ab, GADab, IAA, ICA) in type 1 diabetes: combinatorial islet autoantibody workshop. *Diabetes* 1998; **47**: 1857–1866.

42. Bingley PJ, Bonifacio E, Williams AJK *et al.* Prediction of IDDM in the general population. Strategies based on combinations of autoantibody markers. *Diabetes* 1997; **46**: 1701–1710.

43. Gale EAM, Bingley PJ. Can we really predict IDDM? *Diabetes* 1993; **42**: 213–220.

44. Canadian–European Randomized Control Trial Group. Cyclosporin-induced remission of IDDM after early intervention: association with enhanced insulin secretion. *Diabetes* 1988; **37**: 1574–1582.

45. Feutren G, Papoz L, Assan R *et al.* Cyclosporin increases the rate and length of remission in insulin-dependent diabetes of recent onset. *Lancet* 1986; **ii**: 119–123.

46. Carel JC, Boitard C, Eisenbarth G *et al.* Cyclosporin delays but does not prevent clinical onset in glucose intolerant pre-type 1 diabetic children. *J Autoimmun* 1996; **9**: 739–745.

47. Gotfredsen CF, Buschard K, Frandsen EK. Reduction of diabetes incidence of BB wistar rats by early prophylactic insulin treatment of diabetes-prone animals. *Diabetologia* 1985; **28**; 933–935.

48. Atkinson MA, Maclaren NK, Luchetta R. Insulitis and diabetes in NOD mice reduced by prophylactic insulin therapy. *Diabetes* 1990; **39**: 933–937.

49. Shah SC, Malone JI, Simpson NE. A randomized trial of intensive insulin therapy in newly diagnosed type 1 insulin-dependent diabetes mellitus. *N Engl J Med* 1989; **320**: 550–554.

50. Peakman M, Hussain MJ, Millward BA *et al.* Effect of initiation of insulin therapy on T-lymphocyte activation in type 1 diabetes. *Diabetic Med* 1990; **7**: 327–330.

51. Zhang ZJ, Davidson L, Eisenbarth G, Weiner HL. Suppression of diabetes in nonobese diabetic mice by oral administration of porcine insulin. *Proc Natl Acad Sci USA* 1991; **88**: 10252–10256.

52. Muir A, Peck A, Clare-Salzler M *et al.* Insulin immunization of nonobese diabetic mice induces a protective insulitis characterized by diminished intraislet interferon-γ transcription. *J Clin Invest* 1995; **95**: 628–634.

53. Hartmann B, Bellmann K, Ghiea I *et al.* Oral insulin for diabetes prevention in NOD mice: potentiation by enhancing Th2 cytokine expression in the gut though bacterial adjuvant. *Diabetologia* 1997; **40**: 902–909.

54. Keller RJ, Eisenbarth GS, Jackson RA. Insulin prophylaxis in individuals at high risk of type 1 diabetes. *Lancet* 1993; **341**: 927–928.

55. Fuchtensbusch M, Rabl W, Grassle B *et al.* Delay of type 1 diabetes in high risk, first degree relatives by parenteral insulin administration: the Schwabing Insulin Prophylaxis Pilot Trial. *Diabetologia* 1998; **41**: 536–541.

56. Skyler JS, Marks JB. Immune intervention in type 1 diabetes mellitus. *Diabetes Rev* 1993; **1**: 15–42.

57. Dulin WE, Wyse BM, Kalamazoo MS. Studies on the ability of compounds to block the diabetogenic activity of streptozotocin. *Diabetes* 1969; **18**: 459–466.

58. Lazarow A. Protection against alloxan diabetes. *Anat Rec* 1947; **97**: 353.

59. Pociot F, Reimers JI, Andersen HU. Nicotinamide – biological actions and therapeutic potential in diabetes prevention. IDIG Workshop, Copenhagen, Denmark, 4–5 December 1992. *Diabetologia* 1993; **36**: 574–576.

60. Cetkovic-Cvrlje M, Sandler S, Eizirik DL. Nicotinamide and dexamethasone inhibit IL-1 induced nitric oxide production by RINn5F cells without decreasing mRNA expression for nitric oxide synthase. *Endocrinology* 1993; **133**: 1739–1743.

61. Heller B, Wang ZQ, Wagner EF *et al.* Poly(ADP-ribose) polymerase dependent and independent toxicity of oxygen radicals and nitric oxide in murine islet cells. *J Biol Chem* 1995; **270**: 11176–11180.

62. Mandrup-Poulsen T, Reimers JI, Andersen HU *et al.* Nicotinamide treatment in the prevention of insulin-dependent diabetes mellitus. *Diabetes Metab Rev* 1993; **9**: 295–309.

63. Pozzilli P, Kolb H, Browne PD. The Nicotinamide Trialists. Meta-analysis of nicotinamide treatment in patients with recent-onset IDDM. *Diabetes Care* 1996; **19**: 1357–1363.

64. Elliott RB, Chase HP. Prevention or delay of Type 1 (insulin-dependent) diabetes mellitus in children using nicotinamide. *Diabetologia* 1991; **34**: 362–365.

65. Elliott RB, Pilcher CC, Fergusson DM, Stewart AW. A population based strategy to prevent insulin-dependent diabetes using nicotinamide. *J Pediatr Endocrinol Metab* 1996; **9**: 501–509.

66. Bingley PJ, the ICARUS group. Interactions of age, islet cell antibodies, insulin autoantibodies and first-phase insulin response in predicting risk of progression to IDDM in ICA+ relatives. *Diabetes* 1996; **45**: 1720–1728.

67. Lampeter EF, Klinghammer A, Scherbaum *et al.* (The DENIS Group). The Deutsche Nicotinamide Intervention Study: an attempt to prevent type 1 diabetes. *Diabetes* 1998; **47**: 980–984.

68. Yagi H, Mitsunobu M, Kishimoto Y *et al.* Possible mechanism of the preventive effect of BCG against diabetes in NOD Mouse. *Cellular Immunology* 1991; **138**: 142–149.

69. Shehadeh N, Calcinaro F, Bradley BJ *et al.* Effect of adjuvant therapy on development of

diabetes in mouse and man. *Lancet* 1994; **343**: 706–707.

70. Pozzilli P. BCG vaccine in insulin-dependent diabetes mellitus. *Lancet* 1997; **349**: 1520–1521.

71. Dahlquist G, Gothefors L. The cumulative incidence of childhood diabetes mellitus in Sweden unaffected by BCG-vaccination. *Diabetologia* 1995; **38**: 873–874.

72. Parent M, Siemiatycki J, Menzies R *et al*. Bacille Calmette-Guerin Vaccination and incidence of IDDM in Montreal, Canada. *Diabetes Care* 1997; **20**: 767–772.

73. Ashtonrickardt PG, Bandeira A, Delaney JR *et al*. Evidence for a differential avidity model of T-cell selection in the thymus. *Cell* 1994; **76**: 651–663.

74. Scollay R, Butcher EC, Weissman IL. Thymus cell migration. Quantitative aspects of cellular traffic from the thymus to the periphery in mice. *Eur J Immunol* 1980; **10**: 210–211.

75. Smith H, Chen I, Kubo R, Tung KSK. Neonatal thymectomy results in a repertoire enriched in T cells deleted in the adult thymus. *Science* 1989; **245**: 749–752.

76. Georgiou HM, Lagarde AC, Bellgrau D. T cell dysfunction in the diabetes-prone BB rat: A role for thymic migrants that are not T cell precursors. *J Exp Med* 1988; **167**: 132–148.

77. Reich E, Sherwin RS, Kanagawa O, Janeway CAJ. An explanation for the protective effect of the MHC class II I-E molecule in murine diabetes. *Nature* 1989; **341**: 326–328.

78. Kaufman DL, Clare-Salzler M, Tian J *et al*. Spontaneous loss of T-cell tolerance to glutamic acid decarboxylase in murine insulin-dependent diabetes. *Nature* 1993; **366**: 69–72.

79. Tisch R, Yang X, Singer SM *et al*. Immune response to glutamic acid decarboxylase correlates with insulitis in non-obese diabetic mice. *Nature* 1993; **366**: 72–75.

80. French MB, Allison J, Cram DS *et al*. Transgenic expression of mouse proinsulin prevents diabetes in nonobese diabetic mice. *Diabetes* 1997; **46**: 34–37.

81. Mossman TR, Cherwinski H, Bond MW *et al*. Two types of murine helper T-cell clone. Definition according to lymphokine activities and secreted proteins. *J Immunol* 1986; **136**: 2348–2357.

82. Katz JD, Benoist C, Mathis D. T helper subsets in insulin-dependent diabetes. *Science* 1995; **268**: 1185–1188.

83. Shehadeh N, LaRosa F, Lafferty KJ. Altered cytokine activity in adjuvent inhibition of autoimmune diabetes. *J Autoimmun* 1993; **6**: 291–300.

84. Foulis AK, McGill M, Farquharson MA. Insulitis in type 1 (insulin-dependent) diabetes mellitus in man: macrophages, lymphocytes, and interferon-gamma containing cells. *J Pathol* 1991; **164**: 97–103.

85. Hussain MJ, Peakman M, Gallati H *et al*. Elevated serum levels of macrophage-derived cytokines precede and accompany the onset of IDDM. *Diabetologia* 1996; **39**: 60–69.

86. Kallman BA, Huther M, Tubes M *et al*. Systemic bias of cytokine production toward cell-mediated immune regulation in IDDM and toward humoral immunity in Graves' disease. *Diabetes* 1997; **46**: 237–243.

87. Herold KC, Bluestone JA, Montag AG *et al*. Prevention of autoimmune diabetes with nonactivating anti-CD3 monoclonal antibody. *Diabetes* 1992; **41**: 385–391.

88. Hayward AR, Shriber M. Reduced incidence of insulitis in NOD mice following anti-CD3 injection: Requirement for neonatal injection. *J Autoimmun* 1992; **5**: 59–67.

89. Maki T, Ichikawa T, Blanco R, Porter J. Long-term abrogation of autoimmune diabetes in nonobese diabetic mice by immunotherapy with anti-lymphocyte serum. *Proc Natl Acad Sci USA* 1992; **89**: 3434–3438.

90. Hutchings P, O'Reilly L, Parish NM *et al*. The use of non-depleting anti-CD4 monoclonal antibody to re-establish tolerance to beta cells in NOD mice. *Eur J Immunol* 1992; **22**: 1913–1918.

91. Chatenoud L, Thervet E, Primo J, Bach JF. Anti-CD3 antibody induces long-term remission of overt autoimmunity in non-obese diabetic mice. *Proc Natl Acad Sci USA* 1993; **9**: 1123–1127.

92. Bach JF. Strategies in the immunointervention of insulin-dependent diabetes mellitus. *Ann NY Acad Sci* 1993; **69**: 63–64.

93. Hahn HJ, Kuttler B, Laube F, Emmrich F. Anti-CD4 therapy in recent-onset IDDM. *Diabetes Metab Rev* 1993; **9**: 323–328.

94. Horneff G, Burmester GR, Emmrich F, Kalden JR. Treatment of rheumatoid arthritis with an anti-CD4 monoclonal antibody. *Arthritis Rheum* 1991; **34**: 129–140.

95. Vialettes B, Vague P. Treatment of diabetes by monoclonal antibodies. Lessons from a pilot study using anti-IL-2 receptor MoAb in recently diagnosed diabetic patients. *Diabetes Prev Ther* 1991; **5**: 21–22.

96. Pennline KJ, Roquegaffney E, Monahan M. Recombinant human IL-10 prevents the onset of diabetes in the nonobese diabetic mouse. *Clin Immunol Immunopathol* 1994; **71**: 169–175.

97. Rapoport M, Jaramillo A, Zipris D *et al.* Interleukin 4 reverses T cell proliferative unresponsiveness and prevents the onset of diabetes in non-obese diabetic mice. *J Exp Med* 1993; **17**: 887–899.

98. McFarland HF. Complexities in the treatment of autoimmune disease. *Science* 1996; **274**: 2037–2038.

99. Trembleau S, Penna G, Bosi E *et al.* Interleukin 12 administration induces T helper 1 cells and accelerates autoimmune diabetes in NOD mice. *J Exp Med* 1995; **181**: 817–821.

100. Leonard JP, Waldburger KE, Goldman SJ. Prevention of experimental autoimmune encephalitis by antibodies against interleukin-12. *J Exp Med* 1995; **181**: 381–386.

101. Neurath MF, Fuss I, Kelsall BL *et al.* Antibodies to interleukin 12 abrogate established experimental colitis in mice. *J Exp Med* 1995; **182**: 1281–1290.

102. Trentham DE. Immunotherapy and other novel therapies. *Curr Opin Rheumatol* 1991; **3**: 369–372.

103. Elliot MJ, Maini RN, Feldmann M *et al.* Randomised double-blind comparison of chimeric monoclonal antibody to tumour necrosis factor α (cA2) versus placebo in rheumatoid arthritis. *Lancet* 1994; **344**: 1104–1110.

104. Wells HG. Studies on the chemistry of anaphylaxis. III. Experiments with isolated proteins, especially those of hen's egg. *J Infect Dis* 1911; **9**: 147–151.

105. Schwartz RH. A cell culture model for T lymphocyte clonal anergy. *Science* 1990; **248**: 1349–1356.

106. Weiner HL, Friedman A, Millar A *et al.* ORAL TOLERANCE: immunological mechanisms and treatment of animal and human-specific autoimmune diseases by oral administration of autoantigens. *Ann Rev Immunol* 1994; **12**: 809–837.

107. Chen Y, Inobe J, Marks R *et al.* Peripheral deletion of antigen-reactive T cells in oral tolerance. *Nature* 1995; **376**: 177–180.

108. Lohmann T, Scherbaum WA. T-cell autoimmunity to glutamic-acid decarboxylase in human insulin-dependent diabetes-mellitus. *Hormone Metabolic Res* 1996; **28**: 357–360.

109. Lohmann T, Halder T, Morgenthaler NG *et al.* T cell responses to a novel autoantigen IA2 in IDDM patients and healthy controls. *Diabetologia* 1997; **40**: 327–330.

110. Daniel D, Wegmann DR. Protection of non-obese diabetic mice from diabetes by intranasal or subcutaneous administration of insulin peptide B-(9-23). *Proc Natl Acad Sci USA* 1996; **93**: 956–960.

111. Harrison LC, Dempsey-Collier M, Kramer DR, Takahashi K. Aerosol insulin induces regulatory CD8 gamma delta T cells that prevent murine insulin-dependent diabetes. *J Exp Med* 1996; **184**: 2156–2174.

112. Tian JD, Atkinson MA, Clare-Salzer M *et al.* Nasal administration of glutamate-decarboxylase (GAD65) peptides induces TH2 responses and prevents murine insulin-dependent diabetes. *J Exp Med* 1996; **183**: 1561–1567.

113. Elliott JF, Qin HY, Bhatti S *et al.* Immunization with the larger isoform of mouse Glutamic Acid Decarboxylase (GAD67) prevents autoimmune diabetes in NOD mice. *Diabetes* 1994; **43**: 1494–1499.

114. Tian J, Atkinson M, Clare-Salzer M *et al.* GAD based immunotherapies for murine IDDM (abstr). *Autoimmunity* 1995; **21**(1): 68.

115. Elias D, Cohen IR. Treatment of autoimmune diabetes and insulitis in NOD mice with heat-shock-protein-60 peptide p277. *Diabetes* 1995; **44**: 1132–1138.

116. Bertrand S, de Paepe M, Vigeant C, Yale J. Prevention of adoptive transfer in BB rats by prophylactic insulin treatment. *Diabetes* 1992; **41**: 1273–1277.

117. Thivolet CH, Goillet E, Bedossa P *et al.* Insulin prevents adoptive transfer of diabetes in the autoimmune non-obese diabetic mouse. *Diabetologia* 1991; **34**: 314–319.

118. Weiner HL, Mackin GA, Matsui M *et al.*
     Double-blind pilot trial of oral tolerization
     with myelin antigens in multiple sclerosis.
     Science 1993; **259**: 1321–1324.
119. Sieper J, Kary S, Sorensen H *et al.* Oral type-II
     collagen treatment in early rheumatoid arthritis
     – a double blind placebo-controlled random-
     ized trial. *Arthritis Rheum* 1996; **39**: 41–51.
120. Skolnick AA. First Type 1 diabetes prevention
     trials. *JAMA* 1997; **278**: 1101.
121. Gale EAM, Bingley PJ. Can we prevent
     IDDM? *Diabetes Care* **17**: 339–344.
122. Harrison LC, Colman PG, Dean B *et al.*
     Increase in remission rate in newly diagnosed
     Type 1 diabetic subjects treated with
     Azathioprine. *Diabetes* 1985; **34**: 1306–1308.
123. Moore WP, Gale EAM, The ENDIT group.
     Feasibility of a multinational diabetes preven-
     tion trial in first degree relatives of a child with
     IDDM (abstr). *Diabetologia* 1997; **40**: 67.

4

Glucotoxicity: a role for protein kinase C activation?

Douglas Kirk Ways and George King

Role of metabolic derangements in mediating glucotoxicity

The Diabetes Control and Complications Trial conclusively demonstrated that intensive glycemic control reduced the risk of developing and slowed the progression of diabetic retinopathy, neuropathy, and nephropathy in patients with Type 1 diabetes.[1] A similar beneficial effect of intensified glycemic control on reducing the development and progression of microvascular disease was also observed in patients with Type 2 diabetes.[2] Most recently, the United Kingdom Prospective Diabetes Study (UKPDS) demonstrated a beneficial effect of intensified glycemic control on the development of microvascular complications in patients with Type 2 diabetes.[3,4] These data establish the deleterious effects of hyperglycemia on the onset and progression of microvascular diabetic complications. While the role of hyperglycemia in diabetic complications has been demonstrated, the mechanisms by which hyperglycemia causes these complications have yet to be fully elucidated.

Aberrations in multiple metabolic pathways have been proposed to participate in the pathogenesis of chronic diabetic complications. Enhanced flux through the polyol pathway, myoinositol depletion, enhanced expression of transforming growth factor β (TGF β),

increased expression of vascular endothelial growth factor (VEGF)/vascular permeability factor (VPF), decreased Na^+–K^+-ATPase activity, altered cellular redox, formation of advanced glycation end-products (AGEs), oxidative stress, deficiencies in γ-linolenic acid, altered eicosanoid production, and protein kinase C (PKC) activation have been proposed as potential pathways for mediating the development and progression of chronic microvascular diabetic complications. It seems unlikely that a single mechanism would be responsible for all the chronic complications of diabetes. It may be that specific metabolic abnormalities will be predominately responsible for the etiology of certain complications, while different metabolic aberrations may initiate the development of, or play a role in, the progression of other complications. It is also possible that a significant amount of cross-talk, and even synergy, may exist among these metabolic derangements, initiating or leading to the progression of diabetic complications.

Potential role of PKC activation in glucotoxicity

Preclinical data implicate the inappropriate, glucose-induced activation of members of the PKC gene family as being involved in transducing the signal between hyperglycemia and the development and progression of micro- and macrovascular complications of diabetes. PKC activity has been shown to be activated in cells cultured under hyperglycemic conditions such as glomeruli,[5] mesangial cells,[6,7] endothelium,[8] vascular smooth muscle cells,[9,10] and adipocytes.[11] PKC activity is also increased in diabetic animal tissues such as the glomerulus,[5,12] proximal tubule,[13] skeletal muscle,[14] liver,[15] aorta,[8] and heart.[8,16] PKC is a gene family that lies on a variety of intracellular signal transduction pathways.[17] The gene family is divided into three subfamilies: conventional (α, $\beta1$ $\beta2$, γ), novel (ϵ, δ, θ, μ, η), and atypical (λ, ι). Once activated, PKCs catalyze the transfer of the terminal phosphate group from adenosine triphosphate to a protein. Phosphorylation of proteins can modulate their functional activity and is a common mechanism by which to regulate cellular events.[17]

It is hypothesized that the activation of individual PKC isoforms may selectively elicit specific cellular responses.[17,18] Thus, the activation of an individual PKC isoform may produce one cellular response while activation of another PKC isoform could elicit a different cellular response. This hypothesis implies that the inappropriate activation of an individual PKC isoform could produce a specific cellular response or induce a distinct pathological state(s).

Activation of multiple PKC isoforms, including the α, $\beta1$, $\beta2$, δ, and ϵ isoforms, has been demonstrated in cultured cells exposed to hyperglycemic conditions as well as in preclinical models of diabetes.[8,12,19] A single PKC β gene exists that is alternatively spliced into two isoforms, $\beta1/\beta2$, that differ in their carboxyl-terminal amino acids. While the functional consequences associated with PKC β mRNA splice variants are not yet fully understood, differences in the subcellular localization of the splice variants may provide a mechanism for diversity in cell signalling.[20] The $\beta2$ splice

variant is increased in most tissues derived from diabetic animals,[8,21] except for glomerulus, in which the $\beta1$ variant is also increased.[12] While these findings implicate members of the PKC gene family as potential mediators of hyperglycemia-induced cellular abnormalities, they do not conclusively implicate an individual isoform as being singularly responsible for these abnormalities. A role for PKC β in mediating certain dysfunctions associated with diabetes has been demonstrated by experiments utilizing a selective inhibitor of this isoform.[12,22–25]

Activation of PKC in diabetes – diacylglycerol, AGEs, and oxidation

Members of the conventional and novel PKC subfamilies are activated by diacylglycerol.[17] Exposure of cultured cells to hyperglycemic conditions enhances the *de novo* synthesis of diacylglycerol.[6,11,26] Increases in diacylglycerol occur days after exposure to hyperglycemic conditions and are maintained in diabetic dogs for at least a 5-year period.[26,27] Hyperglycemia-induced increases in diacylglycerol are generated from glycolytic intermediates that are stepwise acylated to phosphatidic acid and ultimately to diacylglycerol.[26] Thus, diabetes-induced increases in intracellular glucose flux elevate intracellular diacylglycerol concentrations which in turn lead to activation of conventional and novel members of the PKC gene family. Occupation of receptors for advanced glycation end-products by AGEs also increases diacylglycerol production and activates PKC.[28,29] Oxidative stress occurs in diabetes.[30] Mild oxidation activates PKC.[31] The salutary effects of vitamin E on diabetes-induced vascular dysfunction could be due to the antioxidant effects of this vitamin.[19,32,33] Alternatively,

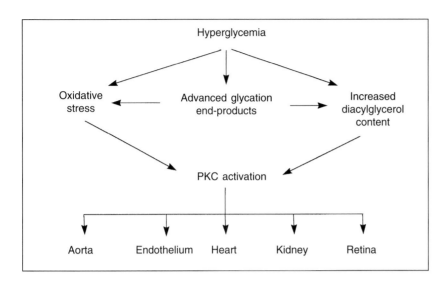

Fig. 4.1
Potential mechanisms of PKC activation in response to hyperglycemia.

vitamin E could exert its effects on diabetic vascular dysfunction by stimulating diacylglycerol kinase, which would reduce diacylglycerol levels and diminish PKC activation stimulated by hyperglycemia.[32] In either case, the effects of vitamin E could be mediated via a PKC-dependent mechanism. Thus, increases in diacylglycerol content, either by increases in *de novo* synthesis or enhanced formation induced by AGEs as well as oxidative activation, are potential mechanisms by which PKC is activated by hyperglycemia (*Fig. 4.1*).

Potential PKC-dependent mechanisms underlying the development of chronic diabetic complications

Role of PKC in vascular dysfunction

Vascular dysfunction is a prominent feature of diabetic retinopathy, nephropathy, neuropathy, and erectile dysfunction. Hyperglycemia-induced damage to the retinal vasculature is thought to be responsible for the onset and progression of diabetic retinopathy to a more severe, sight-threatening stage. Alterations in glomerular hemodynamics are thought to contribute to the initiation and perhaps the progression of the chronic glomerular injury associated with diabetes. Elevation in urinary albumin excretion is believed to reflect glomerular and endothelial cell damage, which is associated with the development of diabetic nephropathy and its progression to end-stage renal disease. Endoneurial blood flow is decreased in preclinical models of diabetes.[34,35] Neuronal ischemia has been postulated to be involved in the pathogenesis of neuropathy in patients with diabetes.[36] Decreases in endothelium-dependent vasorelaxation and Na+–K+-ATPase activity also impair vascular smooth muscle relaxation and interfere with the veno-occlusion that is required for normal erectile function.[37,38]

The endothelium regulates many facets of blood vessel function. The endothelium can regulate vascular function through the production and release of nitric oxide (NO).[39] NO opposes the vasoconstrictive effects of catecholamines, serotonin, and the products of activated platelets.[40] Acute exposure of arteries from normal animals to hyperglycemia decreases vasodilation in response to acetylcholine, ADP, and histamine.[37] In preclinical models, diabetes is associated with attenuated endothelium-dependent vasodilation.[41] In patients with diabetes, endothelium-dependent vasodilation is diminished in angiographically normal coronary arteries,[42] forearm resistance vessels,[43] and peripheral conduit vessels.[44] Patients with Type 2 diabetes have impaired vasodilation to both endogenous and exogenous NO.[45] Thus, diabetes disrupts endothelial NO activity which could lead to vascular dysfunction.

Exposure of endothelial cells to hyperglycemia activates PKC,[8] which reduces NO activity by decreasing transcription of endothelial cell NO synthase[46,47] and by phosphorylating NO synthase, which leads to a decrease in its intrinsic activity.[48,49] PKC inhibitors augment NO release in response to physiological agonists, and PKC activation impairs agonist-induced NO release.[50] In retinal microvascular endothelial cells, hyperglycemia-induced decreases in NO release are partially abrogated by PKC inhibition.[51] Oral administration of LY333531, an orally bioavailable PKC inhibitor with a high degree of specificity for PKC β, to streptozocin (STZ)-treated diabetic rats attenuates decreases in endothelium- and NO-dependent vasodilation of the mesenteric vasculature.[52,53]

Vascular Na+–K+-ATPase activity is reduced in diabetes.[54] Reduction in the activity of this enzyme is associated with vascular dysfunction.[38] PKC β activation has been postulated to mediate hyperglycemia-induced decreases in Na+–K+-ATPase activity.[55] Another study showed that PKC β inhibition abrogated diabetes-induced decreases in retinal vascular Na+–K+-ATPase activity.[56]

These salutary changes in NO and Na+–K+-ATPase signal transduction are associated with amelioration of the abnormal vascular function associated with diabetes. PKC β inhibition has been shown to prevent and reverse diabetes-induced abnormalities in blood flow in retinal, renal, and endoneurial vascular beds.[22,53,57] Normalization of renal hemodynamics was associated with a reduction in albuminuria.[22] Normalization of endoneurial blood flow was associated with amelioration of diabetes-induced decreases in sensory and motor nerve conduction velocities.[53,57] These data suggest that PKC β inhibition could favorably alter the course of complications that have a vascular basis as their etiology, such as retinopathy, neuropathy, nephropathy, and erectile dysfunction (*Fig. 4.2*).

Role of PKC in TGF β overexpression

Although the precise mechanisms by which diabetes induces mesangial expansion have yet to be fully elucidated, increasing evidence points to a role for TGF β in the pathogenesis of this pathological process.[58–60] TGF β is a prosclerotic cytokine released by a variety of cells.[58] TGF β increases the synthesis and reduces the breakdown of extracellular proteins such as Type IV collagen, laminin, and fibronectin.[61–63] Administration of TGF β to normal rodents induces mesangial fibrosis and/or expansion.[64,65] TGF β is increased in cultured renal cells exposed to hyperglycemic conditions and in the kidneys of diabetic animals, as well as in patients with diabetes.[66–70] A role for TGF β in the mesangial expansion is substantiated by the ability of TGF β-neutralizing antibodies to inhibit mesangial expansion in a rodent model of

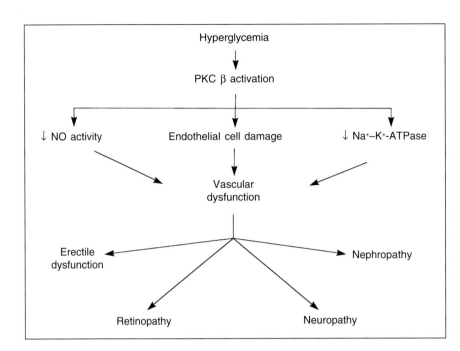

Fig. 4.2
PKC β activation and vascular dysfunction is implicated in the development of multiple diabetic complications.

diabetes.[71] A positive correlation between glycosylated hemoglobin levels in patients with diabetes and the renal content of TGF β mRNA has been observed.[72] Thus, overexpression of TGF β is an attractive candidate for mediating the mesangial expansion that is thought to be an important step in the progression of nephropathy to end-stage renal disease.

A decrease in trabecular smooth muscle content and an increase in corpus cavernosal connective tissue of males with erectile dysfunction have been observed.[73,74] The increase in connective tissue relative to that of smooth muscle content is thought to contribute to erectile dysfunction by reducing the elasticity of the fibroelastic penile frame.[75] Overexpression of TGF β has been implicated in mediating the enhanced production of connective tissue in the corpus cavernosum.[76] Thus, TGF β-induced increases in corpus cavernosal connective tissue content could

contribute to erectile dysfunction observed in males with diabetes.

Cardiovascular disease in patients with diabetes is a significant problem. In the Framingham study, males with diabetes had a fivefold greater incidence of heart failure than males without diabetes, and women with diabetes had twice the incidence of developing heart failure than women without diabetes.[77] The presence of cardiac dysfunction, as exemplified by a reduction in ventricular compliance, suggests the existence of a unique type of diabetic cardiomyopathy.[78] The pathology of diabetic cardiomyopathy shows a pattern of left ventricular hypertrophy associated with increases in Type VI collagen and interstitial fibrosis.[79] Thus, cardiac dysfunction associated with diabetes displays histologic evidence of inappropriate fibrosis and an excess of extracellular matrix accumulation similar to that seen in other organs of patients with diabetes.

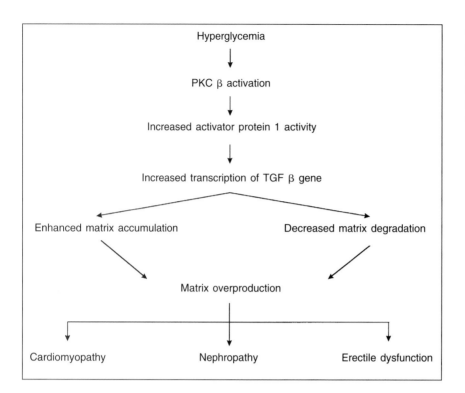

Hyperglycemia

↓

PKC β activation

↓

Increased activator protein 1 activity

↓

Increased transcription of TGF β gene

Enhanced matrix accumulation   Decreased matrix degradation

Matrix overproduction

Cardiomyopathy   Nephropathy   Erectile dysfunction

Fig. 4.3
Activation of PKC β by hyperglycemia stimulates TGF β overexpression and extracellular matrix accumulation.

PKC activity is increased in the kidney and heart of patients with diabetes.[8,12,22] PKC activation can regulate gene expression by activating transcription factors c-*fos* and c-*jun*. Exposure of cultured mesangial cells to hyperglycemic conditions induces c-*fos* and c-*jun* expression and activity.[80] Via an interaction with the activator protein 1 response element, c-*fos* and c-*jun* regulate gene expression.[81,82] The TGF β gene contains activator protein 1 sites in the promoter that are positively regulated by PKC activation.[83,84] TGF β expression as well as that of Type α1(IV) collagen and fibronectin are increased in the glomeruli of diabetic rodents.[12] Oral administration of a PKC β inhibitor completely blocked the increase in mRNA expression of TGF β, Type α1(IV) collagen, laminin, and fibronectin in the glomeruli of diabetic animals.[12] Transgenic mice that specifi-

cally overexpress PKC β2 in the cardiomyocyte develop myocardial fibrosis that is accompanied by an increase in collagen Types α1(IV) and α1(VI), as well as enhanced expression of TGF β.[23] Myocardial fibrosis and hypertrophy were ameliorated by oral administration of a PKC β inhibitor in these transgenic mice.[23] These data demonstrate that PKC β activation is associated with diabetes-induced increases in TGF β expression. Inhibition of PKC β expression normalizes TGF β expression and reduces the enhanced extracellular matrix accumulation and fibrosis due to diabetes or the direct overexpression of PKC β. This information indicates that PKC β activation may be involved in the fibrotic processes that contribute to end-stage diabetic renal disease and potentially to erectile dysfunction in males with diabetes and to diabetic cardiomyopathy (*Fig. 4.3*).

Role of PKC in enhancing vascular permeability and stimulating neovascularization

Diabetic retinopathy is a major cause of blindness in industrialized nations. A majority of the visual loss suffered by patients with diabetes can be attributed to diabetic macular edema and the sequelae of proliferative diabetic retinopathy.

Possible mechanisms responsible for diabetic macular edema include hyperglycemia-induced activation of PKC β and increased expression of VEGF/VPF. Overexpression of PKC β in cultured endothelial cells significantly increases endothelial cell permeability in response to PKC activation.[85] Intravitreal instillation of phorbol esters, agents that directly activate conventional and novel members of the PKC gene family, causes a prompt and significant increase in retinal permeability.[24] Hyperglycemia is associated with increased phosphorylation of connexin-43 and disruption of gap junctional intercellular communication in cultured vascular smooth muscle cells.[86] Hyperglycemia-induced disruption of gap junctional intercellular communication is abrogated by PKC inhibition.[86] Thus, hyperglycemia-induced activation of PKC would be predicted to enhance directly vascular permeability, possibly by altering intercellular gap junction function.

VEGF/VPF is a potent cytokine that stimulates vascular leakage.[87] VEGF/VPF is modestly increased in nonproliferative retinopathy,[88–90] and to a greater extent, in proliferative diabetic retinopathy.[91] While hypoxia stimulates VEGF/VPF expression, hyperglycemia also stimulates production of this factor by vascular smooth muscle cells.[92] Glucose-induced stimulation of VEGF/VPF expression is antagonized by PKC inhibition, suggesting that PKC activation may also mediate at least a portion of diabetes-induced increases in VEGF/VPF expression.[92] PKC activation increases expression of a receptor, KDR, to which VEGF/VPF binds.[93] Occupation of the KDR receptor by VEGF/VPF stimulates the increased permeability and neovascular effects of VEGF/VPF. Thus, hyperglycemia-induced activation of PKC could amplify VEGF/VPF signalling by increasing the KDR receptor number.

Intravitreal injection of VEGF/VPF activates PKC isoforms in the retina which include PKC β.[24] Intravitreal injection of VEGF/VPF induces a rapid increase in retinal permeability in nondiabetic rats, as assessed by vitreous fluorophotometry.[24] Administration of a PKC β inhibitor blocks the ability of VEGF/VPF to increase retinal vascular permeability.[24] In addition to these mechanisms, glycated albumin has been demonstrated to enhance vascular permeability, and this effect is blocked by a PKC β inhibitor.[94] Thus, a PKC inhibitor blocking glucose-induced increases in VEGF/VPF expression, as well as inhibiting the ability of VEGF/VPF to induce increases in retinal permeability and blocking AGE-induced increases in permeability, would be predicted to be of benefit in reducing the progression of macular edema to sight-threatening macular edema.

VEGF/VPF stimulates endothelial cell proliferation and neovascularization.[87] Elevations in the levels of VEGF/VPF in patients with proliferative diabetic retinopathy suggest the involvement of this cytokine in this disease.[91] Upon binding to the KDR receptor, VEGF/VPF activated phospholipase C γ and stimulated diacylglycerol production in cultured endothelial cells.[95] VEGF/VPF-induced generation of diacylglycerol activated members of the conventional and novel PKC gene family in the retina and in cultured endothelial cells.[24,95] PKC β inhibition antagonized VEGF/VPF-stimulated increases in endothelial cell growth, an essential

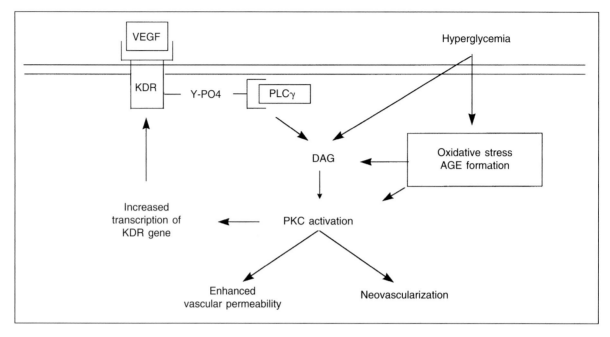

Fig. 4.4
*Role of hyperglycemia-induced activation of PKC
β in enhancing VEGF/VPF signal transduction.*

step in the neovascularization process.[95] The role of PKC in ischemia-induced neovascularization has been examined using an *in vivo* porcine branched retinal vein occlusion model of retinal ischemia.[96] VEGF/VPF is thought to play a prominent role in the hypoxia-driven neovascularization associated with this model.[97] Oral administration of a PKC β inhibitor immediately after retinal vein occlusion induced by photodynamic therapy significantly diminished neovascularization.[25] Thus, by interfering with VEGF/VPF signal transduction, it is predicted that PKC inhibition could retard the progression of VEGF/VPF-dependent neovascular states such as proliferative diabetic retinopathy (*Fig. 4.4*).

Summary

In preclinical models of diabetes, PKC is activated by the *de novo* synthesis of diacylglycerol in organs that develop the chronic complications of diabetes. The ability of AGEs and oxidative stress also to activate PKC suggests that PKC activation could serve as a common pathway linking the varied metabolic derangements that have been postulated to be involved in the development of diabetic complications. Hyperglycemia-induced activation of PKC β is associated with vascular dysfunction. Inhibition of PKC β ameliorates the vascular dysfunction associated with diabetes. Vascular dysfunction has been implicated in the devel-

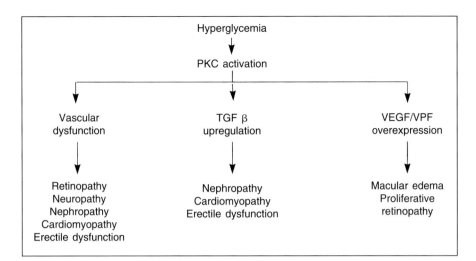

Fig. 4.5
Potential role for PKC activation in the mechanisms leading to the development of diabetic complications.

opment and progression of diabetic retinopathy, nephropathy, neuropathy, and erectile dysfunction (*Fig. 4.5*). Hyperglycemia-induced activation of PKC stimulates expression of TGF β. Overexpression of TGF β has been implicated as a mechanism responsible for the progression of diabetic nephropathy, erectile dysfunction in males with diabetes, and diabetic cardiac dysfunction (*Fig. 4.5*). Hyperglycemia-induced PKC activation stimulates VEGF/VPF production. PKC β also lies on the VEGF/VPF signalling pathway that stimulates increases in vascular permeability and promotes neovascularization. Thus, PKC activation is involved in the mechanisms that have been implicated in the pathogenesis of diabetic macular edema and proliferative diabetic retinopathy (*Fig. 4.5*).

References

1. The Diabetes Control and Complications Trial Research Group. The effect of intensive treatment of diabetes on the development and progression of long-term complications in insulin-dependent diabetes mellitus. *N Engl J Med* 1993; **329**: 977–986.
2. Ohkubo Y, Kishikawa, H, Araki E *et al*. Intensive insulin therapy prevents the progression of diabetic microvascular complications in Japanese patients with non-insulin-dependent diabetes mellitus: a randomized prospective 6-year study. *Diabetes Res Clin Pract* 1995; **28**: 103–117.
3. UK Prospective Diabetes Study (UKPDS) Group. Intensive blood-glucose control with sulphonylureas or insulin compared with conventional treatment and risk of complications in patients with type 2 diabetes (UKPDS 33). *Lancet* 1998; **352**: 837–853.
4. UK Prospective Diabetes Study (UKPDS) Group. Effect of intensive blood-glucose control with metformin on complications in overweight patients with type 2 diabetes (UKPDS 34). *Lancet* 1998; **352**: 854–865.
5. Craven PA, DeRubertis FR. Protein kinase C is activated in glomeruli from streptozotocin diabetic rats. Possible mediation by glucose. *J Clin Invest* 1989; **83**: 1667–1675.
6. Ayo SH, Radnik R, Garoni JA *et al*. High glucose increases diacylglycerol mass and activates protein kinase C in mesangial cell cultures. *Am J Physiol* 1991; **261**: F571–F577.
7. Studer RK, Craven PA, DeRubertis FR. Role for protein kinase C in the mediation of increased

fibronectin accumulation by mesangial cells grown in high-glucose medium. *Diabetes* 1993; **42**: 118–126.

8. Inoguchi T, Battan R, Handler E *et al*. Preferential elevation of protein kinase C isoform β2 and diacylglycerol levels in the aorta and heart of diabetic rats: differential reversibility to glycemic control by islet cell transplantation. *Proc Natl Acad Sci USA* 1992; **89**: 11059–11063.

9. Williams B, Tsai P, Schrier RW. Glucose-induced downregulation of angiotensin II and arginine vasopressin receptors in cultured rat aortic vascular smooth muscle cells. Role of protein kinase C. *J Clin Invest* 1992; **90**: 1992–1999.

10. Williams B, Schrier RW. Characterization of glucose-induced *in situ* protein kinase C activity in cultured vascular smooth muscle cells. *Diabetes* 1992; **41**: 1464–1472.

11. Ishizuka T, Hoffman J, Cooper DR *et al*. Glucose-induced synthesis of diacylglycerol de *novo* is associated with translocation (activation) of protein kinase C in rat adipocytes. *FEBS Lett* 1989; **249**: 234–238.

12. Koya D, Jirousek MR, Lin Y-W *et al*. Characterization of protein kinase C β isoform activation on the gene expression of transforming growth factor-β, extracellular matrix components, and prostanoids in the glomeruli of diabetic rats. *J Clin Invest* 1997; **100**: 115–126.

13. Hise MK, Mehta PS. Characterization and localization of calcium/phospholipid-dependent protein kinase C during diabetic renal growth. *Endocrinology* 1988; **123**: 1553–1558.

14. Saha AK, Kurowski TG, Colca JR, Ruderman NB. Lipid abnormalities in tissues of the KKAy mouse: effects of pioglitazone on malonyl-CoA and diacylglycerol. *Am J Physiol* 1994; **267**: E95-E101.

15. Considine RV, Nyce MR, Allen LE *et al*. Protein kinase C is increased in the liver of humans and rats with non-insulin-dependent diabetes mellitus: an alteration not due to hyperglycemia. *J Clin Invest* 1995; **95**: 2938-2944.

16. Xiang H, McNeill JH. Protein kinase C activity is altered in diabetic rat hearts. *Biochem Biophys Res Comm* 1992; **187**: 703-710.

17. Nishizuka Y. Protein kinase C and lipid signaling for sustained cellular responses. *FASEB J* 1995; **9**: 484–496.

18. Dekker LV, Palmer RH, Parker PJ. The protein kinase C and protein kinase C related gene families. *Curr Opin Struct Biol* 1995; **5**: 396–402.

19. Kunisaki M, Bursell S-E, Clermont AC *et al*. Vitamin E prevents diabetes-induced abnormal retinal blood flow via the diacylglycerol-protein kinase C pathway. *Am J Physiol* 1995; **269**: E239–E246.

20. Blobe GC, Stribling S, Obeid LM, Hannun YA. Protein kinase C isoenzymes: regulation and function. *Cancer Surv* 1996; **27**: 213–248.

21. Shiba T, Inoguchi T, Sportsman JR *et al*. Correlation of diacylglycerol level and protein kinase C activity in rat retina to retinal circulation. *Am J Physiol* 1993; **265**: E783–E793.

22. Ishii H, Jirousek MR, Koya D *et al*. Amelioration of vascular dysfunctions in diabetic rats by an oral PKC β inhibitor. *Science* 1996; **272**: 728–731.

23. Wakasaki H, Koya D, Schoen FJ *et al*. Targeted overexpression of protein kinase C beta 2 isoform in myocardium causes cardiomyopathy. *Proc Natl Acad Sci USA* 1997; **94**: 9320–9325.

24. Aiello LP, Bursell S-E, Clermont A *et al*. Vascular endothelial growth factor-induced retinal permeability is mediated by protein kinase C *in vivo* and suppressed by an orally effective beta-isoform-selective inhibitor. *Diabetes* 1997; **46**: 1473–1480.

25. Danis RP, Bingaman DP, Jirousek M, Yang Y. Inhibition of intraocular neovascularization caused by retinal ischemia in pigs by PKCβ inhibition with LY333531. *Invest Ophthalmol Vis Sci* 1998; **39**: 171–179.

26. Craven PA, Davidson CM, DeRubertis FR. Increase in diacylglycerol mass in isolated glomeruli by glucose from *de novo* synthesis of glycerolipids. *Diabetes* 1990; **39**: 667–674.

27. Xia P, Inoguchi T, Kern TS *et al*. Characterization of the mechanism for the chronic activation of diacylglycerol-protein kinase C pathway in diabetes and hypergalactosemia. *Diabetes* 1994; **43**: 1122–1129.

28. Chappey O, Dosquet C, Wautier MP, Wautier JL. Advanced glycation end products, oxidant stress and vascular lesions. *Eur J Clin Invest* 1997; **27**: 97–108.

29. Yamauchi T, Igarashi M, Brownlee M *et al.* Activation of diacylglycerol and protein kinase C in aortic smooth muscle cells by oxidants and advanced glycation products. *Diabetes* 1998; **47(S1)**: A372.

30. Baynes JW. Role of oxidative stress in development of complications in diabetes. *Diabetes* 1991; **40**: 405–412.

31. Konishi H, Tanaka M, Takemura Y *et al.* Activation of protein kinase C by tyrosine phosphorylation in response to H_2O_2. *Proc Natl Acad Sci USA* 1997; **94**: 11233–11237.

32. Koya D, Lee I-K, Ishii H, Kanoh H, King GL. Prevention of glomerular dysfunctions in diabetic rats by treatment with d-α-tocopherol. *J Am Soc Nephrol* 1997; **8**: 426–435.

33. Bursell S, Clermont A, Aiello L *et al.* Vitamin E treatment normalizes retinal blood flow and improves renal function in IDDM patients: results of a double masked crossover clinical trial. *Diabetes* 1998; **47(S1)**: A100.

34. Cameron NE, Cotter MA, Low PA. Nerve blood flow in early experimental diabetes in rats: relation to conduction deficits. *Am J Physiol* 1991; **261**: E1–E8.

35. Hotta N, Kakuta H, Fukasawa H *et al.* Effect of niceritrol on streptozocin-induced diabetic neuropathy in rats. *Diabetes* 1992; **41**: 587–591.

36. Dyck P. Hypoxic neuropathy: does hypoxia play a role in diabetic neuropathy? The 1988 Robert Wartenberg lecture. *Neurology* 1989; **39**: 111–118.

37. Tesfamariam B, Brown ML, Deykin D, Cohen RA. Elevated glucose promotes generation of endothelium-derived vasoconstrictor prostanoids in rabbit aorta. *J Clin Invest* 1990; **85**: 929–932.

38. Gupta S, Sussman I, McArthur CS *et al.* Endothelium-dependent inhibition of Na+–K+ ATPase activity in rabbit aorta by hyperglycemia. Possible role of endothelium-derived nitric oxide. *J Clin Invest* 1992; **90**: 727–732.

39. DeMey JG, Claeys M, Vanhoutte PM. Endothelium-dependent inhibitory effects of acetylcholine, adenosine triphosphate, thrombin and arachidonic acid in the canine femoral artery. *J Pharmacol Exp Ther* 1982; **222**: 166–173.

40. Furchgott RF, Vanhoutte PM. Endothelium-derived relaxing and contracting factors. *FASEB J* 1989; **3**: 2007–2018.

41. Pieper GM, Gross GJ. Oxygen free radicals abolish endothelium-dependent relaxation in diabetic rat aorta. *Am J Physiol* 1988; **255**: H825–H833.

42. Nitenberg A, Valensi P, Sachs R *et al.* Impairment of coronary vascular reserve and ACh-induced coronary vasodilation in diabetic patients with angiographically normal coronary arteries and normal left ventricular systolic function. *Diabetes* 1993; **42**: 1017–1025.

43. Johnstone MT, Creager SJ, Scales KM *et al.* Impaired endothelium-dependent vasodilation in patients with insulin-dependent diabetes mellitus. *Circulation* 1993; **88**: 2510–2516.

44. Clarkson P, Celermajer DS, Donald AE *et al.* Impaired vascular reactivity in insulin-dependent diabetes mellitus is related to disease duration and low density lipoprotein cholesterol levels. *J Am Coll Cardiol* 1996; **28**: 573–579.

45. Williams SB, Cusco JA, Roddy MA *et al.* Impaired nitric oxide-mediated vasodilation in patients with non-insulin-dependent diabetes mellitus. *J Am Coll Cardiol* 1996; **27**: 567–574.

46. Harrison DG, Inoue N, Ohara Y, Fukai T. Modulation of endothelial cell nitric oxide synthase expression. *Jpn Circ J* 1996; **60**: 815–821.

47. Kuboki K, Jiang Y, Takahara N *et al.* Mechanism of insulin's effect on endothelial nitric oxide synthase (eNOS) expression *in vivo* and *in vitro*. *Diabetes* 1998; **47(S1)**: A24.

48. Bredt DS, Ferris CD, Snyder SH. Nitric oxide synthase regulatory sites. Phosphorylation by cyclic AMP-dependent protein kinase, protein kinase C, and calcium/calmodulin protein kinase; identification of flavin and calmodulin binding sites. *J Biol Chem* 1992; **267**: 10976–10981.

49. Hirata K, Kuroda R, Sakoda T *et al.* Inhibition of endothelial nitric oxide synthase activity by protein kinase C. *Hypertension* 1995; **25**: 180–185.

50. Hecker M, Luckhoff A, Busse R. Modulation of endothelial autacoid release by protein kinase C: feedback inhibition or non-specific attenuation of receptor-dependent cell activation? *J Cell Physiol* 1993; **156**: 571–578.

51. Chakravarthy U, Hayes RG, Stitt AW *et al.*

Constitutive nitric oxide synthase expression in retinal vascular endothelial cells is suppressed by high glucose and advanced glycation end products. *Diabetes* 1998; **47**: 945–952.

52. Jirousek MR, Gillig JR, Gonzalez CM *et al.* (S)-13-[(dimethylamino)methyl]-10,11,14,15-tetrahydro-4,9;16,21-dimetheno-1H,13H-dibenzo[e,k]pyrrolo[3,4-h][1,4,13]-oxadiazacyclohexadecene-1,3(2H)-d ione (LY333531) and related analogues: isozyme selective inhibitors of protein kinase Cβ. *J Med Chem* 1996; **39**: 2664–2671.

53. Cameron N, Jack A, Ways D, Cotter M. Effects of the protein kinase C β inhibitor on nerve and vascular function in diabetic animals. *Diabetologia* 1998; **41(Suppl. 1)**: A54.

54. Winegrad AI. Banting lecture 1986. Does a common mechanism induce the diverse complications of diabetes? *Diabetes* 1987; **36**: 396–406.

55. Xia P, Kramer RM, King GL. Identification of the mechanism for the inhibition of Na+, K+-adenosine triphosphatase by hyperglycemia involving activation of protein kinase C and cytosolic phospholipase A2. *J Clin Invest* 1995; **96**: 733–740.

56. Kowluru RA, Jirousek MR, Stramm L *et al.* Abnormalities of retinal metabolism in diabetes or experimental galactosemia: V. Relationship between protein kinase C and ATPases. *Diabetes* 1998; **47**: 464–469.

57. Nakamura J, Koh N, Hamada Y *et al.* Effect of protein kinase C-β inhibitor on diabetic neuropathy in rats. *Diabetes* 1998; **47(S1)**: A70.

58. Epstein FH. Mechanisms of disease. *N Engl J Med* 1994; **331**: 1286–1291.

59. Craven PA, Studer RK, Negrete H, DeRubertis FR. Protein kinase C in diabetic nephropathy. *J Diabetes Complications* 1995; **9**: 241–245.

60. Sharma K, Ziyadeh FN. Hyperglycemia and diabetic kidney disease. The case for transforming growth factor-β as a key mediator. *Diabetes* 1995; **44**: 1139–1146.

61. MacKay K, Striker LJ, Stauffer JW *et al.* Transforming growth factor β. Murine glomerular receptors and responses of isolated glomerular cells. *J Clin Invest* 1989; **83**: 1160–1167.

62. Suzuki S, Ebihara I, Tomino Y, Koide H. Transcriptional activation of matrix genes by transforming growth factor beta 1 in mesangial cells. *Exp Nephrol* 1993; **1**: 229–237.

63. Nakamura T, Miller D, Ruoslahti E, Border WA. Production of extracellular matrix by glomerular epithelial cells is regulated by transforming growth factor-β1. *Kidney Int* 1992; **41**: 1213–1221.

64. Terrell TG, Working PK, Chow CP, Green JD. Pathology of recombinant human transforming growth factor-β1 in rats and rabbits. *Int Rev Exp Pathol* 1993; **34**: 43–67.

65. Isaka Y, Fujiwara Y, Ueda N *et al.* Glomerulosclerosis induced by *in vivo* transfection of transforming growth factor β or platelet-derived growth factor gene into the rat kidney. *J Clin Invest* 1993; **92**: 2597–2601.

66. Yamamoto T, Nakamura T, Noble NA *et al.* Expression of transforming growth factor β is elevated in human and experimental diabetic nephropathy. *Proc Natl Acad Sci USA* 1993; **90**: 1814–1818.

67. Bollineni JS, Reddi AS. Transforming growth factor-β1 enhances glomerular collagen synthesis in diabetic rats. *Diabetes* 1993; **42**: 1673–1677.

68. Shankland SJ, Scholey JW, Ly H, Thai K. Expression of transforming growth factor-β1 during diabetic renal hypertrophy. *Kidney Int* 1994; **46**: 430–442.

69. Sharma K, Ericksen M, Goldfarb S, Ziyadeh FN. Up-regulation of kidney transforming growth factor-β (TGF-β) gene expression in two rodent models of spontaneous diabetes mellitus. *J Am Soc Nephrol* 1992; **3**: 766.

70. Ziyadeh FN, Sharma K, Ericksen M, Wolf G. Stimulation of collagen gene expression and protein synthesis in murine mesangial cells by high glucose is mediated by autocrine activation of transforming growth factor-β. *J Clin Invest* 1994; **93**: 536–542.

71. Sharma K, Guo J, Jin Y *et al.* Anti-TGFβ antibody attenuates renal hypertrophy and matrix expression in diabetic mice. *J Am Soc Nephrol* 1994; **5**: 972.

72. Iwano M, Kubo A, Nishino T *et al.* Quantification of glomerular TGF-beta 1 mRNA in patients with diabetes mellitus. *Kidney Int* 1996; **49**: 1120–1126.

73. Jevtich MJ, Khawand NY, Vidic B. Clinical significance of ultrastructural findings in the corpora cavernosa of normal and impotent men. *J Urol* 1990; **143**: 289–293.

74. Mersdorf A, Goldsmith PC, Diederichs W *et al.* Ultrastructural changes in impotent penile tissue: a comparison of 65 patients. *J Urol* 1991; **145**: 749–758.

75. Nehra A, Hall SJ, Basil G *et al.* Systemic sclerosis and impotence: a clinicopathological correlation. *J Urol* 1995; **153**: 1140–1146.

76. Moreland RB, Traish A, McMillin MA *et al.* PGE1 suppresses the induction of collagen synthesis by transforming growth factor beta 1 in human corpus cavernosum smooth muscle. *J Urol* 1995; **153**: 826–834.

77. Kannel WB, Hjortland M, Castelli WP. Role of diabetes in congestive heart failure: the Framingham study. *Am J Cardiol* 1974; **34**: 29–34.

78. Raman M, Nesto RW. Heart disease in diabetes mellitus. *Endocrinol Metab Clin North Am* 1996; **25**: 425–438.

79. Bell DS. Diabetic cardiomyopathy. A unique entity or a complication of coronary artery disease? *Diabetes Care* 1995; **18**: 708–714.

80. Kreisberg JI, Radnik RA, Ayo SH *et al.* High glucose elevates c-fos and c-jun transcripts and proteins in mesangial cell cultures. *Kidney Int* 1994; **46**: 105–112.

81. Franza BR, Rauscher FJ, Josephs SF, Curran T. The Fos complex and Fos-related antigens recognize sequence elements that contain AP-1 binding sites. *Science* 1988; **239**: 1150–1153.

82. Chiu R, Boyle WJ, Meek J *et al.* The *c*-Fos protein interacts with *c*-Jun/AP-1 to stimulate transcription of AP-1 responsive genes. *Cell* 1988; **54**: 541–552.

83. Akhurst RJ, Fee F, Balmain A. Localized production of TGF-β mRNA in tumour promoter-stimulated mouse epidermis. *Nature* 1988; **331**: 363–365.

84. Kim S-J, Denhez F, Kim KY *et al.* Activation of the second promoter of the transforming growth factor-β1 gene by transforming growth factor-β1 and phorbol ester occurs through the same target sequences. *J Biol Chem* 1989; **264**: 19373–19378.

85. Nagpala PG, Malik AB, Vuong PT, Lum H. Protein kinase C β1 overexpression augments phorbol ester-induced increase in endothelial permeability. *J Cell Physiol* 1996; **166**: 249–255.

86. Kuroki T, Inoguchi T, Umeda F *et al.* High glucose induces alteration of gap junction permeability and phosphorylation of connexin-43 in cultured aortic smooth muscle cells. *Diabetes* 1998; **47**: 931–936.

87. Ferrara N, Houck K, Jakeman L, Leung DW. Molecular and biological properties of the vascular endothelial growth factor family of proteins. *Endocr Rev* 1992; **13**: 18–32.

88. Elliot D, Amin RH, Frank RN *et al.* Vascular endothelial growth factor (VEGF) expression in retinal Muller cells and optic nerve glial cells in non-proliferative diabetic retinopathy. *Invest Ophthalmol Vis Sci* 1996; **37**: 573a.

89. Foreman D, Williams G, Boulton ME, McLeod D. VEGF distribution in proliferative diabetic retinopathy. *Invest Ophthalmol Vis Sci* 1996; **37**: 4455a.

90. Kunz M, Merges C, McLeod DS, Lutty GA. Vascular endothelial growth factor/vascular permeability factor (VEGF) in diabetic retinopathy. *Invest Ophthalmol Vis Sci* 1996; **37**: 571a.

91. Aiello LP, Avery RL, Arrigg PG *et al.* Vascular endothelial growth factor in ocular fluid of patients with diabetic retinopathy and other retinal disorders. *N Engl J Med* 1994; **331**: 1480–1487.

92. Williams B, Gallacher B, Patel H, Orme C. Glucose-induced protein kinase C activation regulates vascular permeability factor mRNA expression and peptide production by human vascular smooth muscle cells *in vitro*. *Diabetes* 1997; **46**: 1497–1503.

93. Aiello L, Hata Y, Duh E *et al.* Expression of vascular endothelial growth factor (VEGF) and its receptor KDR are regulated by basic fibroblast growth factor (bFGF) through PKC, MAPK and Sp1 dependent mechanisms. *Diabetes* 1998; **47**: A39.

94. Ido Y, Chang K, Smith S, Tilton R *et al.* Vascular dysfunction in granulation tissue induced by glycated albumin is prevented by antibodies against vascular endothelial growth factor and by a selective inhibitor of the β isoform of protein kinase C. *Diabetes* 1998; **47(S1)**: A24.

95. Xia P, Aiello L, Ishii H *et al.* Characterization of vascular endothelial growth factor's effect on the activation of protein kinase C, its isoforms, and endothelial cell growth. *J Clin Invest* 1996; **98**: 2018–2026.

96. Danis RP, Yang Y, Massicotte SJ, Boldt HC. Preretinal and optic nerve head neovascularization induced by photodynamic venous thrombosis in domestic pigs. *Arch Ophthalmol* 1993; 111: 539–543.

97. Miller JW, Adamis AP, Shima DT *et al.* Vascular endothelial growth factor/vascular permeability factor is temporally and spatially correlated with ocular angiogenesis in a primate model. *Am J Pathol* 1994; 145: 574–584.

5

Advanced glycation end-products: impact on diabetic complications

Alan W Stitt and Helen Vlassara

Introduction

Prolonged exposure to hyperglycemia is now recognized as the primary causal factor in the majority of diabetic complications.[1,2] Indeed, glucose has a wide range of reversible effects on normal cell function that reflect the transient nature of hyperglycemia.[3,4] Significantly, many of the effects of hyperglycemia are irreversible and can cause progressive, cumulative cell dysfunction. This is highlighted by the observation that retinal vascular lesions in diabetic dogs progress during a 2.5-year period of euglycemia following a period of severe hyperglycemia.[5] This suggests that long-lived, permanent abnormalities rather than transient, acute abnormalities are of pivotal importance in diabetic complications. Among the irreversible changes which occur as a direct result of hyperglycemia is the formation of advanced glycation end-products (AGEs), which have a range of chemical, cellular, and tissue effects, and act as mediators, not only of diabetic complications but also of widespread changes associated with aging.

The growing recognition of the importance of AGEs within the context of human disease is best illustrated by the exponential rise in AGE-related publications within the medical research literature over recent years (*Fig. 5.1*). The following chapter will review aspects of this literature, focusing on the role that

advanced glycation plays in the initiation and progression of diabetic complications. We will outline known AGE-mediated cellular abnormalities and how these may impact on the organ dysfunction observed in diabetic patients. We will also review current attempts to alleviate the effects of these products and speculate about novel therapeutic interventions.

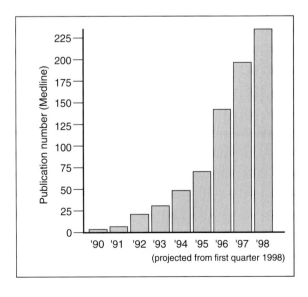

Fig. 5.1
AGEs in the scientific literature over the last 8 years.

Biochemistry of AGE formation

AGEs form via non-enzymatic glycation (NEG) reactions between reducing sugars and ε-amino groups or N-terminal amino acids. These reactions have a preference for lysine and arginine amino acids, although they can occur on free amine-containing lipids and DNA and proceed spontaneously via a complex series of chemical rearrangements to yield reactive products with varying properties, e.g. crosslinking, pigmentation, and fluorescence[6] (*Fig. 5.2*). NEG was first described in detail around the turn of the century by Louis Camille Maillard, who predicted that it could have an important impact on medicine.[7] Unfortunately, the Maillard reaction was not recognized by medical researchers even after its 'rediscovery' by food scientists nearly 50 years later, who realized that NEG reaction products were implicated in nutritional bio-availability, food flavor and aroma.[8,9] Only in the last 20 years has the pathophysiological significance of this ubiquitous reaction emerged as an important field of medical interest.

In biological systems, NEG can proceed when reducing sugars react with free amino groups, forming Schiff base adducts and Amadori products (*Fig. 5.2*). In fact, ambient glucose itself is among the least reactive sugars within biological systems, whilst other sugars, many of

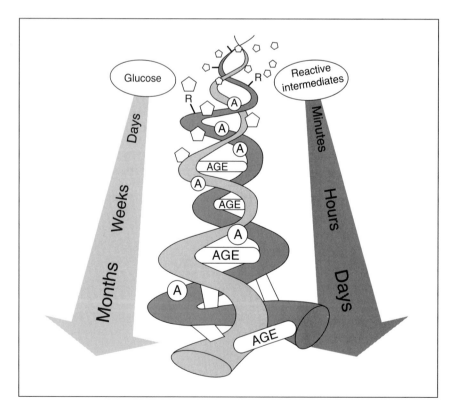

Fig. 5.2
Schematic diagram illustrating the course of AGE formation on a hypothetical fibrilar protein. Open chain sugars or glycolytic intermediates (pentose ring) react with amino groups (R) to form Schiff bases and Amadori products (A), and eventually AGEs. Glucose may take several weeks to culminate in AGE formation, leading to irreversible crosslink formation between protein fibrils or oxidative products. Reactive glycolytic intermediates such as methylglyoxal or 3-deoxyglucosone take much less time to form AGEs.

which are located intracellularly, such as glucose-6-phosphate and glyceraldehyde-3-phosphate, are much more reactive and participate in NEG at a proportionally faster rate[10,11] (*Fig. 5.2*). In any case, the chemically unstable Schiff bases and Amadori products are freely reversible and therefore reach an equilibrium, which is proportional to the amount of free sugar. Amadori product 'steady-state' is reached over a period of approximately 28 days. An understanding of NEG kinetics *in vivo* led to the conceptualization of glycosylated hemoglobin A1c (HbA1c) by Cerami *et al.* and to the eventual development of the clinical assays which measure Amadori product formation on the Hb A1 amino-terminal valine of the β-chain over a 28-day period.[12,13] Although not of major pathological significance, HbA1c levels provide a useful correlative indicator of cumulative exposure of native hemoglobin to hyperglycemia and associated risk for diabetic complications.[13] It should be noted, however, that in diabetic individuals the levels of Amadori products are usually no more than two- to threefold higher than in their non-diabetic counterparts. This reflects the reversible nature of these products and the equilibrium which is always reached between modified and non-modified forms of a protein. Hence, Amadori products do not accumulate indefinitely on long-lived macro-molecules and there is no correlation between the formation of these adducts on tissues and diabetic complications.[14]

NEG reactions eventually culminate in the formation of AGEs, some of which are permanent, irreversible chemical rearrangements. The majority of AGEs, however, includes a vast range of precursor molecules, the variable chemical nature of which contributes to the heterogeneous mixture of glycation end-products. For example, the Amadori intermediate can undergo oxidative fragmentation reactions and give rise to irreversible N-ε-carboxymethylated lysine (CML) residues,[15] which can accumulate on the protein to which they are attached, or can lead to the formation of highly reactive dicarbonyl compounds. Dicarbonyls such as 1-, 3-, or 4-deoxyglucosones, glyoxal, and methylglyoxal are highly reactive intermediates, which will in turn react with proteins and propagate intramolecular or intermolecular crosslink formation.[16–18] These pathways are an equally important source of AGEs within the cell and, because they arise from highly reactive 'AGE-intermediates', they can occur very rapidly.[19] It has recently been realized that there is a significant catalytic inter-play between glycation and oxidation reactions arising from the autooxidation of Amadori products yielding 'glycoxidation' products such as N-ε-(carboxymethyl)lysine (CML).[20,21] Other precursor molecules can undergo slow dehydration and condensation reactions to produce irreversibly bound moieties which persist during the lifetime of the amine-containing substrate. Such 'end-products' are structurally and thermodynamically stable, and they represent the terminal phase of the Maillard reaction.

The chemical nature of these biologically important AGEs, as they occur naturally *in vivo*, is largely unknown due to their hetero-geneous and unstable nature; nevertheless, there is a growing population of structurally defined AGE adducts such as pyrroline,[22] pentosidine,[23] CML,[15] and crossline[24] (*Fig. 5.3*). Some AGEs have been found to be elevated in diabetic tissues.[25–28] Others, such as 2-(2-furoyl)-4(5)-furanyl-1*H*-imidazole (FFI)[29] and 1-alkyl-2-formyl-3, 4-glycosyl-pyrrole (AFGP),[30] are well-defined AGE structures formed from *in vitro* reactions (*Fig. 5.3*) but only immuno-histochemically detected *in vivo*. These molecules have been useful as models for AGE structure and function studies, although there is still some controversy over whether these compounds actually occur *in vivo*.[22,31,32]

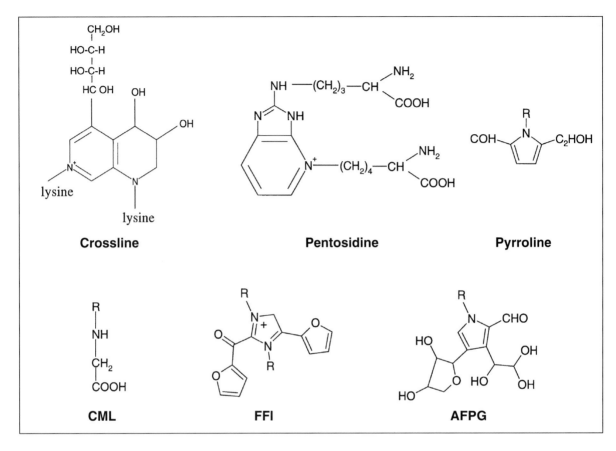

Fig. 5.3
Molecular structures of several advanced glycation end-products.

AGE receptor systems

Early in AGE research it was speculated that a natural receptor-based system existed *in vivo* whereby AGE products could be removed from tissues, thereby limiting their deleterious effects. Work conducted over the last 10 years has led to the recognition of a complex AGE receptor system which plays a critical role in AGE-related biology, as well as in the pathology associated with the complications of diabetes and aging.[33] It was originally demonstrated that AGE-modified proteins are recognized by specific receptors, which are unrelated to previously described scavenger receptor systems.[34] Over recent years, several AGE-binding molecules have been described.

Two AGE-binding proteins, a ~60 kDa (p60) and a ~90 kDa (p90) molecule, isolated from mouse macrophages and rat liver membranes were initially identified.[35,36] p60, Now referred to as AGE-R1, with characteristic membrane-spanning and signal domains, was shown to be homologous to a ~50 kDa component of the

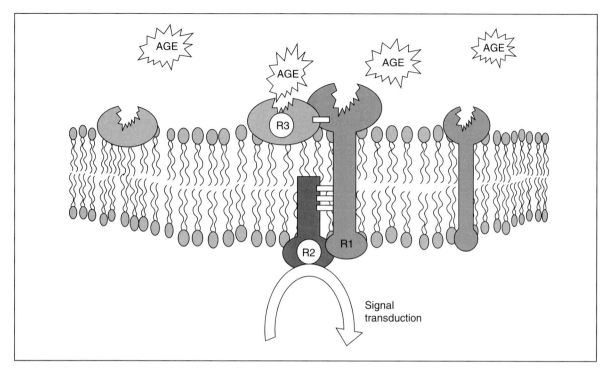

Fig. 5.4
Diagrammatic representation of the AGE–receptor complex. The R1 and R3 components show AGE-binding properties, while the R2 component, which acts as a protein kinase C substrate, may have a role in signal transduction.

oligosaccharyltransferase complex (OST 48), while the p90, also termed AGE-R2, showed complete homology to the protein kinase C (PKC) substrate 80 K-H.[37] Another 32 kDa AGE-binding protein was described soon after with links to the AGE receptor complex (AGE-R), thus described as AGE-R3. This protein, also known as Galectin-3, Mac-2, or carbohydrate-binding protein-35, exhibits high-affinity binding for AGE ligands.[38] AGE binding to AGE-R3 occurs within the 18 kDa C-terminal peptide, and promotes high-molecular-weight complex formation with the AGE ligand and with other membrane-associated receptor molecules on the cell surface (*Fig. 5.4*). The configuration of the assembled components of the AGE-R is not well defined as yet, but it is likely to involve the attack on a thiol–ester of the AGE-R3 component by nucleophilic groups present on AGE proteins. The significance of the participation of high-energy thiol–ester bonds may reflect the need for the efficient attachment and subsequent trafficking to intra-cellular degradative pathways of a heterogeneous class of AGE-modified structures. This receptor complex is identified on many cell types and tissues, including vascular smooth muscle, retinal microvascular pericytes, macrophages, lymphocytes, and renal mesangial cells,[37,39–41] where it appears to mediate tissue-specific changes typical of diabetic vascular complications.

Evidence indicates that AGE-R1 and -R3 are largely responsible for AGE recognition and high-affinity binding. AGE-R2, in its capacity as a substrate for PKC, was shown to be subject to increased phosphorylation in response to AGE albumin.[39] The R2 component of the AGE-R may thus play a critical role in signal transduction associated with cell activation and cytotoxicity associated with AGE-receptor binding.[42–44] The inability of endothelial cells to bind FFI-BSA (a synthetic, model AGE)[39,45] in a manner similar to that of phagocytic cells suggests that the AGE-R of vascular endothelium may have subtle AGE binding/processing capabilities *in vivo*. In certain cells, such as human vascular endothelial cells, gene expression of AGE-R2 and -R3 is upregulated upon exposure to AGEs and more receptor is translocated to the plasma membrane,[39] suggesting differential regulation of the individual receptor components which may be tissue specific.

Other proteins with AGE-binding characteristics have been identified from bovine lung tissue. A novel 35 kDa protein, isolated from bovine lung, has been described as a receptor for AGEs or RAGE.[46] RAGE was cloned, sequenced, and found to be a member of the immunoglobulin superfamily.[47] In common with members of this family, RAGE has the capacity to interact with several other ligands besides AGEs. Its high-affinity binding of amphoterin[48] indicates that the molecule may also serve other functions, including intercellular recognition or as a receptor for certain growth factors. RAGE has been localized in many cells and tissues where it can modulate several AGE-mediated effects.[49–51] Many of the biological functions of RAGE are currently being investigated, but it appears to have a major role in the oxidative stress induced by advanced glycation.[52,53] This is evidenced by its 'downstream' activation of the transcription factor NF-κB, leading to binding to its own promoter region,[54] and VCAM-1 and tissue factor promoters.[55,56] It has been speculated that the extracellular domain of RAGE may be proteolytically cleaved to release a soluble form of the receptor (sRAGE) which may help to bind serum AGEs, limit receptor interaction on cells and ameliorate some of their effects.[53–57]

Together with RAGE, an 80 kDa protein was isolated as an AGE-binding protein and found to be homologous to lactoferrin.[45–47] Another well-characterized immune-defence protein, lysozyme, was also discovered to exhibit significant AGE-binding properties.[58] It was later shown that both lysozyme and lactoferrin bind AGEs via a cysteine-bounded domain 'ABCD' motif. This results in a disruption of their bacteriocidal and agglutination properties.[58]

Other AGE-binding proteins have included the macrophage scavenger receptor, which although not restricted to AGEs, may contribute to cellular changes in the context of atherosclerosis.[59–61] More recently, a novel AGE receptor has been proposed which may show properties somewhat different from those previously described,[62] although the character of this receptor is as yet unelucidated.

It is evident from the above findings that a number of AGE receptors may exist that differ in protein structure, ligand specificity, and modulatory function. Interrelationships between the receptors and how they function when co-expressed in the same cell types remains ill-defined. However, AGE-binding proteins, with or without 'receptor' characteristics, may contribute to the removal, transport, and/or processing of AGE-related adducts, as well as regulation of diverse cellular functions. A recent report suggests that circulating monocytes from diabetic patients may actually express variable levels of AGE receptors compared with their non-diabetic counterparts, which suggests the regulation of these receptors upon exposure to diabetic 'factors', i.e. increased AGE ligands *in vivo*.[63] Furthermore, it could be speculated that variability in AGE-receptor expression between individuals may also underlie genetic differences in susceptibility to specific pathological sequelae between diabetic patients. This may account for the observation that some diabetics develop fewer diabetic complications, despite prolonged history of poor glucose control, compared with others who despite relatively good control suffer severe debilitating disorders.

AGE formation with relevance to biological systems

(a) Endogenous AGEs

(i) Advanced glycation of short-lived molecules

It was thought that AGE formation involves primarily long-lived extracellular proteins as a function of time, and thus represents a form of molecular senescence that has a significant effect on structure and function, especially if the modification occurs at a region crucial for activity of a given macromolecule. It is now clear that AGEs occur on short-lived molecules such as circulating plasma proteins and lipids in the bloodstream at significantly elevated levels in diabetic patients and in patients with impaired renal clearance.[64,65] It is also recognized that they can form very rapidly on short-lived cytoplasmic proteins and nucleic acids. Indeed, it has been demonstrated that intracellular AGEs may form at a rate of up to 14-fold faster in high (30 mM) glucose conditions.[66] Such AGE modification of short-lived proteins

is known to disrupt molecular conformation, alter enzymatic activity, reduce degradative capacity, and result in abnormal recognition by receptors[67–70] (see *Table 5.1*).

The pathological significance of AGE modification is well illustrated in the glycation of lipids and lipoproteins, as in the case of apoprotein B (ApoB) and low-density lipoprotein (LDL).[71] Dyslipidemic changes are evident in diabetic patients and are characterized by increased levels of LDL, which greatly predispose these patients to atherosclerosis, with subsequent increased risk for coronary heart disease and stroke. Advanced glycation of the lipid component of LDL occurs concomitantly with LDL oxidation *in vitro*.[71] Furthermore, the presence of amino groups on phospholipids such as phosphatidylethanolamine and phosphatidylserine provides appropriate sites with which glucose can react with lipid amines to form AGEs.[72] Oxidation/reduction reactions occurring normally during glycation can oxidize fatty acid residues, independently of transition metals or exogenous free-radical-generating systems.[72] Significantly, LDL oxidation follows formation of AGE–LDL, while both occur as a function of glucose concentration and are inhibited by co-incubation with the AGE inhibitor, aminoguanidine.[72] It is apparent, therefore, that amine–glucose interactions are spontaneous and natural in *in vivo* pathways leading to fatty acid oxidation products.

The ApoB component of LDL is a relatively large protein with many potential lysine and arginine AGE modification sites, although the predominant site of such modification has been found distally to the N-terminus of the LDL-receptor-binding domain.[71] AGE-ApoB levels are up to fourfold higher in diabetic patients.[72,73] The pathophysiological implications of this AGE modification have been demonstrated in a study in which AGE–LDL

Table 5.1
A range of macromolecules and the mechanisms by which they are affected by glycation.

Glycated macromolecule(s)	Effects of glycation	Reference(s)
Albumin	Altered conformation	180
β-Amyloid peptide	Aggregation, crosslinking reduced solubility	70
Antithrombin III	Reduced affinity to heparin	181
BM proteins	Reduced cell adherence charge alteration, reduced heparin binding, abnormal 3-D aggregation	69, 85, 86
Crystallins (lens)	Reduced solubility, disappearance of γ crystalin, crosslinkinbg	182, 183
Fibrinogen	Less degradable by pepsin	67, 184
bFGF	Reduced mitogenic activity	167
Insulin	Reduced hormone action	186
IGF-1 binding protein-3	Reduced modulatory effect on IGF-1	187
Lipoproteins	Reduced metabolic properties, reduced receptor recognition	73, 185
β2-microglobulin	Acceleration of β2-microglobulin amyloidosis, stimulate TNF α, IL-6	57, 188
Nitric oxide synthase	Reduced enzymatic activity	156
Ribonuclease	Enzymatic inactivation	68
Superoxide dismutase	Enzymatic inactivation	67, 189
Tubulin (monomeric)	Reduced microtubule formation	190

was injected into transgenic mice expressing the human LDL receptor, in which the modification delayed LDL clearance as compared with native LDL.[73] This suggested that advanced glycation of ApoB can lead to hyperlipoproteinemia and thus actively contribute to atherosclerosis by reducing LDL clearance and facilitating AGE uptake into the vessel wall via AGE-receptor interactions.[74,75]

(ii) Advanced glycation of long-lived molecules
The rate of formation of AGEs is greater than first order. This implies that even modest glycemia or hyperglycemia can result in significant accumulation of AGEs on long-lived macromolecules with time and duration of diabetes.[76–78] This is well illustrated in the case of certain long-lived proteins such as those of

the eye. For example, the progressive post-translational modification of lens crystallins by glucose-derived AGEs explains the premature browning and cumulative crosslinking occurring in the diabetic lens.[79,80] It is now well established that progressive AGE formation on lens crystallins accounts for a significant proportion of lenticular opacification, and subsequently cataractous lenses during aging and diabetes.[81,82] In addition, the collagen network of the human vitreous gel contains increased levels of AGEs and AGE-mediated crosslinking in diabetics (*Fig. 5.5*).[83] The process can be reproduced *ex vivo* using the presence of high glucose concentrations and can be effectively prevented in the presence of the AGE inhibitor aminoguanidine.[83] Also, vitreous AGE levels show a significant correlation with age, suggesting that they may play a major role in diabetes- and age-related vitreous alterations, which has implications for posterior vitreal detachments (PVDs) and progression of proliferative diabetic retinopathy.[83]

The proteins composing the extracellular matrix (ECM) and vascular basement membranes (BM) are amongst the longest lived in the body and are highly susceptible to AGE modification. Functionally, AGE-mediated crosslinks in BM are known to cause reduced solubility and a decrease in enzymatic digestion.[84,85] In addition, AGE formation has been shown to impair the geometrically ordered self-assembly of BM proteins, thereby preventing appropriate component interactions, and causing structural and functional abnormalities. For example, AGE modification of laminin, vitronectin, and collagen can seriously alter molecular charge characteristics, upset the ability to form precisely assembled three-dimensional matrix aggregates and thus to disrupt biological attachment sites, which enable cells to adhere to their substrates.[69,86–88]

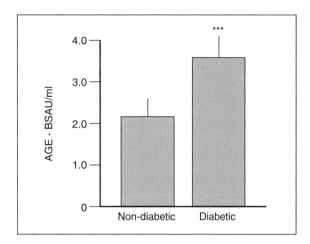

Fig. 5.5
*Comparison of AGE immunoreactivity in vitreous specimens from diabetic and non-diabetic patients. Vitreous samples were matched according to age, since it has been shown that AGEs correlate with age in the normal vitreous humor *** p <0.005.*

Moreover, the impaired matrix binding of heparin sulfate proteoglycan to AGE-modified collagen, laminin, and fibronectin significantly reduces the polyanionic nature of BM,[89,90] seriously altering their charge-mediated properties. Therefore, AGE accumulation on vascular BM of diabetics may have serious pathogenic consequences.

(iii) DNA–AGE interactions as a basis for diabetic embryopathy

The primary amino groups of nucleotides are less-reactive nucleophiles than ϵ-amino groups of lysine and arginine in the process of Maillard reactions. Nonetheless, nucleic acids can react with reducing intracellular sugars to form Amadori and AGE products with characteristic fluorescent and spectral properties.[91] AGE formation on DNA can cause single-strand breaks in genomic DNA with serious teratogenic effects.[91-93] Lee *et al.*[94] further demonstrated this *in vivo* by placing 3–4-day-old mouse embryos transgenic for the *lac*I, *lac*I+ reporter gene in the uterine horns of pseudo-pregnant diabetic and control mice. Through analysis of the *lac*I transgene, it was found that the mice gestated in the diabetic environment had a greater than twofold higher mutation rate, when compared with their non-diabetic counterparts.[94] More recent *in vitro* studies confirmed that AGEs can cause the mobilization of a genomic element, an 853 bp insertion designated INS-1, which is transposed into the genome and may account for AGE-induced insertional mutations.[95]

Teratogenic effects may also be promoted in diabetes by enhanced glycation of histone proteins, which have a vital structural role in maintaining nucleosomes and hence DNA integrity. Intracellular sugars such as glucose-6-phosphate and ADP-ribose have been shown to react strongly with amino groups on histones where they can cause crosslinking *in vitro*[96,97] as well as *in vivo*.[98]

Maternal diabetes has been associated with congenital malformations and increased foetal mortality and morbidity.[99] It is estimated that there is a two- to threefold higher incidence of perinatal infant fatalities with insulin-dependent diabetic mothers, due to congenital malformations in the fetus.[100] Most studies show a generalized increase in malformations involving multiple-organ systems, although the teratogenic mechanisms are largely unknown. From the presented evidence it would appear that AGE-mediated DNA damage is a significant factor in the teratogenicity effects observed during diabetic pregnancy. Congenital abnormalities are not increased in short-term, pregnancy-induced hyperglycemia, however, they do appear to correlate with poor glycemic control over a long time period, even before conception.[101] This, together with the marked reduction in fetal abnormalities with effective management of hyperglycemia during pregnancy has added further evidence for the involvement of AGEs in diabetic embryopathy.

(iv) Degradative mechanisms for removal of AGE-modified molecules

Although AGEs accumulate on long-lived macromolecules, there are potentially important systems which serve to remove senescent molecules and degrade existing AGE crosslinks on tissues. These degradative mechanisms are conducted largely through extracellular proteolysis and by scavenger cells, such as circulating and tissue macrophages, which recognize AGE moieties via AGE receptors. It is also becoming clear that mesenchymal cells such as vascular endothelium or mesangium may have an important role in AGE removal. This function may account in part for the increased endocytic activity of vascular endothelium under conditions of hyperglycemia *in vivo* and high glucose *in vitro*.[102,103] Generally, AGE-modified molecules are recognized and internalized by cell-surface receptor-mediated endocytosis, degraded intracellularly and subsequently released as AGE peptides (or low-molecular-weight AGEs), recently described as 'second generation AGEs'.[104] These include reactive intermediates with high crosslinking or oxidative reactivity;[65,105,106] however, their effects are normally limited by renal excretion.[104] The efficiency of this AGE removal system varies as a function of renal clearance. It is significant that kidney dysfunction, as in the case of diabetic nephropathy, results in a failure to reduce circulating AGEs, thus accounting for the marked elevation of serum AGE levels observed in such patients.[64,65] This negative feedback mechanism may also explain in part why patients with end-stage renal disease (ESRD) suffer from acceleration of extrarenal vascular damage.[107]

It is also becoming evident that intracellular protective systems exist to limit the accumulation of reactive AGE intermediates. One such system involves the degradative glyoxalase enzymes, which can metabolize the reactive dicarbonyl methylglyoxal to *S*-D-lactoylglutathione, in the presence of reduced glutathione as a co-factor. The utility and efficiency of such systems was supported in studies where glyoxalase-1 expression was upregulated by gene transfection in endothelial cells, resulting in significant inhibition of AGE-mediated cell abnormalities such as increased endocytosis.[108]

(b) Exogenous sources of AGEs

Recent studies suggest that AGEs may be introduced to biological systems from exogenous sources and have a significant impact on disease mechanisms. One such source is tobacco smoke-derived AGEs. The curing of tobacco evokes the Maillard reaction cascade, leading to AGE formation. It was established that tobacco is processed in the presence of sugars, leading to derivatives which, upon combustion, generate reactive AGE species. These species, also termed 'glycotoxins', are carried in smoke for inhalation, absorbed through the lungs, and readily transferred onto serum proteins such as lipoproteins.[109] Thus, AGE-apoprotein B and total serum AGE levels in cigarette smokers have been found to be significantly higher than those in non-smokers.[109] Correspondingly, smokers, and especially diabetics who smoke, show high AGE levels in their arteries[110,111] and lenses[111] (*Fig. 5.6*).

Exogenous AGEs may also be absorbed through the intestinal wall in the form of reactive dietary glycotoxins.[112] This results in transient elevation of circulating AGE peptides, which are rapidly normalized by most healthy individuals. However, patients with diabetic nephropathy are less capable of excreting these glycotoxins. Consequently they tend to remain in the circulation at higher levels and for longer intervals.[112] It has thus been suggested that certain foods with inherently high AGE levels may pose a significant environmental risk, especially to diabetic patients with advanced nephropathy.[112]

The role of AGEs in diabetic vascular complications

(a) AGEs in macroangiopathy

Diabetics are more likely than non-diabetics to develop serious cardio- and cerebrovascular disease and suffer a greatly increased risk of stroke or myocardial infarction.[113–115] Plaque formation is the pathophysiological hallmark of the atherosclerotic process, but the interactions between blood-borne proteins, cytokines, growth factors, and different cell types which contribute to the formation of advanced lesions is extremely complex and multifactorial.[116] Atheromatous plaque formation in diabetics may be largely indistinguishable from that occurring in non-diabetics, although the distribution of plaques may be different, and diabetic lesions characteristically show an increased focal medial calcification.[115] Accumulation of lipids and lipoproteins in the vessel wall leading to the formation of fatty streaks is an important step in the formation of advanced atherosclerotic lesions. It has been widely speculated that oxidative modification of LDL *in vivo* results in its reduced recognition by the LDL receptor, leading to increases in serum LDL levels and enhanced uptake of the modified lipoprotein by scavenger receptors on macrophages and vascular smooth muscle cells. Chemical modification of the ApoB component of LDL has been shown to interfere with its recognition by the LDL receptor[117,118] and lead

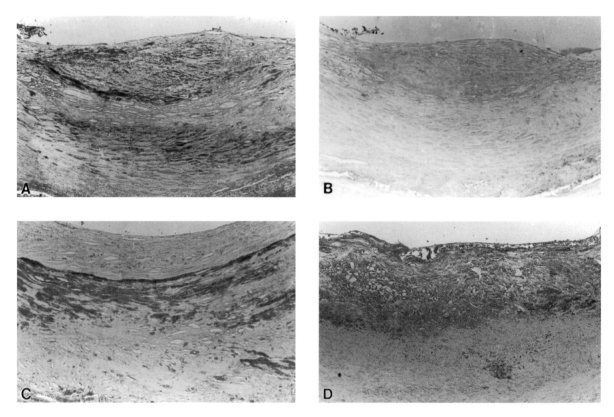

Fig. 5.6
Coronary arteries stained for AGE immunoreactivity. (a) Smoking/non-diabetic patient showing AGEs within the atherosclerotic plaque. (b) Non-immune serum control from adjacent section. (c) Non-smoking/diabetic patient with AGE immunoreactivity in the vessel wall, especially within the innermost layers of the plaque. (d) Smoking/diabetic patient showing very elevated levels of AGE immunoreactivity. Staining appears to be of greater intensity and is more widespread in comparison with other groups.

to abnormally high levels of circulating LDL.[119,120] As mentioned earlier in the chapter, advanced glycation of LDL is a physiologically relevant modification which can occur concomitantly with oxidation of LDL *in vitro*.[72] Indeed, AGEs are now recognized as having an important role in the formation and acceleration of atherosclerotic lesions even in normoglycemic patients,[75] but especially in diabetics[121,122] and more so in diabetics with renal insufficiency.[123]

AGEs have been detected within atherosclerotic lesions in both extra- and intracellular locations.[75,123–126] We have recently reported a significant correlation between serum AGE-ApoB and AGE levels in the vessel wall of carotid arteries from non-diabetic patients with occlusive disease, requiring endarterectomy.[75] A similar correlation was also demonstrated between serum AGE–LDL and AGE immunoreactivity in histological sections from these patients.[75] Significantly, both AGE-R1 and

AGE-R2 were identified in the cellular components of atherosclerotic lesions, with a distribution pattern consistent with the AGE immunoreactivity in the same series.[74,75]

Vascular endothelium expresses receptors for AGEs,[37,39] and it is likely that AGE–LDL can be transcytosed by the endothelium and lead directly to the accumulation of AGEs in the vessel wall. In addition, it has been speculated that intracellular accumulation of AGEs may promote phenotypic conversion of smooth muscle cells and foam cell formation within the atherosclerotic plaque.[126] This is consistent with the diffuse pattern of AGE deposition and endocytosis by endothelium, smooth muscle cells, and macrophages.[33,60,127] It also suggests that the process begins early, persists during the entire atheroma formation, and would be expected to be accelerated during diabetes.

With significance to diabetic atherosclerosis, hypertension, renal impairment, and male impotence, AGE adducts residing in vessel walls are known to interfere with endothelium-derived nitric oxide synthase[128] and the vasodilatory action of nitric oxide (NO·). AGEs react directly to inactivate NO·-mediated vasodilatation[129] while AGE-infused non-diabetic animals show diabetic-like disruption of vasorelaxation processes.[130] Endothelial dysfunction leading to enhanced procoagulant activity may result from exposure of endothelial cells to AGEs *in vitro*.[131] Furthermore, vascular endothelial cells react to AGEs by causing down-regulation of the anticoagulant thrombomodulin[45] and promotion of transendothelial migration by monocytes.[43] Vlassara *et al.*[132] reported an accelerated atherogenic potential in AGE-infused rabbits, characterized by a significant increase in expression of vascular cell adhesion molecule-1 (VCAM-1) and intracellular adhesion molecule-1 (ICAM-1) on the endothelial surface of the rabbit aorta. These AGE-induced changes were markedly accelerated in animals placed on a cholesterol-rich diet.[132] Taken together, it is apparent that AGEs cause significant dysfunctional changes to the macrovascular endothelium in ways that can potentiate vessel wall atherogenesis, hypertension, or prothrombiotic events.

(b) AGEs in microangiopathy

Diabetic microangiopathy is a broad term that describes dysfunctional changes in microvascular beds in which endothelium and associated mural cells are progressively damaged, resulting in capillary occlusion, ischemia, and organ failure. While these abnormalities are most obviously manifested in the kidneys and retina of diabetics, microangiopathy can occur in a wide range of tissues. In fact, damage to the microvasculature is now becoming recognized as a major pathogenic factor in diabetic peripheral nerves leading to neuropathy.[133,134] Recently, AGEs have been implicated in the pathogenesis of diabetic microangiopathy.[135–137] However, their role in diabetic nephropathy and retinopathy is still under intense investigation.

(i) In vivo *evidence*

Diabetic nephropathy is characterized by increased glomerular BM thickening[138] and mesangial extracellular matrix (ECM) deposition, followed by mesangial hypertrophy and diffuse and nodular glomerulosclerosis.[139] Loss of glomerular function is accompanied by a reduction in filtration capacity, culminating in complete renal failure.[140] Structural changes in the glomerulus during diabetes are accompanied by several biochemical abnormalities, including the accumulation of AGEs. Immunohistochemical studies of kidney from normal and diabetic rats have suggested that glomerular BM, mesangium, podocytes, and renal tubular cells accumulate high levels of AGEs

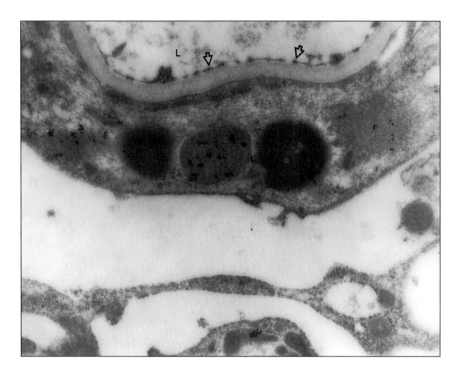

Fig. 5.7
AGE immunoreactivity in the glomerular podocyte cell from a 6-month-old diabetic rat. AGEs appear localized to the lysosomal compartments within the cell. L, lumen of the glomerulus; arrow, fenestrated endothelium of the glomerular capillary.

(*Fig. 5.7*). Ultrastructural studies have demonstrated BSA–AGE gold conjugate binding to glomerular structures of rats[141] and have indicated that AGE peptides may be reabsorbed by the renal proximal tubular cells.[142] AGE deposition can lead to glomerulosclerosis and widespread dysfunction independent of diabetes.[143–145] This had already been suggested by studies in which normal, non-diabetic animals were administered AGE albumin. In the short term, these treatments reproduced some of the vascular defects associated with clinical diabetic nephropathy such as the induction of BM components (e.g. collagen IV) and the ECM-regulating transforming growth factor-beta (TGF-β).[146] Chronic treatment of non-diabetic animals with AGE albumin resulted in glomerular hypertrophy, BM thickening, mesangial ECM expansion, and albuminuria, all consistent with a glomerulopathy resembling diabetic nephropathy.[33,130]

In diabetic patients with IDDM of 10 years duration, the prevalence of diabetic retinopathy is around 80% and it remains among the leading causes of blindness in the United States.[147] Diabetic retinopathy is principally a disease of the intraretinal blood vessels, which become dysfunctional in response to hyperglycemia, with progressive loss of retinal pericytes and eventually of endothelial cells, leading to capillary closure and widespread retinal ischemia. Similar to other vascular beds in the body, AGEs have been localized in the retinal vessels of diabetics.[40,148] The precise role that these adducts play in the pathogenesis of diabetic retinopathy remains ill-defined, although experimental studies have demonstrated that AGEs may be responsible for some retinal pathology[149,150] and that aminoguanidine can prevent the development of diabetes-associated retinal vascular lesions in rats.[151] Interestingly, aminoguanidine does not prevent the initial phase of experimental diabetic retinopathy in rats,[152] although a secondary intervention study with this drug has been shown to retard disease progression.[153] In diabetic rats, AGEs are not only localized to vascular BMs, but also appear to accumulate in the retinal pericytes after 8 months of diabetes (*Fig. 5.8*).[40] Moreover, when non-diabetic animals are infused with AGE–albumin, these adducts accumulate around and within in the pericytes, co-localize with AGE receptors, and induce BM thickening.[40,150]

(ii) In vitro *evidence*

The ability to culture cells *in vitro* that are specifically affected by AGEs *in vivo* has provided important insight into the action of these adducts, their receptors, and how they contribute to tissue dysfunction in diabetes. For example, renal mesangial cells have been shown to bind AGEs through AGE receptors,[154] and to respond by a receptor-mediated upregulation of mRNA and protein secretion of matrix proteins such as collagen IV and laminin.[155] Also *in vitro*, retinal vascular cells exposed to AGEs show abnormal endothelial nitric oxide synthase (eNOS) expression, which may account for some of the vasoregulatory abnormalities observed in the diabetic vasculature.[156] There are also AGE-mediated dysfunctional growth responses,[44,157–159] which appear to be regulated, at least in part, by AGE receptors.[44] Upregulation of key growth factors by AGE-receptor-mediated mechanisms occurs in many cell types. Many of these AGE effects are of key pathological significance, such as increased synthesis of TGF-β in mesangial cells,[144] vascular endothelial growth factor

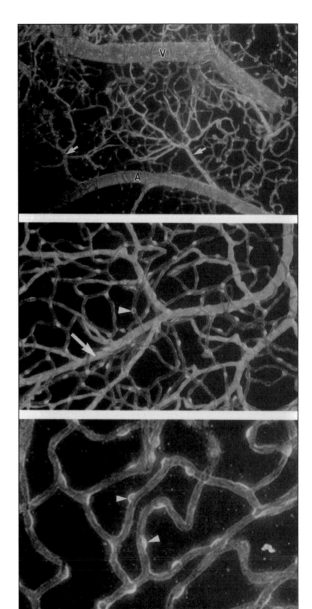

Fig. 5.8
AGE immunoreactivity in an 8-month-old diabetic rat. Progressively higher magnification demonstrates that AGEs seem to occur in all the retinal vessels, including retinal arteries (A), veins (V), and capillary beds. Higher magnification shows preferential localization in the smooth muscle of the retinal arterioles (arrows) and pericytes (arrowheads).

(VEGF) in retinal cells,[160–162] PDGF and IGF-1 by monocytes, and pro-inflammatory cytokines by leukocytes.[42,43,163–165]

Anti-AGE strategies

The interpretation of AGE toxicity has been a key strategy in the prevention of diabetic complications. To date there have been several approaches which seek to (a) prevent AGE formation, (b) reduce AGE effects on cells, and (c) break pre-existing AGE crosslinks.

Amadori product formation is the basis of advanced glycation biochemistry because progression to protein crosslinks requires slow rearrangement of the Amadori to create reactive intermediates that can react with amino groups before the formation of irreversible AGEs. An important pharmacological strategy for the inhibition of this process utilizes the small nucleophilic hydrazine compound aminoguanidine, which is a potent inhibitor of AGE-mediated crosslinking.[166] The terminal amino group of aminoguanidine, by virtue of its low pK_a, reacts specifically with glucose-derived reactive intermediates and prevents crosslinks from forming. Aminoguanidine has been shown by numerous workers to prevent diabetes-related vascular complications in experimental animals.[72,151,167–174] From these extensive studies, it is apparent that aminoguanidine can be used to prevent AGE-mediated tissue damage in animal models of diabetes and aging. In humans, a phase I study of aminoguanidine measured advanced glycation-modified hemoglobin (Hb-AGE) in treated and untreated diabetic subjects and found that it was significantly reduced in the treated group. The mean Hb-AGE value decreased significantly as a result of aminoguanidine therapy (13.8–0.8 U/mg Hb at the initiation of

therapy versus 10.0–0.9 U/mg Hb after 28 days of therapy). HbA_{1c} values were not affected by aminoguanidine treatment, pointing to the specificity of aminoguanidine for inhibition of post-Amadori, advanced glycation reactions. Aminoguanidine and related AGE inhibitors may eventually find widespread use in diabetics or in individuals at risk of age-related vascular sequelae. Development of aminoguanidine is now at phase II/III clinical trials. Other AGE-inhibiting drugs have recently been developed, such as the thiazolidine derivative OPB-9195, which has been shown to prevent the progression of diabetic glomerulosclerosis in diabetic rats.[175]

Prevention of interaction of AGEs with their receptors or other body proteins is a valid therapeutic approach. The use of neutralizing antibodies against glycated albumin has been shown to prevent BM thickening in diabetic db/db mice, despite the fact that the antibodies did not alter the glycemic status of the animals.[150] Likewise, the AGE-binding properties of lysozyme[58] have been used to reduce AGE levels in dialysate from diabetic patients with kidney disease.[176] The protocol involved the capture of *in vivo*-derived AGEs with lysozyme linked to a Sepharose matrix allowing the selective depletion of AGEs from sera or dialysate.[176] Such an approach offers the possibility of reduction of toxic AGE groups from body fluids in patients with renal failure, with or without diabetes.

Recently, a novel therapeutic strategy has been shown to attack the AGE crosslinks formed in biological systems. This is an exciting approach since it would 'break' pre-accumulated AGEs and subsequently clear them via the kidney.[177] Such an AGE crosslink-'breaker' prototype has been described to attack covalent carbon–carbon bonds of dicarbonyl-derived crosslinks *in vitro*.[178] More recently, such an AGE-breaker named ALT-711 was found to be capable of reversing AGE-mediated vascular stiffness and distensibility in diabetic rats.[179]

References

1. Pirart J. Diabetes mellitus and its degenerative complications: prospective study of 4400 patients observed between 1947 and 1973. *Diabetes Care* 1978; **188**: 252–263.

2. The Diabetes Control and Complications Trial Research Group. The effect of intensive treatment of diabetes on the development and progression of long term complications in insulin dependent diabetes mellitus. *N Eng J Med* 1993; **329**: 977–986.

3. Ruderman N, Williamson J, Brownlee M, eds. *Hyperglycemia, Diabetes and Vascular Disease.* New York, Oxford: Oxford University Press, American Physiological Society, 1992.

4. King GL, Kunisaki M, Nishio Y *et al.* Biochemical and molecular mechanisms in the development of diabetic vascular complications. *Diabetes* 1996; **45** (**Suppl. 3**): S105–S108.

5. Engerman RL, Kern TS. Progression of incipient diabetic retinopathy during good glycemic control. *Diabetes* 1987; **36**: 808–812.

6. Baynes JW, Monnier VM, eds. *The Maillard Reaction in Aging, Diabetes, and Nutrition.* *Porg Clin Biol Res* 1989; **304**: 1–410.

7. Maillard LC. Action des acides amines sur les sucres: formation des melanoides par voie methodique. *C R Acad Sci* 1912; **154**: 66–68.

8. Patton AR, Hill EG. Inactivation of nutrients by heating with glucose. *Science* 1948; **107**: 68–69.

9. Ledl F, Schleicher E. New aspects of the Maillard reaction in foods and in the human body. *Angew Chem* 1990; **6**: 565–706.

10. Takagi Y, Kashiwagi A, Tanaka Y *et al.* Significance of fructose-induced protein oxidation and formation of advanced glycation endproducts. *J Diabetes Complications* 1995; **9**: 87–91.

11. Bunn HF, Higgins PJ. Reaction of monosaccharides with proteins: possible evolutionary significance. *Science* 1981; **213**: 222–224.

12. Koenig RJ, Blobstein SH, Cerami A. Structure of carbohydrate of hemoglobin AIc. *J Biol Chem* 1977; **252(9)**: 2992–2997.

13. Cerami A, Stevens VJ, Monnier VM. Role of nonenzymatic glycosylation in the development of the sequelae of diabetes mellitus. *Metabolism* 1979; **28** (**4 Suppl 1**): 431–437.

14. Vishwanath V, Frank KE, Elmets CA *et al.* Glycation of skin collagen in type I diabetes mellitus. Correlation with long-term complications. *Diabetes* 1986; **35**: 916–921.

15. Ahmed MU, Thorpe SR, Baynes JW. Identification of carboxymethyllysine as a degradation product of fructoselysine in glycated protein. *J Biol Chem* 1986; **261**: 8816–8821.

16. Ledl F, Beck J, Sengl M *et al.* Chemical pathways of the Maillard reaction. *Prog Clin Biol Res* 1989; **29**: 23–42.

17. Konishi Y, Hayase F, Kato H. Novel imidazolone compound formed by the advanced Maillard reaction of 3-deoxyglucosone and arginine residues in proteins. *Biosci Biotech Biochem* 1994; **58**: 1953–1955.

18. Hayase F, Konishi Y, Kato H. Identification of the modified structure of arginine residues in proteins with 3-deoxyglucosone, a Maillard reaction intermediate. *Biosci Biotech Biochem* 1995; **59**: 1407–1411.

19. Thornalley PJ. The glyoxalase system: new developments towards characterisation of a metabolic pathway fundamental to biological life. *Biochem J* 1990; **269**: 1–11.

20. Wells-Knecht MC, Thorpe SR, Baynes JW. Pathways of formation of glycoxidation products during glycation of collagen. *Biochemistry* 1995; **34**: 15134–15141.

21. Ahmed MU, Brinkmann Frye E, Degenhardt TP *et al.* N-epsilon-(carboxyethyl)lysine, a product of the chemical modification of proteins by methylglyoxal, increases with age in human lens proteins. *Biochem J* 1997; **324**: 565–570.

22. Njoroge FG, Sayre LM, Monnier VM. Detection of D-glucose-derived pyrrole compounds during Maillard reaction under physiological conditions. *Carbohydr Res* 1987; **167**: 211–220.

23. Miyata S, Monnier V. Immunohistochemical detection of advanced glycosylation end products in diabetic tissues using monoclonal

antibody to pyrroline. *J Clin Invest* 1992; **89:** 1102–1112.

24. Obayashi H, Nakano K, Shigeta H *et al.* Formation of crossline as a fluorescent advanced glycation end product *in vitro* and *in vivo. Biochem Biophys Res Commun* 1996; **226:** 37–41.

25. Sell DR, Nagaraj RH, Grandhee SK *et al.* Pentosidine: a molecular marker for the cumulative damage to proteins in diabetes, aging, and uremia. *Diabetes Metab Rev* 1991; **7:** 239–251.

26. Portero-Otin M, Pamplona R, Bellmunt MJ *et al.* Urinary pyrroline as a biochemical marker of non-oxidative Maillard reactions *in vivo. Life Sci* 1997; **60:** 279–287.

27. Horie K, Miyata T, Maeda K *et al.* Immunohistochemical colocalization of glycoxidation products and lipid peroxidation products in diabetic renal glomerular lesions. Implication for glycoxidative stress in the pathogenesis of diabetic nephropathy. *J Clin Invest* 1997; **100:** 2995–3004.

28. Yamaguchi M, Nakamura N, Nakano K *et al.* Immunochemical quantification of crossline as a fluorescent advanced glycation endproduct in erythrocyte membrane proteins from diabetic patients with or without retinopathy. *Diabet Med* 1998; **15:** 458–462.

29. Pongor S, Ulrich PC, Bencsath FA, Cerami A. Aging of proteins: isolation and identification of a fluorescent chromophore from the reaction of polypeptides with glucose. *Proc Natl Acad Sci USA* 1984; **81:** 2684–2688.

30. Farmer J, Ulrich PC, Bencsath FA, Cerami A. Novel pyyroles from sulfite-inhibited Maillard reactions: insight into the mechanism of inhibition. *J Org Chem* 1988; **53:** 2346–2349.

31. Chang JC, Ulrich PC, Bucala R, Cerami A. Detection of an advanced glycosylation product bound to protein *in situ. J Biol Chem* 1985; **260:** 7970–7974.

32. Lapolla A, Gerhardinger C, Pelli B *et al.* Absence of brown product FFI in nondiabetic and diabetic rat collagen. *Diabetes* 1990; **39:** 57–61.

33. Vlassara H, Bucala R, Striker L. Pathogenic effects of advanced glycosylation endproducts: biochemical, biologic, and clinical implications for diabetes and aging. *Lab Invest* 1994; **70:** 138–151.

34. Vlassara H, Brownlee M, Cerami A. Novel macrophage receptor for glucose-modified proteins is distinct from previously described scavenger receptors. *J Exp Med* 1986; **164:** 1301–1309.

35. Radoff S, Cerami A, Vlassara H. Isolation of surface binding protein specific for advanced glycosylation end products from mouse macrophage-derived cell line RAW 264.7. *Diabetes* 1990; **39:** 1510–1518.

36. Yang Z, Makita Z, Horii Y *et al.* Two novel rat liver membrane proteins that bind advanced glycosylation endproducts: relationship to macrophage scavenger receptor for glucose modified proteins. *J Exp Med* 1991; **174:** 515–524.

37. Li YM, Mitsuhashi T, Wojciehowicz D *et al.* Molecular identity and cellular distribution of advanced glycation endproduct receptors. Relationship of p60 to OST-48 and 80K-H membrane proteins. *Proc Natl Acad Sci USA* 1996; **93:** 11047–11052.

38. Vlassara H, Li YM, Imani F *et al.* Identification of galectin-3 as a high-affinity binding protein for advanced glycation end products (AGE): a new member of the AGE-receptor complex. *Molec Med* 1995; **1:** 634–646.

39. Stitt, AW, He CJ, Vlassara H. Characterization of the advanced glycation endproduct receptor complex in human vascular endothelial cells. *Biochem Biophys Res Commun* 1999; **256:** 549–556.

40. Stitt AW, Li YM, Gardiner TA, Bucala R, Archer DB, Vlassara H. Advanced glycation end products (AGEs) co-localize with AGE receptors in the retinal vasculature of diabetic and of AGE-infused rats. *Am J Pathol* 1997; **150:** 523–531.

41. Li JJ, Dickson D, Hof PR, Vlassara H. Receptors for advanced glycosylation endproducts in human brain: role in brain homeostasis. *Molec Med* 1998; **4:** 46–60.

42. Vlassara H, Brownlee M, Manogue KR *et al.* Cachectin/TNF and IL-1 induced by glucose-modified proteins: role in normal tissue remodeling. *Science* 1988; **240:** 1546–1548.

43. Kirstein M, Aston C, Hintz R, Vlassara H. Receptor-specific induction of insulin-like growth factor I in human monocytes by

advanced glycosylation end product-modified proteins. *J Clin Invest* 1992; **90**: 439–446.

44. Chibber R, Molinatti PA, Rosatto N *et al.* Toxic action of advanced glycation end products on cultured retinal capillary pericytes and endothelial cells: relevance to diabetic retinopathy. *Diabetologia* 1997; **40**: 156–164.

45. Esposito C, Gerlach H, Brett J *et al.* Endothelial receptor-mediated binding of glucose-modified albumin is associated with increased monolayer permeability and modulation of cell surface coagulant properties. *J Exp Med* 1989; **170**: 1387–1407.

46. Schmidt AM, Vianna M, Gerlach M *et al.* Isolation and characterization of two binding proteins for advanced glycosylation end products from bovine lung which are present on the endothelial cell surface. *J Biol Chem* 1992; **267**: 14987–14997.

47. Neeper M, Schmidt AM, Brett J *et al.* Cloning and expression of a cell surface receptor for advanced glycosylation end products of proteins. *J Biol Chem* 1992; **267**: 14998–15004.

48. Hori O, Brett J, Slattery T *et al.* The receptor for advanced glycation endproducts (RAGE) is a cellular binding site for amphoterin. Mediation of neurite outgrowth and co expression of RAGE and amphoterin in the developing nervous system. *J Biol Chem* 1995; **270**: 25752–25761.

49. Brett J, Schmidt AM, Yan SD *et al.* Survey of the distribution of a newly characterized receptor for advanced glycation end products in tissues. *Am J Pathol* 1993; **143**: 1699–1712.

50. Schmidt AM, Crandall J, Hori O *et al.* Elevated plasma levels of vascular cell adhesion molecule-1 (VCAM-1) in diabetic patients with microalbuminuria: a marker of vascular dysfunction and progressive vascular disease. *Br J Haematol* 1996; **92**: 747–750.

51. Hori O, Yan SD, Ogawa S *et al.* The receptor for advanced glycation end-products has a central role in mediating the effects of advanced glycation end-products on the development of vascular disease in diabetes mellitus. *Nephrol Dial Transplant* 1996; **11 (Suppl 5)**: 13–16.

52. Schmidt AM, Hori O, Brett J *et al.* Cellular receptors for advanced glycation end products. Implications for induction of oxidant stress and cellular dysfunction in the pathogenesis of vascular lesions. *Arterioscler Thromb* 1994; **14**: 1521–1528.

53. Wautier JL, Zoukourian C, Chappey O *et al.* Receptor-mediated endothelial cell dysfunction in diabetic vasculopathy. Soluble receptor for advanced glycation end products blocks hyperpermeability in diabetic rats. *J Clin Invest* 1996; **97**: 238–243.

54. Li J, Schmidt AM. Characterization and functional analysis of the promoter of RAGE, the receptor for advanced glycation end products. *J Biol Chem* 1997; **272**: 16498–16506.

55. Schmidt AM, Hori O, Chen JX *et al.* Advanced glycation endproducts interacting with their endothelial receptor induce expression of vascular cell adhesion molecule-1 (VCAM-1) in cultured human endothelial cells and in mice. A potential mechanism for the accelerated vasculopathy of diabetes. *J Clin Invest* 1995; **96**: 1395–1403.

56. Bierhaus A, Illmer T, Kasper M *et al.* Advanced glycation end product (AGE)-mediated induction of tissue factor in cultured endothelial cells is dependent on RAGE. *Circulation* 1997; **96**: 2262–2271.

57. Miyata T, Hori O, Zhang J *et al.* The receptor for advanced glycation end products (RAGE) is a central mediator of the interaction of AGE-beta2microglobulin with human mononuclear phagocytes via an oxidant-sensitive pathway. Implications for the pathogenesis of dialysis-related amyloidosis. *J Clin Invest* 1996; **98**: 1088–1094.

58. Li YM, Tan AX, Vlassara H. Antibacterial activity of lysozyme and lactoferrin is inhibited by binding of advanced glycation-modified proteins to a conserved motif. *Nat Med* 1995; **1**: 1057–1061.

59. Takata K, Horiuchi S, Araki N *et al.* Endocytic uptake of nonenzymatically glycosylated proteins is mediated by a scavenger receptor for aldehyde-modified proteins. *J Biol Chem* 1988; **263**: 14819–14825.

60. Araki N, Higashi T, Mori T *et al.* Macrophage scavenger receptor mediates the endocytic uptake and degradation of advanced

glycation end products of the Maillard reaction. *Eur J Biochem* 1995; **230**: 408–415.

61. Horiuchi S, Higashi T, Ikeda K *et al.* Advanced glycation end products and their recognition by macrophage and macrophage-derived cells. *Diabetes* 1996; **45 (Suppl 3)**: S73–S76.

62. Higashi T, Sano H, Saishoji T *et al.* The receptor for advanced glycation end products mediates the chemotaxis of rabbit smooth muscle cells. *Diabetes* 1997; **46**: 463–472.

63. Festa A, Schmolzer B, Schernthaner G, Menzel EJ. Differential expression of receptors for advanced glycation end products on monocytes in patients with IDDM. *Diabetologia* 1998; **41**: 674–680.

64. Makita Z, Radoff S, Rayfield EJ *et al.* Advanced glycosylation end products in patients with diabetic nephropathy. *N Engl J Med* 1991; **325**: 836–842.

65. Makita Z, Bucala R, Rayfield EJ *et al.* Reactive glycosylation endproducts in diabetic uraemia and treatment of renal failure. *Lancet* 1994; **343**: 1519–1522.

66. Giardino I, Edelstein D, Brownlee M. Nonenzymatic glycosylation *in vitro* and in bovine endothelial cells alters basic fibroblast growth factor activity. A model for intracellular glycosylation in diabetes. *J Clin Invest* 1994; **94**: 110–117.

67. Brownlee M, Vlassara H, Cerami A. Inhibition of heparin-catalyzed human antithrombin III activity by nonenzymatic glycosylation. Possible role in fibrin deposition in diabetes. *Diabetes* 1984; **33**: 532–535.

68. Watkins NG, Thorpe SR, Baynes JW. Glycation of amino groups in protein. Studies on the specificity of modification of RNase by glucose. *J Biol Chem* 1985; **260**: 10629–10636.

69. Tsilibary EC, Charonis AS, Reger LA *et al.* The effect of nonenzymatic glucosylation on the binding of the main noncollagenous NC1 domain to type IV collagen. *J Biol Chem* 1988; **263**: 4302–4308.

70. Vitek MP, Bhattacharya K, Glendening JM *et al.* Advanced glycation end products contribute to amyloidosis in Alzheimer disease. *Proc Natl Acad Sci USA* 1994; **91**: 4766–4770.

71. Bucala R, Mitchell R, Arnold K *et al.* Identification of the major site of apolipoprotein B modification by advanced glycosylation end products blocking uptake by the low density lipoprotein receptor. *J Biol Chem* 1995; **270**: 10828–10832.

72. Bucala R, Makita Z, Koschinsky T *et al.* Lipid advanced glycosylation: pathway for lipid oxidation *in vivo. Proc Natl Acad Sci USA* 1993; **90**: 6434–6438.

73. Bucala R, Makita Z, Vega G *et al.* Modification of low density lipoprotein by advanced glycation end products contributes to the dyslipidemia of diabetes and renal insufficiency. *Proc Natl Acad Sci USA* 1994; **91**: 9441–9445.

74. Stitt AW, Vlassara H, Bucala R. Atherogenesis and advanced glycation: promotion, progression, and prevention. In: Chiorazzi N, Fujio-Numano RG , Ross R, eds. *Atherosclerosis IV.* Annals of the New York Academy of Sciences, Vol 811, 1997: 115–129.

75. Stitt AW, He C, Friedman S *et al.* Elevated AGE-modified ApoB in the sera of euglycemic, normolipidemic patients with atherosclerosis. *Molec Med* 1997; **3**: 617–627.

76. Sell DR, Monnier VM. End-stage renal disease and diabetes catalyze the formation of a pentose-derived crosslink from aging human collagen. *J Clin Invest* 1990; **85**: 380–384.

77. Monnier VM, Cerami A. Nonenzymatic browning *in vivo*: possible process for aging of long-lived proteins. *Science* 1981; **211**: 491–493.

78. Kohn RR, Cerami A, Monnier VM. Collagen aging *in vitro* by nonenzymatic glycosylation and browning. *Diabetes* 1984; **33**: 57–59.

79. Harding JJ, Crabbe MJC. The lens: development proteins, metabolism and cataract. In: Davson H, ed. *The Eye*, Vol 1b. New York: Academic, 1984: 207–492.

80. Stevens VJ, Rouzer CA, Monnier VM *et al.* Diabetic cataract formation: potential role of glycosylation of lens crystallins. *Proc Natl Acad Sci USA* 1978; **75**: 2918–2922.

81. Monnier VM, Stevens VJ, Cerami A. The browning reaction of proteins with glucose. *Arch Biochem* 1979; **24**: 157–178.

82. Matsumoto K, Ikeda K, Horiuchi S *et al.* Immunochemical evidence for increased formation of advanced glycation end products

and inhibition by aminoguanidine in diabetic rat lenses. *Biochem Biophys Res Comm* 1997; **241**: 352–354.

83. Stitt AW, Moore J, Sharkey JA *et al.* Advanced glycation endproducts in vitreous: structural and functional implications for diabetic vitreopathy. *Invest Ophthalmol Vis Sci* 1999; in press.

84. Charonis AS, Tsilibary EC. Structural and functional changes of laminin and type IV collagen after nonenzymatic glycation. *Diabetes* 1992; **41 (Suppl 2)**: 49–51.

85. Knecht R, Leber R, Hasslacher C. Degradation of glomerular basement membrane in diabetes. I. Susceptibility of diabetic and nondiabetic basement membrane to proteolytic degradation of isolated glomeruli. *Res Exp Med* (Berl) 1987; **187**: 323–328.

86. Paul RG, Bailey AJ. Glycation of collagen: the basis of its central role in the late complications of ageing and diabetes. *Int J Biochem Cell Biol* 1996; **28**: 1297–1310.

87. Haitoglou CS, Tsilibary EC, Brownlee M, Charonis AS. Altered cellular interactions between endothelial cells and nonenzymatically glucosylated laminin/type IV collagen. *J Biol Chem* 1992; **267**: 12404–12407.

88. Hammes HP, Weiss A, Hess S *et al.* Modification of vitronectin by advanced glycation alters functional properties *in vitro* and in the diabetic retina. *Lab Invest* 1996; **75**: 325–338.

89. Tarsio JF, Reger LA, Furcht LT. Decreased interaction of fibronectin, type IV collagen, and heparin due to nonenzymatic glycation. Implications for diabetes mellitus. *Biochemistry* 1987; **26**: 1014–1020.

90. Tarsio JF, Reger LA, Furcht LT. Molecular mechanisms in basement membrane complications of diabetes. Alterations in heparin, laminin, and type IV collagen association. *Diabetes* 1988; **37**: 532–539.

91. Bucala R, Model P, Cerami A. Modification of DNA by reducing sugars: a possible mechanism for nucleic acid aging and age-related dysfunction in gene expression. *Proc Natl Acad Sci USA* 1984; **81**: 105–109.

92. Lee AT, Cerami A. Elevated glucose 6-phosphate levels are associated with plasmid

mutations *in vivo*. *Proc Natl Acad Sci USA* 1987; **84**: 8311–8314.

93. Bucala R, Model P, Russel M, Cerami A. Modification of DNA by glucose 6-phosphate induces DNA rearrangements in an Escherichia coli plasmid. *Proc Natl Acad Sci USA* 1985; **82**: 8439–8442.

94. Lee AT, Plump A, DeSimone C *et al.* A role for DNA mutations in diabetes-associated teratogenesis in transgenic embryos. *Diabetes* 1995; **44**: 20–24.

95. Pushkarsky T, Rourke L, Spiegel LA *et al.* Molecular characterization of a mouse genomic element mobilized by advanced glycation endproduct modified-DNA (AGE–DNA). *Molec Med* 1997; **3**: 740–749.

96. Jacobson EL, Cervantes-Laurean D, Jacobson MK. ADP-ribose in glycation and glycoxidation reactions. *Adv Exp Med Biol* 1997; **419**: 371–379.

97. Cervantes-Laurean D, Jacobson EL, Jacobson MK. Glycation and glycoxidation of histones by ADP-ribose. *J Biol Chem* 1996; **271**: 10461–10469.

98. Gugliucci A, Bendayan M. Histones from diabetic rats contain increased levels of advanced glycation end products. *Biochem Biophys Res Comm* 1995; **212**: 56–62.

99. Mills JL. Malformations in infants of diabetic mothers. *Teratology* 1982; **25**: 385–394.

100. Mills JL, Baker L, Goldman AS. Malformations in infants of diabetic mothers occur before the seventh gestational week. Implications for treatment. *Diabetes* 1979; **28**: 292–293.

101. Mills JL, Knopp RH, Simpson JL *et al.* Lack of relation of increased malformation rates in infants of diabetic mothers to glycemic control during organogenesis. *N Engl J Med* 1988; **318**: 671–676.

102. Gardiner TA, Stitt AW, Archer DB. Endocytosis by retinal vascular endothelial cells increases in early diabetes: A quantitative EM study in STZ-diabetic rats. *Lab Invest* 1995; **72**: 439–444.

103. Stitt AW, Chakravarthy U, Archer DB, Gardiner TA. Increased endocytosis of retinal vascular endothelial cells grown in hyperglycaemia is modulated by inhibitors of nonenzymatic glycosylation. *Diabetologia* 1995; **38**: 1271–1275.

104. Vlassara H. Recent progress in advanced glycation end products and diabetic complications. *Diabetes* 1997; **46** (**Suppl 2**): S19–S25.

105. Miyata T, Oda O, Inagi R *et al*. Beta 2–microglobulin modified with advanced glycation end products is a major component of hemodialysis-associated amyloidosis. *J Clin Invest* 1993; **92**: 1243–1252.

106. Miyata T, Inagi R, Iida Y *et al*. Involvement of beta 2-microglobulin modified with advanced glycation end products in the pathogenesis of hemodialysis-associated amyloidosis. Induction of human monocyte chemotaxis and macrophage secretion of tumor necrosis factor-alpha and interleukin-1. *J Clin Invest* 1994; **93**: 521–528.

107. Dolhofer-Bliesener R, Lechner B, Gerbitz KD. Possible significance of advanced glycation end products in serum in end-stage renal disease and in late complications of diabetes. *Eur J Clin Chem Clin Biochem* 1996; **34**: 355–361.

108. Shinohara M, Thornalley PJ, Giardino I *et al*. Overexpression of glyoxalase-1 in bovine endothelial cells inhibits intracellular advanced glycation endproduct formation and prevents hyperglycaemia-induced increases in macromolecular endocytosis. *J Clin Invest* 1998; **101**: 1142–1147.

109. Cerami C, Founds H, Nicholl I *et al*. Tobacco smoke is a source of toxic reactive glycation products. *Proc Natl Acad Sci USA* 1997; **94**: 13915–13920.

110. Founds H, Giordano D, Mitsuhashi T *et al*. Tobacco smoke is a source of advanced glycation endproducts (AGEs): possible role in the accelerated vascular disease of smokers (abstr). *J Invest Med* 1996; **44**: A200.

111. Nicholl ID, Stitt AW, Moore JE, *et al*. Increased levels of advanced glycation endproducts in the lenses and blood vessels of cigarette smokers. *Molec Med* 1998; **4**: 594–601.

112. Koschinsky T, He CJ, Mitsuhashi T *et al*. Orally absorbed reactive glycation products (glycotoxins): an environmental risk factor in diabetic nephropathy. *Proc Natl Acad Sci USA* 1997; **94**: 6474–6479.

113. Lithner F, Asplund K, Eriksson S *et al*. Clinical characteristics in diabetic stroke patients. *Diabets Metab* 1988; **14**: 15–19.

114. Pyorala, K. Diabetes and coronary artery disease: what a coincidence? *J Cardiovasc Pharmacol* 1990; **16**: S8–S14.

115. Ruderman NB, Haudenschild C. Diabetes as an atherogenic factor. *Prog Cardiovasc Dis* 1984; **26**: 273–412.

116. Ross R. The pathogenesis of atherosclerosis: a perspective for the 1990s. *Nature* 1993; **362**: 801–809.

117. Mahley RW, Innerarity TL, Weisgraber KN, Oh SY. Altered metabolism (*in vivo* and *in vitro*) of plasma lipoproteins after selective chemical modification of lysine residues of the apoprotein B. *J Clin Invest* 1979; **64**: 743–750.

118. Mahley RW, Innerarity TL, Pitas RE *et al*. Inhibition of lipoprotein binding to surface receptors of fibroblasts following selective modification of arginyl residues in apoprotein B. *J Biol Chem* 1987; **252**: 7279–7287.

119. Goldstein JL, Ho YK, Basu SK, Brown MS. Binding site on macrophages that mediates uptake and degradation of acetylated low density lipoproteins producing massive cholesterol deposition. *Proc Natl Acad Sci USA* 1979; **76**: 333–337.

120. Fogelman AM, Haberland ME, Seager J *et al*. Factors regulating the activities of the low density lipoprotein receptor and the scavenger receptor on human monocytes macrophages. *J Lipid Res* 1980; **22**: 1131–1141.

121. Palinski W, Koschinsky T, Butler SW *et al*. Immunological evidence for the presence of advanced glycosylation endproducts products in atherosclerotic lesions of euglycemic rabbits. *Arterioscler Thromb Vasc Biol* 1995; **15**: 571–582.

122. Kume S, Takeya M, Mori T *et al*. Immunohistochemical and ultrastructural detection of advanced glycation endproducts in atherosclerotic lesions of human aorta with a novel specific monoclonal antibody. *Am J Pathol* 1995; **147**: 654–667.

123. Nakamura Y, Horii Y, Nishino T *et al*. Immunohistochemical localization of advanced glycosylation endproducts (AGEs) in coronary atheroma and cardiac tissue in diabetes. *Am J Pathol* 1993; **143**: 1649–1656.

124. Sima A, Popov D, Starodub O *et al*. Pathobiology of the heart in experimental diabetes: immunolocalization of lipoproteins,

immunoglobulin G, and advanced glycation endproducts proteins in diabetic and/or hyperlipidemic hamster. *Lab Invest* 1997; **77**: 3–18.

125. Niwa T, Katsuzaki T, Miyazaki S *et al.* Immunohistochemical detection of imidazolone, a novel advanced glycation end product, in kidneys and aortas of diabetic patients. *J Clin Invest* 1997; **99**: 1272–1280.

126. Horiuchi S, Sano H, Higashi T *et al.* Extra- and intracellular localization of advanced glycation end-products in human atherosclerotic lesions. *Nephrol Dial Transplant* 1996; **11 (Suppl 5)**: 81–86.

127. Dobrian A, Lazar V, Tirziu D, Simionescu M. Increased macrophage uptake of irreversibly glycated albumin modified-low density lipoproteins of normal and diabetic subjects is mediated by non-saturable mechanisms. *Biochim Biophys Acta* 1996; **1317**: 5–14.

128. Seftel AD, Vaziri ND, Ni Z *et al.* Advanced glycation end products in human penis: elevation in diabetic tissue, site of deposition, and possible effect through iNOS or eNOS. *Urology* 1997; **50**: 1016–1026.

129. Bucala R, Tracey KJ, Cerami A. Advanced glycosylation products quench nitric oxide and mediate defective endothelium dependent vasodilatation in experimental diabetes. *J Clin Invest* 1991; **87**: 432–438.

130. Vlassara H, Fuh H, Makita Z *et al.* Exogenous advanced glycosylation end products induce complex vascular dysfunction in normal animals: a model for diabetic and ageing complications. *Proc Natl Acad Sci USA* 1992; **89**: 12043–12047.

131. Stern DM, Esposito C, Gerlach H *et al.* Endothelium and regulation of coagulation. *Diabetes Care* 1991; **14**: 160–166.

132. Vlassara H, Fuh H, Donnelly T, Cybulsky M. Advanced glycation endproducts promote adhesion molecule (VCAM-1, ICAM-1) expression and atheroma formation in normal rabbits. *Molec Med* 1995; **1**: 447–456.

133. Dyck PJ, Hansen S, Karnes J *et al.* Capillary number and percentage closed in human diabetic sural nerve. *Proc Natl Acad Sci USA* 1985; **82**: 2513–2517.

134. Vinik AI, Holland MT, Le Beau JM *et al.* Diabetic neuropathies. *Diabetes Care* 1992; **15**: 1926–1975.

135. Soulis Liparota T, Cooper M, Papazoglou D *et al.* Retardation by aminoguanidine of development of albuminuria, mesangial expansion, and tissue fluorescence in streptozotocin induced rat. *Diabetes* 1991; **40**: 1328–1334.

136. Cohen MP. Nonenzymatic glycation: a central mechanism in diabetic microvasculopathy? *J Diabet Complications* 1988; **2**: 214–217.

137. La Selva M, Beltramo E, Passera P *et al.* The role of endothelium in the pathogenesis of diabetic microangiopathy. *Acta Diabetol* 1993; **30**: 190–200.

138. Osterby R. Early phases in the development of diabetic glomerulopathy. *Acta Med Scand* 1975; **574 (Suppl 1)**: 13–77.

139. Osterby R, Anderson MJF, Gundersen HJG *et al.* Quantitative study on glomerular ultrastructure in type I diabetes with incipient nephropathy. *Diab Nephropathy* 1983; **3**: 95–100.

140. Mogensen CE. Renal function changes in diabetes. *Diabetes* 1976; **25 (Suppl 2)**: 872–879.

141. Gugliucci A, Bendayan M. Reaction of advanced glycation endproducts with renal tissue from normal and streptozotocin induced diabetic rats. An ultrastructural study using colloidal gold cytochemistry. *J Histochem Cytochem* 1995; **43**: 591–600.

142. Gugliucci A, Bendayan M. Renal fate of circulating advanced glycation end products (AGE): evidence for reabsorption and catabolism of AGE peptides by renal proximal tubular cells. *Diabetologia* 1995; **39**: 149–160.

143. Makino H, Shikata K, Hironaka K *et al.* Ultrastructure of nonenzymatically glycated mesangial matrix in diabetic nephropathy. *Kidney Int* 1995; **48**: 517–526.

144. Pugliese G, Pricci F, Romeo G *et al.* Upregulation of mesangial growth factor and extracellular matrix synthesis by advanced glycation end products via a receptor-mediated mechanism. *Diabetes* 1997; **46**: 1881–1887.

145. Yamauchi A, Takei I, Makita Z *et al.* Effects of aminoguanidine on serum advanced glycation endproducts, urinary albumin excretion, mesangial expansion, and glomerular basement membrane thickening in Otsuka Long-Evans Tokushima fatty rats. *Diabetes Res Clin Pract* 1997; **34**: 127–133.

146. Yang CW, Vlassara H, Peten EP et al. Advanced glycation end products up-regulate gene expression found in diabetic glomerular disease. Proc Natl Acad Sci USA 1994; 91(20): 9436–9440.

147. Kahn HA, Moorhead HB. Statistics on blindness in the model reporting area, 1969–1970. US Department of Health, Education, and Welfare Publication No. (NIH) 73–427. Washington: US Government Printing Office, 1973.

148. Brownlee M, Vlassara H, Cerami A. Advanced glycosylation end products in tissue and the biochemical basis of diabetic complications. N Engl J Med 1988; 318: 1315–1321.

149. Hammes HP, Wellensiek B, Kloting I et al. The relationship of glycaemic level to advanced glycation end-product (AGE) accumulation and retinal pathology in the spontaneous diabetic hamster. Diabetologia 1998; 41: 165–170.

150. Clements RS Jr, Robison WG Jr, Cohen MP. Anti-glycated albumin therapy ameliorates early retinal microvascular pathology in db/db mice. J Diabetes Comp 1998; 12: 28–33.

151. Hammes HP, Martin S, Federlin K et al. Aminoguanidine treatment inhibits the development of experimental diabetic retinopathy. Proc Natl Acad Sci USA 1991; 88: 11555–11558.

152. Hammes HP, Ali SS, Uhlmann M et al. Aminoguanidine does not inhibit the initial phase of experimental diabetic retinopathy in rats. Diabetologia 1995; 38: 269–273.

153. Hammes HP, Strodter D, Weiss A et al. Secondary intervention with aminoguanidine retards the progression of diabetic retinopathy in the rat model. Diabetologia 1995; 38: 656–660.

154. Skolnik EY, Yang Z, Makita Z et al. Human and rat mesangial cell receptors for glucose modified proteins: potential role in kidney tissue remodelling and diabetic nephropathy. J Exp Med 1991; 174: 931–939.

155. Doi T, Vlassara H, Kirstein M et al. Receptor specific increase in extracellular matrix production in mouse mesangial cells by advanced glycosylation end products is mediated via platelet derived growth factor. Proc Natl Acad Sci USA 1992; 89: 2873–2877.

156. Chakravarthy U, Hayes RG, Stitt AW et al. Constitutive nitric oxide synthase expression in retinal vascular endothelial cells is suppressed by high glucose and advanced glycation end products. Diabetes 1998; 47: 945–952.

157. Preissner KT, Kanse SM, Hammes HP. Integrin chatter and vascular function in diabetic retinopathy. Horm Metab Res 1997; 29: 643–645.

158. Ruggiero-Lopez D, Rellier N, Lecomte M et al. Growth modulation of retinal microvascular cells by early and advanced glycation products. Diabetes Res Clin Pract 1997; 34: 135–142.

159. Kalfa TA, Gerritsen ME, Carlson EC et al. Altered proliferation of retinal microvascular cells on glycated matrix. Invest Ophthalmol Vis Sci 1995; 36: 2358–2367.

160. Lu M, Kuroki M, Amano S et al. Advanced glycation end products increase retinal vascular endothelial growth factor expression. J Clin Invest 1998; 101: 1219–1224.

161. Hirata C, Nakano K, Nakamura N et al. Advanced glycation end products induce expression of vascular endothelial growth factor by retinal Muller cells. Biochem Biophys Res Comm 1997; 236: 712–715.

162. Yamaguishi Si, Yonekura H, Yamamoto Y et al. Advanced glycation end products-driven angiogenesis in vitro. Induction of the growth and tube formation of human microvascular endothelial cells through autocrine vascular endothelial growth factor. J Biol Chem 1997; 272: 8723–8730.

163. Yui S, Sasaki T, Araki N et al. Induction of macrophage growth by advanced glycation end products of the Maillard reaction. J Immunol 1994; 152: 1943–1949.

164. Hasegawa G, Nakano K, Sawada M et al. Possible role of tumor necrosis factor and interleukin-1 in the development of diabetic nephropathy. Kidney Int 1991; 40: 1007–1012.

165. Imani F, Horii Y, Suthanthiran M et al. Advanced glycosylation endproduct-specific receptors on human and rat T-lymphocytes mediate synthesis of interferon gamma: role in tissue remodeling. J Exp Med 1993; 178: 2165–2172.

166. Brownlee M, Vlassara H, Kooney A *et al.* Aminoguanidine prevents diabetes-induced arterial wall protein cross-linking. *Science* 1986; **232**: 1629–1632.

167. Giardino I, Fard AK, Hatchell DL, Brownlee M. Aminoguanidine inhibits reactive oxygen species formation, lipid peroxidation, and oxidant-induced apoptosis. *Diabetes* 1998; **47**: 1114–1120.

168. Panagiotopoulos S, O'Brien RC, Bucala R *et al.* Aminoguanidine has an anti-atherogenic effect in the cholesterol-fed rabbit. *Atherosclerosis* 1998; **136**: 125–131.

169. Nichols K, Mandel TE. Advanced glycosylation endproducts in experimental murine diabetic nephropathy: Effect of islet isografting and of aminoguanidine. *J Lab Invest* 1989; **60**: 486–491.

170. Ellis EN, Good BH. Prevention of glomerular basement membrane thickening by aminoguanidine in experimental diabetes mellitus. *Metabolism* 1991; **40**: 1016–1019.

171. Ido Y, Chang K, Ostrow E *et al.* Aminoguanidine prevents regional blood flow increases in streptozotocin-diabetic rats. *Diabetes* 1990; **39**: 93A.

172. Soulis Liparota T, Cooper M, Papazoglou D *et al.* Retardation by aminoguanidine of development of albuminuria, mesangial expansion, and tissue fluorescence in streptozotocin induced rat. *Diabetes* 1991; **40**: 1328–1334.

173. Edelstein D, Brownlee M. Mechanistic studies of advanced glycosylation endproduct inhibition by aminoguanidine. *Diabetes* 1992; **41**: 26–28.

174. Cho HK, Kozu H, Peyman GA *et al.* The effect of aminoguanidine on the blood retinal barrier in streptozotocin induced diabetic rats. *Ophthalmic Surg* 1991; **22**: 44–47.

175. Nakamura S, Makita Z, Ishikawa S *et al.* Progression of nephropathy in spontaneous diabetic rats is prevented by OPB-9195, a novel inhibitor of advanced glycation. *Diabetes* 1997; **46**: 895–899.

176. Mitsuhashi T, Li YM, Fishbane S, Vlassara H. Depletion of reactive advanced glycation endproducts from diabetic uremic sera using a lysozyme-linked matrix. *J Clin Invest* 1997; **100**: 847–854.

177. Drickamer K. Breaking the curse of the AGEs. *Nature* 1996; **382**: 211–212.

178. Vasan S, Zhang X, Zhang X *et al.* An agent cleaving glucose-derived protein crosslinks *in vitro* and *in vivo*. *Nature* 1996; **382**: 275–278.

179. Wolffenbuttel BH, Boulanger CM, Crijns FR *et al.* Breakers of advanced glycation end products restore large artery properties in experimental diabetes. *Proc Natl Acad Sci USA* 1998; **95**: 4630–4634.

180. Shaklai N, Garlick RL, Bunn HF. Nonenzymatic glycosylation of human serum albumin alters its conformation and function. *J Biol Chem* 1984; **259**: 3812–3817.

181. Brownlee M, Vlassara H, Cerami A. Nonenzymatic glycosylation reduces the susceptibility of fibrin to degradation by plasmin. *Diabetes* 1983; **32**: 680–684.

182. Swamy MS, Abraham EC. Lens protein composition, glycation and high molecular weight aggregation in aging rats. *Invest Ophthalmol Vis Sci* 1987; **28**: 1693–1701.

183. Garlick RL, Mazer JS, Chylack LT Jr *et al.* Nonenzymatic glycation of human lens crystallin. Effect of aging and diabetes mellitus. *J Clin Invest* 1984; **74**: 1742–1749.

184. Krantz S, Lober M, Thiele M, Teuscher E. Properties of *in vitro* nonenzymatically glycated plasma fibrinogens. *Exp Clin Endocrinol* 1987; **90**: 37–45.

185. Witztum JL, Koschinsky T. Metabolic and immunological consequences of glycation of low density lipoproteins. *Prog Clin Biol Res* 1989; **304**: 219–234.

186. Abdel-Wahab YH, O'Harte FP, Ratcliff H *et al.* Glycation of insulin in the islets of Langerhans of normal and diabetic animals. *Diabetes* 1996; **45**: 1489–1496.

187. Cortizo AM, Gagliardino JJ. Changes induced by non-enzymatic glycosylation of IGF-binding protein-3: effects on its binding properties and on its modulatory effect on IGF-I mitogenic action. *J Endocrinol* 1995; **144**: 119–126.

188. Owen WF Jr, Hou FF, Stuart RO *et al.* Beta 2-microglobulin modified with advanced glycation end products modulates collagen synthesis by human fibroblasts. *Kidney Int* 1998; **53**: 1365–1373.

189. Taniguchi N, Arai K, Kinoshita N. Glycation of copper/zinc superoxide dismutase and its inactivation: identification of glycated sites. *Meth Enzymol* 1989; **179**: 570–581.

190. Cullum NA, Mahon J, Stringer K, McLean WG. Glycation of rat sciatic nerve tubulin in experimental diabetes mellitus. *Diabetologia* 1991; **34**: 387–389.

6

Insulin resistance: the prime mover in Type 2 diabetes?

Eleuterio Ferrannini

Introduction

Insulin exerts multiple actions on many cell types. Its anabolic effects on intermediary metabolism are essential for life, for acute insulin lack leads to extreme hyperglycaemia and hyperlipaemia, protein wasting and, ultimately, to ketoacidosis and death. Within this functional pleiotropy, insulin's main control is exerted on the glucose system. In fact, the plasma concentration of glucose, unlike those of lipids or amino acids, is a strongly homeostatic variable, the excursions of which are confined to a very narrow range (3–8 mM) under everyday life conditions. Body glucose stores (less than 2 moles, including tissue glycogen) are small compared with fat or protein reservoirs (e.g. 20 moles of fat mass as triglycerides), yet they are tightly managed, as both hypo- and hyperglycaemia are intolerable to body tissues. Therefore, the ability of pancreatic β-cells to follow glycaemic changes by promptly increasing or decreasing insulin release is key to glucose control.

At the whole-body level, hormone response is the compound result of secretory rate and cellular sensitivity (for protein hormones, distribution throughout body fluids and clearance by degrading tissues are unusual as primary controls of effectiveness). For many protein and non-protein hormones, action is modulated by at least one, often two, hierarchical hormonal feedbacks (e.g. corticotropic-releasing hormone and ACTH for cortisol, gonadotrophin-releasing hormone and gonadotrophins for sex steroids). With this system design, sensitivity is provided by the specific hormone receptors on target tissues as well as on the companion gland of the feedback loop. In the case of insulin, there is no major pituitary or hypothalamic relay: target tissues control secretion directly by determining the level of positive and negative stimuli. Thus, the circulating concentrations of substrates (mostly glucose, but also amino acids, non-esterified fatty acids (NEFA), ketone bodies), that result from insulin action on intermediary metabolism in different tissues feed signals back to the β-cell. Sensitivity gating is provided by insulin receptors on target tissues (and on the β-cell itself) (*Fig. 6.1*). The functional consequences of these different designs are noteworthy. In the usual hormone system, target tissues do not talk back to the secretory units, i.e. they are passive effectors. Therefore, hormone resistance is characterized by generalized hormonal failure in the face of raised concentrations of both the hormone and its releasing factor. For the insulin system, all controlled substrates report to the β-cell on the state of peripheral insulin sensitivity. These multiple inputs are integrated with additional hormonal influences (by gut hormones) to set the output response on a minute-by-minute basis (*Fig. 6.2*). Central nervous system modulation (e.g. through the autonomic nervous system) also occurs, as insulin itself crosses the

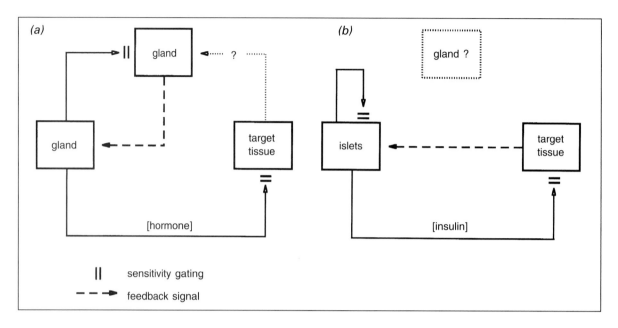

Fig. 6.1
General design of an endocrine system (a), with sensitivity gating at the target tissue and a feedback link between primary and secondary glands. The insulin system (b) lacks a secondary gland, and feedback is provided by direct signalling from target tissues (see text for further explanation).

blood–brain barrier and binds to specific receptors in nuclei of the midbrain.[1] The resulting dynamics of insulin secretion are so complex that the β-cells can be likened to the retina, i.e. a peripheral brain performing highly integrated functions. Current understanding has it that the primary servo-regulated signal for insulin release is the plasma glucose concentration, whilst other substrates and feedbacks play ancillary roles. According to this construct, insulin resistance is *a reduced sensitivity of glucose uptake to insulin stimulation sensed by the β-cell through elevated plasma glucose levels.* Future research may identify additional primary feedback signals (e.g. NEFA), which may become important under some circumstances. At present, however, insulin resistance is defined as defective glucose disposal in the face of raised glucose and insulin concentrations.

Insulin sensitivity is gated not only by the number and affinity of the insulin receptors but also by the functional state of the intracellular signalling pathways that transduce insulin binding to the various effectors (glucose transport, phosphorylation and oxidation, glycogen synthesis, lipolysis, ion exchange, etc.). Importantly, the various insulin effectors are, at least in part, independent of one another.[2] Therefore, a massive reduction in the number of insulin receptors (or the presence of high titres of circulating anti-insulin or anti-insulin-receptor autoantibodies) is associated with a form of insulin resistance that is generalized and extreme (all pathways involved). These are, however, rare cases.[3] More commonly, cellular resistance

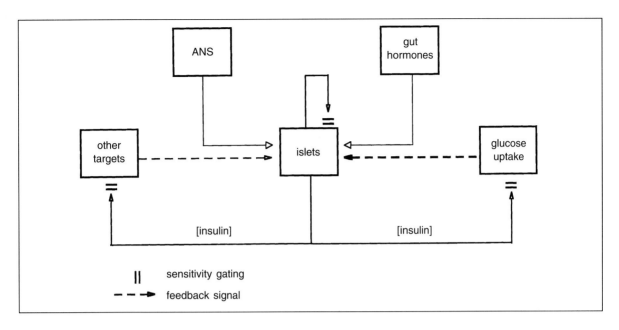

Fig. 6.2
The insulin system includes a negative auto-feedback (insulin receptors on β-cells mediating insulin-induced inhibition of insulin release) and further modulation by gastro-intestinal hormones and the autonomic nervous system (ANS). Though many tissues and substrates are targets for insulin action, the main feedback signal is the plasma glucose concentration (see text for further explanation).

of the glucose pathway is caused by a malfunction of the signal transduction machinery. As a consequence, cellular insulin resistance can be of any degree and is usually incomplete (pathway specific). In addition, resistance in the glucose pathway reinforces the insulin signal to other pathways (e.g. protein turnover) via stimulation of β-cell activity. To the extent that they have preserved their sensitivity, other pathways will be overly stimulated by the compensatory hyperinsulinaemia. The pathophysiological implication of this phenomenon is that, in insulin-resistant states, any abnormality that is found to be associated with defective glucose metabolism, (e.g. dyslipidaemia, higher blood pressure, platelet hypercoagulation, pro-thrombotic changes), theoretically can be due to the insulin resistance itself and/or to the chronic effects of

the attendant hyperinsulinaemia. This is the origin of the *insulin-resistance syndrome.*[4]

With these premises, it is easy to understand why insulin resistance, contrary to other hormone resistances, is a relatively frequent phenomenon in physiology as well as pathophysiology. Thus, puberty and pregnancy are paradigms of physiological impairment of insulin's effect on glucose disposal. In the former case, the compensatory hyperinsulinaemia is conducive to protein anabolism, in the latter glucose is saved up in order to be channelled to the foetus. A number of environmental factors, most notably body weight and physical exercise, impact on insulin sensitivity. Diabetes, on the other hand, is an insulin-resistant state for which a genetic basis of the insulin resistance is suspected.

Measurement of insulin sensitivity in vivo

In *in vitro* systems, insulin action is defined as the dose–response function relating insulin concentrations in the medium with the level of activation of an effector system. As schematized in *Fig. 6.3* (and in analogy to enzyme kinetics), any such function has an approximately sigmoidal shape, indicating saturation kinetics. According to the Michaelis–Menten approximation, the function can be summarized by two parameters: the maximal response (V_{max} or responsiveness) and the sensitivity (K_m), or response at half-maximal hormone concentrations. Strictly speaking, insulin sensitivity is the ratio V_{max}/K_m. For example, the two 'abnormal' curves in *Fig. 6.3* exemplify an isolated defect in sensitivity and a combined defect of sensitivity and responsiveness. As a rule, the latter type of curve indicates a more severe cellular malfunction than the former. Thus, for the dose–response function of glucose

transport, a high K_m would indicate decreased activation of transporters in response to insulin, while a high K_m coupled with a low V_{max} would be compatible with a reduced pool of intracellular transporters.

In vivo, any insulin effect estimated from measurements based on peripheral blood sampling is a compound of multiple tissue responses. Despite this limitation, a number of techniques have been devised to measure insulin sensitivity *in vivo*. Of them (reviewed elsewhere[5]), three can be considered as primary methods, all the others being derivative or surrogate approaches. There is general agreement that the glucose clamp technique, particularly in its euglycaemic version, is the gold standard for the measurement of insulin action. Exogenous insulin is administered in a primed-constant fashion at a rate designed to maintain a pre-set hyperinsulinaemic plateau; simultaneously, the plasma glucose concentration is clamped at the normal fasting (euglycaemic) or any pre-existing (isoglycaemic) level by means

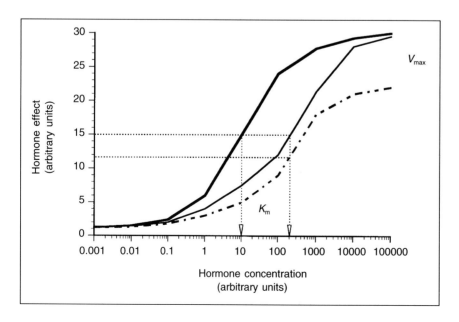

Fig. 6.3
General characteristics of a hormone dose–response curve. The dotted lines identify pairs of curves with the same maximal response (V_{max}) but different sensitivity (K_m) and curves with similar K_m but different V_{max} values (see text for further explanation).

of an exogenous infusion of glucose. By doing this, *in vivo* insulin action is measured under comparable conditions of stimulus (the plasma insulin concentration) and substrate (the plasma glucose concentration). When a steady state is attained, the exogenous glucose infusion rate equals the amount of glucose disposed of by all the tissues in the body, and thus provides a quantitation of overall insulin sensitivity. As shown in *Fig. 6.4*, the time-course of glucose infusion rates during a euglycaemic clamp in non-diabetic subjects shows a quick rise within 40 minutes of starting the

insulin infusion, followed by a gentle upward trend. This general pattern is sensitive to the insulin dose; thus, a higher insulin clamp will produce a steeper initial ascent than a lower insulin infusion. Though the glucose infusion rate never reaches a true steady state, its average value during the final 40–60 minutes of a 2-hour study is a satisfactory index of insulin sensitivity for ordinary purposes. It must be noted that the exogenous glucose infusion rate equals whole-body glucose disposal only when endogenous glucose output is nil; otherwise, total glucose disposal is the

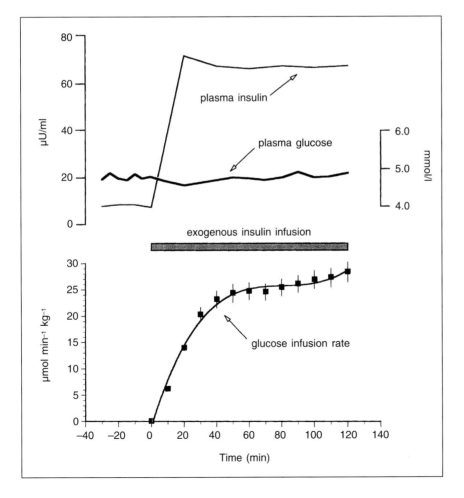

Fig. 6.4
The euglycaemic insulin clamp.

sum of endogenous and exogenous glucose entry. Following insulin administration, endogenous glucose release is effectively suppressed, so that after 30–50 minutes essentially all the glucose metabolized is of exogenous origin. Inhibition of endogenous glucose output is, however, insulin dependent. Therefore, with low insulin-infusion rates (<2.5 pmol min^{-1} kg^{-1}) or in insulin-resistant states, endogenous glucose release must be separately estimated with the use of tracer glucose and the indicator dilution technique.

The clamp method makes it possible to realize any combination of plasma glucose and insulin concentrations; in this way, it has been employed to construct full dose–response curves, and to investigate hypoglycaemic counter-regulation. Importantly, the clamp can be combined with a number of other procedures to enhance the information content of the study. Thus, if tracer glucose is simultaneously used, the inhibitory effect of insulin on endogenous glucose release can be quantitated. By infusing tracers of NEFA (or glycerol) or amino acids, one can assess the influence of insulin on lipolysis and protein breakdown, respectively. When indirect calorimetry[6] is performed during a clamp, the effect of insulin on the pattern of substrate oxidation and the stimulatory action of the hormone on thermogenesis can be measured. In combination with the clamp, positron-emitting tomography (PET) with ^{18}F-deoxy-glucose (FDG) will quantitate regional (e.g. myocardial) insulin-stimulated glucose uptake. Nuclear magnetic resonance (NMR) spectroscopy with ^{13}C-glucose has been used to measure insulin-stimulated glycogen accumulation.[5] Finally, newer insulin actions, such as the ability of the hormone to induce peripheral vasodilatation, to activate the sympathetic nervous system, and to affect the baroreflex control of heart rate, are being explored with the use of the euglycaemic clamp.

The second primary method is the arterio–venous (A–V) balance technique. Here, input–output analysis is applied to a section of the circulation in which the afferent artery (e.g. the brachial and femoral artery for forearm and leg tissues, respectively) and an efferent vein (a deep forearm vein and the femoral vein, respectively) are catheterized. By measuring blood flow, the balance between influx and efflux of substrates or hormones can be quantitated (see ref. 5 for the relevant equations). This technique is tissue-specific and can create more tightly controlled experimental conditions. Like the clamp (with which it can be combined), it is a steady-state method.

The minimal model, a development of the intravenous glucose tolerance test (IVGTT) proposed by Bergman and colleagues,[7] accounts for both insulin and glucose concentrations during the IVGTT in a simplified mathematical model of the glucose–insulin relationships. By using the measured insulin concentration as the input to the model, insulin sensitivity (S_I) is estimated by least-squares fit of the IVGTT glucose concentration profile (which is sampled with high frequency). An inherent limitation of the minimal model analysis of the IVGTT is that it requires a discrete insulin response, i.e. stimulated insulin concentrations that rise detectably and consistently above baseline. Therefore, in insulin-deficient subjects the IVGTT protocol is modified to include an intravenous bolus of tolbutamide – to stimulate endogenous insulin secretion – or a brief exogenous insulin infusion, both administered 20 minutes following the glucose bolus. Owing to the empirical nature of the mathematical model and the non-steady-state conditions of the test, the physiological interpretation of S_I is not unequivocally established. S_I has been considered to represent the ability of insulin to enhance total net glucose disappearance from the extracellular fluid, both by diminishing endogenous glucose production and by augmenting glucose utilization.[7] Both theoretical and experimental results indicate that S_I is a biased estimate of the average slope of the insulin dose–response curve at concentrations below the non-linearity threshold, the bias arising from the model's simplifications. Although S_I has been shown to correlate with the analogous estimate obtained from the glucose clamp over a wide range of insulin sensitivity, in severe insulin resistance the minimal model may yield negative values for S_I.[8] Despite these problems, the clear advantage of the minimal model is that it derives an index of insulin sensitivity and two indices of insulin secretion from a single test.

Insulin actions on glucose metabolism

Following transport across the plasma membrane, glucose is phosphorylated (by hexokinase II in many peripheral tissues, and mostly by glucokinase in the β-cell and the liver) and then channelled through disposal routes. In skeletal muscle and adipose tissue, hexose phosphates can be stored as glycogen or degraded through the glycolytic pathway; the resulting pyruvate can be exported into the extracellular fluids (as such or as lactate) or completely oxidized in the tricarboxylic acid cycle. Several rate-limiting enzymes for intracellular glucose disposition are sensitive to insulin. Thus, the insulin-regulatable glucose carrier protein, GLUT4, is specifically recruited to the plasma membrane from microsomal sites and activated by insulin in a dose-dependent fashion. In *in vivo* studies in the forearm of healthy subjects, using a triple tracer method to measure glucose transport, physiological amounts of insulin under euglycaemic conditions caused a time-dependent stimulation of transmembrane inward glucose transfer, which correlated well with concurrent rates of whole-body glucose disposal.[9] Recent studies using muscle biopsy have documented that insulin enhances glucose phosphorylation by activating hexokinase II (HKII) at doses and in a time-course compatible with the observed stimulation of muscle glucose metabolism.[10] Similar studies have shown that glycogen synthase (GS), a key enzyme in glycogen metabolism that is regulated through phosphorylation–dephosphorylation cycles, is converted into its active form by insulin, again at physiological doses.[11] Finally, phosphofructokinase (PFK), a rate-limiting enzyme for anaerobic glycolysis, and the pyruvate dehydrogenase complex (PDH), which controls pyruvate oxidation, are quite sensitive to insulin. Thus, insulin promotes disposition of plasma glucose by acting at multiple sites, thereby enhancing the overall efficiency of the process. The degree and sequence of activation of these enzymes under physiological circumstances is not known with certainty, but some clues are available. Thus, if the rate of glucose phosphorylation exceeds its rate of transport, free glucose will decrease in the cell cytoplasm. With regard to this, model-based estimates of intracellular free glucose levels in the insulinized human forearm tissues have suggested that transport may lag behind phosphorylation to some extent,[12] but direct evidence for this is still lacking. At the next step, if the transport/phosphorylation ('push' mechanism) does not keep up with the 'pulling' of hexosephosphates up into glycogen or down to pyruvate, intracellular glucose-6-phosphate concentrations will likewise fall under insulin stimulation. In studies employing ^{3}H NMR spectroscopy in humans, Rothman *et al.*[13] were able to show that glucose-6-phosphate concentrations within skeletal muscle drop consistently during a euglycaemic insulin clamp, an indication that

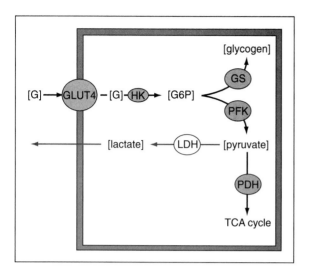

Fig. 6.5

Simplified scheme of the main intracellular routes of glucose disposition in a peripheral target tissue. Substrate concentrations are in brackets, insulin-stimulatable enzymes are inscribed in shaded circles. GLUT4 = isoform 4 of glucose transporter; HK = hexokinase II; GS = glycogen synthase; PFK = phosphofructokinase; PDH = pyruvate dehydrogenase; LDH = lactate dehydrogenase (see text for further explanation).

transport/ phosphorylation sets the pace for the metabolic steps downstream to the hexosephosphate pool (*Fig. 6.5*). Under the same clamp conditions, the systemic blood lactate-to-pyruvate concentration ratio first increases and then returns to baseline values, suggesting that insulin initially stimulates PDH less than PFK, thereby shifting the balance of the lactate dehydrogenase reaction toward lactate. Despite these indications, to reconstruct the temporal pattern of insulin's direct actions on the enzymes of glucose metabolism would require monitoring the intracellular concentration of glucose and its degradation products, as well as enzyme activities from multiple *ex vivo* tissue specimens. *In vivo*, a good approximation of relative glucose flux through the main intracellular disposition routes can be obtained by combining indirect calorimetry with the insulin clamp. As shown in *Fig. 6.6*, net glucose oxidation (by all body tissues) responds to small increments in plasma insulin and saturates quickly, whereas non-oxidative glucose disposal (mostly glycogen

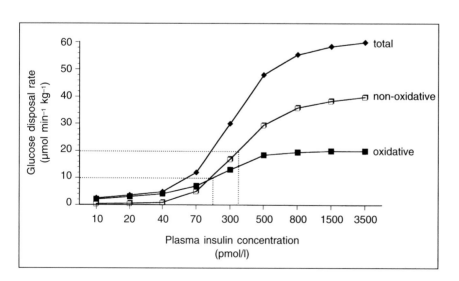

Fig. 6.6

Dose–response curves for total insulin-mediated glucose disposal and its main components, namely glucose oxidation and non-oxidative glucose utilization (mostly, glycogen synthesis). Redrawn from personal data in healthy subjects.

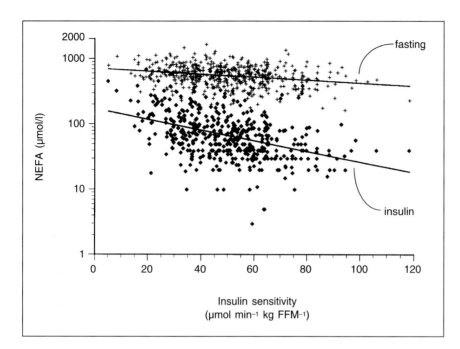

Fig. 6.7

Relationship between insulin sensitivity and plasma NEFA concentrations measured in the fasting state and during a euglycaemic insulin clamp in the non-diabetic cohort of the EGIR study (re-drawn from ref. 14).

synthesis) displays a lower sensitivity (higher K_m), but a higher capacitance. Thus, oxidation is the preferential mode of plasma glucose clearance when plasma insulin rises modestly, while under stronger insulin stimulation plasma glucose disappears predominantly through glycogen deposition.

A further mechanism of insulin sensitivity is represented by the indirect actions of insulin. The most important of these is the ability of insulin to suppress lipolysis through the inhibition of hormone-sensitive lipase (HSL) in adipose tissue, muscle, and liver. As shown in *Fig. 6.7*, in the fasting state, the peripheral plasma concentrations of NEFA are inversely related to insulin sensitivity. Moreover, under the standardized conditions of a euglycaemic insulin clamp, insulin suppresses circulating NEFA in proportion to insulin sensitivity.[14]

Owing to substrate competition, a diminished availability of fatty substrates enhances the usage of glucose by insulin-sensitive tissues via the generation of intracellular signals (low acetyl-coenzyme A/coenzyme A ratio, low citrate, and ATP levels are among the putative messengers).[15] Thus, PDH, PFK, GS, and GLUT4 itself may be de-repressed and collaborate with direct insulin stimulatory effects to promote glucose disposal. The direct versus indirect actions of insulin on glucose metabolism can be inferred from the comparison of the responses of forearm tissues to local insulinization (i.e. the intra-arterial infusion of the hormone) versus the response to systemic insulin administration.[16]

In the liver, glucose phosphorylation (catalysed by glucokinase) is normally exceeded by de-phosphorylation (catalysed by glucose-6-

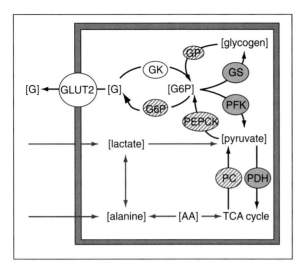

Fig. 6.8
Simplified scheme of the main intracellular routes of glucose synthesis in the liver. Substrate concentrations are in brackets, insulin-sensitive enzymes are inscribed in circles, shaded in the case of stimulation, hatched for an inhibitory action. AA = amino acid; G = glucose; GLUT2 = isoform 2 (non-insulin-sensitive) of glucose transporter; GK = glucokinase; G6P = glucose-6-phosphatase; GP = glycogen phosphorylase; PC = pyruvate carboxylase; PEPCK = phosphoenolpyruvate carboxykinase (see text for further explanation).

phosphatase [G6P]) of glucose-6-phosphate originating from both glycogen breakdown and gluconeogenesis. As a consequence, free intracellular glucose is exported into the extra-cellular space (via GLUT2, a non-insulin-stimulatable glucose carrier) down a concentration gradient. In the fasting state, insulin exerts a tonic inhibitory action on fasting glucose output (GO), thereby balancing the stimulatory influences on GO of glucagon, catecholamines, cortisol, and growth hormone (i.e. the counter-regulatory hormones). In the post-prandial state, insulin readily and effectively suppresses GO by shutting off glycogen breakdown.[11] This is effected through a strong inhibition of glycogen phosphorylase (GP) concomitant with the stimulation of glycogen synthase (GS). Chronic insulinization reduces the expression of key enzymes of the gluconeogenic pathway (e.g. phosphoenolpyruvate carboxykinase [PEPCK]). Also, during acute insulin administration lipolysis is curtailed, thereby limiting the supply of substrate (glycerol) and energy (from hepatic NEFA oxidation) for gluconeogenesis. The time-course and quantitative impact of this 'peripheral' effect on *de novo* glucose synthesis is uncertain. In any case, by inhibiting glucose-6-phosphatase, insulin has the ability to switch glucose-6-phosphate flux away from free glucose and into glycogen, thereby enhancing the overall efficiency of glycogen repletion (*Fig. 6.8*).

By turning off lipolysis, insulin shifts oxidative metabolism from the predominant fat usage of the fasting state to prevalent carbohydrate utilization, as documented by a consistent rise in respiratory quotient (RQ) (*Fig. 6.9*). In this changeover, energy metabolism is stimulated; the associated increment in metabolic rate contributes to diet-induced thermogenesis (DIT).

In sum, insulin control of plasma glucose concentrations is the integrated result of stimulation of glucose uptake and utilization in peripheral tissues, inhibition of glucose output by the liver, and removal of competition by fatty substrates.

Insulin resistance

The pathophysiological features of insulin resistance can be readily deduced from the general scheme of insulin action as above.

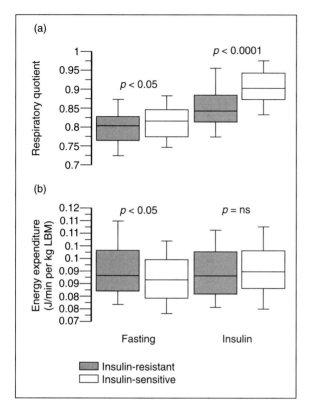

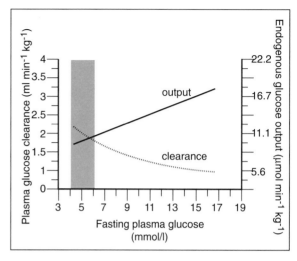

Fig. 6.10
Fasting rates of whole-body plasma glucose clearance and endogenous glucose output as a function of fasting plasma glucose concentration as measured by the tracer glucose technique in a group of volunteers including healthy subjects, individuals with impaired glucose tolerance, and patients with Type 2 diabetes. The shaded area indicates the normal range of fasting glycaemia. Redrawn from ref. 11.

Fig. 6.9
Respiratory quotient (a) and energy expenditure (b) as measured in the fasting state and during a euglycaemic insulin clamp in 322 non-diabetic subjects (the EGIR cohort, see ref. 36). Subjects were subgrouped according to insulin resistance, defined as the lowest decile of M values (insulin-mediated glucose uptake on the clamp) in non-obese subjects (BMI ≤ 25 kg m⁻²).

(a) in the overnight fasted state, plasma glucose clearance is reduced (reflecting impaired glucose uptake by insulin-sensitive tissues), and endogenous GO is insufficiently inhibited by pancreatic insulin flux. The combination of these two defects may be severe enough to cause fasting hyperglycaemia. In a study of a mixed group of volunteeres (healthy subjects, individuals with impaired glucose tolerance and patients with Type 2 diabetes), glucose clearance decreased in a hyperbolic fashion (as expected from the relationship glucose clearance = glucose uptake/plasma glucose concentration), while GO increased in direct proportion to the degree of fasting hyperglycaemia (*Fig. 6.10*). Fasting NEFA concentrations are raised in insulin resistant and/or diabetic subjects, and remain higher than normal following meals.[14] The lower fasting RQ found in insulin-resistant as compared with insulin-sensitive subjects (*Fig. 6.9*) documents a tendency toward enhanced whole-body fat oxidation. Increased drainage of NEFA to the liver stimulates gluconeogenesis, and a higher resting energy output is expended to finance the excess glucose synthesis from protein (*Fig. 6.9*).

(b) under conditions of euglycaemic hyperinsulinaemia, whole-body glucose uptake is reduced in insulin-resistant subjects as a result of a slight decrease in glucose oxidation and a more marked decrease in non-oxidative glucose disposal (glycogen synthesis). Simultaneously, the ability of insulin to suppress endogenous GO is compromised. Thus, the specific ability of insulin to maintain post-prandial glycaemia – by controlling glucose flux through plasma at both the input and the output sites – is lost. This is the picture commonly observed in non-diabetic obese subjects (~50% above ideal body weight) and in non-obese patients with Type 2 diabetes (*Fig. 6.11*). At the cellular level (in particular, in skeletal muscle and fat cells), insulin stimulation of glucose transport and activation of HKII, GS, PFK, and PDH have all been shown to be impaired in resistant patients with Type 2 diabetes.[11] Intracellular signalling of insulin action has been mapped down to fine details in recent years.[17] Thus, phosphorylation

of the intracellular domain of the insulin receptor, phosphorylation of its main substrates (IRS1 and IRS2), and activation of inositol-3-phosphate (I3P)-kinase, a key signal for GLUT4 recuitment, have been shown to be stimulated in human target tissues in response to insulin.[18] The relative contributions of these intracellular messenger molecules to insulin resistance are being actively investigated in *in vitro* systems and in transgenic animal models. Although different actions of insulin are mediated by different intracellular signalling pathways, it is widely accepted that the cellular basis of the insulin resistance of overt Type 2 diabetes involves multiple steps of glucose metabolism (transport, phosphorylation, conversion to glycogen, and oxidation, to name only the most prominent ones) rather than a single defect. An issue that remains currently unresolved is which of these defects is primary, in extent or time sequence, in the natural history of diabetes. A related question is which defect(s) are reversible, by physiological intervention or pharmacologically, and which are intractable.

Under clamp conditions, insulin resistance of lipolysis result in higher circulating NEFA

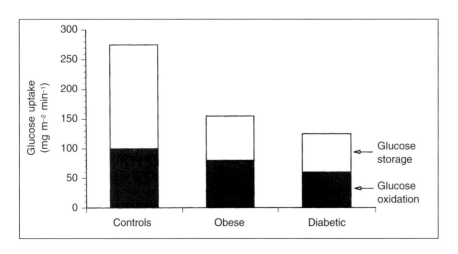

Fig. 6.11
Typical changes in total insulin-mediated glucose uptake and its components, glucose oxidation and glucose storage as glycogen, found in association with obesity and Type 2 diabetes (compiled from personal data).

concentrations (*Fig. 6.7*) and higher rates of lipid oxidation (*Fig. 6.9*). The pathophysiological consequence of this additional insulin resistance is dyslipidaemia. In fact, a larger NEFA flux to the liver throughout the fasting and fed state causes enhanced synthesis and secretion of triglyceride-rich lipid particles, especially intermediate density (IDL) and very low density lipoproteins (VLDL). Altered lipid exchange between different lipoproteins, coupled with accelerated degradation of apolipoprotein A, results in a reduced concentration of circulating high density lipoprotein (HDL)-cholesterol and an enrichment of the low density lipoprotein (LDL) pool with small, dense particles.[19] There emerges the typical dyslipidaemia of insulin-resistant states: high triglycerides, low HDL-cholesterol and an abundance of small, dense LDL particles. The relative contribution of endothelium-bound lipoproteinlipase (LPL) and tissue hormone-sensitive lipase (HSL) to the insulin resistance of lipolysis is imperfectly understood. Insulin appears to stimulate LPL, thereby helping the transfer of NEFA to adipose tissue, and to inhibit HSL, thus restraining the hydrolysis of tissue triglyceride stores. The combined effect of this insulin control is to store away NEFA as fat at a time when carbohydrate is the prevailing substrate to be utilized. Cellular mechanisms, genetic influences, and additional factors (such as adrenergic stimulation and the NEFA concentration itself) involved in insulin actions on lipolysis are under active investigation.

The impaired thermogenesis of insulin resistance also has an important pathophysiological impact. In the long term, in fact, a blunted postprandial thermogenesis may lead to weight gain by reducing heat dissipation. The clinical counterparts of this defect are that: (a) obesity is very often associated with diabetes, (b) weight excess, duration of obesity, and recent weight gain are powerful independent risk factors for

the development of diabetes, and (c) diabetic patients are particularly resistant to weight reduction in response to calorie restriction.

Adaptation to insulin resistance

Under free-living conditions, two mechanisms compensate for insulin resistance of glucose metabolism.

The first is hyperinsulinaemia, which results from increased pancreatic insulin secretion (*Fig. 6.12*). In obese subjects, for example, glucose tolerance is preserved in the face of tissue insulin resistance at the expense of

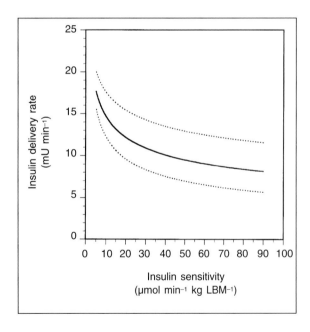

Fig. 6.12
Hyperbolic relationship between insulin sensitivity (as measured on a euglycaemic insulin clamp) and insulin release (estimated as the fasting post-hepatic delivery rate) in the non-diabetic subjects of the EGIR cohort (lines are mean ± 95% confidence intervals, re-drawn from ref. 36).

marked fasting and post-prandial hyperinsulin-aemia. Chronic exposure to high insulin concentrations, however, down-regulates insulin action at the receptor as well as the post-receptor level.[20] Thus, in healthy volunteers, 1 day of experimental, low-degree hyperinsulinaemia has been shown to be sufficient to reduce insulin-mediated glucose disposal in both its components, glucose oxidation and glycogen synthesis.[21]

The second compensatory mechanism is hyperglycaemia itself. By mass action, high extracellular glucose concentrations overcome the block imposed by insulin resistance and force normal – or even supernormal – fluxes of glucose through the cell membrane. Thus, in absolute terms, the hyperglycaemia of overt diabetes is less the consequence of low absolute rates of glucose uptake than raised rates of glucose release. Hyperglycaemia, however, also down-regulates glucose metabolism. Indeed, ample evidence accumulated in recent years has shown that chronic hyperglycaemia is toxic for a number of bodily functions ranging from insulin secretion to turnover of extracellular matrix.[22] One favourite mechanism to explain the toxic effects of hyperglycaemia calls on the enhanced generation of hexosamines from fructose-6-phosphate via the glutamine:fructose-6-phosphate amidotransferase reaction occurring in a variety of tissues.[23] In humans, 1 day of hyperglycaemia produces intense insulin resistance;[24] in experimental animal models, this effect can be reproduced by upregulating the hexosamine pathway.[25] Other intracellular messengers are also imputed of mediating glucose toxicity.[26]

In sum, both hyperinsulinaemia and hyperglycaemia are maladaptive responses. With reference to the scheme in *Fig. 6.1*, the primary insulin–glucose feedback incorporates secondary loops which impose a high cost on the maintenance of glucose tolerance.

Other actions of insulin

Insulin exerts a potent influence on electrolyte metabolism (reviewed in ref. 27). Through the activation of sodium reabsorption by the renal tubules, insulin opposes natriuresis during water diuresis as well as under unrestricted conditions. Renal excretion of uric acid also is reduced by acute insulin administration concomitantly with sodium.[28] On the other hand, insulin is one of the most powerful stimuli for cellular potassium uptake via activation of ATP-dependent, ouabain-inhibitable sodium–potassium exchange.[29] By inducing hypokalaemia, insulin saves potassium from renal excretion and depresses aldosterone secretion, despite a concurrent stimulation of renin synthesis.[27] In smooth muscle cells and platelets, insulin lowers intracellular free calcium concentrations and blunts calcium spikes in response to agonists, thereby opposing vasoconstriction and aggregation, respectively (see ref. 30 for a review). In addition, insulin causes some degree of relaxation of resistance vessels through the release of nitric oxide as well through smooth muscle cell-membrane hyperpolarization.[30] At physiological doses, insulin also stimulates sympathetic activity, as documented by increased heart rate, cardiac output, and circulating noradrenaline concentrations. The simultaneous occurrence of parasympathetic withdrawal and a stress-type neuro-hormonal response has been regarded as evidence that insulin modulates autonomic nervous system activity via direct actions in the central nervous system.[31] In the presence of raised plasma levels of NEFA and glucose, insulin acutely increases the secretion of plasminogen activator inhibitor I (PAI-1), a major factor in fibrinolysis.[30] Recent evidence also suggests that acute insulin administration in physiological doses may reduce the LDL content of vitamin E, thereby rendering these lipoproteins prone to oxidation (Ferrannini E *et al.*, unpublished data). Insulin resistance has been implicated in the microvascular dysfunction that is found in insulin-resistant states such as diabetes, essential hypertension, and dyslipidaemia. Here, the evidence is mixed. Thus, insulin potentiates endothelium-dependent vasodilatation; the effect is, however, similar in healthy volunteers and patients with essential hypertension and endothelial dysfunction.[32] Conversely, endothelial function (assessed as the vasodilatory response to intra-arterial acetylcholine infusion) has been reported to be similar in insulin-sensitive and insulin-resistant subjects.[33] Microalbuminuria, which some investigators view as an index of generalized endothelial dysfunction, is definitely linked with blood pressure and hyperglycaemia, but is arguably an independent correlate of insulin resistance. Thus, the prevalence of microalbuminuria has been found to associate with insulin resistance in one population study[34] but not in another one.[35] Finally, insulin promotes vascular smooth cell proliferation *in vitro*, but whether and to what extent this occurs in hyperinsulinaemic humans remains to be established. Despite gaps of information and understanding, the concept that insulin exerts important actions not directly related to blood glucose and lipid control is gaining consensus.

Perspectives

Insulin sensitivity spans an unusually wide range in humans.[36] This peculiarity can be regarded as the key feature of a primordial physiological system in which euglycaemia, essential for brain function, is to be kept at all costs. Insulin sensitivity is set by numerous effectors in different target tissues. The genetic control of insulin action is therefore very complex even when considering only glucose metabolism. In addition, a large number of acquired factors influence insulin sensitivity; thus, down-regulation of insulin action may occur as an adaptation to physiological events or in response to disease (*Table 6.1*). It is, however, increasingly clear that insulin resistance can be primary with respect to known modulators. In this case, it will

Table 6.1
Conditions associated with insulin resistance.

Type	Condition
Physiological:	Puberty
	Pregnancy
	Bed rest
	Contraceptives
	High-fat diet
Metabolic:	Type 2 diabetes
	Uncontrolled Type 1 diabetes
	Diabetic ketoacidosis
	Obesity
	Severe malnutrition
	Hyperuricaemia
	Insulin-induced hypoglycaemia
	Excessive alcohol consumption
Endocrine:	Thyrotoxicosis
	Hypothyroidism
	Cushing's syndrome
	Pheochromocytoma
	Acromegaly
Non-endocrine:	Essential hypertension
	Chronic uraemia
	Liver cirrhosis
	Rheumatoid arthritis
	Acanthosis nigricans
	Chronic heart failure
	Myotonic dystrophia
	Trauma, burns, sepsis
	Surgery
	Neoplastic cachexia

be interesting to distinguish between genetic make-up and congenital factors (i.e. foetal undernutrition[37]). The interest is justified by the notion that a low level of insulin sensitivity is biologically harmful because it clusters with disturbances of glucose tolerance, lipid metabolism, coagulation, blood pressure homeostasis, and vascular function. Whether (and which) insulin resistance or the attendant hyperinsulinaemia (or both) is the prime mover in the syndrome is a question that remains to be conclusively answered. Hyperinsulinaemia antecedes and predicts some of the components of the insulin-resistance syndrome,[38] but the syndrome could still represent a true cluster of inherently linked functions.

Insulin resistance has double relevance to diabetes. On the one hand, defective insulin action is common in patients with Type 2 diabetes, in whom β-cell function, by definition, fails. This indicates that insulin action and insulin secretion must be interconnected above and beyond the operation of the basic feedback mechanism (*Fig. 6.2*). Again, genetic and acquired interactions are equally possible. The key notion here is that insulin resistance is a powerful independent predictor of diabetes, i.e. β-cell failure. Whether this can simply be explained by pancreatic exhaustion or reflects the deployment of a common programme is unknown. On the other hand, mounting evidence links insulin resistance with the vascular complications of diabetes. Both macro- and microvascular disease can be worsened, if not initiated, by the disturbances associated with the insulin-resistance syndrome. Insulin itself may carry an atherogenic potential.[4] The emerging paradigm (*Fig. 6.13*) views diabetes (at least, the common form of Type 2 diabetes) as part of the insulin-resistance syndrome. While insulin resistance of glucose metabolism is directly related to, and quantitatively accounts for, the hyperglycaemia of diabetes, insulin resistance of other

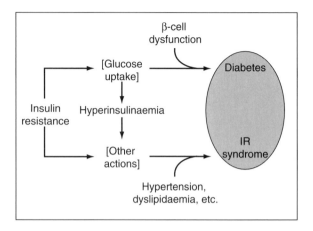

Fig. 6.13

Simplified scheme for the interrelationships between insulin resistance of glucose uptake, insulin action on substrates other than glucose, Type 2 diabetes, and the insulin-resistance (IR) syndrome (see text for further explanation).

pathways, and the hyperinsulinaemia generated in the glucose pathway, explain the other abnormalities of the syndrome. Together with additional genetic influences (predisposition to hypertension, dyslipidaemia, etc.), the insulin-resistance syndrome pushes diabetes into co-morbidity and accelerates the development of vascular disease. In this paradigm, determining what can be stopped or reversed and how to prevent morbidity and mortality is a major task for clinical medicine.

References

1. Schwartz MW, Figlewicz DP, Baskin DG *et al.* Insulin in the brain: a hormonal regulator of energy balance. *Endocr Rev* 1992; **13**: 387–414.
2. Kahn CR, White MP. The insulin receptor and the molecular mechanism of insulin action. *J Clin Invest* 1988; **82**: 1151–1154.

3. Rosen OM. Banting Lecture: structure and function of insulin receptors. *Diabetes* 1989; **38**: 1508–1511.

4. Ferrannini E, Stern MP. Primary insulin resistance: a risk syndrome. In: Leslie RDG, Robbins DC, eds. *Diabetes: Clinical Science in Practice*. Cambridge: Cambridge University Press, 1995: 200–220.

5. Ferrannini E, Mari A. How to measure insulin sensitivity. *J Hypertens* 1998; **16**: 895–906.

6. Ferrannini E. The theoretical bases of indirect calorimetry. A Review. *Metabolism* 1988; **37**: 287–305.

7. Bergman RN, Ider YZ, Bowden CR, Cobelli C. Quantitative estimation of insulin sensitivity. *Am J Physiol* 1979; **236**: E667–E677.

8. Saad MF, Anderson RL, Laws A *et al*. A comparison between the minimal model and the glucose clamp in the assessment of insulin sensitivity across the spectrum of glucose tolerance. *Diabetes* 1994; **43**: 1114–1121.

9. Bonadonna RC, Saccomani MP, Seely L *et al*. Glucose transport in human skeletal muscle: the *in vivo* response to insulin. *Diabetes* 1993; **42**: 191–198.

10. Mandarino LJ, Printz RL, Cusi KA *et al*. Regulation of hexokinase II and glycogen synthase mRNA, protein, and activity in human muscle. *Am J Physiol* 1995; **269**: E701–E708.

11. DeFronzo RA. Pathogenesis of type 2 diabetes: metabolic and molecular implications for identifying diabetes genes. *Diabetes Rev* 1997; **5**: 177–269.

12. Bonadonna RC, Del Prato S, Bonora E *et al*. Roles of glucose transport and glucose phosphorylation in muscle insulin resistance of type 2 (non-insulin-dependent) diabetes mellitus. *Diabetes* 1996; **45**: 915–925.

13. Rothman DL, Shulman RG, Shulman GI. [31]P nuclear magnetic resonance measurements of muscle glucose-6-phosphate: evidence for reduced insulin-dependent muscle glucose transport or phosphorylation activity in non-insulin-dependent diabetes mellitus. *J Clin Invest* 1992; **89**: 1069–1075.

14. Ferrannini E, Camastra S, Coppack SW *et al*. Insulin action and non-esterified fatty acids. *Proc Nutr Soc* 1997; **56**: 753–761.

15. Randle PJ, Garland PB, Hales CN, Newsholme EA. The glucose fatty acid cycle: its role in insulin sensitivity and the metabolic disturbances of diabetes mellitus. *Lancet* 1963; **i**: 785–789.

16. Kelley DE, Mokan M, Simoneau JA, Mandarino LJ. Interaction between glucose and free fatty acid metabolism in human skeletal muscle. *J Clin Invest* 1993; **92**: 91–98.

17. Häring HU, Mehnert H. Pathogenesis of type 2 (non-insulin-dependent) diabetes mellitus: candidates for a signal transmitter defect causing insulin resistance of the skeletal muscle. *Diabetologia* 1993; **36**: 176–182.

18. Klip A, Paquet MR. Glucose transport and glucose transporters in muscle and their metabolic regulation. *Diabetes Care* 1990; **13**: 228–240.

19. Taskinen MR, Nestel PJ. Hypolipidemic agents: their role in diabetes mellitus. In: Alberti KGMM, Zimmet P, DeFronzo RA, eds. *International Textbook of Diabetes Mellitus*, 2nd edn. Chichester: John Wiley & Sons, 1997: 883–898.

20. Cusin I, Terrettaz J, Rohner-Jeanrenaud F *et al*. Hyperinsulinemia increases the amount of GLUT4 mRNA in white adipose tissue and decreases that of muscles: a clue for increased fat depot and insulin resistance. *Endocrinology* 1990; **127**: 3246–3248.

21. Del Prato S, Leonetti F, Simonson DC *et al*. Effect of sustained physiologic hyperinsulinaemia and hyperglycaemia on insulin secretion and insulin sensitivity in man. *Diabetologia* 1994; **37**: 1025–1035.

22. Rossetti L, Giaccari A, DeFronzo RA. Glucose toxicity. *Diabetes Care* 1990; **13**: 610–630.

23. McClain DA, Crook ED. Hexosamines and insulin resistance. *Diabetes* 1996; **45**: 1003–1009.

24. Yki-Järvinen H, Helve H, Koivisto VA. Hyperglycemia decreases glucose uptake in type 1 diabetes. *Diabetes* 1987; **36**: 892–896.

25. Rossetti L, Hawkins M, Chen W *et al*. *In vivo* glucosamine infusion induces insulin resistance in normoglycemic but not in hyperglycemic conscious rats. *J Clin Invest* 1995; **96**: 132–140.

26. Spiegelman BM, Hotamisligil GS. Through thick and thin: wasting, obesity, and TNF-α. *Cell* 1993; **73**: 625–627.

27. Ferrannini E. The phenomenon of insulin resistance: its possible relevance to hypertensive

disease. In: Laragh JH, Brenner BM, eds. *Hypertension: Pathophysiology, Diagnosis, and Management*, 2nd edn. New York: Raven Press, 1995: 2281–2300.

28. Quiñones Galvan A, Natali A, Baldi S *et al.* Effect of insulin on uric acid excretion in humans. *Am J Physiol* 1995; **268**: E1–E8.

29. Ferrannini E, Taddei S, Santoro D *et al.* Independent stimulation of glucose metabolism and Na/K exchange by insulin in the human forearm. *Am J Physiol* 1988; **255**: E953–E957.

30. Ferrannini E. Insulin and blood pressure. In: Reaven GM, Laws A, eds. *Contemporary Endocrinology: Insulin Resistance*. Totowa, NJ: Humana Press Inc., 1999; in press.

31. Muscelli E, Emdin M, Natali A *et al.* Cardiac effects of insulin in humans: influence of obesity. *J Clin Endocrinol Metab* 1998; **83**: 2084–2090.

32. Taddei S, Virdis A, Mattei P *et al.* Effect of insulin on acetylcholine-induced vasodilation in normotensive subjects and patients with essential hypertension. *Circulation* 1995; **92**: 2911–2918.

33. Natali A, Taddei S, Quiñones Galvan A *et al.* Insulin sensitivity, vascular reactivity, and clamp-induced vasodilatation in essential hypertension. *Circulation* 1997; **96**: 849–855.

34. Mykkanen L, Zaccaro DJ, Wagenknecht LE *et al.* Microalbuminuria is associated with insulin resistance in nondiabetic subjects: the insulin resistance atherosclerosis study. *Diabetes* 1998; **47**: 793–800.

35. Jager A, Kostense PJ, Nijpels G *et al.* Microalbuminuria is strongly associated with NIDDM and hypertension, but not with the insulin resistance syndrome: the Hoorn Study. *Diabetologia* 1998; **41**: 694–700.

36. Ferrannini E, Natali A, Bell P *et al.* Insulin resistance and hypersecretion in obesity. *J Clin Invest* 1997; **100**: 1166–1173.

37. Phillips DIW. Insulin resistance as a programmed response to fetal undernutrition. *Diabetologia* 1996; **39**: 1119–1122.

38. Haffner SM, Valdez RA, Hazuda HP *et al.* Prospective analysis of the insulin resistance syndrome (Syndrome X). *Diabetes* 1992; **41**: 715–722.

7

Impaired glucose tolerance and Type 2 diabetes: a role of obesity and leptin?

Asjid Qureshi and Peter Kopelman

Introduction

As with many diseases of multifactorial aetiology, the various aetiological contributors to the development of impaired glucose tolerance (IGT) and Type 2 diabetes remain incompletely defined. Despite many possibilities being proposed through clinical observation and research, few have been so consistently linked with the development of Type 2 diabetes as obesity. This relationship has been demonstrated irrespective of age, gender, and race. Since the diagnostic criteria remain non-uniform amongst researchers, the true extent of the association may not yet have been fully realized. The strength of this relationship has been recognized by the World Health Organization, who, in 1985, described obesity to be the single most important risk factor in the development of Type 2 diabetes. Some researchers have shown a 40-fold increase in the risk of developing Type 2 diabetes over a 14-year period for women who became overweight compared with those who remained at a more normal weight.[1] In other populations, more modest figures still suggest a strong relationship; the Framingham study showed a weight 40% or more above that expected, doubles the risk of developing Type 2 diabetes.[2] In an analysis of six prospective studies which researched the risk factors involved in the transition from IGT to Type 2 diabetes, Edelstein and colleagues concluded that in all studies, measures of obesity were consistently positively associated with the incidence of Type 2 diabetes.[3]

Diabetes and obesity independently predispose to a varied number of pathological states. Diabetes among men aged 35–64 years increases the risk of heart failure fourfold. In such cases, obesity is a further independent risk factor in addition to high-density lipoprotein (HDL) plasma concentration, proteinuria, intraventricular conduction delay, and non-specific cardiac repolarization abnormalities.[4,5] The risk of microalbuminuria is enhanced by obesity.[6,7] Atherosclerosis, hypertension, and stroke mortality are increased by the combination of diabetes and obesity .[8–11] The incidence of 'minor' ailments seem also to be increased by the combination of gout,[12] non-alcoholic steatohepatitis,[13] and gallbladder disease in females under the age of 45 years.[14]

It is not only the overall degree of adiposity that seems to relate to Type 2 diabetes but also the regional distribution of adipose tissue. Indeed, many have shown this to be the more important determinant. It is well established that visceral or central adiposity particularly predisposes to metabolic and cardiovascular complications. Once again, the strength of this relationship is evident despite the non-standardized methods that exist amongst researchers to assess fat distribution, from simple anthropometric measurements such as waist circumference, to abdominal CT scanning. Two studies, which used the waist-to-hip ratio (WHR) to assess fat distribution, demonstrated a closer relationship between fat distribution and the prevalence of IGT than between the overall degree of adiposity and IGT.[15,16] In contrast, other studies of selected communities, such as Pima Indians, have demonstrated overall adiposity to be the greater risk.[15]

An insight into the pathophysiological mechanisms linking obesity and Type 2 diabetes is gained by the study of differences of function between adipose tissue located at different body sites. In particular, visceral adipocytes have a greater lipolytic activity than do subcutaneous adipocytes. The underlying mechanisms for this is the differences in adrenergic adrenoceptors and insulin receptor function at these sites that result in a greater ability of visceral fat to mobilize free fatty acids (FFAs). Visceral fat is unique by its portal venous drainage and as a result exposes the liver to high concentrations of free fatty acids. These stimulate gluconeogenesis, triglyceride synthesis, and inhibition of insulin breakdown,[17] resulting in hyperglycaemia, hyperlipidaemia, and hyperinsulinaemia, features commonly seen in association with central obesity.

The importance of fat distribution is further emphasized when obesity and co-morbidities are studied in various ethnic populations. In populations such as South Asians, where a predisposition to central adiposity has been demonstrated, an increased prevalence of coronary heart disease, glucose intolerance, hyperinsulinaemia, and hypertriglycerideaemia is observed.[18] In such groups, increasing WHR is correlated with glucose intolerance and increased blood pressure, plasma insulin, and triglyceride levels. In contrast, Afro-Caribbean populations, with less abdominal adiposity, have a similarly high prevalence of diabetes yet a reduced risk of heart disease.

Role of adipocyte

The body requires energy for maintenance of cellular function, synthesis of tissues, generation of heat, and locomotor function. Energy is derived in the form of adenosine triphosphate (ATP) from substrates such as glucose, triacylglycerols (TAGs), FFAs, ketone bodies, and amino acids. The two most important sources of energy utilized by the body over any extended period of time are protein from skeletal muscle and fat from adipose tissue. Since a similar weight of adipose tissue releases almost nine times as much energy as an equivalent weight of skeletal muscle, adipose tissue provides the more efficient way for the body to store energy. This energy is stored in the form of TAG in the adipocyte. As the stores of TAG accumulate, the adipocyte enlarges in size. A point is eventually reached which is apparently dependent on factors such as age, gender, and nutrition,[19] when the adipocyte divides into two cells. The size of any one adipocyte is dependent on the balance of influx of triglycerides and efflux of FFA and glycerol. It is the hydrolysis of TAGs that releases FFAs. A number of hormones play a critical role in the balance of lipogenesis and lipolysis in adipose tissue. These include insulin, glucocorticoids, and sex hormones.

The hydrolysis of TAG-releasing FFAs is dependent on hormone-sensitive lipase (HSL). The major lipolysis-regulating hormones are insulin and the catecholamines. Insulin suppresses HSL activity by reducing adipocyte cyclic AMP levels and so suppressing fat mobilization. Under normal circumstances, this suppression occurs even at very low concentrations of insulin. In addition, insulin activates lipoprotein lipase (LPL) in the post-prandial phase. This enzyme is found in capillary endothelial cells and releases FFAs from TAGs, chylomicrons, and very-low-density lipoproteins. LPL activity may be enhanced by glucagon and adrenaline, and decreased by noradrenaline, ethinyloestradiol, testosterone, progesterone, and prolactin.[20]

Catecholamines have a dual action: they inhibit lipolysis via α_2 adrenoreceptors, while they enhance lipolysis via β adrenoreceptors. It is the regional variations in the actions of catecholamines and insulin that result in differences in lipolysis rates in visceral and subcutaneous adipose tissues. A higher activity of β adrenoceptors, a lower activity of α adrenoceptors, and a decreased insulin receptor affinity and signal transduction are found in visceral adipocytes, resulting in a greater rate of lipolysis than that in subcutaneous adipocytes.

Elevated FFA levels in the portal circulation result in increased hepatic insulin resistance, and increase hepatic glucose output and promote gluconeogenesis. Excess circulating FFAs result in tissue lipid accumulation, insulin resistance, and reduced glucose uptake in skeletal muscle and contribute to β-cell dysfunction. In rodents, increased FFA availability has been shown to result in β-cell apoptosis.[21] FFAs are also known to increase insulin resistance in skeletal muscle through several mechanisms. One such mechanism is the FFA-induced decrease in intracellular free CoA/acylCoA that inhibits the stimulatory effect of insulin on glycolysis, glucose transport across the cell membrane, and glycogen storage.[22] In subjects at risk of developing Type 2 diabetes, very early defects in both glycogen storage ability and FFA oxidation capacity have been demonstrated in skeletal muscle, defects which can impair fuel utilization and increase fat storage.

Obesity is also characterized by an increased rate of cortisol production. Cortisol both enhances lipid accumulation and reduces mobilization. Its ability to enhance lipolytic activity is achieved through various mechanisms. It enhances the activity of LPL in the presence of insulin *in vivo* and also inhibits the anti-lipolytic action of insulin.[23] In subjects with visceral obesity, visceral adipocyte expression of glucocorticoid receptors is higher than in subcutaneous adipocytes.[24]

Important sex hormones for adipocyte function include dehydroepiandrosterone (DHEA), 17-hydroxy progesterone, and testosterone. Serum androgen levels are inversely related to fasting plasma glucose and are predictive of central obesity 10–15 years later.[25] Testosterone positively autoregulates the expression of β-adrenergic receptors, thereby enhancing lipolytic sensitivity.[26] Indirect evidence suggests that these additional hormonal factors contribute to lipolysis preferentially occurring in visceral rather than subcutaneous fat. This accentuates the proportion of systemic FFAs originating from visceral adipocytes,[27,28] with a consequential rise in the concentration of FFAs in the portal circulation and further detrimental actions on the liver with dyslipidaemia and hyperinsulinaemia.[17]

Leptin

The word leptin is derived from the Greek word leptos, meaning thin. Leptin, the product of the obesity (ob) gene, was first described in rodent models of genetic obesity, with its deficiency in the ob/ob mouse being characterized by obesity, hyperinsulinaemia, and infertility. Leptin administration in such mice results in a reversal of these features. The db/db mouse, which shares similar metabolic aberrations to the ob/ob mouse, is by contrast hyperleptinaemic. In the db/db mice the metabolic alterations are a consequence of hypothalamic leptin receptor abnormalities which are genetically linked to the diabetes (db) locus on chromosome 4.[29] Leptin administration in such animals is ineffective. The precise role of leptin in humans is uncertain, but the identification of leptin receptors in many different organs throughout the body suggests a potential involvement of leptin in many different body systems. Its effects on various components of carbohydrate metabolism and its interplay with hormones such as insulin and glucocorticoids raises the possibility that leptin is involved in the link between obesity and Type 2 diabetes.

Leptin in animal models of obesity

The lipostatic theory of body weight control has been debated for over 40 years, with many proposed mechanisms postulating a feedback pathway from adipose tissue to the hypothalamus to regulate the overall adiposity. Until the discovery of leptin, no factor had been identified. The ob/ob mouse is leptin-deficient as a consequence of being homozygous for either one of two genetic mutations on mouse chromosome 6. The first mutation blocks transcription, whereas the second results in a defective and therefore inactive protein product. Both genetic abnormalities result in a deficiency of biologically active leptin which, in turn, is associated with hyperphagia, reduced brown adipose tissue (BAT) activity, obesity, hyperinsulinaemia, insulin resistance, and infertility. This presumably explains why there is such a widespread distribution of leptin receptors in various tissues.

It is through the hypothalamus that a deficiency of leptin results in many of the abnormalities seen in the ob/ob mouse.

Intracerebroventricular and intraperitoneal injections of leptin in deficient mice result in a remarkable reversal of many of the observed abnormal features, with a marked reduction in hyperphagia, increased energy expenditure, improved insulin resistance, a reduction in insulin levels, and an improvement in fertility. In contrast, weight reduction alone through dietary means is not associated with an improvement in fertility.

The hypothalamus is believed to be leptin's most important central site of action, although receptors are found in various other parts of the brain. It acts through more than one pathway, and provides a stimulatory effect on some while inhibiting others. Possible mediators of the central effects of leptin include neuropeptide Y (NPY), galanin, melanin-concentrating hormone, neurotensin, and proopiomelanocortin.[30-32] Leptin decreases the biosynthesis and transport of NPY in the brain. NPY is a 36-amino-acid peptide, first isolated in 1982,[33] which plays an important role in rodent energy homeostasis and the development of obesity. It is found extensively in the central and peripheral nervous systems, and in particular abundance in the hypothalamus.[34] Centrally administered exogenous NPY in rodents is a potent stimulator of feeding, acting through the paraventricular and perifornical lateral hypothalamus.[35] NPY neurones of the hypothalamic arcuate (ARC) nucleus project to the paraventricular nuclei (PVN) and dorsomedial nuclei (DMN), and are involved in the control of energy balance, in contradistinction to leptin, by stimulating feeding and inhibiting thermogenesis. In addition to its central actions, NPY reduces heat production in BAT through decreased sympathetic drive and decreased uncoupling protein (UCP) activity (*Fig. 7.1*). NPY has a dual effect on insulin secretion from the pancreas: it increases pancreatic insulin secretion via the vagus nerve

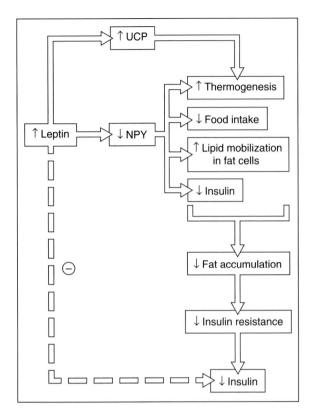

Fig. 7.1
Postulated interactions between leptin, neuropeptide Y (NPY), and uncoupling proteins (UCP) in rodent models. ↑ = increased; ↓ = decreased.

and reduces insulin release by a direct effect on the pancreas.[36,37] NPY further stimulates lipid accumulation in fat cells through increased glucose utilization and lipoprotein lipase activity in white adipose tissue (WAT). Overactivity of NPY neurones could therefore result in obesity, and this appears to be the case in some rodent models of obesity such as the obese Zucker (fa/fa) rat, and ob/ob and db/db mice. Importantly, leptin treatment in ob/ob mice decreases NPY gene expression in the ARC nucleus.[38,39] No such effect is seen in the db/db mouse. NPY-induced obesity results in raised

circulating leptin concentrations, which suggests the existence of a feedback mechanism with leptin and the NPY-ergic ARC–PVN neurones interacting in a homeostatic loop to regulate body fat mass and energy balance.[40]

Leptin's ability to alter thermogenesis and consequently energy expenditure is also mediated through UCPs. UCPs reside in the membrane of BAT mitochondria and act as ion channels, dissipating the proton gradient formed during mitochondrial respiration. This activity results in the exothermic movement of protons through the inner mitochondrial membrane, uncoupled from ATP synthesis, liberating energy as heat as opposed to the formation of stored energy in the form of ATP. Leptin increases energy expenditure in rodents through increasing BAT and skeletal muscle UCP levels.[41,42]

A number of different uncoupling proteins exist, varying in their tissue distribution and operational properties. UCP1 is found in the inner membrane of BAT mitochondria. It is activated by the sympathetic nervous system via noradrenaline, and FFAs enhance its energy-dissipating capacity. Dietary intake and the cold stimulate BAT and UCP1 activity. UCP2 is found in skeletal muscle and WAT in addition to BAT. UCP2 may play a role in leptin-induced lipolysis.[43] Leptin increases UCP2 mRNA by more than 10-fold in epididymal, retroperitoneal, and subcutaneous fat tissue of normal rats, but not of leptin-receptor-defective obese rats.[44] UCP3 is found in skeletal muscle and adipose tissue. Factors regulating UCP3 activity include β_3-adrenergic agonists, dexamethasone, leptin, and diet, with all of these factors being potentially diabetogenic. These regulators of activity seem to affect muscle and BAT to differing extents.[45] There is indirect evidence for the existence of a negative feedback loop between UCP and leptin.[46]

There are particular problems in extrapolating from rodents to humans when considering the association between leptin and Type 2 diabetes. First, a model truly equivalent to human Type 2 diabetes in genetic and phenotypical abnormalities does not exist. Secondly, models most frequently used with clinical features similar to those seen in human Type 2 diabetes often have contrasting genetic abnormalities of either leptin or the leptin receptor. For example, ob/ob and db/db mice and Zucker (fa/fa) rat are obese and insulin resistant. However, the ob/ob mouse has a leptin gene abnormality, and the db/db mouse and Zucker rats have leptin receptor abnormalities. To date, neither leptin nor leptin receptor gene abnormalities have been convincingly associated with Type 2 diabetes in humans. However, a number of rodent studies do provide an insight into the links between leptin and Type 2 diabetes.

Various studies suggest that leptin has 'diabetogenic' properties by reducing glucose-stimulated insulin secretion from the pancreas and impairing glycogen synthesis. The discovery of leptin receptor mRNA in β-cells of rat pancreatic islets suggests the existence of a potentially important relationship between leptin and insulin secretion.[47] In rats, leptin influences the glucose-stimulated insulin secretion from the pancreas; administration of increasing doses of leptin results in a bell-shaped dose–response inhibition of glucose-stimulated insulin secretion by pancreatic islets. This interaction of leptin with glucose-related insulin secretion occurs acutely, with an immediate reversal on withdrawal of leptin. The effectiveness of leptin in influencing this process is dependent on the glucose level. Longer-term exposure to inhibitory levels of leptin reduces both insulin secretion and transcription.[48] Leptin has additionally been shown to impair several other metabolic actions of insulin: Muller and colleagues have demonstrated that leptin is able to impair insulin's ability to stimulate glucose transport, glycogen synthase, lipogenesis and protein synthesis. This inhibition is fully reversed once leptin is withdrawn.[49]

If one assumes that leptin plays a major role in the development of insulin resistance and glucose intolerance, it is surprising that deficiency or resistance to leptin rather than hypersecretion is the characteristic of rodent models of obesity and diabetes. Moreover, treatment of the leptin-deficient ob/ob mouse with leptin results in a marked lowering of plasma insulin concentration and increased glucose disposal.[50] This raises questions about the diabetogenic properties of leptin and/or its deficiency.

Leptin in human obesity

In humans, leptin is synthesized predominantly in mature white adipocytes, is secreted into the circulation, and acts both centrally and peripherally. Leptin crosses the blood–brain barrier through a saturable transport mechanism and has actions on the hypothalamus, choroid plexus, ARC nuclei, PVN, and DMN which are likely to involve the control of appetite and energy expenditure. As in rodent models, leptin is believed to act centrally through mediators such as NPY. However, findings have not been entirely consistent with those in rodent models. Obese women with elevated leptin levels have been found also to have elevated levels of plasma NPY when compared with an equivalent lean control group.[51] NPY levels are twofold higher in human cerebrospinal fluid (CSF) than in plasma. However, studies have found no direct relationship between NPY concentration in CSF and leptin CSF levels.[52] Moreover, molecular studies have failed to link

NPY and NPY-Y1/Y5 receptors with the development of human obesity.[53]

Numerous classes of leptin receptors exist and are found peripherally in many tissues of the body (skeletal muscle, ovaries, testis, bronchioles, blood vessels, liver, adipose tissue, thyroid gland, adrenals, haemopoetic system, and pancreas), suggesting an extensive role for leptin in various bodily systems.

As with many other hormones, serum leptin levels follow a diurnal pattern of variation and peak in the early hours of the morning. There is a distinct gender difference, with higher levels occurring in adult females. The lower level in males is believed to be a consequence of testosterone-mediated inhibition of leptin production. At a very young age, leptin levels are similar in boys and girls, but levels diverge with increasing age. Levels also vary between racial groups, tending to be lower in African women than in Caucasian women of similar age, weight, and adipose tissue mass.[54] Leptin levels in humans have repeatedly been shown to correlate with body mass index (BMI) and the degree of adiposity. The relationship between leptin levels and BMI is exponential, whereas that between leptin levels and measures of degree of adiposity appears more linear. Factors that influence serum leptin levels in the short term include hormones such as insulin, and dietary intake. Despite these short-term changes, leptin appears more to be a chronic marker of adiposity in humans. Only in very rare cases has human obesity been linked to a congenital deficiency in leptin,[55] and although the two individuals were insulin resistant, they were not diabetic.

The importance of BAT in the development of obesity varies from species to species. In humans it seems to be of importance in the neonate after which its role declines. The role of UCP 1 in humans is thought to be of significantly less importance than it is in rodents. However, two homologues of UCP 1, UCP 2,

and UCP 3, may be important. UCP 2 is found widely in different tissues (WAT, skeletal muscle, heart, liver, kidney, and the immune system), and UCP 3 is found in skeletal muscle. Possible genetic associations between UCP 2, UCP 3, and aspects of human obesity such as resting metabolic rate[56] and BMI[57] have been described in selected populations.

In theory, the hyperleptinaemia found in human obesity could be diabetogenic. This may be particularly relevant at the stage of normal glucose tolerance in individuals predisposed to Type 2 diabetes. Nyholm and colleagues studied 40 first-degree relatives of subjects with Type 2 diabetes and 35 control subjects by assessing insulin resistance (using a hyperinsulinaemic euglycaemic clamp method) and fasting serum leptin. Although all of the subjects had a normal oral glucose tolerance test (OGTT), leptin was found to be significantly increased in the group with relatives with Type 2 diabetes.[58] Other studies have also supported a relationship between insulin resistance and leptin by demonstrating a positive correlation between fasting serum insulin and leptin levels independent of BMI, WHR, and age.[59] It is possible that prolonged exposure to high levels of leptin may contribute to insulin resistance and thereby play a role in the progression to IGT. However, insulin is known to stimulate leptin production in humans and a counter-argument is that elevated leptin levels are simply a consequence of hyperinsulinaemia.[60] This does not appear to be the case in hyperinsulinaemic individuals with impaired glucose tolerance because leptin levels tend to decline with time.[61] A possible explanation is that the decline in leptin is an attempt to further enhance insulin secretion by reducing leptin-mediated inhibition of pancreatic insulin secretion. This requires the existence of a feedback mechanism, which has not yet been defined, and for leptin's anti-insulin effects still to be effective despite the relative reduction in its secretion. Subjects with poorly controlled Type 2 diabetes have leptin levels 30% lower than levels in normoglycaemic individuals.[61] Weight loss in Type 2 diabetes is accompanied by improved β-cell responsiveness to glucose-stimulated insulin secretion.[62] Thus, the improved pancreatic secretion could be partly mediated by the fall in leptin levels occurring in these individuals.[63] This supports the suggestion that although leptin is low in Type 2 diabetes, it still plays an important inhibitory role on pancreatic insulin secretion.

The precise role of leptin in the development of Type 2 diabetes is poorly defined and requires further research. However, the properties of leptin suggest that it may play an important role in the progression from normal glucose tolerance to poorly controlled Type 2 diabetes at particular stages.

From obesity to IGT to Type 2 diabetes

A genetic predisposition to obesity, through as yet poorly defined genetic abnormalities, combined with environmental factors such as highly calorific diets and sedentary lifestyles, will result in obesity. Obesity is associated with raised leptin levels and insulin resistance, and the latter is particularly true of visceral obesity.[64] Insulin resistance is of essential importance in the development of IGT and Type 2 diabetes. As mentioned earlier, insulin resistance and raised leptin levels have been shown to exist prior to the onset of IGT in susceptible subjects. Fasting insulin levels have also been demonstrated to be higher in non-diabetic members of certain populations at high risk of developing Type 2 diabetes, such as the Pima Indians and Hispanic Americans.[65–67] Elevated leptin levels, with its anti-insulin effects, may contribute to the devel-

opment of insulin resistance, particularly at this stage of normoglycaemia.

Both obesity and Type 2 diabetes have multi-factorial aetiologies. Genetically, both are polygenic, and it is likely that the presence of a number of abnormal genes predispose an individual to either obesity and/or Type 2 diabetes. The β$_3$-adrenergic receptor is expressed in visceral fat and is a regulator of resting metabolic rate, thermogenesis, and lipolysis. A Trp64Arg mutation of the β$_3$-adrenergic receptor has been described and studied in relation to both obesity and Type 2 diabetes. However, studies have failed to demonstrate convincingly a link between this mutation and obesity or Type 2 diabetes.[68–70] Other gene variants studied include UCP2, the human glucose transporter gene (GLUT1), and carboxypeptidase E, all of which have failed to show an association with obesity and Type 2 diabetes.[71–74] The ob gene in humans has also been studied using microsatellite markers but no association has been found.[75]

As has been described, obesity is associated with an increased rate of FFA turnover/unit lean body mass,[76] with greater lipolytic activity and FFA turnover in visceral fat compared with subcutaneous fat. This results in the liver being exposed to higher levels of FFAs, which leads to increasing hepatic and systemic insulin resistance, reduced glucose storage, and increased hepatic glucose output, and adversely affects lipid profiles. Under normal circumstances, the liver removes 40% of insulin secreted by the pancreas. Insulin reduces FFA levels by suppressing lipolysis and enhancing FFA re-esterification. Insulin resistance therefore results in a reduced ability to suppress FFA release,[77] with rising FFA levels further impairing insulin sensitivity, thus creating a vicious cycle of events (*Fig. 7.2*). Rising FFA levels may be of particular importance in the post-prandial phase, when FFA levels are usually

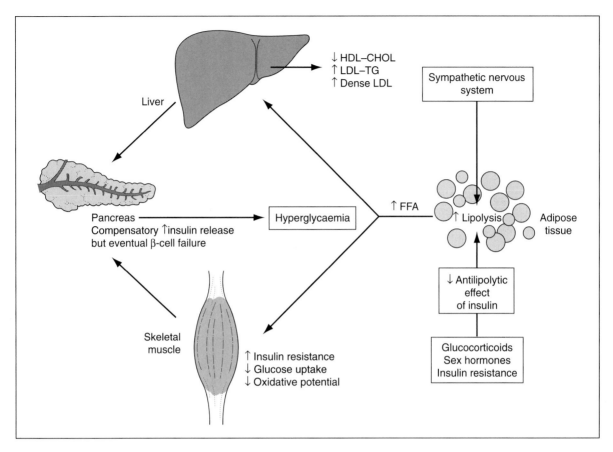

Fig. 7.2
Schematic outline of alterations in metabolic pathways which result in impaired glucose tolerance and, eventually, Type 2 diabetes mellitus. ↑ = increased; ↓ = decreased.

suppressed. At this time, raised FFA levels will impair the utilization of glucose and reduce insulin sensitivity in skeletal muscle. It has been proposed that 25% of insulin's ability to suppress hepatic glucose output is due to a direct effect of insulin via the portal vein, but that most of the effect is explained by an indirect mechanism, partly involving FFAs.[78]

During the stages of normal and impaired glucose tolerance in the presence of insulin resistance, decompensation of glucose control is prevented by pancreatic insulin hypersecretion. Obese individuals with insulin resistance and a normal glucose tolerance achieve normal blood glucose levels during an OGTT, since pancreatic secretion of insulin is able to respond to a state of insulin resistance with compensatory hyperinsulinaemia.[79,80] In obese subjects, and those with subclinical diabetes, weight loss is associated with a reduction in insulin secretion rates, presumably as a result of improvements in insulin sensitivity.[62]

	Normal OGTT in slim	Obese but normal OGTT	IGT	NIDDM
Insulin sensitivity	normal	resistant	resistant	resistant
Insulin production	normal	increased	increased	decreased
Glucose	normal	normal	↑	↑↑

Table 7.1
Features associated with the progression from normal glucose tolerance to IGT and subsequently NIDDM.

At the transition from IGT to Type 2 diabetes, a decline in β-cell production of insulin is seen. Suspected mediators of the decline in β-cell function may include FFAs, triglycerides, amylin (islet amyloid polypeptide, IATP), glucose, and, as discussed, leptin. In rodent models, an excess of triglycerides results in significant triglyceride stores in the islets and subsequent inhibited glucose-induced insulin secretion. This is in part through reduced glucokinase activity in the islets.[81]

Despite a relative reduction in leptin levels and poor β-cell function in poorly controlled Type 2 diabetes, leptin's inhibition of pancreatic insulin secretion in response to a glucose load appears to be of significant importance. Subjects with established Type 2 diabetes show improved β-cell responsiveness to glucose when weight loss is achieved,[62] which may be explained by the accompanying reduction in serum leptin. *Table 7.1* summarizes the progression from obesity to Type 2 diabetes.

References

1. Colditz GA, Willett WC, Stamfer MJ *et al.* Weight as a risk factor for clinical diabetes in women. *Am J Epidemiol* 1990; **132**: 501–513.
2. Wilson PW, Anderson KM, Kannel WB. Epidemiology of diabetes mellitus in the elderly. The Framingham Study. *Am J Med* 1986; **80(5A)**: 3–9.
3. Edelstein SL, Knowler WC, Bain RP *et al.* Predictors of progression from impaired glucose tolerance to Type II diabetes: an analysis of six prospective studies. *Diabetes* 1997; **46**: 701–710.
4. DiBianco R. The changing syndrome of heart failure: an annotated review as we approach the 21st century. *J Hypertens Suppl* 1994; **12(4)**: S73–S87.
5. Eriksson H, Wilhelmsen L, Caidahl K, Svardsudd K. Epidemiology and prognosis of heart failure. *Z Kardiol* 1991; **80 (Suppl 8)**: 1–6.
6. Esmatjes E, Castell C, Gonzalez T *et al.* Epidemiology of renal involvement in Type II diabetics (Type II diabetes) in Catalonia. The Catalan Diabetic Nephropathy Study Group. *Diabetes Res Clin Pract* 1996; **32(3)**: 157–163.
7. Mogensen CE, Poulsen PL. Epidemiology of microalbuminuria in diabetes and in the background population. *Curr Opin Nephrol Hypertens* 1994; **3(3)**: 248–256.
8. Schettler G. Epidemiology and clinical aspects of atherosclerosis. *Langenbecks Arch Chir* 1975; **339**: 153–160.
9. Keller JB. NHLBI workshop panel discussion: a scientific perspective. *Public Health Rep* 1996; **111 (Suppl 2:)** 71–73.
10. Plans P, Tesserras R, Pardell H, Salleras L. Epidemiology of arterial hypertension in the adult population of Cataluna. *Med Clin (Barc)* 1992; **98(10)**: 369–372.

11. Gillum RF. The epidemiology of stroke in Native Americans. *Stroke* 1995; **26**(3): 514–521.

12. Drabo PY. Epidemiological, clinical and evolutive aspects of gout in the internal medicine department at Ouagadougou (Burkina Faso). *Bull Soc Pathol Exot* 1996; **89**(3): 196–199.

13. Sheth SG, Gordon FD, Chopra S. Non-alcoholic steatohepatitis. *Ann Intern Med* 1997; **126**(2): 137–145.

14. Hanis CL, Ferrell RE, Tulloch BR, Schull WJ. Gallbladder disease epidemiology in Mexican Americans in Starr County, Texas. *Am J Epidemiol* 1985; **122**(5): 820–829.

15. Knowler WC, Petit DJ, Saad MF *et al.* Obesity in the Pima Indians: its magnitude and relationship with diabetes. *Am J Clin Nutr* 1991; **53**: 1543S-1551S.

16. McKeigue PM, Pierpoint T, Ferries JE, Marmot MG. Relationship of glucose intolerance and hyperinsulinaemia to body fat pattern in the south Asians and Europeans. *Diabetologia* 1992; **35**: 785–791.

17. Frayn KN, Williams CM, Arner P. Are increased plasma non-esterified fatty acid concentrations a risk marker for coronary heart disease and other chronic diseases? *Clin Sci* 1996; **90**: 243–253.

18. McKeigue PM, Shah B, Marmot MG. Relationship of central obesity and insulin resistance with diabetes prevalence and cardiovascular risk in South Asians. *The Lancet* 1991; **337**: 382–386.

19. Frayn KN, Williams CM, Arner P. Are increased plasma non-esterified fatty acid concentrations a risk marker for coronary heart disease and other chronic diseases? *Clin Sci* 1996; **90**: 243–253.

20. Julve J, Robert MQ, Llobera M, Peinado-Onsurbe J. Hormonal regulation of lipoprotein lipase activity from 5-day-old rat hepatocytes. *Molec Cell Endocrinology* 1996; **116**(1): 97–104.

21. Shimabukuro M, Zhou YT, Levi M, Unger RH. Fatty acid-induced beta cell apoptosis: a link between obesity and diabetes. *Proc Natl Acad Sci USA* 1998; **95**(5): 2498–2502.

22. Brun JF, Bringer J, Raynaud E *et al.* Interrelation of visceral fat and muscle mass in non insulin-dependent diabetes (Type II): practical implications. *Diabete Metab* 1997; **23** (**Suppl 4:**) 16–34.

23. Cigolini M, Smith U. Human adipose tissue in cuture. VIII. Studies on the insulin-antagonistic effect of glucocorticoids. *Metabolism* 1979; **28**: 502–510.

24. Bjorntorp P. Etiology of metabolic syndrome. In: Bray GA, Bouchard C, James WPT, eds. *Handbook of Obesity*. New York: Marcel Dekker, 1998: 573–600.

25. Khaw K-T, Barret-Connor E. Fasting plasma glucose levels and endogenous androgens in non-diabetic postmenopausal women. *Clin Sci* 1991; **80**: 199–203.

26. Xu X, De Pergola G, Bjorntorp P. Testosterone increases lipolysis and the number of beta-adrenoceptors in male rat adipocytes. *Endocrinology* 1991; **128**: 379–382.

27. Rebuffe-Scrive M, Krotkiewski M, Elfverson J, Bjorntorp P. Muscle and adipose tissue morphology and metabolism in Cushing's syndrome. *J Clin Endocrinol Metab* 1998; **67**: 1122–1128.

28. Rebuffe-Scrive M, Anderson B, Olbe L, Bjorntorp P. Metabolism of adipose tissue in intraabdominal depots of non-obese men and women. *Metabolism* 1989; **38**: 453–461.

29. Chen H, Charlat O, Tartaglia LA *et al.* Evidence that the diabetes gene encodes the leptin receptor: identification of a mutation in the leptin receptor gene in db/db mice. *Cell* 1996; **84**(3): 491–495.

30. Sahu A. Evidence suggesting that galanin (GAL), melanin-concentrating hormone (MCH), neurotensin (NT), proopiomelanocortin (POMC) and neuropeptide Y (NPY) are targets of leptin signaling in the hypothalamus. *Endocrinology* 1998; **139**(2): 795–798.

31. Qu D, Ludwig DS, Gammeltoft S *et al.* A role for melanin-concentrating hormone in the central regulation of feeding behavior. *Nature* 1996; **380**: 243–247.

32. Broberger C, Landry M, Wong H *et al.* Subtypes Y1 and Y2 of the neuropeptide Y receptor are respectively expressed in pro-opiomelanocortin- and neuropeptide-Y-containing neurons of the rat hypothalamic arcuate nucleus. *Neuroendocrinology* 1997; **66**(6): 393–408.

33. Tatemoto K, Carlquist M, Mutt V.

Neuropeptide Y. A novel brain peptide with structural similarities to peptide YY and pancreatic polypeptide. *Nature* 1982; **296**: 659–660.

34. Dryden S, Frankish H, Wang Q, Williams G. Neuropeptide Y and energy balance: one way ahead for the treatment of obesity? *Eur J Clin Invest* 1994; **24**: 293–308.

35. Stanley BG, Magdalin W, Seirafi A *et al.* The perifornical area: the major focus of a patchily distributed hypothalamic neuropeptide Y sensitive feeding system(s). *Brain Res* 1993; **604**: 304–317.

36. Moltz JH, McDonald JK. Neuropeptide Y: Direct and indirect action on insulin secretion in the rats. *Peptides* 1985; **6**: 1155–1159.

37. Opara EC, Burch WM, Taylor IL, Akwari OE. Pancreatic hormone response to neuropeptide Y (NPY) perfusion *in vitro. Regul Pept* 1991; **34**: 225–233.

38. Stephens TW, Basinski M, Bristow PK *et al.* The role of neuropeptide Y in the antiobesity action of the obese gene product. *Nature* 1995; 377: 530–532.

39. Schwartz MW, Baskin DG, Bukowski TR *et al.* Specificity of leptin action on elevated blood glucose levels and hypothalamic neuropeptide Y gene expression in ob/ob mice. *Diabetes* 1996; 45: 531–535.

40. Wang Q, Bing C, Al-Barazanji K *et al.* Interactions between leptin and hypothalamic neuropeptide Y neurones in the control of food intake and energy homeostasis in the rat. *Diabetes* 1997; **46**: 335–341.

41. Scarpace PJ, Matheny M, Pollock BH, Tumer N. Leptin increases uncoupling protein expression and energy expenditure. *Am J Physiology* 1997; **273**(1 Pt 1): E226–E230.

42. Liu Q, Bai C, Chen F *et al.* Uncoupling protein-3: a muscle-specific gene upregulated by leptin in ob/ob mice. *Gene* 1998; **207**: 1–7.

43. Qian H, Hausman GJ, Compton MM *et al.* Leptin regulation of peroxisome proliferator-activated receptor-gamma, tumor necrosis factor, and uncoupling protein-2 expression in adipose tissues. *Biochem Biophys Res Comm* 1998; **246**(3): 660–667.

44. Zhou YT, Shimabukuro M, Koyama K *et al.* Induction by leptin of uncoupling protein-2 and enzymes of fatty acid oxidation. *Proc Natl Acad Sci USA* 1997; **94**: 6386–6390.

45. Gong DW, He Y, Karas M, Reitman M. Uncoupling protein-3 is a mediator of thermogenesis regulated by thyroid hormone, beta3–adrenergic agonists, and leptin. *J Biol Chem* 1997; **272**: 24129–24132.

46. Mantzoros CS, Frederich RC, Qu D *et al.* Severe leptin resistance in brown fat deficient uncoupling protein promoter driven diphtheria toxin A mice despite suppression of hypothalamic neuropeptide Y and circulating corticosterone concentrations. *Diabetes* 1998; **47**: 230–238.

47. Kieffer TJ, Heller RS, Habener JF. Leptin receptors expressed on pancreatic beta cells. *Biochem Biophys Res Comm* 1996; **224**: 522–527.

48. Pallett AL, Morton NM, Cawthorne MA, Emilsson V. Leptin inhibits insulin secretion and reduces insulin mRNA levels in rat isolated pancreatic islets. *Biochem Biophys Res Comm* 1997; **238**: 267–270.

49. Muller G, Ertl J, Gerl M, Preibisch G. Leptin impairs metabolic actions of insulin in isolated rat adipocytes. *J Biol Chem* 1997; **272**: 10585–10593.

50. Kulkarni RN, Wang ZL, Wang RM *et al.* Leptin rapidly suppresses insulin release from insulinoma cells, rat and human islets and, *in vivo,* in mice. *J Clin Invest* 1997; **100**: 2729–2736.

51. Baranowska B, Wasilewska-Dziubinska E, Radzikowska M *et al.* Neuropeptide Y, galanin, and leptin release in obese women and in women with anorexia nervosa. *Metab Clin Exp* 1997; **46**: 1384–1389.

52. Dotsch J, Adelmann M, Englaro P *et al.* Relation of leptin and neuropeptide Y in human blood and cerebrospinal fluid. *J Neurol Sci* 1997; **151**: 185–188.

53. Roche C, Boutin P, Dina C *et al.* Genetic studies of neuropeptide Y and neuropeptide Y receptors Y1 and Y5 regions in morbid obesity. *Diabetologia* 1997; **40**: 671–675.

54. Nicklas BJ, Toth MJ, Goldberg AP, Poehlman ET. Racial differences in plasma leptin concentrations in obese postmenopausal women. *J Clin Endocrinol Metab* 1997; **82**: 315–317.

55. Montague CT, Farooqi IS, Whitehead JP *et al.* Congenital leptin deficiency is associated with severe early-onset obesity in humans. *Nature* 1997; **387**: 903–908.

56. Bouchard C, Perusse L, Chagnon YC *et al.*

Linkage between markers in the vicinity of the uncoupling protein 2 gene and resting metabolic rate in humans. *Hum Molec Genet* 1997; **6**: 1887–1889.

57. Cassell PG, Neverova M, Janmohammed S *et al.* A possible association between UCP2 and obesity in a South Indian population. *Int J Obesity* 1998; **22 (Suppl 3)**: S7.

58. Nyholm B, Fisker S, Lund S *et al.* Increased circulating leptin concentrations in insulin-resistant first-degree relatives of patients with non-insulin-dependent diabetes mellitus: relationship to body composition and insulin sensitivity but not to family history of non-insulin-dependent diabetes mellitus. *Eur J Endocrinol* 1997; **136**: 173–179.

59. Zimmet PZ, Collins VR, De Courten MP *et al.* Is there a relationship between leptin and insulin sensitivity independent of obesity? A population-based study in the Indian Ocean nation of Mauritius. Mauritius NCD Study Group. *Int J Obes Relat Metab Disord* 1998; **22**: 171–177.

60. Malmstrom R, Taskinen MR, Karonen SL, Yki-Jarvinen H. Insulin increases plasma leptin concentrations in normal subjects and patients with Type II diabetes. *Diabetologia* 1996; **39**: 993–996.

61. Clement K, Lahlou N, Ruiz J *et al.* Association of poorly controlled diabetes with low serum leptin in morbid obesity. *Int J Obes Relat Metab Disord* 1997; **21**: 556–561.

62. Polonsky KS, Gumbiner B, Ostrega D *et al.* Alterations in immunoreactive proinsulin and insulin clearance induced by weight loss in Type II diabetes. *Diabetes* 1994; **43**: 871–877.

63. Jenkins AB, Markovic TP, Fleury A, Campbell LV. Carbohydrate intake and short-term regulation of leptin in humans. *Diabetologia* 1997; **40**: 348–351.

64. Kissebah AH, Vydelingum N, Murray R. Relation of body fat distribution to metabolic complications of obesity. *J Clin Invest* 1982; **54**: 254–260.

65. Boyko EJ, Keane EM, Marshall JA, Hamman RE. Higher insulin and C-peptide concentrations in Hispanic population at high risk for Type II diabetes. *Diabetes* 1991; **40**: 509–515.

66. Haffner SM, Stern MP, Hazuda HP *et al.* Hyperinsulinaemia in a population at high risk for non-insulin-dependent diabetes mellitus. *New Engl J Med* 1986; **315**: 220–224.

67. Haffner SM. Hyperinsulinaemia as a possible etiology for the high prevalence of non-insulin dependent diabetes in Mexican Americans. *Diabetes Metab* 1987; **13**: 337–344.64.

68. Buettner R, Schaffler A, Arndt H *et al.* The Trp64Arg polymorphism of the beta 3-adrenergic receptor gene is not associated with obesity or type 2 diabetes mellitus in a large population-based Caucasian cohort. *J Clin Endocrin Metab* 1998; **83**: 2892–2897.

69. Silver K, Walston J, Wang Y *et al.* Molecular scanning for mutations in the beta 3-adrenergic receptor gene in Nauruans with obesity and noninsulin-dependent diabetes mellitus. *J Clin Endocrin Metab* 1996; **81**: 4155–4158.

70. Elbein SC, Hoffman M, Barrett K *et al.* Role of the beta 3-adrenergic receptor locus in obesity and noninsulin-dependent diabetes among members of Caucasian families with a diabetic sibling pair. *J Clin Endocrin Metab* 1996; **81**: 4422–4427.

71. Kubota T, Mori H, Tamori Y *et al.* Molecular screening of uncoupling protein 2 gene in patients with noninsulin-dependent diabetes mellitus or obesity. *J Clin Endocrin Metab* 1998; **83**: 2800–2804.

72. Urhammer SA, Dalgaard LT, Sorensen TI *et al.* Mutational analysis of the coding region of the uncoupling protein 2 gene in obese NIDDM patients: impact of a common amino acid polymorphism on juvenile and maturity onset forms of obesity and insulin resistance. *Diabetologia* 1997; **40**: 1227–1230.

73. Baroni MG, D'Andrea MP, Capici F *et al.* High frequency of polymorphism but no mutations found in the GLUT1 glucose transporter gene in NIDDM and familial obesity by SSCP analysis. *Hum Genet* 1998; **102**: 479–482.

74. Utsunomiya N, Ohagi S, Sanke T *et al.* Organization of the human carboxypeptidase E gene and molecular scanning for mutations in Japanese subjects with NIDDM or obesity. *Diabetologia* 1998; **41**: 701–705.

75. Stirling B, Cox NJ, Bell GI *et al.* Identification of microsatellite markers near the human ob gene and linkage studies in NIDDM-affected sib pairs. *Diabetes* 1995; **44**: 999–1001.

76. Campbell PJ, Carlson MG, Nurjhan N. Fat

metabolism in human obesity. *Am J Physiol* 1994; **266**: E600–E605.

77. Coppack SW, Evans RD, Fisher RM *et al.* Adipose tissue metabolism in obesity: lipase action *in vivo* before and after a mixed meal. *Metabolism* 1992; **41**: 264–272.

78. Bergman RN. New concepts in extracellular signaling for insulin action: the single gateway hypothesis. *Recent Prog Hormone Res* 1997; **52**: 359–385.

79. Golay A, Felber J-P. Evolution from obesity to diabetes. *Diabetes Metab* 1994; **20**: 3–14.

80. Lemieux S, Despres JP. Metabolic complications of visceral obesity: contribution to the aetiology of Type 2 diabetes and implications for prevention and treatment. *Diabetes Metab* 1994; **20**: 375–393.

81. Man ZW, Zhu M, Noma Y *et al.* Impaired beta-cell function and deposition of fat droplets in the pancreas as a consequence of hyper-triglyceridemia in OLETF rat, a model of spontaneous Type 2 diabetes. *Diabetes* 1997; **46**: 1718–1724.

8

Diabetic dyslipidemia: metabolic and epidemiological aspects

Francine V van Venrooij, Ronald Stolk, Manuel Castro Cabezas and D Willem Erkelens

Introduction

The burden of vascular disease in diabetes mellitus, both Types 1 and 2, is massive. Type 2 diabetes mellitus in particular carries a high risk of macrovascular disease, which does not differ from atherosclerosis in subjects without diabetes. This macroangiopathy does not only lead to cardiovascular diseases such as myocardial infarction and peripheral artery disease, but also increases the severity of other disorders such as renal failure by atherosclerotic renal artery stenosis, and aggravates functional changes such as ischemic cerebral damage on top of metabolic diabetic encephalopathy.

It has been shown that all classical modifiable cardiovascular risk factors (hypertension, smoking, and hyperlipidemia) play a role in the atherogenesis of diabetic patients. It appears that dyslipidemia contributes the most of these three. First, the pathogenesis of Type 2 diabetes and dyslipidemia are interconnected, and it is to be expected that optimal glucose regulation improves dyslipidemia. Secondly, options for modification of dyslipidemia with the aim to reduce atherosclerotic events are available. In this respect, the outcome of the United Kingdom Prospective Diabetes Study (UKPDS) is important. Since intensive blood glucose control and intensive hypertension treatment influence microangiopathic complication much more than they do macroangiopathic complications, lipid modification remains a potentially successful alternative for atherosclerosis prevention.

In this chapter on diabetic dyslipidemia we set out to look at dyslipidemia from two apparently different angles, that is: metabolism and epidemiology; metabolism to stress the unique lipoprotein modifying mechanisms in diabetes, and epidemiology to support widely applicable therapeutic options.

In the end these two subjects converge: they supply the knowledge and understanding of the metabolic background for the lipoprotein abnormalities that are observed in diabetes mellitus.

Metabolism of diabetic dyslipidemia

Hypertriglyceridemia

Hypertriglyceridemia is the key characteristic of diabetic dyslipidemia (*Table 8.1*).[1-5] Insulin resistance seems to be the common basis, although many mechanisms may contribute to hypertriglyceridemia. Free fatty acid (FFA) release from the adipose tissue is effectively

Table 8.1
Diabetic dyslipidemia.

VLDL-C ↑, VLDL-TG ↑
Plasma triglyceride ↑
HDL-C ↓
Lipoprotein lipase subnormal
Hepatic lipase ↑
Small dense LDL ↑
HDL_3–C > HDL_2–C

suppressed by insulin in non-diabetics. This mechanism is impaired in insulin resistance. Overproduction of very-low-density lipids (VLDL) may occur, caused by the increased flux of FFAs to the liver (*Fig. 8.1*). The resulting raised plasma triglyceride concentrations can be explained by an increased hepatic VLDL production and impaired catabolism of these triglyceride-rich (TG-rich) particles. The defect in VLDL-triglyceride metabolism is, in part, a consequence of subnormal lipoprotein lipase (LPL) activity in the adipose tissue of diabetic patients.[6] Acute insulin infusion in non-diabetics suppresses effectively the production of large $VLDL_1$ particles in the liver, with no effect on $VLDL_2$ particles, leading to decreased secretion of VLDL.[7] $VLDL_1$ suppression by insulin in diabetic patients may be impaired,[8] increasing hypertriglyceridemia.

Hypertriglyceridemia contributes to abnormalities in the composition of LDLs and high-density lipoproteins (HDLs).[4,9] The increased residence time of TG-rich particles allows for a longer exposure to the action of cholesterol ester transfer protein (CETP), facilitating the transfer of cholesterol from HDL and LDL to VLDL, and chylomicrons in exchange for triglyceride. Thus, in the presence of any increased concentration of TG-rich lipoproteins, exchange of triglyceride for cholesterol

ester leads to enrichment of LDL and HDL with triglyceride, while remnants of triglyceride-rich lipoproteins become enriched with cholesteryl esters. Hepatic lipase (HL) is often increased in Type 2 diabetes mellitus,[10] and this enzyme acts not only on VLDL but also on triglyceride-rich LDL and HDL, depleting the particles of triglycerides by hydrolysis. This results in both dense, small LDL and dense, small HDL_3 particles in the circulation.

Hypertriglyceridemia may have further atherogenic and thrombogenic effects besides its contribution to an atherogenic lipid profile. It may cause endothelial cell dysfunction in the artery wall,[11] stimulating the recruitment of macrophages in the subendothelium. Hypertriglyceridemia may promote the synthesis of thrombogenic mediators, suppressing local plasmin synthesis and accelerating intra-arterial fibrin deposition.[1,12,13]

Modified LDL and HDL

The predominance of small, dense LDL particles is associated with the risk of myocardial infarction and coronary artery disease (CAD) in the general population.[14,15] The density pattern has been called pattern B, in contrast to pattern A of large bouyant LDL. Austin *et al.* suggested that LDL size is partly genetically determined. Prevailing triglyceride levels seem to have a strong environmental influence on LDL size.[16–18] Serum triglyceride levels are the major determinant of LDL size when raised above 1.7 mmol/l, and facilitate the formation of small, dense LDL as described above (*Fig. 8.2*).[19]

A preponderance of small, dense LDL is associated with insulin resistance; serum triglyceride concentration increases this association.[20–23] In diabetic subjects there is a two-fold increase in pattern B (*Fig. 8.3*),[23] and this aspect is more pronounced in women than in men.[24,25] Small, dense LDL particles are more

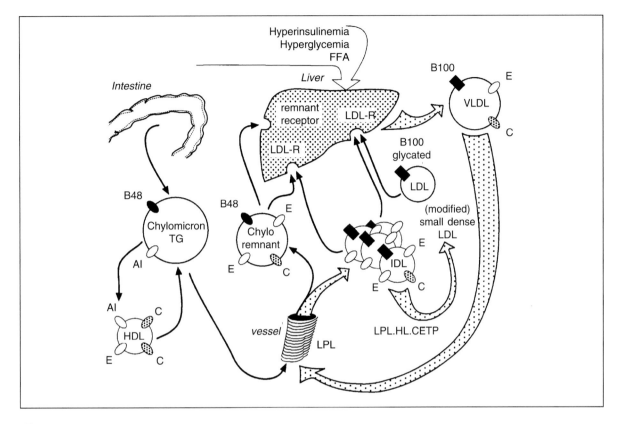

Fig. 8.1

Schematic representation of abnormalities in lipoprotein metabolism in Type 2 diabetes mellitus. Hepatic overproduction of VLDL particles is promoted by increased supply of glucose, FFAs and lipoprotein remnants. Chronic hyperinsulinemia has lost the inhibitory tone on VLDL secretion. Increased competition occurs between VLDL and chylomicrons in the common lipolytic pathway at the level of lipoprotein lipase. Suboptimal lipolysis occurs as a result of low LPL activity or mass, increased inhibitory action of FFA and, possibly, glycation of apo C-II. Delayed elimination of chylomicron remnants may result from increased competition with VLDL remnants (IDL), decreased expression of remnant receptors, and impaired interaction with hepatic receptors (decreased ligand properties of LPL and glycation of apo E). Increased production of atherogenic cholesterolester-enriched remnants and small dense LDL results from the prolonged residence time in the circulation. Relative cholesterol depletion and TG enrichment of HDL particles is due to increased cholesterolester transfer activity.

easily oxidized and may contain less antioxidant.[26-29] This enhanced susceptibility to oxidation may be related to the fatty acid composition of LDL.[30]

Another important modification of LDL in diabetes is glycation.[31,32] The presence of elevated blood glucose levels causes apolipoprotein B molecules to become glycated at the lysine residues, which are located exactly in the binding domain of apo B_{100}. The interaction between apo B_{100} and the LDL receptor is inhibited, forcing LDL into an alternative

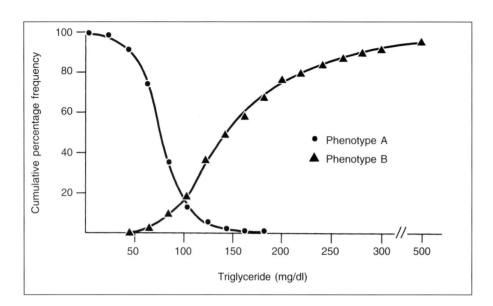

Fig. 8.2
Variation in triglyceride level corresponds to LDL pattern. (Adapted from Austin et al., with permission.[16a])

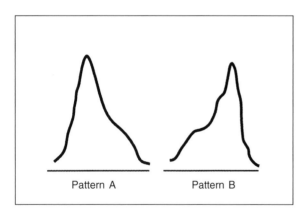

Fig. 8.3
LDL profile by gradient gel electrophoresis. (Adapted from M.A. Austin, with permission.)

catabolic pathway.[33] Free radical formation is induced by glycation and increases susceptibility of LDL to oxidation, a process that has been been called 'glycoxidation'.[34]

The composition of LDL in Type 2 diabetics shows an increase in the cholesteryl ester (CE) to free cholesterol (FC) ratio. Net mass CE

transfer is accelerated.[35] This abnormal LDL has impaired capacity to downregulate cellular cholesterol synthesis.[36]

Normally LDL is removed from the circulation by the LDL receptor that recognizes apo B_{100} as a ligand. Modified LDL particles, by size, oxidation or glycation, are thought to be poor ligands for the receptor, resulting in enhanced removal by the non-receptor-mediated pathway.[37] This scavenger pathway is thought to be 'activated' in the diabetic state, clearing modified LDL at a high rate and thus accumulating intracellular cholesterol in an unregulated way. The scavenger pathway does not downregulate *de novo* synthesis of cholesterol in the cell, nor is the scavenger receptor downregulated by cellular cholesterol accumulation.[38]

Particle size and lipoprotein concentration are important factors for clearance of lipoproteins into the arterial wall. Small LDL particles enter the arterial wall at a faster rate,[39] and the interaction with arterial wall proteoglycans is enhanced.[40,41] Massive storage of cholesterol in the cell leads to the transition of macrophages to lipid-loaded foam cells that in turn promote the various stimuli that trigger the formation of atherosclerotic plaques.

Low HDL cholesterol levels are closely associated with hypertriglyceridemia.[9] Since LPL activity is decreased and lipolysis is impaired in Type 2 diabetes, fewer surface remnants become available to create nascent HDL particles. In addition, the HDL particles become enriched in triglyceride due to the prolonged exposure to CETP.[42] The triglyceride-enriched HDL is cleared faster from the circulation than normal HDL. Both mechanisms may lead to a lower absolute number of circulating HDL particles.[9]

Cholesterol efflux is impaired in Type 2 diabetes.[43] High HL activity hydrolyses the triglycerides in the HDL core, which causes small, dense HDL_3 to predominate at the expense of the larger and cholesteryl-ester-rich HDL_2. Phospholipid transfer protein (PLTP) may be lowered in diabetes. PLTP promotes the conversion of nascent HDL into larger HDL_2 particles.[44] HDL, in particular HDL_2, is associated with less atherosclerotic manifestations in epidemiological surveys. Small HDL_3 particles are lipid poor compared with larger particles. The implication is that HDL particles are lipid depleted in CAD (HDL_3), and thus less efficient vehicles of reverse cholesterol transport.[42] The smaller particle also appears to affect binding with the major HDL protein, apo A-I, in a negative way. Apo A-I dissociates from the smaller, lipid-poor HDL and is filtered by the kidney.[9] A low level of lipoproteins containing both apo A-I and apo A-II (LpA-I:A-II) has been reported as the most significant lipoprotein marker of CAD among Type 2 diabetic men.[45] Low levels of apo A-I have been measured in well-controlled male diabetic patients.[46] In subjects without diabetes, a high level of LpA-I particles is considered an important protective factor against CAD.[47]

Post-prandial dyslipidemia

In most studies on plasma lipids and lipoproteins as risk factors for atherosclerosis, plasma is analysed after an overnight fast. At this time, abnormalities in post-prandial lipoprotein metabolism cannot be detected. This is unfortunate, since humans are in the non-fasting state during most of their lives. The post-prandial state can be considered as an atherogenic condition, characterized by elevated concentrations of remnant particles.[48–50] Post-prandial hyperlipidemia is exaggerated in the insulin-resistant state.[51]

After each meal, the intestine synthesizes chylomicrons (with apo B_{48} as structural protein) which are converted into chylomicron remnants by the action of LPL. At the same time, the liver produces VLDLs (containing apo B_{100} as structural protein) which compete with chylomicrons for the action of LPL, the so-called 'common metabolic pathway of triglyceride-rich particles'.[52] This competition between TG-rich particles may lead to enhanced post-prandial lipemia in conditions like Type 2 diabetes mellitus in which overproduction of VLDL is occurring.

Hydrolysis of VLDLs by LPL results in the formation of intermediate-density lipoproteins (IDLs), which are further converted into LDLs by hepatic lipase. Since chylomicrons are the preferred substrate for LPL, the relative clearance defect of VLDLs occurs in the post-prandial period.

In Type 2 diabetes, decreased clearance of VLDLs may be impaired due to decreased LPL activity,[53] but changed composition of VLDLs may also play a role.[54] In general, VLDLs in Type 2 diabetes are large and triglyceride enriched, with increased concentrations of apo C and apo E. A shift in the apo C to apo E ratio may result in decreased uptake by the liver, mediated by allosteric hindrance with hepatic receptors. It is still not clear whether prolonged post-prandial lipemia in diabetes is a consequence of competition for the same removal mechanisms between VLDL and chylomicrons, or whether diabetes *per se* affects chylomicron clearance directly.[6,52,55,56] For example, Lewis *et al.* found that post-prandial lipemia was enhanced in Type 2 diabetic subjects only if fasting hypertrigly-ceridemia was present.[57] In contrast, Syvänne *et al.* have shown that post-prandial lipemia in well-controlled diabetic patients with relatively normal fasting plasma triglyceride concentrations is significantly enhanced in comparison with matched controls without diabetes.[56] These authors found that post-prandial lipemia could not discriminate between diabetic patients *with* and those *without* CAD. Therefore, the relationship between post-prandial lipemia and coronary artery disease in Type 2 diabetes is still not settled, and future studies should address this issue.

Decreased clearance of TG-rich particles may lead to modified lipoproteins in the circulation which may easily become trapped in the subendothelial space. These 'trapped' remnants interact with proteoglycans and finally are avidly taken up by monocytes and macrophages, resulting in foam cells and, therefore, the initiation of the atherosclerotic plaque.[58] Chylomicron remnants *in vitro* are especially effective in increasing cholesterol esterification and cholesterol ester accumulation in cells.[59]

A different consequence of increased residence time of remnants in the circulation is the enhanced opportunity to interact with other lipoproteins by the action of CETP[60] and PLTP.[61] Modifications of LDLs and HDLs may have profound effects on the metabolism of these lipoproteins. For example, modified HDL particles may result in decreased binding to the HDL receptor, as demonstrated by Bierman and co-workers,[59] and thereby in impaired

ability to act as a cholesterol acceptor. Moreover, glycation of collagen in diabetes may also play an important role in binding potentially atherogenic lipoproteins,[62] and this may be enhanced, especially in the post-prandial state, when chylomicron remnants traverse through the vascular wall.[63]

Impaired glycemic control is associated with hyperlipidemia that is already present in the fasting state. Since fasting triglyceride concentrations largely influence post-prandial lipemia,[1,6,52,57] uncontrolled diabetes is associated with enhanced post-prandial lipemia. Therefore, improved metabolic control usually improves fasting and post-prandial lipemia in Type 2 diabetes. Therapeutic options for modulating post-prandial lipemia are in the first place dietary interventions and lifestyle modifications, as recommended by several authors (for review see refs. 1 and 6). Pharmacological interventions with sulfonyl-ureum derivatives, metformin, acarbose, insulin, fibrates, and HMG-CoA reductase inhibitors have been shown to improve post-prandial lipemia.[1,6,51,64] At present, it is not known whether improved post-prandial lipemia in Type 2 diabetes will result in prolonged survival or decreased morbidity.

The atherogenic lipoprotein phenotype as expressed above in diabetic patients carries a high risk of premature cardiovascular risk.[65] Studies in insulin-resistant people have shown that the atherogenic lipoprotein phenotype already exists in the prediabetic state.[66,67] The risk of total cholesterol level for CAD is strongly influenced by the prevailing levels of HDL and triglycerides. Low HDL and high triglyceride concentrations add up to a high cholesterol level as risk factors. The presence of high triglyceride levels and low HDL cholesterol levels in diabetic patients elevates the risk for atherosclerotic events even when total cholesterol levels are between 5.0 and

6.5 mmol/l. Treatment strategy in diabetic patients thus should aim at aggressive triglyceride lowering to slow exchange of lipids by CETP and to increase HDL formation, even in patients with total cholesterol levels in the normal range for subjects without diabetes.[4,65,66]

Epidemiology of diabetic dyslipidemia

Cardiovascular disease and risk factors

The leading cause of morbidity and mortality in patients with diabetes mellitus is cardiovascular disease (CVD).[68] Especially in diabetes mellitus Type 2, these so-called macrovascular complications are more important than the 'typical' diabetic or microvascular complications (retinopathy, nephropathy, and neuropathy). The age-adjusted relative risk of death from CVD for diabetic patients ranges from 1.5 to 4, depending on the definitions used.[69] The incidence of fatal and non-fatal CVD events are two to 20 times higher in diabetic patients compared with subjects without diabetes of the same age. This difference decreases with increasing age. In addition, the prognosis of CVD is worse in diabetic patients.[68]

Diabetes, or hyperglycemia, is usually accompanied by other metabolic cardiovascular risk factors in the same patient. This clustering of risk factors has been referred to as Syndrome X,[70] the deadly quartet,[71] and the insulin-resistance syndrome.[72] Risk factors involved in this clustering are, among others, raised glucose and insulin, lowered HDL cholesterol, raised triglycerides, increased PAI-1, raised factor VII and fibrinogen levels, obesity, increased abdominal fat, and hypertension. Several studies have found that dyslipi-

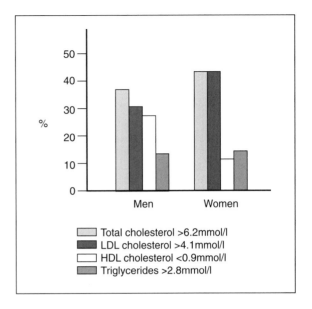

Fig. 8.4
Prevalence of dyslipidemia in diabetes mellitus Type 2. Age: 20–74 years. Second National Health and Nutrition Examination Survey, 1976–1980.

demia is more severe in women than in men with diabetes.[73,74] This difference is already present in newly diagnosed patients. At the baseline examination of the UKPDS, a study in more than 3,800 patients with newly diagnosed diabetes mellitus Type 2, the mean total cholesterol levels in men and women were 5.5 mmol/l (SD 1.1) and 5.8 (SD 1.2), HDL-cholesterol levels were 1.01 mmol/l (SD 0.24) and 1.09 (SD 0.25), whereas the geometric mean of triglycerides was 1.8 mmol/l (1 SD interval 1.1–3.1) and 1.8 (SD 1.1–2.9), respectively.[73] *Fig. 8.4* presents the prevalence of dyslipidemia in patients with diabetes mellitus Type 2 from the population-based NHANES II.[75] This gender difference is in accordance with the greater risk of CVD in women with diabetes than in diabetic men.[68,76]

Variable	Cut point upper tertile	Hazard ratio
LDL cholesterol	3.89 mmol/l	2.26 (1.70–3.00)
HDL cholesterol	1.15 mmol/l	0.55 (0.41–0.73)
HbA1c	7.5%	1.52 (1.15–2.01)
Systolic blood pressure	142 mmHg	1.82 (1.34–2.47)
Smoking	current	1.41 (1.06–1.88)

Values are hazard ratios with the 95% confidence interval for the upper tertile, adjusted for all other variables, age, and gender.

Table 8.2
Risk for coronary artery disease in the 3,055 newly diagnosed diabetes patients in the UKPDS.[80]

Risk of dyslipidemia

The importance of hyperglycemia for the development of microvascular complications has been shown in both observational and intervention studies in patients with diabetes mellitus.[77,78] A number of follow-up studies did not find a relationship between glycemia or duration of diabetes and the incidence of CVD. Also, the recently completed UKPDS, a randomized trial aiming to intensify glucose control in patients with newly diagnosed diabetes mellitus Type 2, did not find that intensive glucose lowering decreased the incidence of atherosclerotic diseases or mortality.[78] Indeed, several authors have challenged the accepted association between hyperglycemia and CVD.[69,79]

In contrast, the roles of the 'classical' CVD risk factors do not differ between diabetic and non-diabetic subjects. The risk factors for the incidence of coronary artery disease during 10 years of follow-up in the UKPDS are given in *Table 8.2*.[80] In the univariate analyses, triglycerides were also significantly associated with coronary artery disease, but due to the strong correlation with HDL cholesterol it was not included in the final multivariate model. In this study the strongest risk factor in patients with newly diagnosed diabetes was LDL cholesterol, similar to the general population. However, as discussed previously, in diabetes patients LDL cholesterol may be more pathogenic, owing to the presence of small dense lipoprotein particles and (glyc)oxidation. Also, the 12-year follow-up of diabetic subjects screened for the MRFIT study indicated that similar risk factors predict CVD in subjects with and without diabetes.[81]

Only a few follow-up studies have been published in which a more extensive assessment of lipids and lipoprotein fractions was performed at baseline.[82] In the Paris Prospective Study, the strongest predictor for the incidence of cardiovascular disease during the follow-up period of 11 years in subjects with glucose intolerance (impaired glucose tolerance or diabetes) was the triglyceride level.[2] Patients with triglycerides higher than 1.5 mmol/l had a relative risk of 3.3 ($p < 0.01$). However, HDL cholesterol was not measured in this study. A follow-up study among 313 diabetic patients in East Finland showed that low HDL cholesterol, mainly the HDL_2 fraction, and high triglycerides were the only independent risk factors for the incidence of coronary heart disease after 7 years.[83] Low HDL (<0.9 mmol/l) was associated with a relative risk of 3.9 ($p < 0.001$), whereas the

Study	Number	LDL lowering (%)	CVD decrease (%)
4S[88]	202	38	55 ($p < 0.01$)
CARE[89]	586	27	25 ($p < 0.05$)
Helsinki Heart Study[90]	135	61	60 (NS)

Table 8.3
Lipid-lowering trials reporting on diabetic patients.

relative risk of a higher concentration of triglycerides (>2.3 mmol/l) was 2.2 ($p = 0.001$). A consistent finding in all follow-up studies is that total cholesterol is not an independent risk factor for CVD in diabetic patients, after adjustment for triglycerides.[5] Therefore, triglyceride level is a stronger predictor of future CVD in diabetes than is total cholesterol. HDL cholesterol may be a more powerful predictor, but there are only limited data available on this association.

Lipid lowering in diabetes

Nutritional intervention is recommended as the first step in the treatment of diabetic dyslipidemia.[84] The current recommendations suggest weight loss and decreased consumption of saturated fats, which are similar to the recommendations for non-diabetics with dyslipidemia. Usually lifestyle interventions are not sufficient to lower adequately serum lipid levels. There are a number of different drugs available to treat dyslipidemia. All types of medication have been shown to lower effectively serum levels of cholesterol and triglycerides in patients with diabetes.[85] Today the recommended drugs are HMG-CoA reductase inhibitors (statins) to lower LDL cholesterol and fibrates for the treatment of elevated triglycerides. However, the ultimate goal of using these drugs is not to lower serum lipids,

but to reduce the incidence of CVD and death, which might be beyond the effect on cholesterol.[86]

Currently, a number of clinical trials to study the effect of lipid lowering on the incidence of CVD are being conducted in diabetic patients. It will take a few years before these results become available. However, the study populations of some large clinical trials have included patients with diabetes mellitus. The reported results on these subgroups are summarized in *Table 8.3*.

The Scandinavian Simvastatin Survival Study (4S study) is a secondary prevention trial in patients with a history of myocardial infarction. Total cholesterol had to be between 5.5 and 8.0 mmol/l at baseline, and serum triglycerides lower than or equal to 2.5 mmol/l. The study included 4,444 subjects, who were followed for an average period of 5.4 years.[87] In a *post-hoc* analysis, the effect of lipid lowering in the 202 patients with diabetes mellitus was investigated.[88] This is the first study to show a reduction of the risk of new cardiovascular events by lipid lowering in diabetic patients. Owing to the exclusion criteria, these patients are not representative of diabetic patients in the general population. However, the risk in the placebo group was still 1.7 times higher in those with diabetes than in those without. The reduction in risk of coronary heart disease death or non-fatal myocardial infarction was 55% (95% confidence interval

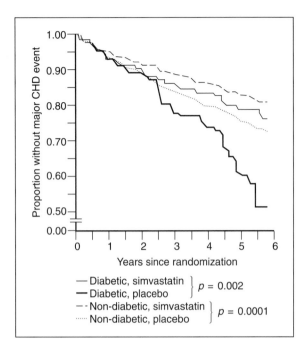

Fig. 8.5
Kaplan–Meier survival curves for the possibility of remaining free of a major CHD event during follow-up in non-diabetic and diabetic patients treated with placebo or simvastatin in the 4S study. (Adapted from Pyörälä et al.,[88] with permission from the authors.)

(CI) 24–73%), which was greater than the reduction in the non-diabetic population (32%, 95% CI 23–40%). In *Fig. 8.5*, the corresponding Kaplan–Meier curves are given. Also, the reduction of total mortality was greater in the diabetic subgroup, although this did not reach statistical significance due to the small number (*n* = 29): 43% (95% CI –8–70%) *vs* 29% (95% CI 13–42%).

The other published secondary prevention trial using a statin (pravastatin) is the CARE study (Cholesterol and Recurrent Events trial).[89] The total study population was 4,159 patients, including 586 patients with diabetes mellitus. The reduction of fatal or non-fatal

coronary heart disease was 25% in subjects with diabetes (95% CI 0–43%), which was similar to the results in the whole study population (24%, 95% CI 9–36%). The authors hypothesized that the smaller effect observed in CARE compared with that in the the 4S study was due to the lower baseline LDL levels in CARE. The reduction of LDL was also lower (28 *vs* 34%), which might be related to the differences at baseline.

The Helsinki Heart Study is a primary prevention trial with gemfibrozil. The study population included 135 men with diabetes mellitus.[90] The risk of CVD was reduced with 60%, but this did not reach statistical significance. In the two recently completed primary prevention trials with statins, the West of Scotland Coronary Prevention Study and Air Force/Texas Coronary Atherosclerosis Prevention Study,[91,92] diabetes was an exclusion criterium.

Conclusion

Both metabolic aspects and epidemiology support the notion that hyperlipidemia is a key risk factor for macroangiopathic damage in diabetes mellitus. Dyslipidemia is present in almost all patients with Type 2 diabetes mellitus, usually in combination with other cardiovascular risk factors ('insulin resistance syndrome'). The increased residence time of intestinal- and liver-derived lipoproteins with its metabolic sequelae, low HDL cholesterol, and small, dense LDL aggravate the hyperglycemic intoxication of the vascular wall. Glycation is in this a unique feature of diabetic dyslipidemia. As it were, the diabetic patient is in a continuous post-prandial state with respect to lipid metabolism.

It is of note that at this moment lipid reduction is a reasonably effective tool for reducing the risk of cardiovascular events. The results of intervention studies have shown that lipid lowering is associated with a decreased risk of cardiovascular events. Therefore, adequate management of dyslipidemia may be at least as important as strict glycemic control in diabetic patients.

It is expected that through better understanding of the pathophysiologic mechanisms and treatment options, diabetic dyslipidemia can be diagnosed and treated with the sole aim of reducing the atherosclerotic events in this particularly vulnerable, large patient group.

References

1. Lewis GF, Steiner G. Hypertriglyceridemia and its metabolic consequences as a risk factor for atherosclerotic cardiovascular disease in non-insulin-dependent diabetes mellitus. *Diabetes Metab Rev* 1996; **12**: 37–56.
2. Fontbonne A, Eschwege E, Cambien F *et al.* Hypertriglyceridaemia as a risk factor of coronary heart disease mortality in subjects with impaired glucose tolerance or diabetes. Results from the 11-year follow-up of the Paris Prospective Study. *Diabetologia* 1989; **32**: 300–304.
3. Assmann G, Schulte H. The prospective cardiovascular Münster (PROCAM) study: Prevalence of hyperlipidemia in persons with hypertension and/or diabetes mellitus and the relationship to coronary heart disease. *Am Heart J* 1988; **116**: 1713–1724.
4. Taskinen MR, Lahdenperä S, Syvänne M. New insights into lipid metabolism in non-insulin-dependent diabetes mellitus. *Ann Med* 1996; **28**: 335–340.
5. Syvänne M, Taskinen MR. Lipids and lipoproteins as coronary risk factors in non-insulin-dependent diabetes mellitus. *Lancet* 1997; **350** (**Suppl 1**): SI20–S123.
6. De Man FH, Cabezas MC, Van Barlingen HH *et al.* Triglyceride-rich lipoproteins in non-insulin-dependent diabetes mellitus: post-prandial metabolism and relation to premature atherosclerosis. *Eur J Clin Invest* 1996; **26**: 89–108.
7. Malmström-R, Packard CJ, Caslake MJ *et al.* Effects of Insulin and acipimox on VLDL1 and VLDL2 apolipoprotein B production in normal subjects. *Diabetes* 1998; **47**: 779–787.
8. Malmström-R, Packard CJ, Caslake MJ *et al.* Defective regulation of triglyceride metabolism by insulin in the liver in NIDDM. *Diabetologia* 1997; **40**: 454–462.
9. Ginsberg HN. Diabetic dyslipidaemia: basic mechanisms underlying the common hypertriglyceridemia and low HDL cholesterol levels. *Diabetes* 1996; **45** (**Suppl 3**): S27–S30.
10. Harno K, Nikkila EA, Kuusi T. Plasma HDL-cholesterol and postheparin plasma hepatic endothelial lipase (HL) activity: relationship to obesity and non-insulin dependent diabetes (NIDDM). *Diabetologia* 1980; **19**: 281.
11. Creager MA, Selwyn A. When 'normal' cholesterol levels injure the endothelium. *Circulation* 1997; **96**: 3255–3257.
12. Mennen LI, Schouten EG, Grobbee DE, Kluft C. Coagulation factor VII, dietary fat and blood lipids: a review. *Thromb Haemost* 1996; **76**: 492–499.
13. Väisänen S, Baumstark MW, Penttilä I *et al.* Small, dense LDL particle concentration correlates with plasminogen activator inhibitor type-1 (PAI-1) activity. *Thromb Haemost* 1997; **78**: 1495–1499.
14. Lamarche B, Tchernof A, Moorjani S *et al.* Small, dense low-density lipoprotein particles as a predictor of the risk of ischemic heart disease in men. Prospective results from the Quebec Cardiovascular Study. *Circulation* 1997; **95**: 69–75.
15. Gylling H, Miettinen TA. Cholesterol absorption and lipoprotein metabolism in type II diabetes mellitus with and without coronary artery disease. *Atherosclerosis* 1996; **126**: 325–332.
16. Lahdenperä S, Syvänne M, Kahri J, Taskinen MR. Regulation of low-density lipoprotein particle size distribution in NIDDM and coronary disease: importance of serum triglycerides. *Diabetologia* 1996; **39**: 453–461.
16a. Austin MA, King MC, Vranizan KM, Krauss RM. Atherogenic lipoprotein phenotype. A proposed genetic marker for coronary heart disease risk. *Circulation* 1990; **82**: 495–506.
17. Stampfer MJ, Krauss RM, Ma J *et al.* A prospective study of triglyceride level, low-density lipoprotein particle diameter, and risk

of myocardial infarction. *JAMA* 1996; **276**: 882–888.

18. Packard CJ, Shepherd J. Lipoprotein heterogeneity and apolipoprotein B metabolism. *Arterioscler Thromb Vasc Biol* 1997; **17**: 3542–3556.

19. Lahdenperä S, Syvänne M, Kahri J, Taskinen MR. Regulation of LDL particle size distribution in NIDDM and coronary disease: importance of serum triglycerides. *Diabetologia* 1996; **39**: 453–461.

20. Reaven GM, Chen YD, Jeppesen J *et al*. Insulin resistance and hyperinsulinemia in individuals with small, dense low density lipoprotein particles. *J Clin Invest* 1993; **92**: 141–146.

21. Tan KCB, Cooper MB, Ling KLE *et al*. Fasting and postprandial determinants for the occurence of small dense LDL species in non-insulin-dependent diabetic patients with and without hypertriglyceridaemia: the involvement of insulin, insulin precursor species and insulin resistance. *Atherosclerosis* 1995; **113**: 273–287.

22. Mykkanen L, Haffner SM, Rainwater DL *et al*. Relationship of LDL size to insulin sensitivity in normoglycemic men. *Arterioscler Thromb Vasc Biol* 1997; **17**: 1447–1453.

23. Feingold KR, Grunfeld C, Pang M *et al*. LDL subclass phenotypes and triglyceride metabolism in non-insulin-dependent diabetes. *Arterioscler Thromb* 1998; **12**: 1496–1502.

24. Caixas A, Ordonez Llanos J, de Leiva A *et al*. Optimization of glycemic control by insulin therapy decreases the proportion of small dense LDL particles in diabetic patients. *Diabetes* 1997; **46**: 1207–1213.

25. Haffner SM, Mykkanen L, Stern MP *et al*. Greater effect of diabetes on LDL size in women than in men. *Diabetes Care* 1994; **17**: 1164–1171.

26. Yoshida H, Ishikawa T, Nakamura H. Vitamin E/lipid peroxide ratio and susceptibility of LDL to oxidative modification in non-insulin-dependent diabetes mellitus. *Arterioscler Thromb Vasc Biol* 1997; **17**: 1438–1446.

27. Fuller CJ, Chandalia M, Garg A *et al*. RRR-alpha-tocopheryl acetate supplementation at pharmacologic doses decreases low-density-lipoprotein oxidative susceptibility but not protein glycation in patients with diabetes mellitus. *Am J Clin Nutr* 1996; **63**: 753–759.

28. Reaven P. Dietary and pharmacologic regimens to reduce lipid peroxidation in non-insulin-dependent diabetes mellitus. *Am J Clin Nutr* 1995; **62**: 1483S-1489S.

29. Nourooz-Zadeh J, Rahimi A, Tajaddini-Sarmadi J *et al*. Relationships between plasma measures of oxidative stress and metabolic control in NIDDM. *Diabetologia* 1997; **40**: 647–653.

30. Dimitriadis E, Griffin M, Owens D *et al*. Oxidation of low-density lipoprotein in NIDDM: its relationship to fatty acid composition. *Diabetologia* 1995; **38**: 1300–1306.

31. Sobenin IA, Tertov VV, Orekhov AN. Atherogenic modified LDL in diabetes. *Diabetes* 1996; **45** (**Suppl 3**): S35–S39.

32. Lyons TJ. Glycation and oxidation: a role in the pathogenesis of atherosclerosis. *Am J Cardiol* 1993; **71**: 26B–31B.

33. Kortlandt W, Benschop C, van Rijn H, Erkelens DW. Glycated low density lipoprotein catabolism is increased in rabbits with alloxan-induced diabetes mellitus. *Diabetologia* 1992; **35**: 202–207.

34. Lopes Virella MF, Virella G. Cytokines, modified lipoproteins, and arteriosclerosis in diabetes. *Diabetes* 1996; **45** (**Suppl 3**): S40–S44.

35. Elchebly M, Porokhov B, Pulcini T *et al*. Alterations in composition and concentration of lipoproteins and elevated cholesteryl ester transfer in non-insulin-dependent diabetes mellitus (NIDDM). *Atherosclerosis* 1996; **123**: 93–101.

36. Owens D, McBrinn S, Collins P *et al*. The effect of low density lipoprotein composition on the regulation of cellular cholesterol synthesis: a comparison in diabetic and non-diabetic subjects. *Acta Diabetol* 1993; **30**: 214–219.

37. Kramer-Guth A, Quaschning T, Galle J *et al*. Structural and compositional modifications of diabetic low-density lipoproteins influence their receptor-mediated uptake by hepatocytes. *Eur J Clin Invest* 1997; **27**: 460–468.

38. Hamilton CA. Low-density lipoprotein and oxidised low-density lipoprotein: Their role in the development of atherosclerosis. *Pharmacol Ther* 1997; **74**: 55–72.

39. Bjornheden T, Babyi A, Bondjers G, Wiklund O. Accumulation of lipoprotein fractions and subfractions in the arterial wall, determined in an *in vitro* perfusion system. *Atherosclerosis* 1996; **123**: 43–56.

40. Anber V, McConnell M, Shepherd J, Packard CJ. Interaction of very-low-density, intermediate-density, and low-density lipoproteins with human arterial wall proteoglycans. *Arterioscler Thromb Vasc Biol* 1997; **17**: 2507–2514.

41. Anber V, Griffin BA, McConnell M *et al.* Influence of plasma lipid and LDL-subfraction profile on the interaction between low density lipoprotein with human arterial wall proteoglycans. *Atherosclerosis* 1996; **124**: 261–271.

42. Syvänne M, Ahola I, Lahdenperä S *et al.* High density lipoprotein subfractions in non-insulin-dependent diabetes mellitus and coronary artery disease. *J Lipid Res* 1995; **36**: 573–582.

43. Syvänne M, Castro G, Dengremont C *et al.* Cholesterol efflux from Fu5AH hepatoma cells induced by plasma of subjects with or without coronary artery disease and non-insulin-dependent diabetes: importance of LpA-I:A-II particles and phospholipid transfer protein. *Atherosclerosis* 1996; **127**: 245–253.

44. Elchebly M, Pulcini T, Porokhov B *et al.* Multiple abnormalities in the transfer of phospholipids from VLDL and LDL to HDL in non-insulin-dependent diabetes. *Eur J Clin Invest* 1996; **26**: 216–223.

45. Syvänne M, Kahri J, Virtanen KS, Taskinen MR. HDLs containing apolipoproteins A-I and A-II (LpA-I:A-II) as markers of coronary artery disease in men with non-insulin dependent diabetes mellitus. *Circulation* 1995; **92**: 364– 370.

46. Cavallero E, Brites F, Delfly B *et al.* Abnormal reverse cholesterol transport in controlled type II diabetic patients. Studies on fasting and postprandial LpA-I particles. *Arterioscler Thromb Vasc Biol* 1995; **15**: 2130–2135.

47. Fruchart J, De Geitere C, Delfly B, Castro G. Apolipoprotein A-I-containing particles and reverse cholesterol transport: evidence for connection between cholesterol efflux and atherosclerosis risk. *Atherosclerosis* 1994; **110**: S35–S39.

48. Cohn JS. Postprandial lipid metabolism. *Curr Opin Lipidol* 1994; **5**: 185–190.

49. Meyer E, Westerveld HT, de Ruyter-Meijstek FC *et al.* Abnormal postprandial apolipoprotein B-48 and triglyceride responses in normolipidemic women with greater than 70% stenotic coronary artery disease. *Atherosclerosis* 1996; **124**: 221–235.

50. Karpe F, Steiner G, Uffelman K *et al.* Postprandial lipoproteins and progression of coronary atherosclerosis. *Atherosclerosis* 1994; **106**: 83–97.

51. Coppack SW. Postprandial lipoproteins in non-insulin-dependent diabetes mellitus. *Diabetic Medicine* 1997; **14**: S67–S74.

52. Brunzell JD, Hazzard WR, Porte DJ, Bierma EL. Evidence for a common, saturable, triglyceride removal mechanism for chylomicrons and very low density lipoproteins in man. *J Clin Invest* 1973; **52**: 1578–1585.

53. Taskinen MR. Lipoprotein lipase in diabetes. *Diabetes Metab Rev* 1987; **3**: 551–570.

54. Howard BV, Howard WJ. Dyslipidaemia in non-insulin-dependent diabetes mellitus. *Endocr Rev* 1994; **15**: 263–274.

55. Howard BV. Lipoprotein metabolism in diabetes. *Curr Opin Lipidol* 1994; **5**: 216–220.

56. Syvänne M, Hilden H, Taskinen MR. Abnormal metabolism of postprandial lipoproteins in patients with non-insulin-dependent diabetes mellitus is not related to coronary artery disease. *J Lipid Res* 1994; **35**: 15–26.

57. Lewis GF, O'Meara NM, Soltys PA *et al.* Fasting hypertriglyceridemia in non-insulin-dependent diabetes mellitus is an important predictor of postprandial lipid and lipoprotein abnormalities. *J Clin Endocrinol Metab* 1998; **72**: 934–944.

58. O'Brien KD, Olin KL, Alpers CE *et al.* Comparison of apolipoprotein and proteoglycan deposits in human coronary atherosclerotic plaques. Colocalization of biglycan with apolipoproteins. *Circulation* 1998; **98**: 519–527.

59. Bierman EL. Atherogenesis in diabetes. *Arterioscler Thromb* 1992; **12**: 647– 656.

60. Dullaart RPF, Groener JEM, Erkelens DW. Cholesteryl ester transfer between lipoproteins. *Nutr Metab* 1991; **14**: 329–343.

61. Riemens SC, van Tol A, Sluiter WJ, Dullaart RPF. Plasma phospholipid transfer protein activity is related to insulin resistance: impaired acute lowering by insulin in obese type II diabetic patients. *Diabetologia* 1998; **41**: 929–934.

62. Brownlee M, Vlassara H, Cerami A. Nonenzymatic glycosylation of products on collagen covalently trap low-density lipoprotein. *Diabetes* 1985; **34**: 938–941.

63. Proctor SD, Mamo JCL. Retention of fluorescent-

labelled chylomicron remnants within the intima of the arterial wall. Evidence that plaque cholesterol may be derived from post-prandial lipoproteins. *Eur J Clin Invest* 1998; **28**: 497–503.

64. Syvänne M, Vuorinen-Markkola H, Hilden H, Taskinen MR. Gemfibrozil reduces postprandial lipemia in non-insulin-dependent diabetes mellitus. *Arterioscler Throm* 1993; **13**: 286–295.

65. Packard CJ. LDL subfractions and atherogenicity: an hypothesis from the University of Glasgow. *Curr Med Res Opin* 1996; **13**: 379–390.

66. Haffner SM. The prediabetic problem: development of non-insulin-dependent diabetes mellitus and related abnormalities. *J Diabetes Complications* 1997; **11**: 69–76.

67. Haffner SM. Management of dyslipidaemia in adults with diabetes. *Diabetes Care* 1998; **21**: 160–178.

68. Wingard DL, Barrett Connor EL. Heart disease and diabetes. In: Harris MI, Cowie CC, Stern MP *et al*. eds. *Diabetes in America*, 2nd edn. Bethesda: US Govt Printing Office, 1995: 429–448.

69. Nathan DM, Meigs JB, Singer DE. The epidemiology of cardiovascular disease in type 2 diabetes mellitus: how sweet it is . . . or is it? *Lancet* 1998; **350** (**Suppl 1**): SI4–SI8.

70. Reaven GM. Banding lecture. Role of insulin resistance in human disease. *Diabetes* 1988; **37**: 1595–1607.

71. Kaplan NM. The deadly quartet. Upper-body obesity, glucose intolerance, hypertriglyceridemia, and hypertension. *Arch Intern Med* 1989; **149**: 1514–1520.

72. Despres JP. Abdominal obesity as important component of insulin-resistance syndrome. *Nutrition* 1993; **9**: 452–459.

73. UKPDS. Plasma lipids and lipoproteins at diagnosis of NIDDM by age and sex. *Diabetes Care* 1997; **20**: 1683–1687.

74. Stolk RP, Pols HA, Lamberts SW *et al*. Diabetes mellitus, impaired glucose tolerance, and hyperinsulinemia in an elderly population. The Rotterdam Study. *Am J Epidemiol* 1997; **145**: 24–32.

75. Cowie CC, Harris MI. Physical and metabolic characteristics of persons with diabetes. In: Harris MI, Cowie CC, Stern MP *et al*. eds.

Diabetes in America, 2nd edn. Bethesda: US Govt Printing Office, 1995: 117–164.

76. Barrett Connor EL, Cohn BA, Wingard DL, Edelstein SL. Why is diabetes mellitus a stronger risk factor for fatal ischemic heart disease in women than in men? The Rancho Bernardo Study. *JAMA* 1991; **265**: 627–631.

77. Klein R, Klein BE, Moss SE *et al*. Glycosylated hemoglobin predicts the incidence and progression of diabetic retinopathy. *JAMA* 1988; **260**: 2864–2871.

78. UKPDS. Intensive blood-glucose control with sulphonylureas or insulin compared with conventional treatment and risk of complications in patients with type 2 diabetes (UKPDS 33). *Lancet* 1998; **352**: 837–853.

79. Barrett-Connor E. Does hyperglycemia really cause coronary heart disease? *Diabetes Care* 1997; **20**: 1620–1623.

80. Turner RC, Millns H, Neil HAW *et al*. Risk factors for coronary aretry disease in non-insulin dependent diabetes mellitus: United Kingdom prospective diabetes study (UKPDS: 23). *Br Med J* 1998; **316**: 823–828.

81. Stamler J, Vaccaro O, Neaton JD, Wentworth D. Diabetes, other risk factors, and 12-yr cardiovascular mortality for men screened in the Multiple Risk Factor Intervention Trial. *Diabetes Care* 1993; **16**: 434–444.

82. Laakso M. Lipids and lipoproteins as risk factors for coronary heart disease in non-insulin-dependent diabetes mellitus. *Ann Med* 1996; **28**: 341–345.

83. Laakso M, Lehto S, Penttila I, Pyorala K. Lipids and lipoproteins predicting coronary heart disease mortality and morbidity in patients with non-insulin-dependent diabetes. *Circulation* 1993; **88**: 1421–1430.

84. Franz MJ, Horton ES, Sr, Bantle JP *et al*. Nutrition principles for the management of diabetes and related complications. *Lancet* 1994; **344**: 1383–1389.

85. Garber AJ, Vinik AI, Crespin SR. Detection and management of lipid disorders in diabetic patients. A commentary for clinicians. *Diabetes Care* 1992; **15**: 1068–1074.

86. Vaughan CJ, Murphy MB, Buckley BM. Statins do more than just lower cholesterol. *Lancet* 1996; **348**: 1079–1082.

87. Scandinavian Simvastatin Survival Study

Group. Randomised trial of cholesterol lowering in 4444 patients with coronary heart disease: the Scandinavian Simvastatin Survival Study (4S). *Lancet* 1994; **344**: 1383–1389.

88. Pyörälä K, Pedersen TR, Kjekshus J *et al.* Cholesterol lowering with simvastatin improves prognosis of diabetic patients with coronary heart disease. A subgroup analysis of the Scandinavian Simvastatin Survival Study (4S). *Diabetes Care* 1997; **20**: 614–620.

89. Goldberg RB, Mellies MJ, Sacks FM *et al.* Cardiovascular events and their reduction with pravastatin in diabetic and glucose-intolerant myocardial infarction survivors with average cholesterol levels. Subgroup analyses in the cholesterol and recurrent events (CARE) trial.

Circulation 1998; **98**: 2513–2519.

90. Koskinen P, Manttari M, Manninen V *et al.* Coronary heart disease incidence in NIDDM patients in the Helsinki Heart Study. *Diabetes Care* 1992; **15**: 820–825.

91. Shepherd J, Cobbe SM, Ford I *et al.* Prevention of coronary heart disease with pravastatin in men with hypercholesterolemia. West of Scotland Coronary Prevention Study Group. *N Engl J Med* 1995; **333**: 1301–1307.

92. Downs JR, Clearfield M, Weis S *et al.* Primary prevention of acute coronary events with lovastatin in men and women with average cholesterol levels: results of AFCAPS/TexCAPS. Air Force/ Texas Coronary Atherosclerosis Prevention Study. *JAMA* 1998; **279**: 1615–1622.

9

Endothelial dysfunction

John Cockcroft and Jonathan Goodfellow

Diabetes: a vascular disease

Until recently, diabetes has been viewed as an essentially endocrine disease. However, although the risk of developing specific complications of diabetes such as retinopathy, nephropathy, and neuropathy is clearly associated with the degree and duration of hyperglycaemia, the relationship of diabetes with macrovascular disease is poorly understood.[1] Atherosclerosis occurs earlier in diabetics, and is both more severe and more generalized than in non-diabetics.[2] This has lead some researchers to consider diabetes as a 'vascular disease' – indeed, diabetes seems to induce 'premature vascular ageing'. Exactly why diabetes should promote atherogenesis is unclear. Some excess risk may be related to the association of diabetes with other risk factors, including hyperlipidaemia and hypertension in the 'metabolic syndrome'.[3] However, there is mounting evidence that disruption of normal endothelial function and increased vascular stiffness may play an important role.[4] In this chapter we will focus on the evidence for endothelial dysfunction associated with diabetes and the methods used for its assessment. We will also review the emerging concept of vascular stiffness and its possible relationship to endothelial dysfunction. Finally we will discuss novel therapeutic strategies for cardiovascular risk reduction in diabetes using endothelial function as a surrogate end-point.

A better understanding of the mechanisms involved in atherogenesis associated with diabetes offers the exciting prospect of reducing cardiovascular mortality and morbidity in this important patient group.

Introduction

Vascular endothelium

The vascular endothelium is a monolayer of cells which lines the entire vascular tree. For many years it was considered to act as a simple semipermeable membrane facilitating the transfer of molecules across the vessel wall. The seminal discovery in 1980 by Furchgott and Zawadski of the obligatory role of the endothelium in the relaxation response to acetylcholine changed our view of the endothelium and heralded an explosion of interest and research into its functions.[5] Furchgott and Zawadski named the dilator produced by the endothelium in response to acetylcholine endothelium-derived relaxing factor (EDRF). EDRF has subsequently been identified as nitric oxide (NO).[6] A number of other vasodilators have since been shown to depend on the integrity of the vascular endothelium for their activity; these include bradykinin[7] and substance P.[8] Over the past 20 years a large number of vasodilator and vasoconstrictor substances produced by the vascular endothelium have been discovered (*Table 9.1*)[9].

Table 9.1

Functions of the vascular endothelium.

Regulation of haemostasis	Regulation of vascular tone	Regulation of cellular growth	Regulation of metabolism
Anti-thrombotic	Vasodilators	Growth inhibitors	General
NO	NO	NO	lipids
PGI_2	PGI_2	TGFb	insulin
TPA	EDHF		plasma proteins
immunoglobulins			
AT III			
thrombomodulin			
ADP			
Pro-thrombotic	Vasoconstrictors	Growth promoters	Vasoactive
vWf	ET-1 & ET-3	ET-1	ProET-1
TXA_2	TXA_2	PDGF	NA
PGH_2	PGH_2	FGF	5HT
ANG II	ANG II	ANG II	ANG I
	EDCF	IL-1	adenine nucleotides
	superoxide	IGF-1	

NO = nitric oxide; PGI_2 = prostacyclin; TPA = tissue plasminogen activator; AT III = antithrombin III; ADP = adenosine diphosphatase; TGFb = tumour growth factor b; vWf = Von Willibrand factor; TXA_2 = thromboxane A_2; PGH_2 = prostaglandin H_2; ANG II = angiotensin II; EDHF = endothelin-derived hyperpolarizing factor; ET-1 and ET-3 = endothelin 1 and 3; EDCF = endothelium-derived constricting factor; PDGF = platelet-derived growth factor; IL-1 = interleukin 1; Pro ET-1 = pro endothelin-1; NA = noradrenaline; 5HT = 5 hydroxytryptamine; ANG I = angiotensin I; IGF = intimal growth factor; FGF = fibroblast growth factor.

L-arginine/NO pathway

An important component of such endothelium-dependent responses consists of Ca^{2+}-dependent stimulation of a constitutive enzyme, endothelial NO synthase (eNOS), which catalyses conversion of L-arginine to L-citrulline and NO.[10] Once synthesized, NO diffuses to the underlying vascular smooth muscle, where it activates soluble guanylate cyclase, leading to a rise in cyclic GMP and relaxation.[11] eNOS can be competitively inhibited using guanidino-substituted analogues of L-arginine such as N^G-monomethyl-L-arginine (L-NMMA).[11] Inorganic nitrates such as sodium nitroprusside can activate the same effector pathway by providing an inorganic source of NO,[12] and their activity is thus not dependent on the functional integrity of the vascular endothelium. Endothelium-derived NO is important in the regulation of basal vascular tone and hence blood pressure,[13,14] and has a number of antiatherogenic actions. Thus, endothelial cells serve not only as a passive barrier to diffusion between the circulating blood and the underlying vascular smooth muscle, but also as

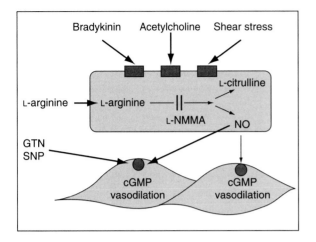

Fig. 9.1

The L-arginine/nitric oxide pathway. Endothelium-dependent vasodilators such as acetylcholine activate a Ca²⁺-dependent constitutive enzyme NO synthase (cNOS) that catalyses conversion of L-arginine to L-citrulline and NO. Once synthesized, NO diffuses to the underlying vascular smooth muscle where it activates soluble guanylate cyclase, leading to a rise in cyclic GMP and relaxation. cNOS can be competitively inhibited using guanidino-substituted analogues of L-argnine such as N^{G}-monomethyl-L-arginine (L-NMMA). Inorganic nitrates such as sodium nitroprusside and organic nitrates such as GTN can activate the same effector pathway by providing a source of NO, and their activity is thus not dependent on the functional integrity of the vascular endothelium.

dynamic modulators of vascular structure and function.[15] The endothelium plays a key role in the regulation of coagulation, lipid transport, immunological reactivity, and vascular tone (*Table 9.1*)[9]. The endothelium participates actively in the regulation of vascular tone both as a sensor and transducer of changes in the circulation and also as a generator of the numerous biological mediators involved. Much interest has therefore focused on the possibility that pathological conditions that are risk factors for cardiovascular disease, including diabetes, hypertension, and hypercholesterolaemia, may involve impairment of the L-arginine/NO pathway. In addition to relaxing vascular smooth muscle, NO also inhibits platelet activation[16] and vascular smooth muscle proliferation,[17] which suggests that impairment of its biosynthesis could predispose to arterial thrombosis and atherosclerosis. The L-arginine/NO pathway may be impaired at a number of sites in cardiovascular disease states. Endothelial dysfunction may lead to a decrease in either basal or stimulated release of NO, or alternatively there may be an increased breakdown of NO. Finally, the underlying vascular smooth muscle may exhibit a decreased sensitivity to the actions of NO. Endothelium-dependent agonists have therefore been widely used to assess the integrity of the L-arginine/NO pathway in a variety of pathological conditions.

The majority of studies assessing endothelial function in human cardiovascular disease have been invasive, involving infusion of endothelium-dependent and independent vasodilators into the coronary or brachial arteries. Recently, non-invasive techniques measuring endothelium-dependent responses to sheer stress have been developed,[18] and studies employing these techniques to investigate endothelial function in cardiovascular disease are reviewed below.

Diabetes mellitus and endothelial dysfunction

Atherosclerosis and microvascular disease are the principal causes of mortality and morbidity in patients with diabetes mellitus.[19–22] Atherosclerosis occurs earlier, and is more severe and widespread in diabetic patients than non-diabetics.[21] It is recognized that the risk of developing the specific complications of diabetes such as retinopathy, nephropathy, and neuropathy is associated with the degree and duration of hyperglycaemia;[1] however, the mechanism(s) underlying the development of macrovascular disease are less well understood. We will briefly review the evidence for vascular endothelial cell dysfunction in diabetic patients and animals.

Animal models of diabetes

It is possible to induce diabetes in experimental animals by selective ablation of the pancreatic beta cells. The commonly used models are the streptozotocin rat and the alloxan rabbit, but there are also some studies using the spontaneously diabetic BB rat. In the vast majority of experiments, investigators have assessed endothelium-dependent relaxation to acetylcholine in large conduit arteries such as aortic ring or strip preparations.

Most studies on diabetic arteries have shown a blunting of the normal relaxation response to acetylcholine.[23-27] This abnormality appears to lie at the level of the endothelium, as responses to nitrovasodilator drugs which act as NO donors were normal. The endothelial abnormality appears not to be a specific muscarinic receptor defect, as responses to histamine and ADP (both non-muscarinic endothelium-dependent agonists) were also abnormal.[23,28] The abnormal relaxation response to acetylcholine may be due to reduced NO synthesis. This mechanism was not directly investigated in the early animal work; however, basal- and acetylcholine-stimulated production of cyclic GMP have been shown to be reduced in diabetic vessels, suggesting reduced NO synthesis.[26] A further possibility is that acetylcholine may stimulate the release of an endothelium-derived constricting factor. Such a mechanism does appear to exist in some,[25] but not all,[23,29] of the animal species studied. Acetylcholine stimulates

release of an endothelium-derived constrictor prostanoid, probably prostaglandin H_2 (PGH_2). The blunted relaxation to acetylcholine can be normalized by cyclooxygenase inhibition or PGH_2/thromboxane A_2 receptor antagonists. The impaired relaxation seen in diabetic vessels may also be normalized by superoxide dismutase, a free radical scavenger, suggesting that PGH_2 acts both as a direct vasoconstrictor and via increased production of superoxide.[30]

Clinical studies

The first evidence of endothelial cell dysfunction in diabetic patients came from an *in vitro* study which demonstrated impaired endothelium-mediated relaxation of penile smooth muscle. The tissue came from insulin-dependent and non-insulin-dependent diabetic patients who had penile implants to treat impotence. Acetylcholine-induced relaxation was blunted in the diabetic patients when compared with non-diabetics. There was no difference between the responses of insulin-dependent and non-insulin-dependent diabetics, and the abnormal response did not correlate with the duration of diabetes. The diabetic patients contained smokers and hypertensives (both independently associated with endothelial dysfunction); however, correcting for these factors did not influence the finding that diabetes was associated with endothelial dysfunction.[31]

Coronary circulation

These investigations are invasive, expensive, and not without risk to the individual. Endothelial function is assessed in the large coronary arteries by measuring diameter changes in response to acetylcholine infusion, and endothelium-independent responses using isosorbide dinitrate or GTN (nitrovasodilators). Coronary vascular reserve (CVR) is used to determine microvascular function; it is the ratio of the coronary artery flow following a maximally vasodilating dose of papaverine (or adenosine) as compared with the resting flow.

One such study in diabetic patients with angiographically normal coronary arteries and normal left ventricular function purported to show impaired coronary vascular reserve and acetylcholine-induced vasodilatation. The diabetic patients in the study comprised six insulin-dependent and five non-insulin-dependent individuals; of these 11 subjects, 10 were treated hypertensives.[32]

Venous occlusion plethysmography

This invasive technique provides an estimation of forearm blood flow and of vascular resistance in the small skeletal muscle arterioles. Endothelium-dependent relaxation has been assessed in several studies in diabetic patients using brachial artery infusions of muscarinic agonists (e.g. acetylcholine, carbachol, or methacholine). The results of these studies in diabetic patients have been variable, and taken at face value present a confusing and apparently contradictory picture.

The studies are briefly described below, taking those involving insulin-dependent diabetic patients first. Halkin *et al.* demonstrated increased basal blood flow and reduced vascular resistance in the diabetic patients, but no abnormality in the response to carbachol or sodium nitroprusside.[33] Smits *et al.* also found no abnormality in the dilator responses.[34] In contrast, Calver *et al.* found a normal response to acetylcholine but a reduced response to sodium nitroprusside.[35] Calver *et al.* also demonstrated a reduced effect of L-NMMA on basal blood flow.[35] Elliot *et al.* reported similar findings, but the abnormal responses were seen only in those diabetic patients with microalbu-

minuria.[36] Finally, Johnstone *et al.* reported abnormal relaxation to methacholine.[37]

In the studies involving non-insulin-dependent diabetic patents, McVeigh *et al.* demonstrated reduced responses to both acetylcholine and GTN, whereas L-NMMA did not influence basal flow in a consistent manner in either diabetic or control subjects.[38]

Some of the variability in the results obtained with venous occlusion plethysmography may be explained by several factors: (1) the choice of muscarinic agonist – this is important as it is now clear that, unlike acetylcholine and carbachol, methacholine does not act via the NO pathway;[39] (2) the length of the forearm is also important in determining the response to acetylcholine, which is rapidly destroyed by cholinesterase;[40] (3) the selection and characterization of diabetic patients is important, e.g. in the study by Elliot *et al.* only those diabetics with microalbuminuria had abnormal responses;[36] and (4) the increased basal blood flow found in diabetics, which may confound the responses to vasoactive drugs.

Therefore, taking the above factors into consideration, the results in insulin-dependent diabetic subjects may be summarized as demonstrating an increased basal blood flow and reduced forearm vascular resistance with normal endothelium-dependent agonist responses and nitrovasodilator responses (apart from Calver *et al.*[35]). There was an impaired vasoconstrictor response to L-NMMA in the diabetic subjects which may be interpreted in one of two ways. There may be reduced NO synthesis in diabetic patients; consequently L-NMMA produces less vasoconstriction because NO-mediated vasodilatation makes less of a contribution to overall forearm vascular tone. Alternatively, NO synthesis may be increased in diabetic patients, thus increasing the amount of L-NMMA required to overcome the dilatation.

In non-insulin-dependent diabetes, the blunted response to acetylcholine suggests either reduced production or release of NO. The reduced response to GTN suggests that the abnormality does not reside solely at the level of the endothelium, and that there may be a selective functional defect in the diabetic vasculature. In the study by McVeigh *et al.* there was no correlation between the blunted responses to acetylcholine and GTN in individual subjects, suggesting the involvement of multiple mechanisms in the abnormal vascular responses to these drugs.[38]

Ultrasonic assessment of flow-mediated dilatation

This technique, which has the advantage of being non-invasive, utilizes the phenomenon of flow-mediated dilatation (FMD). When pulsatile blood flow through an artery is increased, the artery dilates. The phenomenon of FMD has been demonstrated in vessels *in vitro*[41] and *in vivo*,[42] in animals and in humans.[43] FMD has been shown to be an endothelium-dependent phenomenon.[41,42] Shear forces acting via mechanotransduction at the endothelial cell surface stimulate the release of NO, resulting in dilatation. In 1992, Celermajer and colleagues described a simple and elegant method to measure endothelial function in humans.[18] Brachial artery diameter was measured using high-resolution ultrasound under conditions of resting flow, then brachial artery blood flow was increased in order to induce dilatation, the degree of dilatation providing an indication of the functional state of the endothelium. Increased blood flow in the brachial artery was induced by release of a wrist cuff which had been inflated to suprasystolic pressure for 4–5 minutes, thus causing reactive hyperaemia in the hand circulation. The subsequent increase in flow upstream in the brachial artery caused the vessel to dilate, and this was measured using high-resolution ultrasound. Endothelium-independent responses were measured following sublingual glyceryl trinitrate (400 µg). The reproducibility and repeatability of diameter measurements with this technique have been validated.[44] The use of an ultrasonic wall tracking system has further improved the resolution of the diameter measurements, and this technique has also been validated.[45]

Using the latter technique, we have demonstrated in non-insulin-dependent diabetic patients that the normal endothelium-dependent flow-related dilatation and increase in brachial artery distensibility was abolished, whereas the GTN-induced dilatation and increase in distensibility were unimpaired.[46] Clarkson *et al.* have shown impaired FMD in patients with insulin-dependent diabetes and that this impairment correlates with duration of diabetes and also with low density lipoprotein levels.[47] In this study the GTN-induced dilatation was also impaired in diabetics compared with normal subjects.[47]

Arterial stiffness, diabetes mellitus and endothelial function

Cardiovascular disease is the most common cause of death in the diabetic population, and large artery atheromatous disease is a major contributor to the high mortality and morbidity associated with this condition. However, the aetiology and progression of large artery atheromatous disease remains poorly understood. As with other risk factors for cardiovascular disease, diabetes results in increases in arterial stiffness which has been proposed as an important factor both in the initiation and/or progression of atheromatous disease.[4,48] In addition to structural changes, diabetics exhibit abnormalities of endothelial function (as discussed above), resulting in decreased bioavailability of NO, which may also contribute to increased arterial stiffness. Arterial stiffness related to endothelial dysfunction may not only precede clinical evidence of large vessel atheromatous disease, but, unlike arterial stiffness due to structural changes, it is potentially reversible. Current invasive methodologies to assess endothelial function in human vascular beds *in vivo* involve infusion of endothelium-dependent and -independent vasodilators into the coronary or brachial arteries. Interpretation of studies in the coronary vasculature is problematic, since many patients undergoing cardiac catheterization may have coronary artery disease which is not angiographically evident. Perhaps not surprisingly, results of studies using these methodologies have often been conflicting. Techniques such as ultrasonic assessment of FMD, which allow non-invasive, simple, reliable, and reproducible assessment of endothelial function, have the potential to be used in large population studies for detecting endothelial dysfunction and cardiovascular risk at a stage when therapeutic intervention will be of greatest benefit.

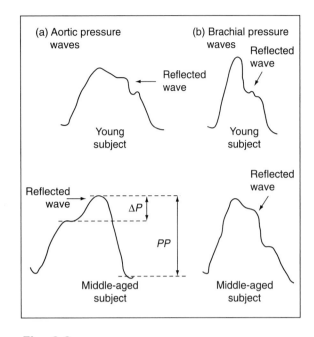

Fig. 9.2

The arterial pressure wave and pulse wave analysis. Schematic representation of arterial pressure waves from (a) ascending aorta and (b) brachial artery. The upper panel depicts wave-forms in a young subject and the lower panel wave-forms in a middle-aged subject. With increasing age, the reflected wave returns earlier from the periphery. In the aorta, this has the effect of increasing systolic pressure, but in the periphery it does not, since it remains in diastole. Augmentation is defined as P/PP, where PP is the pulse pressure and P the difference in height between the first and second systolic peaks. This is normally expressed as a percentage.

Arterial stiffness

Large arteries are compliant structures, and serve to buffer the pressure changes resulting from intermittent ventricular ejection of blood into the aorta. By absorbing a proportion of the energy in systole and releasing it in diastole, peripheral blood flow is smoothed, and diastolic coronary artery flow maintained. Pressure waves are reflected back from the periphery and summate with the forward-going wave to produce the characteristic pressure waveform, the contour of which varies along the vascular tree. Normally, the reflected wave arrives in the central arteries after closure of the aortic valve, and so does not influence central systolic pressure. However, with vascular stiffening, pulse wave velocity (PWV) and the amplitude of the reflected wave both increase, such that the reflected wave arrives earlier and adds to (or augments) central systolic pressure (*Fig. 9.2*). The ratio of this augmentation of central pressure over the pulse pressure is defined as the augmentation index (AIx). These changes are not accurately reflected by conventional sphygmomanometry, because peripheral pressures change much less.[49] This is important as it is central pressure that is the major determinant of left ventricular afterload and the subsequent development of left ventricular hypertrophy,[50,51] which is an independent risk factor for cardiovascular mortality.[52,53] Moreover, increased pressures alter shear stress, accelerating atherogenesis and arteriosclerosis.[4] Such structural changes further increase stiffness, setting up a vicious circle. Interestingly, diabetics have increased left ventricular mass (LVM) compared with non-diabetics, even when correction is made for peripheral blood pressure.[54,55] Increased stiffness leading to higher central pressures may be the mechanism by which diabetes, and other risk factors, predispose to cardiovascular disease.

Pulse wave analysis

O'Rourke and colleagues in Australia have developed the technique of pulse wave analysis (PWA) to record central pressures non-invasively.[56] The system uses the principle of applanation tonometry to record accurately peripheral arterial wave-forms. This involves flattening the curved surface of a pressure-containing structure (such as the radial artery) using a pencil-shaped probe incorporating a micromanometer at its tip (*Fig. 9.3*). When this is achieved, the circumferential stresses in the vessel wall are accurately balanced and the pressure wave-form is accurately recorded. By applying a validated integral transfer function,

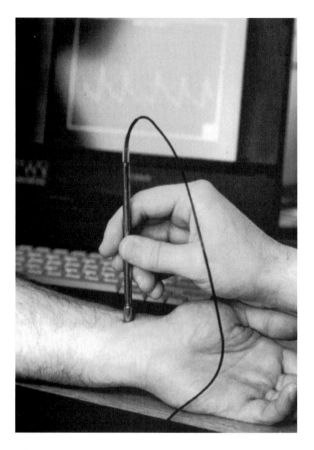

Fig. 9.3
Applanation tonometry. The radial artery is flattened at the wrist using a pencil-shaped probe incorporating a micromanometer at its tip. When this is achieved the circumferential stresses in the vessel wall are accurately balanced and the pressure wave-form is accurately recorded.

the central wave-form can be derived and analysed.[57,58] The derived wave-form is almost identical to that recorded invasively.[57,59] Thus, PWA provides an accurate, non-invasive, easily-applied method with which to measure central pressures and two indices of stiffness: pulse wave velocity (PWV) and AIx.[56] PWA has certain advantages over other techniques which have been applied to assess vascular stiffness.[60] PWV measurements, although a good surrogate marker for vascular stiffness, are only applicable to large arterial segments. Ultrasound techniques[61] are limited by the ability of the operator to image accurately the anterior and posterior walls of the vessel being studied, and thus are only directly applicable to large accessible arteries. It is also an assumption that stiffness determined in these accessible arteries accurately reflects the compliance of the vasculature as a whole. Since the contribution to the AIx made by the reflected wave is a composite of many small wave reflections within the peripheral vasculature, AIx may be a better surrogate marker of whole body compliance than PWV in single arterial beds.[60] Recently, we have shown that the variability in measurement of AIx, using the Sphygmocor apparatus of O'Rourke, is <2 mmHg;[62] lower than most automated sphygmomanometers. Indeed, in our hands, the reproducibility of PWA is better than that recently quoted using an ultrasonic technique to assess dynamic vessel wall properties.[61]

Role of the endothelium

The elastic behaviour of conduit arteries serves to convert pulsatile cardiac ejection into continuous tissue perfusion and thus reduces systolic pressure relative to flow, resulting in reduced workload relative to perfusion (cardiovascular efficiency). It is determined by structural components of the arterial wall, by smooth muscle tone and by transmural pressure. Distensibility ($dV/V.dP$, where V is luminal volume and P is transmural pressure) is a frequently used measure of the elastic behaviour of an artery. It may thus change acutely with changes in smooth muscle tone or in transmural pressure,[63] or chronically with

changes in structure as in ageing,[64,65] hypertension[66] and atherosclerosis.[67] We have demonstrated in humans that conduit artery distensibility may be increased by infusion of acetylcholine (an endothelium-dependent agonist) and increased blood flow.[45,46] When NO activity is impaired, such as in diabetes and chronic heart failure, we have shown the endothelium-dependent changes in distensibility to be reduced,[45,46] with adverse consequences for overall cardiovascular efficiency.

It is unlikely that physical structure alone determines arterial stiffness, since a number of therapeutic interventions can influence vascular stiffness.[68-70] It is likely that vascular stiffness associated with diabetes is due, in part, to decreased bioavailability of NO from the vascular endothelium. Indeed there is accumulating evidence that the endothelium regulates vascular stiffness. The concept that stiffness of the aorta and large vessels is regulated by basal release of NO in the same way as vascular tone in resistance arterioles is further supported by recent animal studies. Anggard's group have measured peripheral pulse pressure wave-forms in rabbits using the technique of photoplethysmography.[71] This involves applying a photopulse sensor to the dorsal surface of the animal's ear. The pulse wave-form obtained is characterized by a dichrotic notch on the descending limb of the wave-form. The relative height of the dichrotic notch, b/a, was recorded (where a is the total amplitude of the wave-form and b is the height of the dichrotic notch). Although the origin of the dichrotic notch is uncertain, it is likely that it represents wave reflection from the periphery in a similar way to the AIx recorded in human subjects using PWA. Indeed, we have recently demonstrated that changes in relative notch height and AIx induced by GTN in human volunteers are the same (unpublished observations). Acute inhibition of eNOS in the rabbit is associated with an increased height of the dichrotic notch.[71] Infusion of acetylcholine, which stimulates endothelial NO release, lowers the dichrotic notch and this can be blocked by eNOS inhibition.[71] Furthermore, in rabbits with hypercholesterolaemia (a condition associated with endothelial dysfunction) the decrease in notch height produced by acetylcholine was blunted compared with normocholesterolaemic controls. This blunted response could be reversed by treating the rabbits with vitamin E.

In humans it has long been recognized that acute administration of glyceryl trinitrate (GTN), which is metabolized to NO within the vascular wall, profoundly alters the pulse pressure wave-form, lowering the dichrotic notch.[72] Although this may be due, in part, to vasodilatation of the peripheral vascular tree, it could equally be explained by decreased stiffness of the large conduit arteries. Recent studies have shown that vasodilator effects of β-adrenergic agonists are mediated in part via the L-arginine/NO pathway.[73] MacCallum et al. have used the technique of photoplethysmography to record peripheral pulse wave-forms from the finger in normal human volunteers. They showed that the relative notch height was decreased both by inhaling the endothelium-dependent agonist salbutamol and sublingual administration of the endothelium-independent agonist GTN.[74] However, when the experiment was repeated during administration of the NO synthase inhibitor L-NMMA, responses to salbutamol but not to GTN were inhibited, suggesting that the change in notch height induced by salbutamol was in some way endothelium dependent.

As previously stated, using FMD and high-resolution vessel wall tracking, we have demonstrated increased arterial stiffness in a group of non-insulin-dependent diabetics with no clinical evidence of vascular disease (Fig. 9.4).[46] Similarly, abnormalities of the pulse

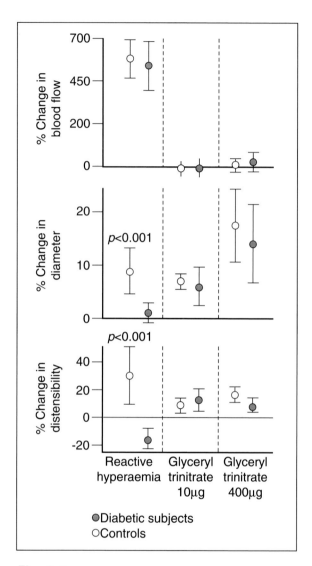

Fig. 9.4
Mean changes in blood flow, diastolic diameter, and distensibility of brachial artery in 12 diabetic subjects and 12 controls during reactive hyperaemia, 10 mg glyceryl trinitrate, and 400 µg glyceryl trinitrate. Bars show 95% confidence intervals.

wave consistent with increased stiffness are detectable early in the course of the disease in asymptomatic patients.[38] Fish oil, known to

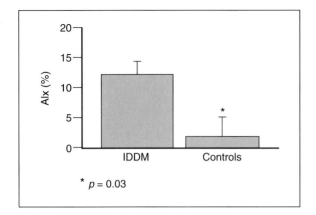

Fig. 9.5
Pecentage augmentation index (AIx) in 21 normotensive subjects with IDDM (age range 19–46 years, mean 32 years) with no clinical evidence of cardiovascular disease and 21 non-diabetic subjects (age range 21–42 years, mean 30 years). AIx was determined by pulse wave analysis from the radial artery. (Wilkinson et al.[81])

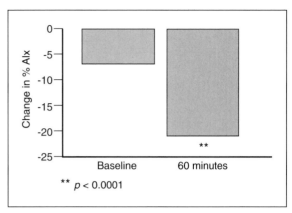

Fig. 9.6
Percentage augmentation index (AIx) in seven healthy volunteers (age range 22–29 years, mean 25 years) at baseline and 60 minutes after an oral glucose load of 75 g. AIx was determined by pulse wave analysis from the radial artery.[154]

improve endothelial function in NIDDM,[75] has also been shown to decrease arterial stiffness.[68] Angiotensin-converting enzyme inhibitors both improve endothelial function[76] and also decrease aortic stiffness,[77] whereas an equal reduction in blood pressure produced by diuretics is without effect.[77] Finally, oestrogen, which increases basal NO release from the endothelium of post-menopausal women,[78] also decreases aortic stiffness.[79] Although it is well documented that vascular stiffness, measured with a variety of techniques, is increased in NIDDM and IDDM,[38,80] until recently, central aortic waveforms have not yet been recorded. We have studied 21 normotensive IDDM subjects with no clinical evidence of cardiovascular disease.[81] AIx was determined from the radial artery pressure wave-form using PWA and compared with the AIx in 21 normotensive

non-diabetic controls. Heart rate, systolic blood pressure, height, and age did not differ significantly between the two groups, but the IDDM patients had a higher mean AIx of $10.8 \pm 9.5\%$ (SD) relative to the controls, $2.2 \pm 15.4\%$ ($p = 0.03$) (*Fig. 9.5*).

The mechanisms underlying endothelial dysfunction in diabetes remain unclear, but hyperglycaemia appears to be more important than insulin resistance.[82] In humans, acute hyperglycaemia attenuates endothelial function in the forearm circulation,[83] but in IDDM endothelial dysfunction correlates best with the degree of chronic hyperglycaemia.[82] Moreover, the development of microalbuminuria and overt cardiovascular disease also correlates with hyperglycaemia. Thus, hyperglycaemia may underlie the endothelial dysfunction found in diabetic patients, and this may lead to increased arterial stiffness, higher central pressures, and ultimately cardiovascular disease. Since acute hyperglycaemia has been shown to attenuate endothelial function as assessed by FMD, we studied changes in AIx in normal subjects following an acute oral glucose load of 75 g. Instead of increasing, as might be predicted if attenuation of endothelial function increased vascular stiffness, AIx actually fell from a baseline value of $-6.7 \pm 17.8\%$ (SD) to a trough of $-20.7 \pm 13.0\%$ 60 minutes following glucose administration (*Fig. 9.6*). These findings suggest that glucose was decreasing vascular stiffness as assessed by PWA. However, the results may equally reflect the fact that insulin release was responsible for the decrease in arterial stiffness and that NIDDM subjects have increased stiffness due to insulin resistance. This may be particularly relevant, as insulin is known to exert some of its vasodilator action via the release of endothelial NO.[84] Support for this hypothesis comes from further studies performed by Yki-Jarvinen and colleagues, who performed euglycaemic hyperinsulinaemic clamps in 10 normal male volunteers.[85] Central aortic pressure waves were synthesized from the radial artery pulse pressure wave-form using applanation tonometry and PWA. During the initial 120 minutes infusion, insulin produced no changes in heart rate, peripheral systolic, or diastolic blood pressure, forearm blood flow, or peripheral resistance. However, AIx was decreased significantly by insulin but not saline. This decrease in AIx is not necessarily due to direct changes in arterial compliance but may represent arterial dilation proximal to resistance vessels,[72] since GTN also decreases AIx without altering PWV or peripheral resistance.[72] Insulin decreases peripheral vascular resistance via an endothelium-dependent mechanism,[84] so it is possible that in this study insulin decreased AIx via arterial dilation. Coupled with the marked temporal dissociation between insulin's effect on AIx and forearm blood flow this suggests that insulin at physiological concentrations may preferentially dilate arteries before arterioles.

Diabetes is known to be associated with increased arterial stiffness.[48] However, whether increased stiffness is a risk factor or marker for cardiovascular disease in this condition remains to be established, and the relationship between vascular stiffness and endothelial function needs to be explored further. Pulse wave analysis offers the potential to screen large diabetic populations and to stratify the individuals at highest cardiovascular risk. Before this goal can be achieved the technique requires validation in the clinical setting and large-scale trials should be undertaken to determine whether arterial stiffness is a better predictor of mortality in a diabetic population than existing risk factors.

Mechanisms of endothelial dysfunction

An understanding of the mechanisms involved in the aetiology of endothelial dysfunction associated with diabetes is vital to the effective targeting of potential therapeutic interventions aimed at improving impaired endothelium-dependent vasoreactivity associated with this condition. The molecular and cellular mechanisms involved in endothelial dysfunction in pathophysiological conditions,[86] and in diabetes in particular,[87] have been reviewed in depth elsewhere. A number of potential causes of endothelial dysfunction in diabetes have been identified, including increased oxidative stress, advanced glycosylated end-products, and concomitant lipid abnormalities.[88]

Oxidative stress and lipid abnormalities

Increased oxidative stress has been suggested as a common pathway mediating atherogenesis across a wide spectrum of pathological conditions which include not only diabetes but also hypertension, hypercholesterolaemia, smoking, and obesity.[89] Recent evidence suggests that contrary to original belief, atheromatous disease is a chronic inflammatory condition and not a degenerative process.[90] Particular interest has focused on oxidized low-density lipoprotein (Ox-LDL), a peroxidation product which damages the endothelium and has potent atherogenic actions, including enhanced uptake by macrophages, leading to cholesterol ester enrichment, and monocyte chemotaxis and cytotoxicity.[91] In diabetics, as discussed above, endothelial damage often precedes the onset of clinically evident atheromatous disease and is associated with impaired endothelial function due to decreased bioavailability of NO. NO, in addition to being a potent vasodilator, has a number of antiatherogenic actions.[92] Whether endothelial dysfunction initiates the atheromatous process or is simply a marker for more generalized endothelial damage remains controversial. However, oxidative stress mediates both processes.[89] In diabetes, this is supported by a number of findings. First, Ox-LDL is a more potent inhibitor of endothelium-dependent relaxation than native LDL.[93] Secondly, it has also been shown that the native LDL from men with NIDDM is more potent at inhibiting endothelial-dependent relaxation than LDL from normal controls.[94] Thirdly, LDL from individuals with NIDDM or IDDM causes cholesterol accumulation in cultured intimal aortic cells. Taken together, these studies suggest that there are qualitative abnormalities of LDL in subjects with diabetes. Indeed, the LDL particles in subjects with insulin resistance or NIDDM are smaller, denser, and more susceptible to oxidation than those from non-diabetics.[95] Furthermore, diabetic subjects have been shown to be under increased oxidative stress[96] in the face of decreased antioxidant defences,[97]

and to have increased circulating levels of antibodies to Ox-LDL.[97] Ox-LDL may impair the L-arginine/NO pathway at a number of points in diabetes: at the level of signal transduction,[98] by down-regulating expression of eNOS,[99] and by interacting directly with NO to decrease its bioavailability. In addition to Ox-LDL, other free radicals such as superoxide may also impair endothelial function by reacting with NO to form peroxynitrite.[100] Increased free radical activity may occur as a result of either increased production or inadequate antioxidant defences. Interestingly, *in vitro* LDL cholesterol has been shown to uncouple the electron transport chain within eNOS so that instead of generating NO, the enzyme generates increasing amounts of superoxide.[101] Increasing concentrations of the substrate for NO production, L-arginine, were shown to recouple the enzyme,[101] providing an explanation as to why L-arginine has been shown to reverse endothelial dysfunction in both hypercholesterolaemia[102] and diabetes.[103] Tetrahydrobiopterin (THB) is an essential cofactor for the binding of L-arginine to eNOS.[104] In the absence of THB, the enzyme is uncoupled, transferring electrons to molecular oxygen and generating a superoxide anion.[104] An interesting feature of THB is the fact that it is capable of both generating and scavenging oxygen-free radicals, and recent studies suggest that it may be deficient in conditions such as diabetes[105] and hypercholesterolaemia.[106] Indeed, THB has been shown to restore impaired endothelium-dependent dilation in the forearm vascular bed of hypercholesterolaemic subjects,[106] although this has not, as yet, been demonstrated in diabetics.

Advanced glycosylation end-products (AGEs)

Endothelial cells express receptors for AGEs, which are involved in their internalization within the cell in diabetes.[107] AGEs may then impair endothelial function by modifying LDL cholesterol either by oxidation or glycosylation, or via a direct quenching effect on NO.[108]

Therapeutic interventions

Antioxidant vitamins

Vitamin E

As discussed above, oxidant stress and increased levels of Ox-LDL may be involved in the genesis of endothelial dysfunction associated with diabetes. Vitamin E is lipophilic and, when incorporated into the LDL particle, inhibits its oxidation.[95] Vitamin E also decreases oxidative stress by acting synergistically with NO to scavenge free radicals.[109] Since vitamin E levels are reduced in diabetic individuals[97] and oxidative stress is enhanced,[97,110] dietary supplementation with vitamin E is a logical approach to reducing the incidence of atheromatous vascular complications associated with diabetes.[95]

Two recent studies have addressed the issue of vitamin E supplementation in the secondary prevention of CHD. In an uncontrolled trial, Hodis et al.[111] demonstrated that oral supplements of at least 100 IU per day of vitamin E reduced progression of coronary atheroma in patients on cholesterol-lowering therapy. Most recently, CHAOS (Cambridge Heart AntiOxidant Study)[112] demonstrated a 47% reduction in death and non-fatal myocardial infarction in patients with angiographically proven CHD who took 400 or 800 IU of vitamin E daily. The latter study included a few patients with diabetes, and it is not possible to ascertain whether this group would have benefited more from antioxidant therapy.

Vitamin E supplementation prevents abnormalities of aortic and coronary artery endothe-

lium-dependent relaxation in the streptozotocin-diabetic rat.[113,114] In humans, insulin resistance is associated with endothelial dysfunction,[82] although the two are not necessarily causally related. Vitamin E supplementation has been shown to improve insulin resistance in healthy human subjects.[115] Interestingly, the novel insulin-sensitising drug, troglitazone, which contains the vitamin E moiety, is an antioxidant,[116] and, in addition to improving insulin resistance, has also been shown to lower blood pressure in normotensive glucose-intolerant subjects,[117] possibly by increasing the bioavailability of NO. However, despite the rationale for using vitamin E in humans and the encouraging data from animal studies, the results from studies of vitamin E supplementation in human cardiovascular disease states have been somewhat disappointing, with no improvement in endothelial function seen post myocardial infarction,[118] in hypercholesterolaemia,[119] and in hypercholesterolaemics with coronary artery disease,[102] despite evidence that at the doses used LDL oxidation was inhibited.[119] Our own studies in uncomplicated NIDDM subjects showed no improvement in endothelial function following 8 weeks supplementation with 1600 IU of vitamin E.[120] Recently, in an animal model of IDDM, vitamin E has been shown to reduce lipid peroxidation but impair vascular function in small arteries,[121] raising the possibility of differential effects of the vitamin based on dose and arterial bed studied. Despite no clear evidence that vitamin E improves endothelial function in humans, there is equally no evidence that it is harmful. Indeed, in the CHAOS study vitamin E reduced non-fatal heart attacks by 77%[112] but there was an increase in cardiovascular deaths.

Vitamin C

In contrast to vitamin E, direct intra-arterial infusion of pharmacological doses of vitamin C improves endothelial function in the forearm vascular bed not only in diabetics[122] but also in a number of other cardiovascular disease states associated with increased oxidative stress, including hypertension,[123] hypercholesterolaemia[70] and heart failure.[124] An intravenous bolus of vitamin C has also been shown to reduce blood pressure in subjects with diabetes,[125] again suggesting that vitamin C may be exerting its hypotensive effect via increasing bioavailability of NO. This is supported by the fact that oral vitamin C supplementation has also been shown to lower blood pressure. Despite this, there are as yet no published studies which look at oral vitamin C supplementation and cardiovascular end-points. Although antioxidant therapy offers potential benefits and the case for examination of the relationship between antioxidants and vascular disease in the general population has been made,[126,127] current evidence is insufficient to recommend intervention trials targeted specifically at diabetic subjects. However, diabetics should be actively recruited into future studies which examine the relationship between atheroma, oxidative stress, and anti-oxidants.

Fish oil

Epidemiological evidence supports the therapeutic potential of dietary marine fish oil in patients with coronary heart disease.[129] Recently, Goode and colleagues studied the effect of marine fish oil in hypercholesterolaemic subjects and demonstrated an improvement in small artery endothelial function *in vitro* following 3 months therapy with maxepa capsules.[129] *In vivo* human studies have also shown a beneficial effect of fish oil on endothelial function in hypercholesterolaemic subjects.[130] In NIDDM, abnormalities of the pulse wave consistent with increased stiffness are detectable early in the course of the disease

in asymptomatic patients.[38] Fish oil both improves endothelial function in NIDDM[75] and decreases arterial stiffness.[68]

L-arginine

The possible protective role of arginine on endothelial function in diabetes has recently been reviewed.[105] Decreased plasma arginine concentrations have been demonstrated in both diabetic animals[113] and humans.[131] Acute administration of the NO precursor L-arginine has been shown to reverse impaired dilator responses to acetylcholine both in animal preparations[132] and *in vivo* in the human coronary microcirculation.[133] Similar results have been obtained in the human forearm vascular bed of hypercholesterolaemic men, where infusion of L-arginine acutely reverses the decreased dilator response to acetylcholine in men with[102] and without[134] coronary disease. In cholesterol-fed rabbits, dietary supplementation with L-arginine is effective not only in preventing endothelial dysfunction but also the development of atherosclerosis.[135] A recent study in humans has also shown that supplementation with L-arginine improves endothelium-dependent dilatation in young adults with hypercholesterolaemia,[136] although as yet there is no evidence that arginine prevents the development of atherosclerosis in such subjects. However, endothelial dysfunction in young patients with IDDM did not improve following intravenous administration of L-arginine, perhaps indicating the different underlying pathophysiologies.[137]

Angiotensin-converting enzyme (ACE) inhibitors

ACE inhibitors reverse abnormalities of endothelium-dependent vascular relaxation in animal models of hypertension[138] and hypercholesterolaemia,[139] and in humans with hypertension and atheromatous disease.[76,140] In spontaneously hypertensive rats, acute and chronic treatment with an ACE inhibitor improved vascular endothelial dysfunction. Hydrallazine, despite similar anti-hypertensive effects, had no effect on endothelial dysfunction.[138] In humans with hypertension, treatment with captopril or nifedipine achieved similar reductions in blood pressure, but only the ACE inhibitor improved endothelium-dependent vasodilatation.[140]

Improvements of endothelium-dependent vasodilatation following ACE inhibition have now been reported in the human coronary circulation.[76] The Trial on Reversing ENdothelial Dysfunction (TREND) examined the effect of ACE inhibition on endothelial function in patients with several risk factors for cardiovascular disease and angiographically proven coronary atherosclerosis. At baseline, acetylcholine, infused directly into the coronary arteries, produced a paradoxical constriction, although responses to the endothelium-independent vasodilator GTN were unaffected. Patients were then randomized to receive the ACE inhibitor quinapril or placebo. Following 6 months treatment with quinapril, responses to GTN were unchanged, but there was a significant reversal of the constrictor response to acetylcholine (from 14.3% at baseline to 2.3% at follow-up). Responses in the placebo group did not change significantly (9.4–10.5%). Interestingly, the effect of ACE inhibition was similar in magnitude to that of cholesterol reduction in similar studies.[141] These studies included few patients with diabetes and, as yet, little is known about the effects of ACE inhibitors on the endothelial dysfunction associated with this condition.

ACE inhibitors have a number of properties that may increase the bioavailability of endothelium-derived NO. Bradykinin is produced by endothelial cells[142] and stimulates NO release.[143] Systemic ACE inhibition elevates circulating levels of bradykinin[144] and enhances the vasodilator response to exogenous bradykinin in the human forearm vascular bed.[145] Preserved vasodilator responses to bradykinin have been demonstrated in vessels from insulin-dependent diabetic animals and humans,[28] despite blunted responses to acetylcholine. In hypercholesterolaemia, the endothelial defect becomes more generalized.[146] These studies suggest that acetylcholine and bradykinin stimulate NO release via different signal transduction mechanisms,[147] and provide a promising mechanism by which ACE inhibitors may improve endothelial dysfunction in diabetes.

Angiotensin II (AII) increases superoxide production from vascular smooth muscle cells in culture by up-regulating the actions of NADH and NADPH oxidases.[148] Superoxide reacts with NO to form peroxynitrite[149] and so reduces local NO bioavailibility. Removal of NO from the constrictor/dilator equilibrium in vessels may cause excess constrictor influence and an inability of the vasculature to respond to physiological stimuli to NO production. In diabetes, superoxide-mediated NO destruction may occur more rapidly since diabetes is associated with an increase in circulating oxygen-derived free radicals.[30] AII also up-regulates the production of the vasoconstrictors endothelin 1 and PGH_2. This will further exacerbate the problem of reduced NO availability by enhancing the opposing constrictor influences. ACE inhibition reduces local AII levels, and so may increase NO availability and decrease vasoconstrictor influences.

To date, only two studies have examined the effect of ACE inhibition on endothelial function in patients with diabetes.[150,151] Both these studies used small numbers of subjects and no control groups. Chronic ACE inhibition for 6 months had no effect on methacholine-induced vasodilatation in the forearm vascular bed,[150] though the same researchers had previously questioned the use of methacholine as a reliable endothelium-dependent agonist.[152] A second group studied uncomplicated patients with IDDM and failed to demonstrate enhanced endothelium-dependent vasodilatation, as assessed by flow-mediated changes in brachial artery diameter, following 5 weeks therapy with an ACE inhibitor.

Conclusions

Diabetes is a condition which despite improved management and control remains associated with excess cardiovascular mortality. The discovery of the L-arginine/NO pathway and the antiatherogenic properties of NO have stimulated the hypothesis that abnormalities of this pathway may be in part responsible for the increased atherogenic tendency seen in diabetes. Subsequent research has indeed demonstrated endothelial dysfunction, characterized by decreased bioavailability of NO in both IDDM and NIDDM, although the mechanisms involved are heterogeneous and remain to be further clarified. Despite this, a number of therapeutic strategies are currently being evaluated to improve endothelial function in diabetes with the expectation that the successful agents will be evaluated in large end-point studies. For the future, the interaction of insulin with blood vessels at various levels, such as the production of NO, vasodilatation, and stimulation of vascular smooth muscle growth, opens up a new and exciting avenue for continued research. For, despite decades of successful research, diabetes remains as it always has been, a disease of blood vessels, not muscle.[153]

References

1. UKPDS. United Kingdom prospective diabetes study group. UK prospective study 33: intensive blood glucose control with sulphonylureas or insulin compared with conventional treatment and risk of complications in patients with type 2 diabetes. *Lancet* 1998; **352**: 837–853.
2. Keen H, Jarett RJ. The WHO multinational study of vascular disease in diabetes: 2 Macrovascular disease prevalence. *Diabetes Care* 1979; **2**: 187–195.
3. Reaven GM. Role of insulin resistance in human disease. *Diabetes* 1988; **37**: 1595–1607.
4. Arnett DK, Evans GW, Riley WA. Arterial stiffness: a new cardiovascular risk factor? *Am J Epidemiol* 1994; **140**: 669–682.
5. Furchgott RF, Zawadzki JV. The oligatory role of endothelial cells in the relaxation of arterial smooth muscle by acetylcholine. *Nature* 1980; **288**: 373–376.
6. Palmer RMJ, Ferrige AG, Moncada S. Nitric oxide release accounts for the biological activity of endothelium derived relaxing factor. *Nature* 1987; **327**: 524–526.
7. Cherry PD, Furchgott RF, Zawadzki JV, Jothianandan D. Role of endothelial cells in relaxation of isolated arteries by bradykinin. *Proc Natl Acad Sci USA* 1982; **79**: 2106–2110.
8. Furchgott RF. Role of endothelium in responses of vascular smooth muscle. *Circ Res* 1983; **53**: 557–573.
9. Vane JR, Anggard EE, Botting RM. Regulatory functions of the vascular endothelium. *N Engl J Med* 1990; **323**: 27–36.
10. Palmer RMJ, Ashton DS, Moncada S. Vascular endothelial cells synthesise nitric oxide from L-arginine. *Nature* 1988; **333**: 664–666.
11. Palmer RMJ, Moncada S. A novel citrulline-forming enzyme implicated in the formation of nitric oxide by endothelial cells. *Biochem Biophys Res Comm* 1989; **158**: 348–352.
12. Smith RP, Kurszyna H. Nitroprusside causes cyanide poisoning via reaction with haemoglobin. *J Pharmacol Exp Ther* 1974; **191**: 557–563.
13. Vallance P, Collier J, Moncada S. Effects of

endothelium-derived nitric oxide on peripheral arteriolar tone in man. *Lancet* 1989; ii: 997–1000.

14. Haynes WG, Noon JP, Walker BR, Webb DJ. Inhibition of nitric oxide synthesis increases blood pressure in healthy humans. *J Hypertens* 1993; **11**: 1375–1380.

15. Dzau VJ, Gibbons GH. Endothelium and growth factors in vascular remodeling and hypertension. *Hypertension* 1991; **18** (**Suppl III**): III-115–III-121.

16. Radomski MW, Palmer RMJ, Moncada S. Endogenous nitric oxide inhibits human platelet adhesion to vascular endothelium. *Lancet* 1987; ii: 1057–1058.

17. Garg UC, Hassid A. Nitric oxide-generating vasodilators and 8-bromocyclic guanosine monophosphate inhibit mitogenesis and proliferation of cultured rat vascular smooth muscle cells. *J Clin Invest* 1989; **83**: 1774–1777.

18. Celermajer DS, Sorenson KE, Gooch VM *et al.* Non-invasive detection of endothelial dysfunction in children and adults at risk of atherosclerosis. *Lancet* 1992; **340**: 1111–1115.

19. Kannel WB, McGee DL. Diabetes and cardiovascular disease: The Framingham study. *JAMA* 1978; **241**: 2035–2038.

20. Ruderman NB, Haudenschild C. Diabetes as an atherogenic factor. *Prog Cardiovasc Disease* 1984; **26**: 373–412.

21. Keen H, Jarrett R. The WHO multinational study of vascular disease in diabetes: 2 Macrovascular disease prevalence. *Diabetes Care* 1979; **2**: 187–195.

22. Panzram G. Mortality and survival in Type 2 (non-insulin-dependent) diabetes mellitus. *Diabetalogia* 1987; **30**: 123–131.

23. Oyama Y, Kawasaki H, Hattori Y, Kanno M. Attenuation of endothelium-dependent relaxation in aorta from diabetic rats. *Eur J Pharmacol* 1986; **131**: 75–78.

24. Durante W, Sen AK, Sunhara FA. Impairment of endothelium-dependent relaxation in aortae from spontaneously diabetic rats. *Br J Pharmacol* 1988; **94**: 463–468.

25. Tesfamariam B, Jakubowski JA, Cohen RA. Contraction of diabetic rabbit aorta caused by endothelium-derived PGH_2–TXA_2. *Am J Physiol* 1989; **257**: H1327–H1333.

26. Kamata K, Miyata N, Kasuya Y. Impairment of endothelium dependent relaxation and changes in cyclic GMP in aorta from streptozotocin-induced diabetic rats. *Br J Pharmacol* 1989; **97**: 614–618.

27. Kappagoda T, Jayleody L, Rajote R *et al.* Endothelium-dependent relaxation to acetylcholine in the aorta of STZ-diabetic rat and BB-diabetic rat. *Clin Invest Med* 1989; **12**: 187–193.

28. Poston L, Taylor PD. Endothelium-mediated vascular function in insulin-dependent diabetes mellitus. *Clin Sci* 1995; **88**: 245–255.

29. Gebremedhin D, Kotai MS, Pogatsa G *et al.* Influence of experimental diabetes on the mechanical responses of canine coronary arteries: role of endothelium. *Cardiovasc Res* 1988; **22**: 537–544.

30. Tesfamariam B, Cohen RA. Free-radicals mediate endothelial-cell dysfunction caused by elevated glucose. *Am J Physiol* 1992; **263**: H321–H326.

31. De Tejada IS, Goldstein I, Azadzoi K *et al.* Impaired neurogenic and endothelium-mediated relaxation of penile smooth muscle from diabetic men with impotence. *N Engl J Med* 1989; **320**: 1025–1030.

32. Nitenburg A, Valensi P, Sachs R *et al.* Impairment of coronary vascular reserve and ACh-induced coronary vasodilation in diabetic patients with angiographically normal coronary arteries and normal left ventricular systolic function. *Diabetes* 1993; **42**: 1017–1025.

33. Halkin A, Benjamin N, Doktor HS *et al.* Vascular responsiveness and cation exchange in insulin dependent diabetes. *Clin Sci* 1991; **81**: 223–232.

34. Smits P, Kapama JA, Jacobs MC *et al.* Endothelium-dependent vascular relaxation in patients with Type 1 diabetes. *Diabetes* 1993; **42**: 148–153.

35. Calver A, Collier J, Vallance P. Inhibition and stimulation of nitric oxide in the human forearm arterial bed of patients with insulin-dependent diabetes. *J Clin Invest* 1992; **90**: 2548–2554.

36. Elliott TG, Cockcroft JR, Groop P-H *et al.* Inhibition of nitric oxide synthesis in forearm vasculature of insulin-dependent diabetic

patients: blunted vasoconstriction in patients with microalbuminuria. *Clin Sci* 1993; **85:** 687–693.

37. Johnstone MT, Creager SJ, Scales KM *et al*. Impaired endothelium-dependent vasodilation in patients with insulin dependent diabetes mellitus. *Circulation* 1993; **88:** 2510–2516.

38. McVeigh G, Brennan G, Hayes R *et al*. Vascular abnormalities in non-insulin dependent diabetes mellitus identified by arterial waveform analysis. *Am J Med* 1993; **95**.

39. Chowienczyk PJ, Cockcroft JR, Ritter JM. Differential inhibition by N^G-monomethyl-L-arginine of vasodilator effects of acetylcholine and methacholine in human forearm. *Br J Pharmacol* 1993; **110:** 736–738.

40. Chowienczyk PJ, Cockcroft JR, Ritter JM. Blood flow responses to intra-arterial acetylcholine in man: effects of basal flow and conduit vessel length. *Clin Sci* 1994; **87:** 45–51.

41. Kuo L, Davies MJ, Chilian WM. Endothelium-dependent, flow-induced dilation of isolated coronary arterioles. *Am J Physiol* 1990; **259:** H1063–H1070.

42. Pohl U, Holtz J, Busse R, Bassenge E. Crucial role of the endothelium in the vasodilator response to flow *in vivo*. *Hypertension* 1985; **8:** 37–44.

43. Drexler H, Zeiher A, Wollschlager H *et al*. Flow-dependent coronary artery dilatation in humans. *Circulation* 1989; **80:** 466–474.

44. Sorenson KE, Celermajer DS, Speiglehalter DJ *et al*. Non invasive measure of human endothelium-dependent arterial responses: accuracy and reproducability. *Br Heart J* 1995; **74:** 247–253.

45. Ramsey MW, Goodfellow J, Jones CJH *et al*. Endothelial control of arterial distensibility is impaired in chronic heart failure. *Circulation* 1995; **92:** 3212–3219.

46. Goodfellow J, Ramsey MW, Luddington LA *et al*. Endothelium and inelastic arteries: an early marker of vascular dysfunction in non-insulin dependent diabetes. *Br Med J* 1996; **312:** 744–745.

47. Clarkson P, Celermajer DS, Donald AE *et al*. Impaired vascular reactivity in insulin-dependent diabetes mellitus is related to disease duration and low density lipoprotein choles-

terol levels. *J Am Coll Cardiol* 1996; **28:** 573–579.

48. Glasser SP, Arnett DK, McVeigh GE *et al*. Vascular compliance and cardiovascular disease. Risk factor or a marker? *Am Heart J* 1997; **10:** 1175–1189.

49. O'Rourke MF, Safar M, Dzau V. *Arterial Vasodilatation: Mechanisms and Therapy*. London: Edward Arnold, 1993.

50. O'Rourke MF, Kelly RP. Wave reflection in the systemic circulation and its implications in ventricular function. *J Hypertens* 1993; **11:** 327–337.

51. Saba PS, Roman MJ, Pini R *et al*. Relation of arterial pressure waveform to left ventricular and carotid anatomy in normotensive subjects. *J Am Coll Cardiol* 1993; **22:** 1873–1880.

52. Levy D, Garrison R, Savage DD *et al*. Prognostic implications of echocardiographically determined left ventricular mass in the Framingham heart study. *N Engl J Med* 1990; **332:** 1561–1566.

53. Bikkina M, Levy D, Evans JC *et al*. Left ventricular mass and risk of stroke in an elderly cohort. The Framingham Heart Study. *JAMA* 1994; **272:** 33–36.

54. Kimball T, Daniels S, Khoury P *et al*. Cardiovascular status in young patients with insulin-dependent diabetes mellitus. *Circulation* 1994; **357:** 357–361.

55. Lee M, Gardin JM, Smith V-E *et al*. Diabetes mellitus and echocardiographic left ventricular function in free-living elderly men and women. The Cardiovascular Health Study. *Am Heart J* 1997; **133:** 36–43.

56. O'Rourke MF, Gallagher DE. Pulse wave analysis. *J Hypertens* 1996; **14 (Suppl 5):** S147–S157.

57. Karamanoglu M, O'Rourke MF, Avolio AP, Kelly RP. An analysis of the relationship between central aortic and peripheral upper limb pressure waves in man. *Eur Heart J* 1993; **14:** 160–167.

58. Chen CH, Nevo E, Fetics B *et al*. Estimation of central aortic pressure waveform by mathematical transformation of radial tonometry pressure – validation of generalised transfer function. *Circulation* 1997; **95:** 1827–1836.

59. O'Rourke MF, Lei J, Gallagher DE, Avolio

AP. Determination of the ascending aorta pressure wave augmentation from the radial artery pressure pulse contour in humans. *Circulation* 1995; **92** (**Suppl 1**): 1–745.

60. Cockcroft JR, Wilkinson IB. Vessel wall properties and cardiovascular disease. *J Hum Hypertens* 1998; **12**: 343–344.

61. Van den Berkmortel F, Wollersheim H, van Langen H, Thein T. Dynamic vessel wall properties and their reproducibility in subjects with increased cardiovascular risk. *J Hum Hypertens* 1998; **12**: 345–350.

62. Wilkinson IB, Fuchs S, Jansen I *et al.* The reproducibility of augmentation index measured using applanation tonometry. *J Hypertens* 1998; **16** (**Suppl 2**): S20.

63. Cox RH. Mechanics of canine iliac artery smooth muscle *in vitro. Am J Physiol* 1976; **230**: 462–470.

64. Kelly R, Haward C, Avolio A, O'Rourke MF. Noninvasive determination of age-related changes in the human arterial pulse. *Circulation* 1989; **80**: 1652–1659.

65. Learoyd BM, Taylor MG. Alterations of age in the viscoelastic properties of human arterial walls. *Circulation Res* 1966; **18**: 278–292.

66. Ting C-T, Brin KP, Lin SJ *et al.* Arterial hemodynamics in hypertension. *J Clin Invest* 1986; **78**: 1462–1471.

67. Hirai T, Sasayama S, Kawasaki T, Yagi S. Stiffness of systemic arteries in patients with myocardial infarction: a noninvasive method to predict severity of coronary atherosclerosis. *Circulation* 1989; **80**: 78–86.

68. McVeigh G, Brennan G, Cohn J *et al.* Fish oil improves arterial compliance in non-insulin-dependent diabetes mellitus. *Arterioscler Thromb* 1994; **14**: 1425–1429.

69. Ting C-T, Yang T-M, Chen J-W *et al.* Arterial hemodynamics in human hypertension effects of angiotensin converting enzyme inhibition. *Hypertension* 1993; **22**: 839–846.

70. Ting HH, Timimi FK, Haley EA *et al.* Vitamin C improves endothelium-dependent vasodilation in forearm resistance vessels of humans with hypercholesterolaemia. *Circulation* 1997; **95**: 2617–2622.

71. Klemsdahl O, Andersson TLG, Matz J *et al.* Vitamin E restores endothelium-dependent vasodilatation in cholesterol-fed rabbits *in*

vivo measurements by photoplethysmography. *Cardiovasc Res* 1994; **28**: 1397–1402.

72. Yaginuma T, Avolio A, O'Rourke M *et al.* Effect of glyceryl trinitrate on peripheral arteries alters left ventricular hydraulic load in man. *Cardiovasc Res* 1986; **20**: 153–160.

73. Dawes M, Chowienczyk PJ, Ritter JM. Effects of inhibition of the L-arginine/NO pathway on beta-adrenergic mediated vasodilatation in human forearm vasculature. *Circulation* 1997; **95**: 2293–2297.

74. MacCallum H, Chowienczyk PJ, Dawes M *et al.* Effect of inhaled salbutamol on the digital volume pulse wave in healthy men. *Br J Clin Pharmacol* 1998; **45**: 197.

75. McVeigh GE, Brennan GM, Johnston GD *et al.* Dietary fish oil augments nitric oxide production or release in patients with type 2 (non-insulin-dependent) diabetes mellitus. *Diabetologia* 1993; **36**: 33–38.

76. Mancini GBJ, Henfy GC, Macaya C *et al.* Angiotensin-converting enzyme-inhibition with quinapril improves endothelial vasomotor dysfunction in patients with coronary artery disease – the TREND (trial on reversing endothelial dysfunction) study. *Circulation* 1996; **94**: 258–265.

77. Breithaupt-Grogler K, Leschinger M, Belz GG *et al.* Influence of antihypertensive therapy with cilazipril and hydrochlorthiazuide on the stiffness of the aorta. *Cardiovasc Drugs Ther* 1996; **10**: 49–57.

78. Krishnankutty S, Jennings GL, Funder JW, Komesaroff PA. Estrogen enhances basal nitric oxide release in the forearm vasculature in perimenopausal women. *Hypertension* 1996; **28**: 330–334.

79. Chelsky R, Wilson RA, Morton MJ *et al.* Rapid alteration of ascending aortic compliance following treatment with pergonal. *Circulation* 1990; **82**: 111.

80. Jensen-Urstad J, Reichard P, Rosors J *et al.* Early atherosclerosis is retarded by improved long-term glucose control in patients with IDDM. *Diabetes* 1996; **45**: 1253–1258.

81. Wilkinson IB, Hupperetz PC, van Thoor CJ *et al.* Increased arterial stiffness in patients with insulin-dependent diabetes mellitus. *Diabetic Med* 1998; **15** (**Suppl 1**): 107.

82. Makimattila S, Virkamaki A, Groop P *et al.*

Chronic hyperglycaemia impairs endothelial function and insulin sensitivity via different mechanisms in insulin-dependent diabetes mellitus. *Circulation* 1996; **94**: 1276–1282.

83. Williams SB, Goldfine AB, Timimi FK *et al.* Acute hyperglycaemia attenuates endothelium-dependent vasodilation in humans *in vivo*. *Circulation* 1998; **97**: 1695–1701.

84. Steinberg HO, Brechtel G, Johnson A *et al.* Insulin-mediated skeletal muscle vasodilation is nitric oxide dependent. *J Clin Invest* 1994; **94**: 1172–1179.

85. Westerbacka J, Wilkinson I, Cockcroft J *et al.* Diminished wave reflection in the aorta. A novel physiological action of insulin on large blood vessels. *Hypertension* 1999; **33**: 1118–1122.

86. Harrison DG. Cellular and molecular mechanisms of endothelial cell dysfunction. *J Clin Invest* 1997; **100**: 2153–2157.

87. Tribe RM, Poston L. Oxidative stress and lipids in diabetes: a role in endothelium vasodilator function? *Vasc Med* 1996; **1**: 195–206.

88. Chowienczyk PJ, Watts GP. Endothelial dysfunction, insulin resistance and non-insulin diabetes. *Endocrinol Metab* 1997; **4**: 225–232.

89. Alexander RW. Hypertension and the pathogenesis of atherosclerosis. Oxidative stress and the mediation of arterial inflammatory response: a new perspective. *Hypertension* 1995; **25**: 155–161.

90. Berliner JA, Navab M, Fogelman AM *et al.* Atherosclerosis: basic mechanisms, oxidation, inflammation, and genetics. *Circulation* 1995; **91**: 2488–2496.

91. Witztum JL, Steinberg D. Role of oxidized low density lipoprotein in atherogenesis. *J Clin Invest* 1991; **88**: 1785–1792.

92. Cooke JP, Tsao PS. Is NO an endogenous antiatherogenic molecule? *Arterioscler Thromb* 1994; **14**: 653–655.

93. Jacobs M, Plane F, Bruckdorfer KR. Native and oxidized low-density lipoproteins have different inhibitory effects on endothelium-derived relaxing factor in rabbit aorta. *Br J Pharmacol* 1990; **100**: 21–26.

94. McNeill KL, Fontana L, Ritter JM *et al.* Inhibitory effects of low-density lipoprotein on endothelium-dependent relaxation are exaggerated in men with NIDDM. *Diabetic Med* 1998; **15 (Suppl 1)**: A4.

95. Reaven P. Dietary and pharmacologic regimens to reduce lipid peroxidation in non-insulin-dependent diabetes mellitus. *Am J Clin Nutr* 1995; **62**: 1483S-1489S.

96. Gopaul NK, Anggard EE, Mallet AI *et al.* Plasma 8–epi-PGF$_{2\alpha}$ levels are elevated in individuals with non-insulin dependent diabetes mellitus. *FEBS Lett* 1995; **368**: 225–229.

97. Sundaram RK, Bhaskar A, Vijayalingam S *et al.* Antioxidant status and lipid peroxidation in type II diabetes mellitus with and without complications. *Clin Sci* 1996; **90**: 255–260.

98. Liao JK, Clark SL. Regulation of G protein α_2 subunit expression by oxidised low-density lipoprotein. *J Clin Invest* 1995; **95**: 1457–1463.

99. Liao JK, Shin WS, Lee WY, Clark SL. Oxidised low density lipoprotein decreases the expression of endothelial nitric oxide synthase. *J Biol Chem* 1995; **2270**: 319–324.

100. Halliwell B. Free radicals, antioxidants and human disease: curiosity, cause, consequence. *Lancet* 1994; **344**: 721–724.

101. Pritchard KA, Groszek L, Smalley DM *et al.* Native low-density lipoprotein increases endothelial cell nitric oxide synthase generation of superoxide anion. *Circ Res* 1995; **77**: 510–517.

102. Chowienczyk PJ, Kneale BJ, Brett SE *et al.* Lack of effect of vitamin E on L-arginine-responsive endothelial dysfunction in patients with mild hypercholesterolaemia and coronary artery disease. *Clin Sci* 1998; **94**: 129–134.

103. Chowienczyk PJ, Barnes DJ, Brett SE *et al.* Correction of impaired NO mediated vasodilation by L-arginine in non-insulin-dependent diabetics (Abstr). *Endothelium* 1995; **3**: S95.

104. Pou S, Pou WS, Bredt DS *et al.* Generation of superoxide by purified brain nitric oxide synthase. *J Biol Chem* 1992; **267**: 24173–24176.

105. Pieper GM. Review of alterations in endothelial nitric oxide production in diabetes. Protective role of arginine on endothelial function. *Hypertension* 1998; **31**: 1047–1060.

106. Stroes ES, Koomans HA, de Bruin TW, Rabelink TJ. Vascular function in the forearm of hypercholesterolaemic patients off and on

lipid-lowering medication. *Lancet* 1995; **346:** 467–471.

107. Wautier JL, Wautier MP, Schmidt AM *et al.* Advanced glycosylation end products (AGE's) on the surface of diabetic erythrocytes bind to the vessel wall via a specific receptor inducing oxidant stress in the vasculature: a link between surface-associated AGE's and diabetic complications. *Proc Natl Acad Sci USA* 1994; **91:** 7742–7746.

108. Buchala R, Tracey KJ, Cerami A. Advanced glycosylation end products quench nitric oxide and mediate defective endothelium-dependent vasodilation in experimental diabetes. *J Clin Invest* 1991; **87:** 432–438.

109. Rubbo H, Paler-Martinez A, Freeman BA. Synergistic interactions between nitric oxide and α-tocopherol in antioxidant reactions. *Endothelium* 1995; **3 (Suppl 1):** S10.

110. Collier A, Wilson R, Bradley H *et al.* Free radical activity in type 2 diabetes. *Diabetic Med* 1989; **7:** 27–30.

111. Hodis HN, Mack WJ, LaBree L *et al.* Serial coronary angiographic evidence that antioxidant vitamin intake reduces progression of coronary artery atherosclerosis. *JAMA* 1995; **273:** 1849–1854.

112. Stephens NG, Parsons A, Schofield PM *et al.* Randomised controlled trial of vitamin E in patients with coronary disease: Cambridge heart antioxidant study (CHAOS). *Lancet* 1996; **347:** 781–786.

113. Rösen P, Ballhausen T, Bloch W, Addicks K. Endothelial relaxation is disturbed by oxidative stress in the diabetic rat heart: influence of tocopherol as antioxidant. *Diabetologia* 1995; **38:** 1157–1168.

114. Keegan A, Walbank H, Cotter MA, Cameron NE. Chronic vitamin E treatment prevents defective endothelium-dependent relaxation in diabetic rat aorta. *Diabetologia* 1995; **38:** 1475–1478.

115. Paolisso G, D'Amore A, Giugliano D *et al.* Pharmacologic doses of vitamin E improve insulin action in healthy subjects and non-insulin-dependent diabetic patients. *Am J Clin Nutr* 1993; **57:** 650–656.

116. Dandona P, Khurana U, Aljada A *et al.* Troglitazone as an antioxidant. *Diabetes* 1995; **44:** 57A.

117. Nolan JJ, Ludvik B, Beerdsen P *et al.* Improvement in glucose tolerance and insulin resistance in obese subjects treated with troglitazone. *N Engl J Med* 1994; **331:** 1188–1193.

118. Elliott TG, Barth JD, Mancini GBJ. Effects of vitamin E on endothelial function in men after myocardial infarction. *Am J Cardiol* 1995; **76:** 1188–1192.

119. Gilligan DM, Sack MN, Guetta V *et al.* Effect of antioxidant vitamins on low density lipoprotein oxidation and impaired endothelium-dependent vasodilation in patients with hypercholesterolaemia. *J Am Coll Cardiol* 1994; **24:** 1611–1617.

120. Gazis AG, White DJ, Page SR, Cockcroft JR. Oral vitamin E does not improve endothelial function in subjects with type 2 diabetes. *Diabetic Med* 1998; **15 (Suppl 1):** A2.

121. Palmer AM, Thomas CR, Gopaul N *et al.* Dietary antioxidant supplementation reduces lipid peroxidation but impairs vascular function in small mesenteric arteries of the streptozotocin rat. *Diabetologia* 1998; **41:** 148–156.

122. Timimi FK, Ting HH, Haley EA *et al.* Vitamin C endothelium-dependent vasodilation in patients with insulin-dependent diabetes mellitus. *J Am Coll Cardiol* 1998; **31:** 552–557.

123. Taddei S, Virdis A, Ghiadoni L *et al.* Vitamin C improves endothelium-dependent vasodilation by restoring nitric oxide activity in essential hypertension. *Circulation* 1998; **97:** 2222–2229.

124. Hornig B, Arakawa N, Kohler C, Drexler H. Vitamin C improves endothelial function of conduit arteries in patients with chronic heart failure. *Circulation* 1998; **97:** 363–368.

125. Ceriello A, Giugliano D, Quatraro A, Lefebvre PJ. Anti-oxidants show an anti-hypertensive effect in diabetic and hypertensive subjects. *Clin Sci* 1991; **81:** 739–742.

126. Oliver MF. Antioxidant nutrients, atherosclerosis, and coronary heart disease. *Br Heart J* 1996; **73:** 299–301.

127. Cockcroft JR, Chowienczyk PJ. Beyond cholesterol reduction in coronary heart disease: is vitamin E the answer? *Heart* 1996; **76:** 293–294.

128. Ascherio A, Rimm EB, Stampfer MJ *et al.* Dietary intake of marine n-3 fatty acids, fish

intake and the risk of coronary disease among men. *N Engl J Med* 1995; **332**: 977–982.

129. Goode GK, Garcia S, Heagerty AM. Dietary supplementation with marine fish oil improves *in vitro* small artery endothelial function in hypercholesterolaemic patients: a double-blind placebo-controlled study. *Circulation* 1997; **96**: 2802–2807.

130. Chin JPF, Dart AM. Therapeutic restoration of endothelial function in hypercholesterolaemic subjects: effect of fish oils. *Clin Exp Pharmacol Physiol* 1994; **21**: 749–755.

131. Hagenfeldt L, Dahlquist G, Persson B. Plasma amino acids in relation to metabolic control in insulin-dependent diabetic children. *Acta Paediatr Scand* 1989; **794**: 278–282.

132. Cooke JP, Andon NA, Girerd XJ *et al.* Arginine restores cholinergic relaxation of hypercholesterolaemic rabbit thoracic aorta. *Circulation* 1991; **83**: 1057–1062.

133. Drexler H, Zeiher AM, Meinzer K, Just H. Correction of endothelial dysfunction in coronary microcirculation of hypercholesterolaemic patients by L-arginine. *Lancet* 1991; **338**: 1546–1550.

134. Chowienczyk PJ, Watts GF, Cockcroft JR *et al.* Sex differences in endothelial function in normal and hypercholesterolaemic subjects. *Lancet* 1994; **344**: 305–306.

135. Cooke JP, Singer AH, Tsao P *et al.* Antiatherogenic effects of L-arginine in the hypercholesterolaemic rabbit. *J Clin Invest* 1992; **90**: 1168–1172.

136. Clarkson P, Adams MR, Powe AJ *et al.* Oral L-arginine improves endothelium-dependent dilatation in hypercholesterolaemic young adults. *J Clin Invest* 1996; **97**: 1989–1994.

137. Thorne S, Mullen MJ, Clarkson P *et al.* Early endothelial dysfunction in adults at risk from atherosclerosis: differnet responses to L-arginine. *JACC* 1998; **32**: 110–116.

138. Clozel M, Kuhn H, Hefti F. Effects of angiotensin converting enzyme inhibitors and of hydrallazine on endothelial function in hypertensive rats. *Hypertension* 1990; **16**: 532–540.

139. Becker RHA, Wiemer G, Linz W. Preservation of endothelial function by ramipril in rabbits on a long-term atherogenic diet. *J Cardiovasc Pharmacol* 1991; **18** (s2): S110–S115.

140. Hirooka Y, Imaizumi T, Masaki H *et al.* Captopril improved impaired endothelium-dependent vasodilatation in hypertensive patients. *Hypertension* 1992; **20**: 175–180.

141. Anderson TJ, Meredith IT, Yeung AC *et al.* The effect of cholesterol-lowering and antioxidant therapy on endothelium-dependent coronary vasomotion. *N Engl J Med* 1995; **332**: 488–493.

142. Wiemer G, Scholkens BA, Becker RHA, Busse R. Ramiprilat enhances endothelial autocoid formation by inhibiting breakdown of endothelium-derived bradykinin. *Hypertension* 1991; **18**: 558–563.

143. Cockcroft JR, Chowienczyk PJ, Brett SE, Ritter JM. Effect of N-G–monomethyl-L-arginine on kinin-induced vasodilation in the human forearm. *Br J Clin Pharmacol* 1994; **38**: 307–310.

144. Pellacani A, Brunner HR, Nussberger J. Plasma kinins increase after angiotensin-converting enzyme-inhibition in human subjects. *Clin Sci* 1994; **87**: 567–574.

145. Benjamin N, Cockcroft JR, Collier JG *et al.* Local inhibition of converting enzyme and vascular responses to angiotensin and bradykinin in the human forearm. *J Physiol* 1989; **412**: 543–555.

146. Casino PR, Kilcoyne CM, Cannon RO *et al.* Impaired endothelium-dependent vascular relaxation in patients with hypercholesterolaemia extends beyond the muscarinic receptors. *Am J Cardiol* 1995; **75**: 40–44.

147. Flavahan NA. Atherosclerosis or lipoprotein-induced endothelial dysfunction. *Circulation* 1992; **85**: 1927–1938.

148. Griendling KK, Minieri CA, Ollerenshaw JD, Alexander RW. Angiotensin II stimulates NADH and NADPH oxidase activity in cultured vascular smooth muscle cells. *Circ Res* 1994; **74**: 1141–1148.

149. Huie RE, Padjama S. The reaction of NO with superoxide. *Free Rad Res Comm* 1993; **18**: 195–199.

150. Bijlstra PJ, Smits P, Lutterman JA, Thien T. Effect of long-term angiotensin-converting enzyme inhibition on endothelial function in patients with the insulin resistance sydrome. *J Cardiovasc Pharmacol* 1995; **25**: 658–664.

151. Smulders RA, Lambert J, Aarsen M *et al*. The effect of ACE-inhibition on endothelial function in uncomplicated insulin-dependent diabetic subjects. *Diabetologia* 1995; **38**: A49.

152. Rongen GA, Smits P, Thien T. N(G)-mono-methyl-L-arginine reduces the forearm vaso-dilator response to acetylcholine but not methacholine in humans. *J Cardiovasc Pharmacol* 1993; **22**: 884–888.

153. Yki-Jarvinen H, Utriainen T. Insulin-induced vasodilatation: physiology or pharmacology? *Diabetologia* 1998; **41**: 369–379.

154. Wilkinson IB, Hupperetz TC, van Thoor CJ *et al*. Acute hyperglycaemia reduces central aortic pressure in healthy subjects. *Br J Clin Pharm* 1998; **46**: 289.

10

New targets for the prevention and treatment of diabetic nephropathy

Paula Chattington and Mark Cooper

Introduction

The pathophysiology involved in the initiation and progression of diabetic nephropathy has been gradually delineated over the past 20 years.[1] With the recent improved understanding of the complex interactions between metabolic and haemodynamic factors, and the mediating role of cytokines and growth factors, new targets for the prevention and treatment of diabetic nephropathy are now available.

Assessing renal function

With the evolution of diabetic nephropathy, patients progress from normoalbuminuria to microalbuminuria and eventually onto overt proteinuria. Microalbuminuria is often referred to as incipient nephropathy; it is defined as a urinary albumin excretion of between 20 and 200 µg/min on an overnight sample, or between 30 and 300 mg per day on a 24-hour urine specimen.[2] A convenient method for routine use is assessment of the albumin/creatinine ratio on an early morning urine sample, with a cut-off for microalbuminuria taken as >2.5 mmol/mg creatinine for men and >3.5 mmol/mg creatinine for women, in the absence of a urinary tract infection. With the advent of Micral-II test strips, microalbuminuria can be reliably detected but not quantified in a spot urine test.[3]

Pathophysiology of diabetic renal disease

Nephromegaly with expansion of the mesangial matrix and hyperfiltration have long been recognized as early features of diabetes, and correlate to poor metabolic control.[4] Hyperfiltration is an early feature of diabetes mellitus, with a glomerular filtration rate (GFR) raised by between 20 and 40% on the initial diagnosis of Type 1 diabetes and between 10 and 17% in Type 2 diabetes.[5] GFR is maintained during the period of microalbuminuria until just prior to the onset of proteinuria. The rate of decline is predominantly influenced by blood pressure and to a lesser extent by glycaemic control. The rate of fall in GFR is positively correlated to the glomerular basement membrane thickness and interstitial volume fraction.[6]

Microalbuminuria is closely linked to rising blood pressure[7] and antecedent hyperfiltration, and this combination has been postulated to be predictive of later renal disease,[8] but this has not been a universal finding.[9] Microalbuminuria is not only associated with renal involvement, but is clearly linked to vascular disease and retinopathy.[10] Microalbuminuria represent a population at high risk for the subsequent development of diabetic nephropathy, retinopathy, and cardiovascular disease.[11,12]

Table 10.1

Complications associated with albumin excretion rate (AER) in Type 1 diabetes mellitus.[19]

Condition	Normoalbuminuria (%)	Microalbuminuria (%)	Macroalbuminuria (%)
Proliferative retinopathy	12	28	58
Blindness	1.4	5.6	10.6
Peripheral neuropathy	21	31	50
Arterial hypertension	19	30	65

Micropuncture studies in animal models of diabetes have shown that even in the absence of systemic hypertension, the glomerulus in diabetes is exposed to elevated pressure.[13] This glomerular capillary hypertension can be ameliorated by angiotensin-converting enzyme (ACE) inhibition,[13] with an associated decrease in proteinuria and a reduction in both glomerulosclerosis and tubulointerstitial injury.[14] This class of drugs may act on a cytokine-dependent pathway, primarily involving transforming growth factor-β (TGF-β).[14] TGF-β has a prosclerotic effect on extracellular matrix formation. It has been demonstrated that this growth factor is angiotensin II-dependent *in vitro*, and overexpression of TGF-β in the diabetic kidney can be prevented by ACE inhibition.[14]

Diabetes is a state of chronic hyperglycaemia that leads to the formation of advanced glycation end-products (AGEs) which accumulate in various organs, including the kidney.[15] Aminoguanidine inhibits AGE formation and reduces AGE accumulation in the kidney. This has been associated with a reduction in albuminuria and mesangial expansion.[15] Clinical studies are now underway which are evaluating the role of agents such as aminoguanidine in diabetic

nephropathy.[16] The thiazolium compound, phenacylthiazolium bromide (PTB), has been shown to cleave the crosslinks in preformed AGEs and may, therefore, have a role in the treatment of established diabetic renal disease.[17]

The polyol pathway has also been implicated in the development of diabetic nephropathy. Aldose reductase inhibitors inhibit this pathway, but experimental and clinical studies have shown variable results. Protein kinase C activity is increased in diabetic glomeruli, and an inhibitor of the β-II isoform of protein kinase C, LY333531, prevents hyperfiltration and albuminuria in diabetic rats.[18] This provides an alternative approach for the prevention and treatment of diabetic nephropathy.

Type 1 diabetes

Nephropathy remains a major cause of morbidity and mortality in Type 1 diabetic subjects. Furthermore, diabetic nephropathy is the major cause of end-stage renal disease (ESRD) in the Western world. Approximately 50% of diabetic subjects in ESRD programmes have Type 1 diabetes. The presence of either

Complication	Type 1 diabetes	Type 2 diabetes
Prevalence microalbuminuria	10–25%	15–25%
Incidence proteinuria[21]	0.5–3% a year	1–2% a year
Prevalence of proteinuria[21]	15–20%	10–25%

Cumulative incidence of proteinuria[20]	Years from diagnosis	Type 1 diabetes	Type 2 diabetes
	3	–	3%
	5	3%	–
	10	5.2%	6%
	15	8.6%	10%
	20	28%	28%
	25	46%	56%

Table 10.2
Prevalence and incidence of diabetic renal disease.

incipient (microalbuminuria) or overt diabetic nephropathy is closely associated with an increased risk of other conditions, as shown in prospective studies by Parving's group (*Table 10.1*).[19]

Type 2 diabetes

The incidence of diabetic renal disease in Type 2 diabetes is highly dependent on ethnic origin (see later) and family history of hypertension or diabetic nephropathy. Although it has previously been assumed that Type 2 diabetes is less commonly associated with diabetic nephropathy, this has been clearly shown not to be true. Indeed, in Type 2 diabetic subjects with a long duration of diabetes mellitus, similar rates of complications are observed when compared with Type 1 subjects (*Table 10.2*).[20,21] Furthermore, as there is at least a fivefold increase in prevalence for Type 2 when compared with Type 1 diabetes mellitus, Type 2 patients now contribute a similar number of patients on ESRD programmes.[22]

Diabetic nephropathy is associated with a significant excess morbidity and mortality, and this is related primarily to cardiovascular disease rather than to renal dysfunction. A patient with Type 2 diabetes with nephropathy has a relative risk (RR) of between 3 and 6 for mortality with a RR of 5–10 for a myocardial infarction when compared with age-matched, normotensive, normoalbuminuric, Type 2 patients.[21] The risks of stroke, peripheral vascular disease, amputations, and blindness also increase significantly.[21]

Type 2 diabetes is often associated with other clinical features, including hypertension, obesity (especially truncal), dyslipidaemia (including hypertriglyceridaemia, reduced high-density lipid (HDL) cholesterol concentrations), and insulin resistance. This constellation is also known as the metabolic syndrome or syndrome X.[23] These patients have significantly increased cardiovascular morbidity and mortality. Therefore, treatment aimed at renal protection must take account of concomitant conditions, and any screening should identify other risk factors such as hypertension and dyslipidaemia.

Ethnicity

There is a wide ethnic variation in the incidence of diabetes and in the development of diabetic nephropathy. In the USA, ESRD is between two- and sixfold higher in Afro-Americans after adjustment for the prevalence of diabetes, the increased risk being predominantly observed in the Type 2 diabetic population.[24] Mexican-Americans with Type 2 diabetes have been shown to have a 4.5–6.6-fold increase in diabetes-related ESRD when compared with non-Hispanic white diabetic subjects.[25]

Hypertension

Definition of hypertension

The diagnostic criteria for hypertension in diabetes have been changed from 160/95 mmHg (1983 WHO) to 140/90 (1993 JNC-V, WHO, and Australian Hypertension Consensus Statement 1994) and more recently to 130/85 mmHg (1997, JNC-VI).[26] These blood pressure (BP) readings should be exceeded on two separate occasions with the patient rested. The Joint National Committee (JNC) on prevention, detection, evaluation, and treatment of high blood pressure, issues guidelines to provide guidance for primary care clinicians in the USA, on appropriate BP targets and therapeutics for different patient groups. The new JNC-VI criteria imply that many patients previously classified as normotensive should now be re-classified as hypertensive. The JNC-VI report also recommends a therapeutic goal of <125/75 mmHg in the presence of renal disease.[26]

Using JNC-V (BP >140/90 mmHg) criteria, the proportions of Type 1 diabetic subjects having hypertension attending a Danish diabetes clinic were 42, 52, and 79% in normo-, micro-, and macroalbuminuric subjects, respectively. In Type 2 diabetes, the proportions were 71 normo-, 90 micro-, and 93% of macroalbuminuric patients.[27] These prevalence rates will be even higher if one takes account of the current definition of hypertension in diabetes (>130/85 mmHg), recently published by JNC-VI.

In a range of studies, elevation of blood pressure has been shown to correlate closely with the later development of diabetic nephropathy. Indeed, in a recent epidemiological analysis of Type 2 diabetic patients in the United Kingdom Prospective Diabetes Study (UKPDS), blood pressure correlated closely with the development of a range of diabetic vascular complications.[28] The HOT (hypertension optimal treatment) Study explored the role of intensive blood pressure reduction in hypertensive subjects, a significant proportion of whom had diabetes. The greatest cardiovascular protection was seen in this subgroup of 1,500 diabetic patients, with a 51% reduction in major cardiovascular events in the group with intensified hypotensive therapy.[29] Those in the lowest blood pressure target group were more likely to be on multiple antihypertensive agents, making interpretation of the role of blood pressure reduction *per se* rather difficult. The contribution of a specific renoprotective effect of some of the classes of antihypertensive agents, such as ACE inhibitors, to the decrease in cardiovascular mortality and morbidity in this study cannot be excluded.

Clinical implications of hypertension in diabetes

Hypertension is approximately twice as common in diabetic patients when compared to age-matched non-diabetic subjects.[30] The association is probably due to an interaction between inherited factors and the metabolic abnormalities of diabetes. Diabetes, particularly when associated with hypertension, is characterized by expanded plasma volume, raised peripheral vascular resistance, increased arteriolar reactivity, and low plasma renin activity. With the development of nephropathy, the renal ability to excrete excess sodium and fluid is reduced, probably contributing to worsening of hypertension with increasing albuminuria.

Hypertension is a major contributor to large vessel disease, especially in Type 2 diabetes. It is probable that the level of albuminuria reflects the degree of macrovascular risk. Macroalbuminuria in Type 1 patients confers a 30-fold increase in mortality, mostly from cardiovascular disease.[31] In both Type 1 and 2 diabetes, hypertension is associated with an increase in vascular-related mortality, of which approximately 70% is due to coronary heart disease and 30% due to cerebrovascular disease. In Type 2 diabetes with concomitant hypertension, there is a four- to fivefold increase in mortality when compared with normotensive Type 2 diabetic patients.[32]

Diurnal rhythm

Hypertensive non-diabetic patients who lack the normal nocturnal decline in blood pressure (non-dippers) have an increased incidence of cardiovascular complications. Previous work has shown that the nocturnal fall in BP is less in Type 1 diabetic patients than in age-matched controls. In a group of Type 1 and 2 diabetic subjects with persistent proteinuria secondary to diabetic nephropathy, ambulatory blood pressure monitoring was performed and patients classified as dippers (mean sleeping systolic and diastolic BP 10% less than awake BP) or non-dippers. In the dipper group the rate of decline of creatinine clearance was –2.9 ml/min/year, compared with –7.9 ml/min/

year in the non-dipper group.[33] There was no significant difference in daytime mean blood pressures, HbA_{1c} or age.[33] These findings suggest that the lack of nocturnal decline in blood pressure may be an additional risk factor for progression of diabetic nephropathy.

Therapeutic options

JNC-VI recommends that a diuretic or a β-blocker or both be chosen as the initial drug for therapy for hypertension in non-diabetic individuals.[26] In diabetic patients without albuminuria, JNC-VI recommends that the choice be made from ACE inhibitors, calcium channel blockers (CCBs), diuretics, and β-blockers, depending on the clinical context.[26] For patients with either micro- or macroalbuminuria, initial therapy should be based on an ACE inhibitor. It is predicted that selective angiotensin II receptor antagonists will ultimately share this indication.

It is widely thought that blood pressure reduction *per se* should not be considered as the only marker of clinical efficacy of antihypertensive therapy in diabetic patients. It has been suggested that certain antihypertensive agents, such as ACE inhibitors, may have additional renoprotective properties, independent of reduction in blood pressure. Furthermore, β-blockers and diuretics have deleterious effects on lipid and glucose parameters[34] that could adversely affect cardiovascular morbidity and mortality. We await further information from ongoing clinical trials, particularly in Type 2 diabetic patients.[35] Therefore, at this stage it is appropriate to endorse ACE inhibitors, β-blockers, and diuretics as primary therapy for patients with diabetes and hypertension, providing that no contraindications exist. ACE inhibitors would be favoured as initial therapy in diabetic subjects with any evidence of renal disease. It has been suggested that CCBs should be used only when ACE inhibitors, β-blockers, and diuretics are unsuccessful in lowering blood pressure.[36] Further studies are needed to determine whether CCBs exert a renoprotective effect in humans, over and above their effects on systemic blood pressure.

Cardiovascular risk reduction in relation to therapeutic agents

Three recent studies; ABCD (Appropriate Blood pressure Control in Diabetes),[37] FACET (Fosinopril vs Amlodipine Cardiovascular Events randomized Trial),[38] and MIDAS (Multicentre Isradipine Diuretic Atherosclerosis Study),[39] have raised the possibility that macrovascular disease does not respond in direct proportion to the degree of BP lowering with certain antihypertensive agents. Several investigators have suggested that CCBs of the dihydropyridine class may be deleterious or at least not as efficacious in reducing cardiovascular events as other antihypertensive agents such as ACE inhibitors.[40] In the ABCD and FACET studies, macrovascular endpoints were observed in a smaller percentage of patients on ACE inhibitors than on CCB. The disparity in cardiovascular events observed between ACE inhibitors and CCBs in the FACET and ABCD studies needs to be viewed with caution, on account of the small size of the study groups and the fact that cardiovascular events were a secondary and not a primary end-point of the study protocol. The HOT Study argues against claims of cardiac damage by CCB, and suggests that the high rates of coronary events noted in the FACET and ABCD studies could reflect superior protection by ACE inhibitors and not damage by CCBs.[29] Furthermore, in the FACET study, the group receiving the combination of ACE inhibitors and CCB did not have increased cardiovascular events when compared with the group receiving ACE inhibitors alone.[38] Nevertheless, in the absence of concurrent control groups, it is not possible to determine whether ACE inhibitors are particularly effective in preventing macrovascular disease or whether the CCBs are in fact harmful.

Recently, the UKPDS reported its findings on aggressive antihypertensive treatment in newly diagnosed, hypertensive, Type 2 diabetic subjects. Randomization to the tight blood pressure control group was associated with a decrease in vascular disease when compared with the group with conventional blood pressure control.[28] Interestingly, no significant difference was observed between the atenolol- and the captopril-treated study groups.[41] This may be due to inadequate power of the study or to the possibility that both agents confer cardiovascular protection.

ACE genotype

The vasoactive hormone, angiotensin II, has been implicated in the initiation and progression of diabetic nephropathy, presumably via haemodynamic and trophic actions within the kidney. Polymorphism of genes relevant to the renin–angiotensin system, such as ACE and the angiotensin (ATI) receptor, have been assessed. Polymorphisms of the ACE gene have been linked to diabetic nephropathy by some investigators and may represent a genetic determinant of the renal response to ACE inhibitor therapy.[42] The D/D genotype confers resistance to the protective effects of ACE inhibitors when measured as the rate of decline in GFR.[42]

Role of sodium restriction

Salt sensitivity (mean arterial pressure increase >3 mmHg on a high salt diet) is present in 43%

of Type 1 diabetics, 50% of those with microalbuminuria, and 37% with normoalbuminuria, compared with 17% of non-diabetic controls.[43] Salt restriction has been reported to prevent hyperfiltration, renal enlargement, and increasing albuminuria in experimental diabetes.[44] In the Melbourne Diabetic Nephropathy Study (MDNS), the reduction in albuminuria in response to the antihypertensive agents was dependent on salt intake.[45] In those patients resistant to the effects of ACE inhibition, in terms of reduction in blood pressure or albuminuria, agents such as diuretics should be considered. The advent of the dual ACE-neutral endopeptidase inhibitors offers another possible therapeutic approach for hypertensive diabetic subjects in the future.[46]

Calcium channel blockers (CCBs)

Dihydropyridine vs *non-dihydropyridine CCBs*

Over the past 10 years, it has been suggested, mainly by Bakris and colleagues, that certain classes of CCB may differ in terms of their effects on progression of diabetic nephropathy.[47] Animal data have suggested that dihydropyridine (nifedipine-like) CCBs effectively reduce arterial pressure yet do not significantly affect proteinuria or prevent the development of glomerular scarring. These agents do not reduce glomerular membrane permeability,[48] and fail to affect the synthesis of key matrix proteins that perpetuate the development of the glomerular scarring. By contrast, the non-dihydropyridine CCBs, such as diltiazem and verapamil, blunt both the rise in proteinuria as well as mesangial matrix expansion and subsequent glomerular scarring. Long-term clinical studies in diabetic

nephropathy show renal protection from treatment with non-dihydropyridine CCBs that is not found with the dihydropyridine class when given at equihypotensive doses.[47]

Role of ACE inhibitors plus CCBs

There is a theoretical case to be made for combining these two therapeutic classes. Angiotensin II is implicated in the development of proteinuria and progression of renal disease. ACE inhibitors reduce the generation of angiotensin II, and CCBs interfere with the action of angiotensin II, particularly at the efferent arteriole. Since clinicians are unable to achieve blood pressure levels that are suggested in the guidelines for diabetic patients with early and overt renal disease, it is likely that multiple drugs will be needed. Bakris has demonstrated in diabetic patients that the combination of lisinopril and diltiazem is more effective than the respective monotherapies.[49] Similar results have been obtained with the combination of lisinopril and verapamil.[50]

Angiotensin II receptor antagonists

Antagonists in this relatively new therapeutic class competitively block the binding of angiotensin to angiotensin II receptors and therefore block the effects of angiotensin more selectively than do ACE inhibitors.[51] These agents reduce angiotensin II-induced vasoconstriction, sodium reabsorption, and aldosterone release, without affecting bradykinin degradation. Angiotensin II receptor antagonists are not associated with cough and are particularly useful in people with an ACE inhibitor-induced cough. Animal studies suggest that the renoprotective effects of these AII receptor antagonists and ACE inhibitors are similar.[52]

Clinical studies on this class of antihypertensive agent are now in progress, and the results keenly awaited.[35]

The role of antihypertensive agents in normotension

It should be noted that many of the studies of antihypertensive agents in supposedly normotensive patients used higher levels of blood pressure to define hypertension than are now recommended. Most of the studies have been carried out in Type 1 diabetic subjects. Fewer patients with Type 2 diabetes are normotensive, and many have significant co-morbidity and concomitant therapy.

Overt nephropathy

In 1989, Parving reported that the ACE inhibitor captopril reduced AER in normotensive Type 1 diabetic subjects.[53] The situation in Type 2 diabetes is less clear, as few proteinuric Type 2 diabetic subjects are truly normotensive.

Microalbuminuria

Type 1 diabetes
Several groups have reported a beneficial effect for ACE inhibitor therapy in normotensive diabetic subjects (Table 10.3). GFR was measured in some of the studies using various techniques. There is a trend for the GFR to remain stable on the ACE inhibitor while continuing to decline in the placebo group in these studies. In many of these studies, the reduction in blood pressure in the treatment arm was modest. This has been interpreted as indicating that the renoprotective effect of ACE inhibitors may be partly independent of their antihypertensive properties, but another poss-ibility is that modest reduction in blood pressure is particularly beneficial in the context of afferent arteriolar vasodilation, as has been observed experimentally in the diabetic kidney.

Type 2 diabetes
In Type 2 normotensive, microalbuminuric diabetic subjects, the rate of renal deterioration is relatively slow. The vast majority of Caucasian diabetic patients with microalbumin-uria are already hypertensive. Conversely, many Asian Type 2 diabetic subjects will be normoten-sive on the current criteria. The studies reported in Table 10.3, show a beneficial effect of ACE inhibitors compared with placebo in this population of normotensive, microalbuminuric, Type 2 diabetic subjects. Whether these data are applicable to the older, more obese, Caucasian population is not yet certain.

Normoalbuminuria

The majority of patients in the EUCLID study were normotensive Type 1 diabetic subjects. In this group, studied over 2 years, there was no clear benefit of ACE inhibitors in preventing the development of microalbuminuria.[54] However, these findings should be interpreted with caution, since the study was of a relatively short duration. At present, there is no evidence that ACE inhibitors are indicated in Type 2 diabetic patients with normotensive and normoalbuminuria.

In the EUCLID study, ACE inhibition was associated with reduced progression of retinopathy,[55] providing evidence of the link between angiotensin II-dependent mechanisms and diabetic retinopathy. Interestingly, in the recent UKPDS, tight blood pressure control was also associated with a reduction in retinopathy.[28] Further studies are required with retinopathy as a primary end-point to confirm the potential benefit of antihypertensive

Table 10.3
Effects of antihypertensive agents on urinary albumin excretion rate (AER) in normotensive, Type 1 and 2 microalbuminuric patients with diabetes.

Study	Type of diabetes	Duration of study	Number	Agent	Change in AER (%)
Viberti et al. 1994[56]	1	2 years	46	Captopril	↓
			46	Placebo	↑
O'Donnell 1993[57]	1	48 weeks	12	Lisinopril	↓ (−50)
			15	Placebo	→
Laffel et al. 1995[58]	1	2 years	67	Captopril	↓ (−36)
			70	Placebo	↑ (+24)
Marre et al. 1988[59]	1	12 months	10	Enalapril	↓
			10	Placebo	↑
Mathiesen et al. 1991[60]	1	4 years	21	Captopril	↓ (−32)
			23	Placebo	↑ (+63)
EUCLID 1997[54]	1	2 years	32	Lisinopril	↓ (−50)
			37	Placebo	↑
Jerums 1997[61]	1	>3 years	13	Perindopril	↓
			9	Nifedipine	↑
			14	Placebo	↑
Crepaldi et al. 1998[62]	1	3 years	32	Lisinopril	↓ (−47)
			26	Nifedipine	↓ (−18)
			34	Placebo	↑ (+35)
Ahmad et al. 1997[63]	2	5 years	52	Enalapril	↓ (−64)
			51	Placebo	↑ (+60)
Sano et al. 1994[64]	2	4 years	12	Enalapril	↓ (−47)
			12	Untreated	→
Ravid et al. 1993[65]	2	5 years	49	Enalapril	→
			45	Untreated	↑ (+152)

therapy and, in particular, agents such as ACE inhibitors and AII receptor antagonists on diabetic retinopathy.

Isolated systolic hypertension

Isolated systolic hypertension (systolic pressure >160 with diastolic <90 mmHg) is common in elderly Type 2 diabetic patients. In the SHEP (Systolic Hypertension in the Elderly Program) study, 10% of participants had diabetes and

derived similar beneficial effects from blood pressure reduction as did the non-diabetic subjects.[66]

Glycaemic control

Type 1 diabetes

In the Diabetes Control and Complications Trial (DCCT), strict glycaemic control, when compared with conventional insulin therapy, gave a reduced mean adjusted risk for the cumulative incidence of microalbuminuria of 34% in those patients initially normoalbuminuric.[67] Albuminuria (AER) decreased by 15% in the first year of treatment only; thereafter, the rates of change for AER in each treatment group stayed at zero. In the secondary prevention arm of the DCCT, intensive therapy in the low microalbuminuric group (20–28 µg/min), was associated with reduced progression of renal disease. The benefit of intensified insulin treatment in those subjects with higher levels of AER was not as readily apparent. It should be noted that the benefits gained in the intensively treated group were at the expense of significantly more hypoglycaemic episodes.

It had been previously considered that once a patient had established nephropathy, glycaemic control had no role in retarding progression in ESRD. However, more recent data have shown a beneficial effect of intensified glycaemic control in macroalbuminuric diabetic subjects, especially if it is combined with good blood pressure control.[68]

Type 2 diabetes

In the Japanese Kumamato study, intensive treatment to improve glycaemic control resulted in a reduced rate of nephropathy.[69] The UKPDS has recently confirmed a close relationship between glycaemic control and vascular complications.[70] In particular, intensified glycaemic control with either sulphonylureas or insulin was associated with a decrease in microvascular events, including retinopathy and albuminuria, with a tendency for a reduction in cardiovascular end-points.[70] Interestingly, metformin was at least as effective, if not superior to, the other hypoglycaemic agents in preventing diabetes-related end-points.[71]

Lipids

Recently, it has been suggested that lipid-lowering therapy may also confer renoprotection in diabetic subjects.[72,73] There are many theoretical reasons for lipids to accelerate renal injury, including activation of cytokine-dependent pathways, and stimulation of macrophage proliferation and recruitment.[74] Several studies have suggested that HMG CoA reductase inhibitors retard the progression of incipient[73] and overt diabetic nephropathy,[72] but these findings have not been universal.[75]

Protein

Several studies involving small numbers of patients have suggested that protein restriction may slow the decline in renal function in patients with diabetic nephropathy. Zeller *et al.* have reported that a low protein diet was associated with a 75% reduction in the rate of decline of the GFR in patients with Type 1 diabetic nephropathy.[76] A meta-analysis of the various trials in diabetic subjects has concluded that there is a beneficial effect on GFR, creatinine clearance, and albuminuria with modest (0.5–0.85 g/kg/day) protein restriction.[77]

References

1. Cooper ME. Pathogenesis, prevention, and treatment of diabetic nephropathy. *Lancet* 1998; **52:** 213–219.
2. Mogensen CE, Keane WF, Bennett PH *et al.* Prevention of diabetic renal disease with special reference to microalbuminuria. *Lancet* 1995; **346:** 1080–1084.
3. Gilbert RE, Akdeniz A, Jerums G. Detection of microalbuminuria in diabetic patients by urinary dipstick. *Diabetes Res Clin Pract* 1997; **35:** 57–60.
4. Mogensen CE, Andersen MJF. Increased kidney

size and glomerular filtration rate in untreated juvenile diabetics. Normalization by insulin treatment. *Diabetologia* 1975; **11**: 221–224.

5. Vora JP, Dolben J, Dean JD *et al*. Renal haemodynamics in newly presenting non-insulin-dependent diabetes mellitus. *Kidney Int* 1992; **41**: 829–835.

6. Rudberg S, Østerby R. Decreasing glomerular filtration rate – an indicator of more advanced diabetic glomerulopathy in the early course of microalbuminuria in IDDM adolescents? *Nephrol Dial Transplant* 1997; **12**: 1149–1154.

7. Poulsen PL, Hansen KW, Mogensen CE. Ambulatory blood pressure in the transition from normo- to microalbuminuria. A longitudinal study in IDDM patients. *Diabetes* 1994; **43**: 1248–1253.

8. Mogensen CE. Hyperfiltration, hypertension and diabetic nephropathy in IDDM patients. *Diabetes Nutr Metab* 1989; **2**: 227–244.

9. Lervang H, Jensen S, Brochner-Mortsensen J, Ditzel J. Early glomerular hyperfiltration and the development of late nephropathy in Type I (insulin-dependent) diabetes mellitus. *Diabetologia* 1988; **31**: 723–729.

10. Gilbert RE, Tsalamandris C, Allen TJ *et al*. Evolving nephropathy and vision-threatening retinal disease in type I diabetes. *J Am Soc Nephrol* 1998; **9**: 85–89.

11. Mogensen CE. Microalbuminuria predicts clinical proteinuria and early mortality in maturity onset diabetes. *N Engl J Med* 1984; **310**: 356–360.

12. Messent JWC, Elliot TG, Hill RD *et al*. Prognostic significance of microalbuminuria in insulin-dependent diabetes mellitus. A twenty-three year follow-up study. *Kidney Int* 1992; **41**: 836–839.

13. Zatz R, Dunn BR, Meyer TW *et al*. Prevention of diabetic glomerulopathy by pharmacological amelioration of glomerular capillary hypertension. *J Clin Invest* 1986; **77**: 1925–1930.

14. Gilbert RE, Cox A, Wu LL *et al*. Expression of transforming growth factor β-1 and type VI collagen in the renal tubulointerstitium in experimental diabetes. *Diabetes* 1998; **47**: 414–422.

15. Soulis T, Cooper ME, Vranes D *et al*. The effects of aminoguanidine in preventing experimental diabetic nephropathy are related to duration of treatment. *Kidney Int* 1996; **50**: 627–634.

16. Wuerth J-P, Bain R, Mecca T *et al*. and the Pimagedine Investigators Group. Baseline data from the Pimagedine Action trials. *Diabetologia* 1997; **40**: A548.

17. Vasan S, Zhang X, Zhang X *et al*. An agent cleaving glucose-derived protein crosslinks *in vitro* and *in vivo*. *Nature* 1996; **382**: 275–278.

18. Ishii H, Jirousek MR, Koya D *et al*. Amelioration of vascular dysfunction in diabetic rats by an oral PKC β inhibitor. *Science* 1996; **272**: 728–731.

19. Parving H-H, Hommel E, Mathiesen ER *et al*. Prevalence of microalbuminuria, arterial hypertension, retinopathy and neuropathy in insulin-dependent diabetic patients. *Br Med J* 1988; **296**: 156–160.

20. Hasslacher C, Ritz E, Wahl P, Michael C. Similar risks of nephropathy inpatients with Type 1 or Type 2 diabetes mellitus. *Nephrol Dial Transplant* 1989; **4**: 859–863.

21. Borch-Johnsen K. The cost of nephropathy in Type II diabetes. *Pharmaco Economics* 1995; **8 (Suppl 1)**: 40–45.

22. Eggers PW. Effects of transplantation on the medicare end-stage renal disease program. *N Engl J Med* 1988; **318**: 223–229.

23. Williams B. Insulin resistance: the shape of things to come. *Lancet* 1994; **344**: 521–524.

24. Cowie CC, Port FK, Wolfe RA *et al*. Disparities in incidence of diabetic end stage renal disease according to race and type of diabetes. *N Engl J Med* 1989; **321**: 1074–1079.

25. Pugh JA, Medina RA, Cornell JC, Basu S. NIDDM is the major cause of diabetic end-stage renal disease. More evidence from a tri-ethnic community. *Diabetes* 1995; **44**: 1375–1380.

26. Joint National Committee on prevention detection and treatment of high blood pressure. The sixth report of the joint national committee on prevention, detection, evaluation and treatment of high blood pressure. *Arch Int Med* 1997; **157**: 2413–2445.

27. Tarnow L, Rossing P, Gall MA *et al*. Prevalence of arterial hypertension in diabetic patients before and after JNC-V. *Diabetes Care* 1994; **17**: 1247–1251.

28. UK Prospective Diabetes Study (UKPDS) Group. Tight blood pressure control and risk of macrovascular and microvascular complications

in Type 2 diabetes: UKPDS 38. *Br Med J* 1998; **317**: 703–713.

29. Hansson L, Zanchetti A, Carruthers SG *et al.* Effects of intensive blood-pressure lowering and low-dose aspirin in patients with hypertension: principle results of the hypertension optimal treatment (HOT) randomised trial. *Lancet* 1998; **351**: 1755–1762.

30. Gilbert RE, Jerums G, Cooper ME. Diabetes and hypertension: prognostic and therapeutic considerations. *Blood Pressure* 1995; **4**: 329–338.

31. Borch-Johnsen K, Andersen PK, Deckert T. The effect of proteinuria on relative mortality in type 1 (insulin-dependent) diabetes mellitus. *Diabetologia* 1985; **28**: 590–596.

32. Dupree EA, Mayer MB. Role of risk factors in the complications of diabetes mellitus. *Am J Epidemiol* 1980; **112**: 100–112.

33. Farmer CKT, Goldsmith DJA, Quinn JD *et al.* Progression of diabetic nephropathy – is diurnal blood pressure rhythm as important as absolute blood pressure level? *Nephrol Dial Transplant* 1998; **13**: 635–639.

34. Gilbert RE, Cooper ME, Krum H. Drug administration in patients with diabetes mellitus. Safety considerations. *Drug Safety* 1998; **18**: 441–455.

35. Rodby RA. Antihypertensive treatment in nephropathy of type II diabetes: role of the pharmacological blockade of the renin–angiotensin system. *Nephrol Dial Transplant* 1997; **12**: 1095–1096.

36. Califf RM, Granger CB. Hypertension and diabetes and the Fosinopril vs Amlodipine Cardiovascular events trial (FACET). More ammunition against surrogate end-points. *Diabetes Care* 1998; **21**: 655–657.

37. Estacio RO, Jeffers BW, Hiatt WR *et al.* The effect of nisoldipine as compared with enalapril on cardiovascular outcomes in patients with non-insulin-dependent diabetes and hypertension. *N Engl J Med* 1998; **338**: 645–652.

38. Tatti P, Pahor M, Byington RP *et al.* Outcome results of the fosinopril vs amlodipine cardiovascular events randomized trial (FACET) in patients with hypertension and NIDDM. *Diabetes Care* 1998; **21**: 597–603.

39. Byington RP, Craven TE, Furberg CD, Pahor M. Isradipine, raised glycosylated haemoglobin and risk of cardiovascular events. *Lancet* 1997; **350**: 1075–1076.

40. Pahor M, Psaty BM, Furberg CD. Treatment of hypertensive patients with diabetes. *Lancet* 1998; **351**: 689–690.

41. UK Prospective Diabetes Study (UKPDS) Group. Efficacy of atenolol and captopril in reducing risk of macrovascular and microvascular complications in type 2 diabetes: UKPDS 39. *Br Med J* 1998; **317**: 713–720.

42. Parving H-H, Jacobsen P, Tarnow L *et al.* Effect of deletion polymorphism of angiotensin converting enzyme gene on progression of diabetic nephropathy during inhibition of angiotensin converting enzyme: observational follow up study. *Br Med J* 1996; **313**: 591–594.

43. Strojek K, Grzeszczak W, Lacka B *et al.* Increased prevalence of salt sensitivity of blood pressure in IDDM with and without microalbuminuria. *Diabetologia* 1995; **38**: 1443–1448.

44. Allen TJ, Waldron MJ, Casley D *et al.* Salt restriction reduces hyperfiltration, renal enlargement, and albuminuria in experimental diabetes. *Diabetes* 1997; **46**: 119–124.

45. Jerums G, Allen TJ, Tsalamandris C, Cooper ME, for the Melbourne Diabetic Nephropathy Study Group. Angiotensin converting enzyme inhibition and calcium channel blockade in incipient diabetic nephropathy. *Kidney Int* 1992; **41**: 904–911.

46. Tikkanen T, Tikkanen I, Rockell M *et al.* Dual inhibition of neutral endopeptidase and angiotensin converting enzyme in rats with hypertension and diabetes mellitus. *Hypertension* 1998; **32**: 778–785.

47. Bakris GL, Copley JB, Vicknair N *et al.* Calcium channel blockers versus other antihypertensive therapies on progression of NIDDM associated nephropathy. *Kidney Int* 1996; **50**: 1641–1650.

48. Smith AC, Toto R, Bakris GL. Differential effects of calcium channel blockers on size selectivity of proteinuria in diabetic glomerulopathy. *Kidney Int* 1998; **54**: 889–896.

49. Bakris GL. Effects of diltiazem or lisinopril on massive proteinuria associated with diabetes mellitus. *Ann Int Med* 1990; **112**: 701–702.

50. Bakris GL, Barnhill BW, Sadler R. Treatment of arterial hypertension in diabetic humans:

Importance of therapeutic selection. *Kidney Int* 1992; **41**: 912–919.

51. Johnston CI. Angiotensin receptor antagonists: focus on losartan. *Lancet* 1995; **346**: 1403–1407.

52. Allen TJ, Cao Z, Youssef S *et al*. The role of angiotensin II and bradykinin in experimental diabetic nephropathy: functional and structural studies. *Diabetes* 1997; **46**: 1612–1618.

53. Parving H-H, Hommel E, Damkjaer NM, Giese J. Effect of captopril on blood pressure and kidney function in normotensive insulin-dependent diabetics with nephropathy. *Br Med J* 1989; **299**: 533–536.

54. The EUCLID Study Group. Randomised placebo-controlled trial of lisinopril in normotensive patients with insulin-dependent diabetes and normoalbuminuria or microalbuminuria. *Lancet* 1997; **349**: 1787–1792.

55. Chaturvedi N, Sjolie AK, Stephenson JM *et al*. Effect of lisinopril on progression of retinopathy in normotensive people with type 1 diabetes. *Lancet* 1998; **351**: 28–31.

56. Viberti GC, Mogensen CE, Groop LC, Pauls JF, for the European Microalbuminuria Captopril Study Group. Effect of captopril on progression to clinical proteinuria in patients with insulin-dependent diabetes mellitus and microalbuminuria. European microalbuminuria study group. *JAMA* 1994; **271**: 275–279.

57. O'Donnell MJ, Rowe BR, Lawson N. Placebo-controlled trial of lisinopril in normotensive diabetic patients with incipient nephropathy. *J Hum Hypertens* 1993; **7**: 327–332.

58. Laffel LM, McGill JB, Gans DJ, for the North American Microalbuminuria study group. The beneficial effect of angiotensin-converting enzyme inhibition with captopril on diabetic nephropathy in normotensive IDDM patients with microalbuminuria. *Am J Med* 1995; **99**: 497–504.

59. Marre M, Chatelier G, Leblanc H *et al*. Prevention of diabetic nephropathy with enalapril in normotensive diabetics with microalbuminuria. *Br Med J* 1988; **297**: 1092–1095.

60. Mathiesen ER, Hommel E, Giese J, Parving H-H. Efficacy of captopril in postponing nephropathy in normotensive insulin-dependent diabetic patients with microalbuminuria. *Br Med J* 1991; **308**: 81–87.

61. Jerums G. Angiotensin-converting enzyme inhibition and calcium-channel blockade in diabetic patients with microalbuminuria. *Nephrology* 1997; **3**: S41.

62. Crepaldi G, Carta Q, Deperrari G *et al*. Effects of lisinopril and nifedipine on the progression to overt albuminuria in IDDM patients with incipient nephropathy and normal blood pressure. *Diabetes Care* 1998; **21**: 104–110.

63. Ahmad J, Siddiqui MA, Ahmad H. Effective postponement of diabetic nephropathy with enalapril in normotensive type 2 diabetic patients with microalbuminuria. *Diabetes Care* 1997; **20**: 1576–1581.

64. Sano T, Kawamura T, Matsumae H *et al*. Effects of long-term enalapril treatment on persistent microalbuminuria in well-controlled hypertensive and normotensive NIDDM patients. *Diabetes Care* 1994; **17**: 420–424.

65. Ravid M, Savin H, Jutrin I *et al*. Long-term stabilizing effect of angiotensin-converting enzyme inhibition on plasma creatinine and on proteinuria in normotensive Type 2 diabetic patients. *Ann Int Med* 1993; **118**: 577–581.

66. Systolic Hypertension in the Elderly Program cooperative research group. Implications of the systolic hypertension in the elderly program. *Hypertension* 1993; **21**: 335–343.

67. The Diabetes Control and Complications (DCCT) research group. Effect of intensive therapy on the development and progression of diabetic nephropathy in the diabetes control and complications trial. *Kidney Int* 1995; **47**: 1703–1720.

68. Alaveras AE, Thomas SM, Sagriotis A, Viberti GC. Promoters of progression of diabetic nephropathy: the relative roles of blood glucose and blood pressure control. *Nephrol Dial Transplant* 1997; **2**: 71–74.

69. Ohkubo Y, Kishikawa H, Araki E *et al*. Intensive insulin therapy prevents the progression of diabetic microvascular complications in Japanese patients with non-insulin-dependent diabetes mellitus: a randomised prospective 6-year study. *Diabetes Res Clin Pract* 1995; **28**: 103–117.

70. UK Prospective Diabetes Study (UKPDS) Group. Intensive blood-glucose control with sulphonylureas or insulin compared with

conventional treatment and risk of complications in patients with Type 2 diabetes (UKPDS 33). *Lancet* 1998; **352**: 837–853.

71. UK Prospective Diabetes Study (UKPDS) group. Effect of intensive blood-glucose control with metformin on complications in overweight patients with Type 2 diabetes (UKPDS 34). *Lancet* 1998; **352**: 854–865.

72. Lam KS, Cheng IK, Janus ED, Pang RW. Cholesterol-lowering therapy may retard the progression of diabetic nephropathy. *Diabetologia* 1995; **38**: 604–609.

73. Tonolo G, Ciccarese M, Brizzi P *et al*. Reduction of albumin excretion rate in normotensive microalbuminuric Type 2 diabetic patients during long-term simvastatin treatment. *Diabetes Care* 1997; **20**: 1891–1895.

74. Park YS, Guijarro C, Kim Y *et al*. Lovastatin reduces glomerular macrophage influx and expression of monocyte chemoattractant protein-1 mRNA in nephrotic rats. *Am J Kidney Dis* 1998; **31**: 190–194.

75. Hommel E, Andersen P, Gall MA *et al*. Plasma lipoproteins and renal function during simvastatin treatment in diabetic nephropathy. *Diabetologia* 1992; **35**: 447–451.

76. Zeller K, Whittaker E, Sullivan L *et al*. Effect of restricting dietary protein on the progression of renal failure in patients with insulin-dependent diabetes mellitus. *N Engl J Med* 1991; **324**: 78–84.

77. Pedrini MT, Levey AS, Lau J *et al*. The effect of dietary protein restriction in the progression of diabetic and nondiabetic renal diseases – a meta-analysis. *Ann Int Med* 1996; **124**: 627–632.

11

The diabetic foot

Edward B Jude and Andrew JM Boulton

Introduction

Foot problems in diabetic patients account for more hospital admissions than any of the other long-term complications of diabetes and also result in increasing morbidity and mortality in diabetic patients.[1] Therefore, understanding the underlying causes and pathogenesis of foot problems may help direct more specific treatment and perhaps improve the outcome of diabetic foot disease.

The 'diabetic foot' encompasses a number of pathologies, including diabetic neuropathy, peripheral vascular disease, Charcot neuroarthropathy, foot ulceration, and osteomyelitis, and the potentially preventable end-point, amputation.[2] Diabetic foot ulceration is traditionally considered to be a consequence of peripheral neuropathy and peripheral vascular disease. Diabetic neuropathy is the most important causative and major contributory factor to foot ulceration in over 80% of cases. A study from King's College Hospital, London, showed that 62% of diabetic foot ulcers were of predominantly neuropathic aetiology, 13% purely vascular and 25% neuroischaemic.[3] In our centre, Thomson *et al.*[4] reported 45% to be of purely neuropathic aetiology, 7% ischaemic, and 45% of mixed aetiology, or in other words nearly 90% had a neuropathic component.

The impact of foot ulceration on patient care and quality of life is enormous, not only in diabetic patients, but also on family members and carers.[5] Approximately 15% of all diabetic patients will develop a foot ulcer during their lifetime.[6] Various studies report the incidence of foot ulceration, the commonest risk factor to amputation, in the range 3–7%.[7-11] A recent multicentre study found that the annual incidence of foot ulceration was 7.2% in diabetic individuals with established neuropathy.[12]

Foot ulceration is an important predisposing factor to amputation, and is present in over 80% of all diabetes-related amputations.[10] Lower-extremity amputation is 15 times more common in the diabetic than in the non-diabetic population. There is also a 50% chance of a diabetic patient with one lower limb amputation developing a serious lesion in the second limb within 2 years.[13]

The cost of diabetic foot ulceration to the health-care services is enormous. It is estimated that in the UK at least 4–5% of the total annual budget is spent on diabetes management. Of this, the expenditure on diabetic foot disease is over £13 million per annum.[14] Preventing foot disease with proper care and education will help reduce the burden on already scarce health-care resources.

Pathogenesis of foot ulceration

Diabetic neuropathy (DN)

Neuropathy is one of the commonest long-term complications of diabetes mellitus, although estimates of the problem have varied widely, depending on the minimal criteria for diagnosis and population involved. Depending on the study and population studied, estimates of prevalence usually vary between 12 and 50%. Incidence and severity also vary with age, duration of diabetes, and glycaemic control, as well as fluctuation in blood glucose, since onset of diabetes. In a large study in the UK, symptomatic neuropathy was present in 28.5% of 6,500 diabetic patients.[15] Similarly, in a multicentre study in Europe, in Type 1 diabetes, the incidence was 28%.[16] However, in the Rochester Study, although only 13% were symptomatic, more than half of the diabetic patients had clinical evidence of neuropathy.[17]

Classification

As the precise aetiopathogenesis of neuropathy remains enigmatic, a classification based on pathogenetic grounds is not possible, so the diverse manifestations are generally classified according to clinical presentation. However, even in this area, a number of classifications exist: examples include the purely clinical, descriptive classification originally proposed by Boulton and Ward[18] (*Table 11.1*), or that based upon potential reversibility together with clinical description proposed by Thomas (*Table 11.2*).[19,20] Most patients, however, will not have any single type but will overlap with features of more than one clinical type of DN, such as chronic sensory polyneuropathy and autonomic neuropathy.

Clinical and electrophysiological assessment of neuropathy

Distal sensorimotor polyneuropathy: Distal sensory peripheral neuropathy is the commonest presentation of diabetic neuropathy. Studies on patients with proven peripheral neuropathy, by neurophysiological testing, have shown that many patients may be symptomatic and an equal number could by asymptomatic. The clinical presentation is extremely variable, ranging from severely painful ('positive') symptoms at one extreme to the completely painless variety, which may present with an insensitive foot ulcer, at the other.[21] Most patients do, at some time in the evolution of their neuropathy, experience symptoms, although these may be 'negative' and might

Polyneuropathy	Mononeuropathy

Sensory
    chronic sensorimotor
    acute/chronic sensory
	Cranial

Autonomic	Isolated peripheral
Amyotrophy	Mononeuritis multiplex
Radicular	Radicular

Table 11.1
Clinical classification of diabetic neuropathies.

Classification	
Rapidly reversible	Hyperglycaemic neuropathy
Symmetrical polyneuropathies	Distal somatic sensorimotor (mainly large fibre) Autonomic Small fibre
Focal/multifocal neuropathies	Cranial Truncal radiculopathies Focal limb Amyotrophy Compression/entrapment
Mixed forms	

Table 11.2
Clinical classification of diabetic neuropathies. Modified from Thomas (1997)[19] and Sima et al[20].

comprise 'numbness' or 'deadness' in the lower limbs. Positive symptoms most commonly include burning pain, altered and uncomfortable temperature perception, paraesthesiae, shooting, stabbing and lancinating pain, hyperaesthesiae, and allodynia. Many patients find the symptoms difficult to describe, but most report them to be extremely uncomfortable, distressing, and prone to nocturnal exacerbation. The feet and lower legs are most commonly affected, although some patients with long-standing neuropathy may experience similar, though less severe, symptoms in the upper limbs.

Although the symptoms are generally sensory, in many cases the signs are sensory and motor, with sensory loss in a stocking and glove distribution, and, to a lesser degree, minor degrees of muscle wasting and, occasionally, weakness. The ankle reflex is often reduced or absent, and the foot skin dry, caused by the frequently associated peripheral autonomic dysfunction. As some patients report no symptoms, distal symmetrical polyneuropathy cannot be excluded without a careful neurological examination.

A detailed neurologic examination cannot be covered in this chapter. Briefly, all modalities of sensation such as touch, pain, temperature, vibration (128 MHz tuning fork), and joint position sense will need to be assessed. Quantitative tests using a biothesiometer for vibration sense, a 10 g Semmes–Weinstein monofilament for pressure perception, or the tactile circumferential discriminator, which also assesses large fibre function,[22] are simple, quick, inexpensive tests that can be carried out in a routine clinic setting and be used for the diagnosis and progression of neuropathy. Studies have shown that diabetic patients with a vibration perception threshold (VPT) of >25 V in the lower limbs are at risk of insensitive foot ulceration (*Fig. 11.1*).[23]

Autonomic neuropathy: Involvement of the autonomic nervous system in diabetes can affect almost any part of the body, resulting in severe symptoms and disability. The main

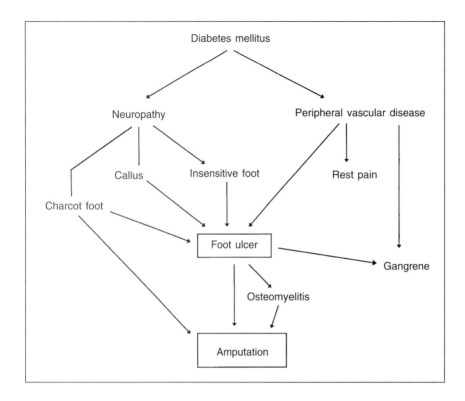

Fig. 11.1
Pathways to foot ulceration and amputation in diabetic patients.

Table 11.3
Clinical features of autonomic neuropathy. Modified from Watkins PJ, Edmonds ME. Autonomic neuropathy, in Alberti KGMM, Zimmet P, DeFronzo RA, eds. International Textbook of Diabetes Mellitus, 1997: 1497–1506.

Cardiovascular	Postural hypotension Neuropathic oedema	Increased peripheral blood flow Tachyarrhythmias
Sweating	Nocturnal sweating Gustatory sweating Dry, fissured feet	
Genito-urinary	Impotence Neurogenic bladder	
Gastro-intestinal	Diarrhoea Gastroparesis	Oesophageal motility Gall bladder emptying
Respiratory	Arrests ?Sudden deaths	?Sleep apnoea
Bone	Charcot joints	Reduced bone density in lower limbs
Eye		Pupillary size reduced

clinical features of autonomic neuropathy are shown in *Table 11.3*. In the following discussion, only impaired autonomic function of the peripheral nerve will be considered.

Peripheral vascular sympathetic denervation causes a peripheral vasodilatation associated with an opening of arteriovenous shunts,[24] resulting in an increase in blood flow to the lower limbs. This damage to the small unmyelinated nerve fibres presents clinically as warm feet with dry skin and bounding pulses, marked venous distention, and, occasionally, neuropathic oedema. Bone blood flow is also increased, leading to activation of osteoclasts and localized osteoporosis,[25,26] which may predispose to the development of Charcot's neuroarthropathy.

Postural hypotension can be a severe disabling consequence of autonomic neuropathy. Symptoms range from mild giddiness on standing up, progressing to a blurring of vision, and, in severe cases, loss of consciousness. Sweating loss is another feature of autonomic neuropathy, resulting in a dry skin which may cause its fissuring, and thus can be a predisposing factor for ulceration.

Electrophysiological studies of peripheral nerve function are the most sensitive, reliable and reproducible measures of nerve function, and will distinguish between axonal degeneration and demyelination, two important pathological aspects of peripheral nerve disease. However, electrophysiology will not diagnose the cause of a neuropathy, and is not necessary in day-to-day clinical practice.

The sural nerve at the ankle is the preferred site for cutaneous nerve biopsy. Biopsy is indicated in very few conditions and is rarely performed.

Treatment

Treatment of DN is far from satisfactory and results are variable. It can be divided into two broad groups: symptomatic relief and treatment that may alter the course and progression of the nerve damage.

Glycaemic control: Of all the known factors, probably the most important is achieving near-normal glycaemic control. Studies have shown that achieving tight glycaemic control delays the onset and slows the progression of DN, as well as providing some symptomatic relief.[27-30]

Drugs: Various drugs have been developed and tried in peripheral neuropathy, with varying results. Aldose reductase inhibitors (ARIs) act by blocking the rate-limiting enzyme in the polyol pathway, but convincing evidence about their efficacy is still lacking. However, if the efficacy of ARIs can be demonstrated in the various ongoing trials, then these agents are likely to slow the progression of neuropathy rather than provide symptomatic relief.[31,32] Alpha lipoic acid,[33] gamma linoleic acid,[27,34] and nerve growth factor[35] probably hold some promise for the treatment of DN in the future. Preliminary studies have demonstrated that parenteral NGF may be beneficial in diabetic neuropathy.[35-37]

Symptomatic treatment consists of drugs such as tricyclics,[38,39] carbamazepine, phenytoin, mexilitine and lignocaine, and topical capsaicin.[40] Traditional therapies such as acupuncture have also been employed with good results in painful neuropathy.[41,42] Although some or all of the above treatments may slow the progression of DN and provide symptomatic relief, the condition progresses relentlessly and ultimately prevention of the complications of DN is of utmost importance.

Peripheral vascular disease (PVD)

Atherosclerosis is the major complication of diabetes mellitus, and several studies indicate that diabetic patients have 2–5 times increased mortality due to the atherosclerosis disease compared with non-diabetic patients.[43] The relative risk of PVD in diabetic patients is even greater.

PVD is the most important cause of amputation in diabetic patients. There is a fivefold increase in the incidence of peripheral vascular disease in diabetes, resulting in a 20- to 50-fold elevation in gangrene.[44–47] In one study, about a quarter of all patients undergoing lower-extremity revascularization surgery were diabetic.[48] Fifty per cent of all patients undergoing amputation have diabetes, and 25% of all expenditure on inpatient care of diabetic patients is spent on the treatment of the diabetic foot.[49,50]

Clinical features

Examination for PVD must begin with palpating the foot pulses. In the Framingham Study, absent foot pulses were found to be 50% more common in diabetic men and women than in the general population.[51] Although the absence of foot pulses is a *sine qua non* of PVD, diabetic patients with peripheral vascular insufficiency do not always have absent foot pulses as a result of medial arterial calcification and the possible presence of more distal vessel disease. Involvement of the microcirculation was demonstrated in a prospective study in which failure of diabetic foot ulcers to heal was predicted by decreases in tissue perfusion in the foot.[52] However, whether this involvement of the microcirculation in patients with foot ulceration is causal or incidental requires further study.

The main clinical features of PVD in diabetic patients is no different to that in the non-diabetic population, and is characterized by calf claudication, foot ulceration, and gangrene, leading to amputation. Ischaemia is a major causative factor in 38–52% of all cases of diabetic foot ulcers, and a predisposing factor to amputation in nearly half of all

diabetes-related amputations. However, in most cases other factors such as neuropathy may be involved, and trauma is usually a triggering factor for ulceration.

Regular assessment of the peripheral circulation is important because in the presence of severe neuropathy, diabetic patients may present late, as claudication may not always be a feature in the diabetic patient. Ankle brachial pressure index (ABPI) is an important bedside clinical measurement for assessing the lower limb circulation. Using Doppler pressures, PVD was found to be 2.5–3 times more common in the diabetic than in non-diabetic subjects.[53] However, arterial calcification is common in diabetic patients, making it difficult to measure the ankle pressures. Because medial arterial calcification does not extend into the digital arteries it is possible to assess perfusion pressure by measuring toe systolic pressure, and this can be expressed as a ratio of pressure recorded from the arm to obtain the toe systolic index.[54]

Peripheral angiography is the gold standard for diagnosing peripheral arterial disease and also for planning management and revascularization. Angiography in the diabetic patient carries an increased risk of precipitating renal insufficiency and occasionally acute renal failure. Post-angiogram renal dysfunction appears to be related to the contrast material and is more likely to occur in a patient whose renal function is already compromised.[55] Distribution of vascular disease in the lower limb is thought to be different in diabetes, with more frequent involvement of vessels below the knee. Strandness *et al.*[56] reported that diabetic patients had more infrapopliteal disease, although King *et al.*[57] found greater involvement of the profunda femoris. In our random study of patients referred for angiography, no difference was seen in proximal disease (iliac, femoro-popliteal vessels) but distal disease (calf vessel) was twice as high in diabetic than non-diabetic patients.[58]

Treatment

Diabetic patients with intermittent claudication, ischaemic ulcers, or gangrene need referral to a vascular surgeon. Medical measures can be implemented, but ultimately revascularization is vital. Medical measures comprise exercise therapy,[59] cessation of smoking,[54] strict glycaemic control, treatment of hypertension and hypercholesterolaemia, and discontinuing beta-blockers and aspirin, all of which are probably most useful in the longer term.[60–63] However, in patients with non-healing foot ulcers, severe ischaemia, and gangrene, surgical intervention is required.

Revascularization is more difficult in the diabetic than the non-diabetic patient owing to more generalized disease of the peripheral circulation and also due to other coexisting problems such as neuropathy, ulceration, and infection. Proximal arterial disease is usually amenable to angioplasty or may require bypass surgery. However, with advances in vascular surgery, distal bypass is now possible and good results have been reported for this procedure resulting in a decline in amputation in the ischaemic diabetic foot.[64–66]

Biomechanical aspects

The most important cause for foot ulceration is loss of 'protective pain sensation', resulting in 'painless' repetitve trauma and tissue injury. However, vertical pressure being applied to the plantar surface of the feet during walking and standing predisposes to ulceration. Patients with peripheral neuropathy and in particular ulcer patients have higher plantar pressures,[67] although high pressures alone in the absence of insensitivity do not lead to ulceration.[68] Neuropathy with altered proprioception and

small muscle wasting leads to alteration in foot shape, clawing of the toes, prominent metatarsal heads, limited joint mobility, and a high arch, all of which result in changes in foot pressures.[69] The more severe deformity of the Charcot foot with joint dislocation and bony deformities also results in increased foot pressures and foot ulceration.

Callus formation

A callus (callosity) is a diffuse area of relatively even thickness, often several millimetres thick, which results from hypertrophy of the stratum corneum. The normal physiological process of keratinization, which maintains the stratum corneum as a protective cover, becomes stimulated to overactivity under the influence of intermittent high foot pressures. This excessive keratinization develops over sites of high pressure loading and results from a combination of increased vertical and shear forces, which presumably stimulate keratinocyte activity, and dryness of the skin due to autonomic neuropathy. Callus formation can increase plantar foot pressures and may cause haemorrhage into the callus, with subsequent ulceration.[70]

Footwear

The provision to patients of specially designed shoes may help reduce abnormal foot pressures, callus formation,[71] and foot ulcers.[72] Inappropriate footwear can be an independent risk factor for ulceration.[73] Uccioli and colleagues,[72] in a randomized study, demonstrated that in patients with previous ulceration, the wearing of therapeutic shoes resulted in a reduced incidence of ulcer relapses or new ulcers compared with those patients wearing normal shoes.

Other risk factors for ulceration

Although one or more of the above factors are necessary in the development of a foot ulcer, other factors play an important role in predicting foot ulceration. Of all the risk factors identified, the most important is a previous history of ulceration or amputation of the other leg.[74] Other risk factors include old age, duration of diabetes, nephropathy, cigarette smoking, social deprivation, and social isolation.[7,10,12,53,70,75-79] Patients with poor knowledge of diabetes and its management are also more at risk of ulceration. In one study, only a quarter of patients with new foot ulcers had considered themselves at risk of foot ulceration, and over two-thirds had never had their feet measured.[74]

Classification and management of diabetic foot ulcers

Classification of foot ulcers is important for prognosis, as well as for choosing aids for their management. The Wagner classification[80] is the most frequently used, and is based on the depth of penetration of the ulcer and the extent of tissue necrosis (*Table 11.4*).

Grade 0 foot

A grade 0 foot has no ulcers but is at risk, and regular examination is essential. Presence of callus under weight-bearing areas is particularly dangerous because this can act like a foreign body and cause ulceration of the underlying skin. Bleeding into a callus can be a predisposing factor to ulceration, and haemorrhage has been demonstrated in diabetic patients with neuropathy. A recent study demonstrated increased capillary fragility in the feet of neuropathic patients with a history of ulceration compared with those of neuropathic control subjects.[81] Removal of callus can prevent foot ulceration by decreasing foot pressure, and patients need regular review by the chiropodist. These patients also need education in proper foot care and follow-up at the foot clinic.

Grade 1 ulcers

These are superficial with full-thickness skin loss, and are commonly of neuropathic aetiology and present under areas of pressure such as the metatarsal heads (*Fig. 11.2*). They may also occur on the toes or, less commonly, at other sites. These ulcers are usually not infected and treatment is directed at debridement and

Table 11.4
Wagner classification of the diabetic foot.

Grade 0	At-risk foot, no ulcer; callus formation, no ulcer
Grade 1	Superficial ulcer – not infected
Grade 2	Deeper ulcer – often infected
Grade 3	Deep ulcer, abscess formation, or bone involvement
Grade 4	Partial gangrene of foot (heel or toe)
Grade 5	Gangrene of whole foot

relieving pressure of the ulcerated area. Pressure relief can be done using a walking plaster cast or scotch cast boot.[82,83] Although this treatment is effective in decreasing pressure, patients should be advised to rest as much as possible, since casting an insensitive limb itself can cause ulcers.[84]

Grade 2 ulcers

These are mostly neuropathic, deeper, often penetrating subcutaneous tissue, with infection but no bony involvement. Wound fluid culture may be required, but diagnosis of infection is often made on clinical evidence of purulent discharge, inflammation, and cellulitis. Diabetic foot infections tends to be polymicrobial in over 70% of patients, and on average three to five organisms are cultured per patient.[85,86] Aerobic gram-positive cocci are most commonly isolated, of which *Staphylococcus aureus* is the most frequent, followed by coagulase-negative staphylococcus, streptococcus species, and enterococci. Of the gram-negative pathogens, *Proteus, E. coli*, and *Pseudomonas*, and anaerobes such as *Bacteroides* may be isolated. The method of obtaining a wound swab is important, and superficial wound swabs have been shown to be inadequate and isolate multiple organism and skin commensals.[87–89] Therefore, deep tissue specimens using a currette should be sent and cultured on anaerobic and aerobic culture media. If infection is suspected, then it is best to use broad-spectrum antibiotics, such as cephalexin, augmentin (amoxycillin and clavulinic acid), or clindamycin, since they cover most common pathogens.[90] Severely infected ulcers with cellulitis may be treated with a combination of one of the above plus a quinolone such as ciprofloxacin. If anaerobic infection is suspected, metronidazole is added to the regimen. However, in more serious, limb-threatening infections, intravenous antibiotics should be initiated immediately with β-lactam plus β-lactamase inhibitor, cefoxitin, or cefotetan. Combination therapy with vancomycin, metronidazole, and aztreonam or fluoroquinolone and clindamycin may be used.[91] The rationale is that the infection is invariably polymicrobial (enteric gram-negative bacteria, gram-positive cocci, and anaerobic). The treatment regimen can be modified once wound fluid culture results are available. Close association with the microbiologist and the infectious disease specialist is essential. Newer treatments, such as platelet-derived growth factor,[92] granulocyte colony-stimulating factor,[93] Dermagraft,[94] and hyperbaric oxygen,[95] have shown improved healing of diabetic foot ulcers in a research setting. However, it must be stressed that no treatment, however effective, would replace regular chiropody, education, and off-loading the ulcer with appropriate footwear.

Grade 3 ulcers

These are diagnosed when there is cellulitis, occasionally with abscess formation, and osteomyelitis. Osteomyelitis is a serious complication of foot ulceration, usually in the setting of a deep penetrating ulcer and failure of the ulcer to heal. Clinically, osteomyelitis should be suspected if on probing the ulcer with a blunt instrument one can reach the bone. Plain X-rays are indicated in any non-healing foot ulcer and can be used to diagnose osteomyelitis in about 70% of cases. Repeat X-rays may help by providing a comparison with previous X-rays. However, in difficult cases, further investigations such as magnetic resonance imaging, three-phase bone scans, and ^{111}In-labelled white scans invariably pick up the majority of cases of osteomyelitis. Conservative treatment of osteomyelitis is usually long term (up to 6 months or longer) with clindamycin or augmentin.[96] Osteomyelitis which is recalcitrant may need referral to an orthopaedic surgeon for debridement or removal of infected bone, or as a last resort for amputation.

Grade 4 lesions

This is diagnosed in the presence of localized gangrene of the toes, part of the heel, or a larger area of the distal foot. Inpatient treatment is required, and complete vascular work-up as described above will be needed. Amputation is usually inevitable, and in a 'dry gangrene' a painless black toe may be left to demarcate and amputate spontaneously. Patients with gangrene of the forefoot and toes usually require a major below-knee amputation following a period of stabilization. This decision is based on the surgeons prognosis, and will depend on the clinical picture and the results of the investigative findings.

Grade 5 lesions

The patient with extensive gangrene of the foot requires urgent hospital admission, control of diabetes and infection, and a major amputation. Such patients are best managed on the surgical ward by a vascular surgeon.

Charcot arthropathy

Charcot arthropathy, a relatively rare but devastating disorder, typically affects the joints of the feet and is seen mainly in diabetic patients with peripheral neuropathy (*Fig. 11.3*). The incidence of clinical neuropathic bone and joint changes in diabetes mellitus has been reported to be from 0.08 to 7.5%.[97] However, radiographic changes in the neuropathic foot

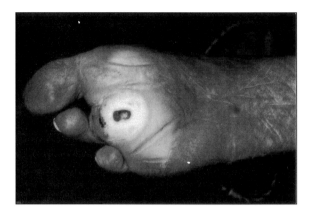

Fig. 11.2
Typical neuropathic ulcer under the third metatarsal head, with callus around the ulcer. Second and fourth toes were amputated for osteomyelitis.

have been found in around 10% of patients, and in over 16% of those with history of neuropathic foot ulceration.[98]

The exact pathogenesis is unclear, but presence of severe peripheral neuropathy, often with autonomic dysfunction, seems to be a prerequisite for the development of a Charcot joint. Trauma to the foot, however trivial, appears to be a precipitating factor leading to the occurrence of joint destruction. Studies have shown increased blood flow to the leg, arteriovenous shunting in diabetic neuropathy, and in one study increased blood flow to and vascularity of the bones of the feet, in particular in patients with a Charcot joint.[25] Reduced bone mineral density in the lower limbs of patients with Charcot foot suggests that osteopaenia may precede or precipitate the development of bone and joint changes.[26]

Clinically, the patient presents with a hot, painless, swollen foot with or without a history of preceding trauma (sometimes the trauma is so trivial that the patient does not recall it).

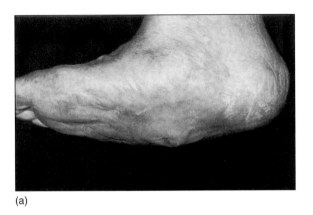

(a)

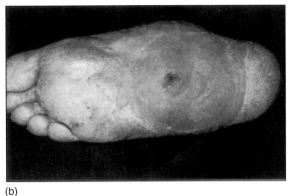

(b)

Fig. 11.3
(a) Charcot arthropathy of the left foot with collapse of the plantar arch and rocker-bottom deformity. (b) Plantar ulceration is seen under the bony deformity.

Some patients may complain of discomfort, in the absence of pain, but the majority are symptom-free. It is usually unilateral, but can be bilateral in about 10% of patients. It is commoner in the older age group (over 60s) but can also occur in the younger patient. Acute Charcot arthropathy may occasionally be mistaken for osteomyelitis or inflammatory arthritis, hence specialized investigations are required in some patients. Plain X-rays reveal bone and joint destruction, fragmentation, and remodelling in advanced cases, but early changes may be subtle or undetectable. The joints frequently involved are those of the phalanges and metatarsals, although involvement of the tarsal bones and ankles are known to occur. Three-phase ^{99m}Tc bisphosphonate bone scans demonstrate an early increase in bone uptake, which is due to the increase in blood flow through the bone that accompanies the active Charcot process. Although radiologically a diagnosis can be made with some confidence, it may be difficult to rule out osteomyelitis, especially in the presence of a foot ulcer. To rule out incidental osteomyelitis, ^{111}In-labelled leucocyte scans and magnetic resonance imaging may be required. The bone turnover markers, bone resorption (deoxypyridinoline crosslinks, carboxy-terminal telopeptide domain of type 1 collagen) and bone formation (bone-specific alkaline phosphatase), are increased in the active Charcot foot.[99,100] However, these markers will not differentiate between Charcot osteoarthropathy and osteomyelitis, since they may be elevated in the latter.

Treatment of this condition is at best difficult and is directed at reducing further the destruction of the joints. Immobilization achieved using a plaster-of-Paris cast (sometimes up to a year),[101] and reduced weight bearing is the best that can be offered at the present time. In some centres, patients are provided with a scotch-cast boot and advised to observe avoidance of weight bearing in the affected foot. Anti-inflammatory drugs such as indomethacin may be prescribed. Immobilization and rest should be continued as long as the Charcot process is active (evidenced by increased skin temperature >2°C over the active joint compared with that site of the uninvolved contralateral foot), following which special custom-fitted shoes with moulded insoles can be worn. The only pharmaceutical treatment tried to date is the bisphosphonate, pamidronate, which acts by reducing osteoclastic activity. In this small, open-labelled study we showed a rapid clinical improvement (as judged by a reduction in foot temperature) and a reduction in alkaline phosphatase.[102] We are now concluding a multicentre double-blind study using pamidronate, which will be completed in 1999. Surgical treatment has no role in the acute Charcot foot, but may be helpful in the quiescent stage for stabilizing the joints of the foot and removing bony deformities, which can be a predisposing factor to foot ulceration. Meanwhile, attention should be paid to the contralateral foot, as this foot is at risk of similar joint changes and nothing could be more devastating than the development of a Charcot arthropathy in the other foot.

Pathways to foot ulceration and amputation

An insensitive foot does not spontaneously ulcerate, but neuropathy serves as a permissive factor (*Fig. 11.1*). A recent multicentre study identified three common causal factors leading to foot ulceration: neuropathy, minor trauma, and foot deformity. This triad was present in two-thirds of patients with foot ulcers,[103] whereas vascular disease was a factor in one-third of foot ulcers. Studies have demonstrated that patients with neuropathy have abnormally high foot pressures and are more susceptible to ulceration. The presence of autonomic neuropathy heightens the risk for ulceration. Autonomic dysfunction leads to dry skin,

fissures, and callus formation, leading to higher pressures, bleeding into the callus, and foot ulceration. Pecoraro and colleagues[10] defined the causal pathways to amputation. The causal sequence of minor trauma, foot ulceration, and poor wound healing was present in 72% of the amputations. Sixty-one per cent of the amputations were attributed to neuropathy and 46% to ischaemia. However, of all the component factors, the most frequent and potentially preventable event was minor trauma, which preceded the onset of ulceration in 87% of patients.

Screening for and prevention of diabetic foot disease

The St Vincent's declaration[104] has stated that a reduction in amputation by 50% must be achieved, and to achieve this goal, diabetologists, vascular surgeons, chiropodists, and orthotists and specialist foot nurses involved in diabetes care must be aware of the impact which foot ulcers have on diabetes care, and prevention is of paramount importance if one is to reduce the incidence of amputation. However, amputation is not an inevitable consequence of vascular disease or neuropathy. Early recognition of the 'at-risk' foot, the prompt institution of preventative measures, and the provision of rapid and intensive treatment of foot complications in multidisciplinary foot clinics have reduced the number of amputations in diabetic patients.[3,4] Screening is important if foot ulceration and amputation are to be prevented. With proper training, screening can be performed by any person in the foot clinic, and the equipment required is easily available, cheap, and simple to use. The most commonly used is the 5.07 Semmes–Weinstein nylon monofilaments. The inability to feel pressure applied on the skin (recommended sites: under the hallux, five metatarsal heads, and the heel) when the monofilament buckles is taken as an important predictor of foot ulceration. Other findings of peripheral neuropathy include reduced or absent vibration (tuning fork or biothesiometer), reduced or absent pin-prick or thermal sensation in the foot, and absent ankle reflexes.[105] The peripheral circulation should be evaluated by palpating for foot pulses and measuring the ABPI (keeping in mind that arterial calcification would give high ABPI in the presence of vascular insufficiency). The foot should be examined for deformities, callus formation, and skin changes. A recent study has shown that diabetic foot screening is not only effective in reducing foot ulceration and amputation, but is also cost-effective in terms of amputations averted.[106]

The mainstay in the prevention of foot ulceration in diabetic patients with neuropathy is threefold: education, removal of callus, and suitable footwear. Many patients with foot ulceration have a poor understanding of foot care, and this includes those who have had previous foot ulcers.[71] Providing the patient with information on foot care and prevention of ulcers can reduce the risk of ulceration and amputation.[7,107,108] In one study, educating each patient for just 1 hour reduced amputation rates by 70% over a period of 2 years as compared with the control group, which did not receive this advice.[106] The general principles of foot-care education are shown in *Table 11.5*. Education should not be restricted to the patients alone, but should also be provided for health-care professionals. The information given to the patients should be simple without medical jargon which

Table 11.5
General principles of foot-care education.

Information given to the patient should be simple and easily understood.

Suggest 'dos' rather than 'don'ts', to encourage a positive approach.

Do:
- Inspect feet daily
- Check shoes (inside and outside) before wearing them
- Have feet measured when buying shoes
- Buy lace-up shoes with plenty of room for toes
- Attend chiropodist regularly
- Keep feet away from heat (fires, radiators, hot-water bottles) and check bath-water temperature before stepping in
- Wear protective footwear when indoors, and avoid barefoot walking

Repeat the advice regularly

Also give advice to family members of the patient

Modified from Boulton AJM, Foot problems in patients with diabetes mellitus, in Pickup JC, Williams G, eds. *Textbook of Diabetes,* Oxford: Blackwell Science, 1997: 58.1–58.20.

the patient would have difficulty understanding, and should be in the language the patient understands. Patients should be advised to inspect their feet daily and must report immediately to the foot clinic at the onset of a foot ulcer. All patients' feet should be examined at each clinic visit and foot care should be reviewed and reinforced with the patient. Regular chiropody and removal of callus has been shown to reduce incidence of ulceration. Footwear should also be inspected to ensure that patients wear correct-fitting shoes and appropriate footwear, and, if necessary, special shoes or 'bespoke' shoes should be prescribed.[72]

Conclusion

Frequent examination of the diabetic foot, identifying the 'at-risk' foot, and follow-up in a specialist multidisciplinary foot clinic are important in the management of diabetic foot problems. Once ulceration develops, regular, frequent visits to the foot clinic for chiropody, debridement, and early diagnosis of infection or other complications will facilitate healing and have been shown to reduce amputations. Although research into newer treatments are ongoing, prevention is of primary importance, for which education, chiropody (for callus removal), and appropriate footwear will reduce the incidence (and recurrence) of foot ulceration.

References

1. Boyko EJ, Ahroni JH, Smith DG, Davignon D. Increased mortality associated with diabetic foot ulcer. *Diabetic Med* 1996; **13**: 967–972.
2. Krans HMJ, Porta M, Keen H et al. *Diabetes care and research in Europe: the St Vincent Declaration Action Programme Implementation Document*, 2nd edn. Copenhagen: WHO, 1995.
3. Edmonds ME. Experience in a multidisciplinary diabetic foot clinic. In: Boulton AJM, Connor H, Ward JD, eds. *The Foot in Diabetes*, 1st edn. Chichester: Wiley, 1987: 121–133.
4. Thomson FJ, Veves A, Ashe H et al. A team approach to diabetic foot care: the Manchester experience. *The Foot* 1991; **1**: 75–82.
5. Williams DRR. The size of the problem: Epidemiological and economic aspects of foot problems in diabetes. In: Boulton AJM, Connor H, Cavanagh PR, eds. *The Foot in Diabetes*, 2nd edn. Chichester, UK: Wiley, 1994: 16–24.
6. Palumbo PJ, Melton LJ. Peripheral vascular disease and diabetes. In: Harris MI, Hamman RF, eds. *Diabetes in America*. NIH Pub. No. 85-1468, XV 1–21. Washington DC; US Govt Printing Office, 1985.
7. Kumar S, Ashe HA, Parnell LN et al. The prevalence of foot ulceration and its correlates in type 2 diabetic patients: a population based study. *Diabetic Med* 1994; **11**: 480–484.
8. Neil HAW, Thompson AV, Thorogood M et al. Diabetes in the elderly: the Oxford Community Diabetes Study. *Diabetic Med* 1989; **6**: 608–613.
9. Moss SE, Klein R, Klein B. The prevalence and incidence of lower extremity amputation in a diabetic population. *Arch Intern Med* 1992; **152**: 610–613.
10. Pecoraro RE, Reiber GE, Burgess EM. Pathways to diabetic limb amputation: basis for prevention. *Diabetes Care* 1990; **13**: 513–521.
11. Verhoeven S, van Ballegooie E, Casparie AF. Impact of late complications in type 2 diabetes in a Dutch population. *Diabetic Med* 1991; **8**: 435–442.
12. Abbott CA, Vileikyte L, Williamson SH et al. Multi-centre study of the incidence and predictive factors for diabetic foot ulceration. *Diabetes Care* 1998; **21**: 1071–1075.
13. Guthner MG. The fate of the second leg in the diabetic amputee. *Diabetes* 1960; **9**: 100–103.
14. Boulton AJM. Foot problems in patients with diabetes mellitus. In: Pickup J, Williams G, eds. *Textbook of Diabetes*, 2nd edn. Oxford: Blackwell Science, 1997: 1–20.

15. Young MJ, Boulton AJM, McLeod AF *et al.* A multicentre study of the prevalence of diabetic peripheral neuropathy in the UK hospital clinic population. *Diabetologia* 1993; **36**: 150–154.

16. Tesfaye S, Stevens LK, Stephenson JM *et al.* The prevalence of diabetic peripheral neuropathy and its relation to glycaemic control and potential risk factors: the EURODIAB IDDM complications study. *Diabetologia* 1996; **39**: 1377–1384.

17. Dyck PJ, Kratz KM, Karnes JL *et al.* The prevalence by staged severity of various types of diabetic neuropathy, retinopathy and nephropathy in a population-based cohort: the Rochester diabetic neuropathy study. *Neurology* 1993; **43**: 817–824.

18. Boulton AJM, Ward JD. Diabetic neuropathies and pain. *Clin Endocrinol Metab* 1986; **16**: 917–931.

19. Thomas PK. Classification, differential diagnosis and staging of diabetic peripheral neuropathy. *Diabetes* 1997; **46** (**Suppl 2**): S54–S57.

20. Sima AAF, Thomas PK, Ishii D *et al.* Diabetic neuropathies. *Diabetologia* 1997; **40** (**Suppl 3**): B74–B77.

21. Young MJ, Jones GC. Diabetic neuropathy: symptoms, signs and assessment. In: Boulton AJM, ed. *Diabetic Neuropathy*. Lancaster: Marius Press, 1997: 41–61.

22. Vileikyte L, Hutchings G, Hollis S *et al.* The tactile circumferential discriminator: a new, simple screening device to identify diabetic patients at risk of foot ulceration. *Diabetes Care* 1997; **20**: 623–626.

23. Young MJ, Breddy JL, Veves A *et al.* The prediction of diabetic foot ulceration using vibration perception thresholds. *Diabetes Care* 1994; **17**: 557–561.

24. Boulton AJM, Scarpello JH, Ward JD. Venous oxygenation in the diabetic foot: evidence of arteriovenous shunting? *Diabetologia* 1982; **22**: 6–8.

25. Edmonds ME, Clarke MB, Newton S *et al.* Increased uptake of bone radiopharmaceutical in diabetic neuropathy. *Q J Med* 1985; **57**: 843–855.

26. Young MJ, Marshall A, Adams JE *et al.* Osteopenia, neurological dysfunction, and the development of Charcot neuroarthropathy. *Diabetes Care* 1995; **18**: 34–38.

27. Boulton AJM. New treatments for diabetic neuropathy. *Curr Opin Endocrinol Diabet* 1996; **3**: 330–334.

28. DCCT Research Group. The effect of intensive treatment of diabetes on the development and progression of long-term complications in insulin-dependent diabetes mellitus. *N Engl J Med* 1993; **329**: 977–986.

29. DCCT Research Group. The effect of intensive diabetes therapy on the development and progression of neuropathy. *Ann Int Med* 1995; **122**: 561–568.

30. Watkins PJ. Treatment for diabetic neuropathy. *Diabetic Med* 1996; **13**: 1007–1008.

31. Pfeifer MA, Schumer MP, Gelber DA. Aldose reductase inhibitors: the end of an era or the need for different trials designs? *Diabetes* 1997; **46** (**Suppl 2**): S82–S89.

32. Nicolucci A, Carinci F, Cavaliere D *et al.* A meta-analysis of trials on aldose reductase inhibitors in diabetic peripheral neuropathy. *Diabetic Med* 1996; **13**: 1017–1026.

33. Ziegler D, Hanefeld M, Ruthnau KJ *et al.* Treatment of symptomatic diabetic peripheral neuropathy with the anti-oxidant alpha-lipoic acid. *Diabetologia* 1995; **38**: 1425–1433.

34. Horrobin DF. Gamma-linolenic acid in the treatment of diabetic neuropathy. In: Boulton AJM, ed. *Diabetic Neuropathy*. Lancaster: Marius Press, 1997: 183–195.

35. Anand P, Terenghi G, Warner G *et al.* The role of endogenous growth factor in diabetic neuropathy. *Nature Med* 1996; **2**: 703–707.

36. Dyck PJ. Nerve growth factor and diabetic neuropathy. *Lancet* 1996; **348**: 1044–1045.

37. Thomas PK. Growth factors and diabetic neuropathy. *Diabetic Med* 1994; **11**: 732–739.

38. Max MB, Culnane M, Schafer SC *et al.* Amitriptyline relieves diabetic neuropathy pain in patients with normal and depressed mood. *Neurology* 1987; **37**: 589–596.

39. Sindrup SH. Antidepressants in the treatment of diabetic neuropathy. *Dan Med Bull* 1994; **41**: 66–67.

40. Zhang WY, Po ALW. The effectiveness of topically applied capsaicin: a meta-analysis. *Eur J Clin Pharmacol* 1994; **46**: 517–522.

41. Ewins DL, Vileikyte L, Borg-Costanzi J *et al.*

Acupuncture: a novel treatment for painful diabetic neuropathy. In: Hotta N, Ward JD, Sima AAF, eds. *Diabetic Neuropathy: New Concepts and Insights.* Amsterdam: Exc Medica, 1995: 405–409.

42. Abuaisha BB, Costanzi JB, Boulton AJM. Acupuncture for the treatment of chronic painful peripheral diabetic neuropathy: a long-term study. *Diabetes Res Clin Pract* 1998; **39**: 115–121.

43. Steiner G. Diabetes and artherosclerosis; epidemiology and intervention trials. In: Woodford FP, Davignon J, Sniderman A, eds. *Atherosclerosis X.* Amsterdam: Elsevier, 1995: 749–752.

44. Kannel WB, McGee DL. Diabetes and glucose tolerance as risk factors for cardiovascular disease. The Framingham Study. *Diabetes Care* 1979; **2**: 120–126.

45. Krolewski AS, Warran JHM, Christlieb AR. Onset, source, complications and prognosis of diabetes mellitus: In: Marble A, Geall LP, Bradley RF *et al.*, eds. *Joslin's Diabetes Mellitus*, 12th edn. Philadelphia: Lea and Febiger, 1985: 251–277.

46. Pyörälä K, Laakso M. Macrovascular disease in diabetes mellitus. In: Mann JI, Pyörälä K, Teuscher E, eds. *Diabetes in Epidemiological Perspectives.* Edinburgh: Churchill Livingstone, 1983: 183–247.

47. WHO Multinational Study of Vascular Disease in Diabetics. Prevalence of small and large vessel disease in diabetic patients from 14 centres. *Diabetologia* 1985; **28 (Suppl)**: 615–640.

48. Farkouh ME, Rihal CS, Gersh BJ *et al.* Influence of coronary heart disease on morbidity and mortality after lower extremity revascularisation surgery: a population based study in Olmsted County, Minnesota (1970–1987). *J Am Coll Cardiol* 1994; **4**: 1290–1296.

49. Levine ME, O'Neal IW. *The Diabetic Foot*, 3rd edn. St Louis, Toronto, London: Mosby, 1983.

50. National Health Interview Survey (NHIS). In: Harris MI, Hamman RF, eds. *Diabetes in America.* NIH Publication No. 85. Washington DC, US Govt Printing Office, 1985: 1468.

51. Abbott RD, Brand FN, Kannel WB. Epidemiology of some peripheral arterial findings in diabetic men and women: experiences from the Framingham study. *Am J Med* 1990; **88**: 376–381.

52. Moriarty KT, Perkins AC, Robinson AM *et al.* Investigating the capillary circulation of the foot with ^{99m}Tc-macroaggregated albumin: a prospective study in patients with diabetes and foot ulceration. *Diabetic Med* 1994; **11**: 22–27.

53. Walters DP, Gatling W, Mullee MA, Hill RD. The prevalence, detection and epidemiological correlates of peripheral vascular disease: a comparison of diabetic and non-diabetic subjects in an English community. *Diabetic Med* 1992; **9**: 710–715.

54. Weitz JL, Byrne J, Claget P *et al.* Diagnosis and treatment of chronic arterial insufficiency of the lower extremities: a critical review. *Circulation* 1996; **94**: 3026–3049.

55. Martin-Paredero V, Dixon SM, Baker JD *et al.* Risk of renal failure after major angiography. *Arch Surg* 1983; **118**: 1417–1420.

56. Strandness DE, Priest RE, Gibbons RE, Seattle MD. Combined clinical and pathological study of diabetic and non-diabetic peripheral artery disease. *Diabetes* 1961; **13**: 366–372.

57. King TA, DePalma RG, Rhodes RS. Diabetes mellitus and atherosclerotic involvement of the profunda femoris artery. *Surg Gynecol Obstet* 1984; **159**: 553–556.

58. Jude EB, Shaw J, Chalmers N, Boulton AJM. Peripheral vascular disease (PVD) in diabetic and non-diabetic patients: a comparison. *Diabetic Med* 1996; **13 (Suppl 7)**: S47.

59. Ernst E, Fialka V. A review of the clinical effectiveness of exercise therapy for intermittent claudication. *Arch Intern Med* 1993; **153**: 2357–2360.

60. Palumbo PJ, O'Fallon WM, Osmundson PJ *et al.* Progression of peripheral occlusive arterial disease in diabetes mellitus. *Arch Intern Med* 1991; **151**: 717–721.

61. Morrish NJ, Stevens LK, Fuller JH *et al.* Risk factors for macrovascular disease in diabetes mellitus: the London follow-up to the WHO multinational study of vascular disease in diabetes. *Diabetologia* 1991; **34**: 590–594.

62. Garg A. Lipid lowering therapy and

macrovascular disease in diabetes mellitus. *Diabetes* 1992; **41 (Suppl 2)**: 111–115.

63. Taskinen MR. Criteria for metabolic control and intervention in diabetes. *Diabetes* 1996; **45 (Suppl 3)**: S120–S122.

64. Cantelmo NL, Snow JR, Menzoian Jo, LoGerfo FW. Successful vein bypass in patients with an ischaemic limb and palpable popliteal pulse. *Arch Surg* 1986; **121**: 217–220.

65. Hurley JJ, Auer AI, Hershey FB *et al.* Distal arterial reconstruction: patency and limb salvage in diabetes. *J Vasc Surg* 1987; **5**: 796–800.

66. LoGerfo FW, Gibbons GW, Pomposelli FB Jr *et al.* Evolving trends in the management of the diabetic foot. *Arch Surg* 1992; **127**: 617–621.

67. Veves A, Murray HJ, Young MJ, Boulton AJM. The risk of foot ulceration in diabetic patients with high foot pressures: a prospective study. *Diabetologia* 1992; **35**: 660–663.

68. Masson EA, Hay EM, Stockley I *et al.* Abnormal foot pressure alone does not cause ulceration. *Diabetic Med* 1989; **6**: 426–428.

69. Boulton AJM. The pathogenesis of diabetic foot problems: an overview. *Diabetic Med* 1996; **13 (Suppl 1)**: S12–S16.

70. Murray HJ, Young MJ, Hollis S, Boulton AJM. The association between callus formation, high pressures and neuropathy in diabetic foot ulceration. *Diabetic Med* 1996; **13**: 979–982.

71. Colagiuri S, Marsden LL, Naidu V, Taylor L. The use of orthotic devices to correct planar callus in people with diabetes. *Diabetes Res Clin Pract* 1995; **28**: 29–34.

72. Uccioli L, Aldeghi A, Faglia E *et al.* Manufactured shoes in the prevention of diabetic foot ulcers. *Diabetes Care* 1995; **18**: 1376–1378.

73. Litzelman DK, Marriott DJ, Vinivor F. The role of footwear in the prevention of foot lesions in patients with NIDDM. *Diabetes Care* 1997; **20**: 156–162.

74. Masson EA, Angle S, Roseman P *et al.* Diabetic foot ulcers – do patients know how to protect themselves? *Pract Diabetes* 1989; **6**: 22–23.

75. Caddick SL, McKinnon M, Payne N *et al.* Hospital admissions and social; deprivation of

76. Chaturvedi N, Stephenson JM, Fuller JH. The relationship between socio-economic status and diabetes control and complications in the EURODIAB IDDM complications study. *Diabetes Care* 1996; **16**: 423.

77. Edmonds M, Boulton A, Buckenham T *et al.* Report of the diabetic foot and amputation group. *Diabetic Med* 1996; **13**: S27–S42.

78. De Sonnaville JJ, Colly LP, Wijkel D, Heine RJ. The prevalence and determinants of foot ulceration in type II diabetic patients in a primary care setting. *Diabetes Res Clin Pract* 1997; **35**: 149–156.

79. Litzelman DK, Marriott DJ, Vinivor F. Independent physiological predictors of foot lesions in patients with NIDDM. *Diabetes Care* 1997; **20**: 1272–1278.

80. Wagner FW. Algorithms of diabetic foot care. In: Levin ME, O'Neal LW, eds. *The Diabetic Foot*, 2nd edn. St Louis: Mosby Yearbook, 1983: 201–302.

81. Brash PD, Foster JE, Vennart W *et al.* Magnetic resonance imaging reveals microhaemorrhages in the feet of diabetic patients with a history of ulceration. *Diabetic Med* 1996; **13**: 973–987.

82. Mueller MJ, Diamond JE, Sinacore DR *et al.* Total contact casting in treatment of diabetic plantar ulcers. Controlled clinical trials. *Diabetes Care* 1989; **12**: 384–388.

83. Burden AC, Jones R, Jones GR *et al.* Use of 'Scotchcast boot' in treating diabetic foot ulcers. *Br J Med* 1983; **286**: 1555–1557.

84. Boulton AJM, Bowker JH, Gadia MT *et al.* Use of plaster casts in the management of diabetic neuropathic foot ulcers. *Diabetes Care* 1986; **9**: 149–152.

85. Wheat LJ, Allen SD, Henry M *et al.* Diabetic foot infections: bacteriologic analysis. *Arch Int Med* 1986; **146**: 1935.

86. Calhoun JH, Cantrell J, Cobos J *et al.* Treatment of diabetic foot infections: Wagner classification therapy and outcome. *Foot Ankle* 1988; **9**: 101.

87. Sharp CS, Bessman AN, Wagner FW *et al.* Microbiology of superficial and deep tissues in infected diabetic gangrene. *Surg Gynecol Obstet* 1979; **149**: 217.

88. Sapico FL, Witte JL, Canawati HN *et al.* The infected foot of the diabetic patient: quantitative microbiology and analysis of clinical features. *Rev Infect Dis* 1984; **6 (Suppl 1)**: S171.

89. Lipsky BA, Pecoraro RE, Wheat LJ. The diabetic foot. Soft tissue and bone infection. *Infect Dis Clin North Am* 1990; **4**: 409–432.

90. Lipsky BA, Pecoraro RE, Larson SA *et al.* Outpatient management of uncomplicated lower-extremity infections in diabetic patients. *Arch Int Med* 1990; **150**: 790–797.

91. Slovenkai MP. Foot problems in diabetes. *Med Clin North Am* 1998; **82**: 949–971.

92. Wieman TJ, Smiell JM, Su Y. Efficacy and safety of a topical gel formulation of recombinant human platelet-derived growth factor-BB (Becaplermin) in patients with chronic neuropathic diabetic ulcers. *Diabetes Care* 1998; **21**: 822–827.

93. Gough A, Clapperton M, Rolando N *et al.* Randomised placebo-controlled trials of granulocyte-colony stimulating factor in diabetic foot ulceration. *Lancet* 1997; **350**: 855–859.

94. Gentzkow G, Iawaski S, Hershon K *et al.* Use of Dermagraft, a cultured human dermis, to treat diabetic foot ulcers. *Diabetes Care* 1996; **19**: 350–354.

95. Faglia E, Favales F, Aldeghi A *et al.* Adjunctive systemic hyperbaric oxygen therapy in the treatment of severe prevalently ischaemic diabetic foot ulcers. *Diabetes Care* 1996; **19**: 1338–1343.

96. Venkatesan P, Lawn S, Macfarlane RM *et al.* Conservative management of osteomyelitis in the foot of diabetic patients. *Diabetic Med* 1997; **14**: 487–490.

97. Sanders LJ, Frykberg RG. Diabetic neuropathic osteoarthropathy: The Charcot foot. In: Frykberg RG, ed. *The High Risk Foot in Diabetes Mellitus.* New York: Churchill Livingstone, 1991; 297–338.

98. Cavanagh PR, Young MJ, Adams JE *et al.* Radiographic abnormalities in the feet of patients with diabetic neuropathy. *Diabetes Care* 1994; **17**: 210–219.

99. Gough A, Abraha H, Purewal TS *et al.* Measurement of markers of osteoclast and osteoblastic activity in patients with acute and chronic diabetic Charcot neuroarthropathy. *Diabetic Med* 1997; **14**: 527–531.

100. Selby PL, Jude EB, Burgess J *et al.* Bone turnover markers in acute Charcot neuroarthropathy. *Diabetologia* 1998; **41 (Suppl 1)**: A275.

101. Sanders LJ, Frykberg RG. Charcot foot. In: Levin ME, O'Neal LW, eds. *The Diabetic Foot*, 5th edn. St Louis: Mosby Yearbook, 1993: 149–180.

102. Selby PL, Young MJ, Adams JE, Boulton AJM. Bisphosphonate: a new treatment for diabetic Charcot neuroarthopathy. *Diabetic Med* 1994; **11**: 14–20.

103. Reiber GE, Vileikyte L, Boyko EJ *et al.* Casual pathways for incident lower extremeity ulcers in patients with diabetes from two settings. *Diabetes Care* 1999; in press.

104. Diabetes Care and Related Research in Europe: The Saint Vincent Declaration. *Diabetic Med* 1990; **7**: 360.

105. Boulton AJM, Gries FA, Jervell JA. Guidelines for the diagnosis and outpatient management of diabetic peripheral neuropathy. *Diabetic Med* 1998; **15**: 508–514.

106. McCabe CJ, Stevenson RC, Dolan AM. Evaluation of a diabetic foot screening and protection programme. *Diabetic Med* 1998; **15**: 80–84.

107. Malone JM, Snyder M, Anderson G *et al.* Prevention of amputation by diabetic education. *Ann J Surg* 1989; **158**: 520–524.

108. Litzelman DK, Slemenda CW, Langefield CD *et al.* Reduction of lower extremity clinical abnormalities in patients with non-insulin dependent diabetes mellitus. *Ann Int Med* 1993; **199**: 36–41.

12

Erectile failure: the complication 'that dare not speak its name'

Julian Shah

Introduction

Erectile dysfunction is one of the commoner afflictions of man, causing both physical and psychological distress. It is well recognized that there is a strong association between erectile dysfunction and diabetes mellitus. Many patients who present to 'impotence clinics' with erectile difficulties are suffering from diabetes mellitus. However, many diabetics do not seek advice, which is readily available to them. The prevalence of impotence in diabetic males is reported to be somewhere between 20 and 89.2%.[1-4] A comparison of impotence in healthy individuals was 16.7%, hypertensives 43.6%, and diabetics 89.2%.[2] In the Massachusetts male ageing study from Feldman et al.[1] the incidence of impotence was 52%. The prevalence appeared to triple between the ages of 40 and 70 years. It is reported, however, that cultural and attitudinal differences in different countries may have an effect on the reporting of the frequency of occurrence of impotence in diabetics.[5] Thus, not withstanding the relative figures, the condition is common and is a cause of distress for patient and partner. Thus, it is important not only to discover the presence of erectile dysfunction in diabetic patients but also to be able to offer advice and treatment, should it be desired.

Aetiology of erectile dysfunction

Erection depends upon the coordination of autonomic neurological function and the efficient vascular components of the penis. It is well recognized that diabetics suffer with both neurological and vascular problems, and it is a combination of these factors which may be responsible for the development of failure to gain an erection or sustain an erection sufficient for sexual activity. Autieri et al.[6] have demonstrated that altered gene expression in tissue from the corpora cavernosa may play a significant part in erectile dysfunction in a patient with neuropathy but not diabetics. Neurological factors are also involved. Ho et al.[7] demonstrated that bulbo-cavernosal reflux latency was prolonged in diabetics, but this could not be used to distinguish between non-neurogenic and neurogenic causes of impotence. It is well recognized that poor metabolic control in diabetics gives rise to higher risks of the complications of erectile dysfunction.[8]

Normal males experience between three and four nocturnal erections during a night's sleep. The frequency of erections and their quality can be measured by nocturnal penile tumescence (NPT) monitoring (*Fig. 12.1*). Nofzinger et al.[9] demonstrated that 70–90% of diabetics

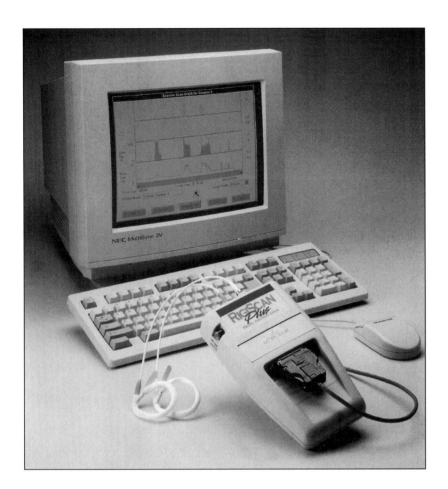

Fig. 12.1
Nocturnal penile tumescence monitoring.

have NPT abnormalities even if they have functioning erections. Yamaguchi and Kumamoto[10] demonstrated that 85% of diabetics have failure to achieve or maintain an erection, and had a decrease in NPT. They commented upon the likelihood of a major organic contribution to erectile dysfunction in diabetics. They also noted that penile vascular disorders were seen in 67.7% of diabetics, particularly those over the age of 60 years. Although neurological factors are commonly implicated in diabetes, the vascular abnormality associated with diabetes appears to play a more convincing primary role, with vascular obstruction causing cavernous arterial insufficiency being the most likely cause.[11,12] Diabetic complications due to poor diabetic regulation have an adverse effect on erectile dysfunction.[13,14] Nitric oxide, which is the known comediator of penile erection,[15] is thought to be reduced in the cavernosa of diabetics and has been demonstrated in a diabetic rat model.[16]

Psychological factors

Although organic causes are undoubtedly present in diabetics, psychological factors may also be present. Takanami *et al.*[17] demonstrated that psychological stress was also present, and that not all patients had diabetic neuropathy or organic impotence. They stated that the psychological stress of being diabetic may contribute to erectile dysfunction. This is contrary to Veves *et al.*,[18] who stated that psychogenic factors were the only cause in 11%, the main cause in 24%, and a contributing cause in 17% of subjects. Marital disharmony, medical treatment, and peripheral vascular disease were the principal factors causing erectile dysfunction in diabetics.

Presentation of diabetic impotence

Erectile dysfunction in diabetics appears to develop approximately 10 years after the onset of diabetes,[12] though there are many examples of patients who develop erectile dysfunction at the time of or soon after the diagnosis of the diabetic condition. Erectile dysfunction presents as impaired morning erections, reduction in spontaneous erections, erectile weakness, and ejaculatory disturbances. A reduction in sexual interest and complete erectile failure may also occur.[2] Schiavi *et al.*[14] showed significant reduction in sexual desire, subjective arousal, erectile capability, and coital frequency. Sexual satisfaction is also reduced in diabetics when compared with controls.

Investigation of impotence

It is important to obtain a clear medical history from patients with diabetes and in particular to discover the nature of the diabetic condition, diabetic control, and associated abnormalities such as peripheral vascular disease and peripheral neuropathy. A history pro forma is valuable in obtaining information about sexual function (*Fig. 12.2*). It is important in specific questioning to avoid offence, and certain questions may be omitted if there is a possibility of embarrassment to the patient. It is important to be aware of racial differences in assessing erectile dysfunction, as some patients may be very sensitive to questions of a personal nature. It is useful when taking the history about erectile dysfunction to discover whether the patient is married, and if so to discover the relationship with the patient's wife. If the patient is not married, it is useful to discover the nature of any sexual relationship. The frequency of coitus and when the last act of sexual intercourse took place should be recorded. The quality of erection, whether it is sustained or not, the quality of orgasm and ejaculation, the frequency of coitus, and the index of satisfaction should all be noted. Clinical examination is generally unremarkable and, even in diabetic patients, often no vascular abnormalities are discovered. However, examination of the penis, feeling for Peyronies plaques, and examination of the scrotum and testicles, along with a rectal examination for men over 40 years of age, should be performed.

Investigations

Most 'routine investigations' do not reveal any abnormality. Plasma glucose should be measured if diabetes is suspected. If the diabetic condition is recognized, the state of the diabetic control should be known. If renal impairment is suspected, serum creatinine should be measured; this is uncommon. Changes in testosterone, LH, and FSH are

Name:	Hosp No:	DOB:	Age:

Address:

Post code: Occupation:

Telephone - Home: Work:

GP: Referred by:

History of erectile dysfunction:

Duration of problem: Onset:sudden/gradual
Quality of erection:normal/moderate/poor/none
Self-stimulated erection:normal/good/poor/none
Early morning erections:yes/no

Married/Single/Partner   Children:

Sexual frequency: Ejaculation:
                                        normal/reduced/absent/retrograde

Libido:normal/reduced/poor

Risk factors: State:
cardiovascular   endocrine
neurological   operations
radiotherapy   trauma

Smoking   Alcohol
Recreational drugs   Body-building drugs

Relationship problems
Psychological events
Major life events

Sexual expectations
Self   Partner

Urinary symptoms: Frequency: Nocturia:
Urgency: yes/no Urge incontinence: yes/no
Stress incontinence: Pads:
Continuous/unconscious incontinence:

Hesitancy: yes/no
Stream-normal/reduced/interrupted/variable
TD/PMD   Emptying: complete/incomplete
Straining: yes/no

Dysuria/infection/haematuria
Pain:renal/bladder/urethral/prostatic/back

Drugs:

Examination

Fig. 12.2
History pro forma.

uncommon. Testosterone should be measured if there is a suggestion of hypogonadism or loss of libido. LH and FSH should be measured if testosterone is low. Prolactin measurement is only necessary if testosterone is low or there is loss of libido.

It is well recognized that a colour Doppler examination of the penis can demonstrate lower cavernosal artery peak blood flow,[19] and NPT monitoring using the RigiScan™ device (*Fig. 12.3*) may be of some assistance in diagnosing psychogenic factors over physical

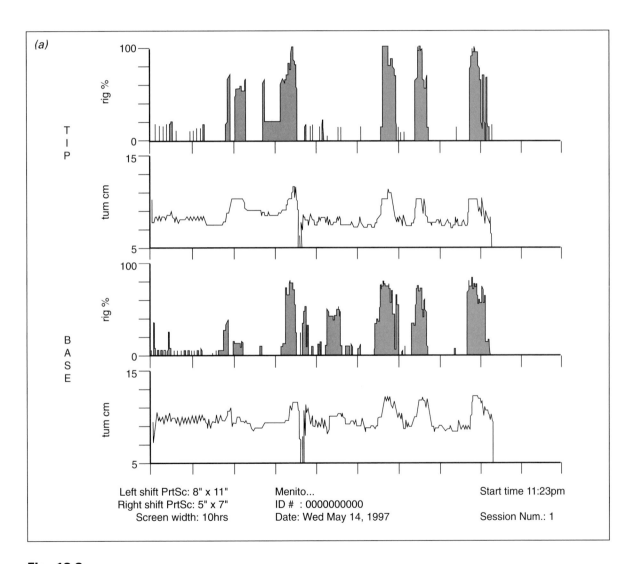

Fig. 12.3
Nocturnal penile tumescence traces, demonstrating (a) regular normal erections in a normal male and (b) NPT in a diabetic male.

Continued

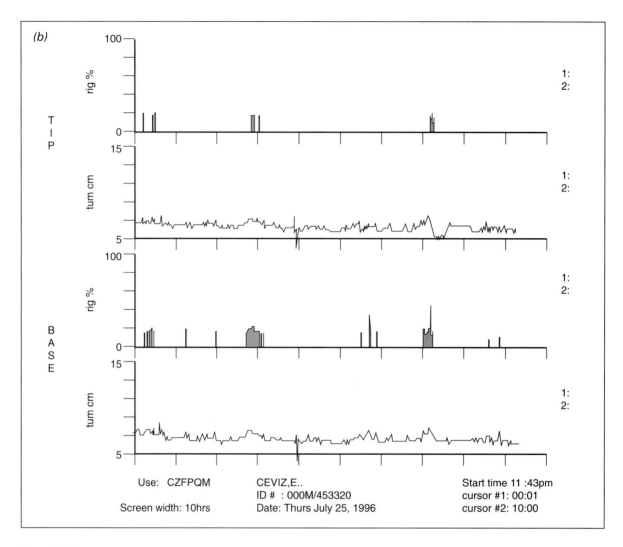

Fig. 12.3
Continued

factors. However, the majority of patients will have a combination of physical and psychological factors, and treatment may be instituted without involving investigations or hospitalization for NPT.

Management

Better diabetic control[20] has been demonstrated to reduce the frequency of impotence in diabetics. Psychological factors are also prevalent in diabetics, as has been previously mentioned. The professional discussion that takes place with the patient during initial consultation may be of benefit in explaining the condition and assisting in improvements in the sexual condition. A full explanation of the treatment options along with the patient's and partner's needs and desires should be taken into consideration. Psychosexual counselling may be of benefit for the suitably motivated patient and, where there are acknowledged psychological factors, can provide benefits to the relationship in addition to the erectile dysfunction. Medical therapy with a pharmacological agent may effectively resolve an erectile difficulty, particularly when the problem has a psychological basis: if confidence is restored normal erectile function may return.

Many patients, however, prefer the ease of medical therapy. Since the discovery of the injection of vasoactive agents into the corpora cavernosa[21] with papaverine, a number of new agents have become available which have benefits over papaverine in reducing the incidence of drug-induced priapism. Prostaglandin E1 and drug mixtures such as phentolamine and VIP are useful agents for intracavernosal injection, producing an erection within 5–15 minutes which is sustained for an hour or more. Montorsi *et al.*[22] have demonstrated that intracavernosal injections are effective and safe in up to 80% of diabetic patients at 18 months. Desvaux and Mimoun,[23] however, found that fewer diabetics experienced success with intracavernosal prostaglandin, with approximately 52.3% having positive results. Vasopotin, a combination of phentolamine and VIP, has been shown to be useful in diabetic patients[24] and may be administered using an injection pen, which has attractions to some patients. Injection therapy is simple to teach and simple to use providing that the patient does not have needle phobia (*Fig. 12.4*). If the patient finds injection therapy

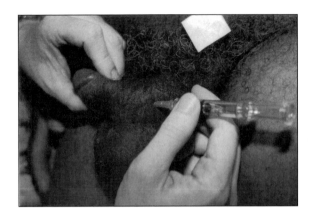

Fig. 12.4
Injection of vasoactive agent.

acceptable, he may continue to use this treatment indefinitely. It is recommended that injections should be used no more than 2–3 times weekly. Injection-related Peyronie's plaques may occur in between 1 and 20% of patients.

The patient should be warned of the risk of persistent erection (priapism), which occurs in 1–5% of patients. Patients should be advised to undertake activity such as running up and down the stairs or cycling, which tends to steal the blood sufficient to make the erection go down. Cooling the penis by taking a cold shower or using an ice-pack may also help. If, in spite of these measures, the erection is persistent, then the patient should seek medical treatment in the local Accident and Emergency Department. A 19–21 gauge butterfly needle is inserted into the corpus on one side and 20–25 ml of blood is aspirated from the penis. Blood may be aspirated from the other side of the penis. If the erection persists, 0.5–1 ml of phenylephrine in a concentration of 200 mcg/ml should be slowly injected into the penis every 5–10 minutes to a maximum dose of 1 mg. Continuous measurement of pulse and blood pressure monitoring should be performed. Pharmacological detumescence will usually take place. If this fails, surgical advice should be sought.

Intra-urethral prostaglandin in the form of MUSE has also been found to be effective in diabetic males (*Fig. 12.5*). The pellet of prostaglandin, which comes in doses from 250 to 1,000 micrograms, is effective in 60% of males in producing an erection. The patients should be advised to massage the penis for 3–10 minutes after the pellet has been placed in the urethra. Intra-urethral burning may be experienced by 30% of patients, but few patients discontinue use of MUSE because of

this effect.[25-27] MUSE is not as effective as intracavernosal injections.

Since the discovery that nitric oxide is a mediator in erectile function, a new phosphodiesterase inhibitor, Sildenafil, has gained worldwide appeal for treating males with erectile dysfunction. Oral Sildenafil taken between 1 and 4 hours before sexual activity has been shown to be effective in males with erectile dysfunction. The drug comes in doses of 25, 50, and 100 mg, with the efficacy increasing with increases in drug dosage.[28-30] Up to 80% of men who have taken Sildenafil have noticed improvements in their erection sufficient for sexual activity. The most frequent side-effects are headache (17%), flushing (15%), heartburn (7%), and visual disturbances (3%). Each of these side-effects is reversible once the drug is stopped. Deaths related to Sildenafil have occurred in patients with heart disease. The use of this agent is contraindicated in patients with angina, a known history of heart disease and concomitant use of glyceryl trinitrate.

Vacuum devices

Mechanical aids may be of use to many men with erectile dysfunction. These devices avoid the need for medication. Some patients find the thought of intrapenile injections distressing, though diabetics who use insulin tend to have fewer aversions than non-diabetics. The vacuum aid (*Fig. 12.6*) is an effective means of providing an erection. A vacuum created around the penis within the cylinder causes tumescence. Once the penis is tumescent, a specially designed ring is slipped onto the base of the penis. This constriction ring maintains the erection whilst sexual intercourse takes place. The erection may be uncomfortable, and the base of the penis is not stable. The ring should be removed within 15–20 minutes to avoid penile ischaemia.

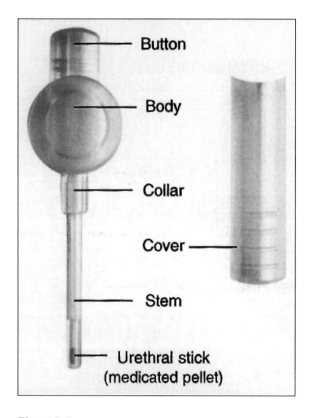

Fig. 12.5
Intra-urethral MUSE.

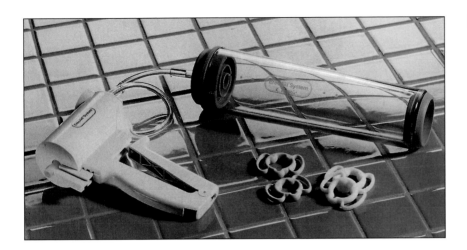

Fig. 12.6
Vacuum aid system.

Ecchymoses and discomfort are the commonest side-effects of constriction therapy. Five out of ten diabetic men have been found to prefer the vacuum constriction device,[31]and Price *et al.*[32] demonstrated that 75% of 44 diabetic men were able to use the device for sexual activity approximately 5.5 times a month. The lack of spontaneity of use affects the use of the vacuum aid in some patients.

Surgery

If the impotent patient fails to respond to conservative measures or has an aversion to the lack of spontaneity that accompanies the majority of medical therapies, surgery may be of benefit in some, provided that the risks and complications are explained.

Prior to the knowledge that nitric oxide was involved in erection and its failure, the condition known as venous leak was commonly thought to be the cause of erectile dysfunction. Venous leak surgery was used for demonstrated venous leakage on cavernosography and shown in one study to be beneficial to 14 of 22 patients at 1 year.[32] This has not, however, been the general experience, with much lower results being reported. Since the advent of Sildenafil, intracavernosal injections, and implants, venous leak surgery has fallen into disfavour. Where a patient requires a surgical operation, the most effective long-term management of erectile dysfunction for a patient who does not respond or does not wish to use either medication or intracavernosal injection is a penile

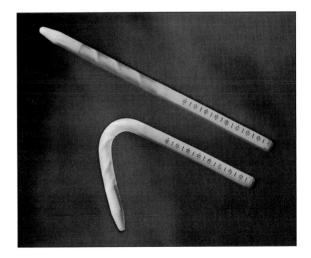

Fig. 12.7
Semi-rigid penile implant.

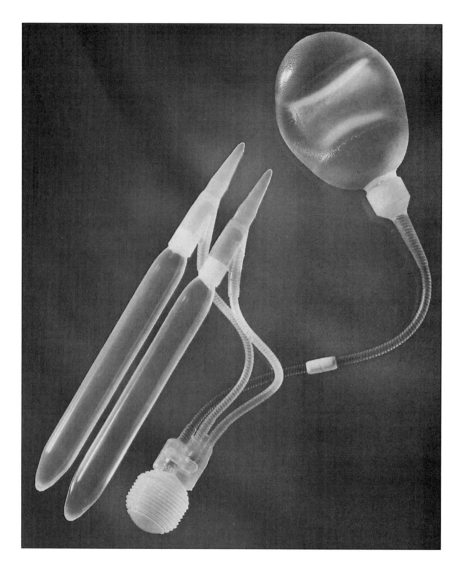

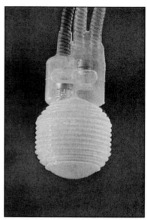

Fig. 12.8
Inflatable penile implant.

implant. There are two principal types of implants, the semi-rigid (*Fig. 12.7*) and the inflatable (*Fig. 12.8*). There have been concerns over the risks of infection in diabetics undergoing implantation of a penile implant. The infection risk is reported to vary between 3 and 8.7%.[34,35] Three diabetic patients have developed gangrene of the penis in association with a penile implant.[36] There has been some argument as to whether or not the presence of glycosylated haemoglobin in the serum indicates increased risk for patients undergoing implants. Wilson *et al.*[35] dispute this, where as Bishop *et al.*[37] state that there is an association. It is important that each patient undergoing the implantation of a penile implant should have careful pre-operative skin preparation to avoid the risks of contamination during the procedure. Appropriate antibiotic prophylaxis is also essential. The initial cost of these devices is high, but benefits outweigh the disadvantages, provided that complications do not arise. Long-term follow-up of patients with implants is advisable, as the late complications of mechanical dysfunction, aneurysm formation in the corpora, and migration do occur, although relatively uncommonly.

Summary

Erectile dysfunction is a common complaint associated with diabetes mellitus, increasing with age and giving rise to considerable psychological and physical distress. Modern methods of clinical management have enabled the majority of patients to gain a recovery to satisfactory sexual functioning. Early control of diabetes with cooperation from the patient should reduce the incidence of erectile dysfunction, but as patients become more aware that treatment is available for them, we shall be seeing increasing numbers of patients presenting for our advice.

References

1. Feldman HA, Goldstein I, Hatzichristou DG *et al*. Impotence and its medical and psychosocial correlates: results of the Massachusetts Male Ageing Study. *J Urol* 1994; **151**: 54–61.
2. El-Rufaie OE, Bener A, Abuzeid MS, Ali TA. Sexual dysfunction among type II diabetic men: a controlled study. *J Psychosomatic Res* 1997; **43**: 605–612.
3. Brunner GA, Pieber TR, Schattenberg S *et al*. Erectile dysfunction in patients with type I diabetes mellitus. *Wien-Med-Wochenschr* 1995; **145**: 584–586.
4. O'Hare JA, Abuaisha F, Geoghegan M. Prevalence and forms of neuropathic morbidity in 800 diabetics. *Ir J Med Sci* 1994; **163**: 132–135.
5. Tesfaye S, Stevens LK, Stephenson JM *et al*. Prevalence of diabetic peripheral neuropathy and its relation to glycaemic control and potential risk factors: the EURODIAB IDDM complications study. *Diabetologia* 1996; **39**: 1377–1384.
6. Autieri MV, Malman A, Christ GJ. Identification of a down-regulated mRNA transcript in corpus cavernosum from diabetic patients with erectile dysfunction. *Int J Impot Res* 1996; **8(2)**: 69–73.
7. Ho KH, Ong BK, Chong PN, Teo WL. The bulbocavernosus reflex in the assessment of neurogenic impotence in diabetic and non-diabetic men. *Ann Acad Med Singapore* 1996; **25**: 558–561.
8. Zonszein J. Diagnosis and management of endocrine disorders of erectile dysfunction. *Urol Clin North Am* 1995; **22**: 789–802.
9. Nofzinger EA, Reynolds CF, Jennings JR *et al*. Results of nocturnal penile tumescence studies are abnormal in sexually functional diabetic men. *Arch Int Med* 1992; **152**: 114–118.
10. Yamaguchi Y, Kumamoto Y. Etiological analysis of male diabetic erectile dysfunction with particular emphasis on findings of vascular and neurological examinations. *Nippon Hinyokika Gakkai Zasshi* 1994; **85**: 1474–1483.
11. Benvenuti F, Boncinelli L, Vignoli GC. Male sexual impotence in diabetes mellitus: vasculogenic versus neurogenic factors. *Neurourol Urodyn* 1993; **12**: 145–151; discussion 152.
12. Wang CJ, Shen SY, Wu CC *et al*. Penile blood flow study in diabetic impotence. *Urol Int* 1993; **50**: 209–212.
13. Bemelmans BL, Meuleman EJ, Doesburg WH *et al*. Erectile dysfunction in diabetic men: the neurological factor revisited. *J Urol* 1994; **151**: 884–889.
14. Schiavi RC, Stimmel BB, Mandeli J, Rayfield EJ. Diabetes mellitus and male sexual function: a controlled study. *Diabetologia* 1993; **36**: 745–751.
15. Ehmke H, Junemann KP, Mayer B, Kummer W. Nitric oxide synthase and vasoactive intestinal polypeptide colocalization in neurons innervating the human penile circulation. *Int J Impot Res* 1995; **7**: 147–156.
16. Vernet D, Cai L, Babbit ML, Murray FT *et al*. Reduction of penile nitric oxide synthase in diabetic BB/WORdp (type I) and BBZ.WORdp (type II) rats with erectile dysfunction. *Endocrinology* 1995; **136**: 5709–5717.

17. Takanami M, Nagao K, Ishii N *et al.* Is diabetic neuropathy responsible for diabetic impotence? *Urol Int* 1997; **58**(3): 181–185.

18. Veves A, Webster L, Chen TF *et al.* Aetiopathogenesis and management of impotence in diabetic males: four years experience from a combined clinic. *Diabet Med* 1995; **12**: 77–82.

19. Kadioglu A, Erdogru T, Karisdag K *et al.* Evaluation of penile arterial system with color Doppler ultrasonography in nondiabetic and diabetic males. *Eur Urol* 1995; **27**: 311–314.

20. Klein R, Klein BE, Lee KE *et al.* Prevalence of self reported erectile dysfunction in people with long term IDDM. *Diabetes Care* 1996; **19**: 135–141.

21. Brindley GS. Pilot experiments on the actions of drugs injected into the human corpus cavernosum penis. *Br J Pharmacol* 1986; **87**: 495–500.

22. Montorsi F, Guazzoni G, Bergamaschi F *et al.* Clinical reliability of multi-drug intracavernous vasoactive pharmacotherapy for diabetic impotence. *Acta Diabetol* 1994; **31**: 1–5.

23. Desvaux P, Mimoun S. Prostaglandin E1 in the treatment of erectile insufficiency. Comparison of efficacy and tolerance based on difference etiologies. *J Urol Paris* 1994; **100**: 17–22.

24. McMahon CG. A pilot study of the role of intracavernous injection of vasoactive intestinal peptide (VIP) and phentolamine mesylate in the treatment of erectile dysfunction. *Int J Impo Res* 1996; **8**: 233–236.

25. Padma-Nathan H, Hellstrom WJ, Kaiser FE *et al.* Treatment of men with erectile dysfunction with transurethral alprostadil. Medicated urethral system for erection (MUSE) study group. *N Engl J Med* 1997; **336**(1): 1–7.

26. Engel JD, McVary KT. Transurethral alprostadil as therapy for patients who withdrew from or failed prior intracavernous injection therapy. *Urology* 1998; **51**: 687–692.

27. Porst H. Transurethral alprostadil with MUSE (medicated urethral system for erection) vs intravcavernous alprostadil – a comparative study in 103 patients with erectile dysfunction. *Int J Impot Res* 1997; **9**(4): 187–192.

28. Boolell M, Gepi-Attee S, Gingell JC, Allen MJ. Sildenafil, a novel effective oral therapy for male erectile dysfunction. *Br J Urol* 1997; **79**: 663–664.

29. Jeremy JY, Ballard SA, Naylor AM *et al.* Effects of sildenafil, a type 5 cGMP phosphadiesterase inhibitor, and papaverine on cyclic GMP and cyclic AMP levels in the rabbit cavernosum *in vitro*. *Br J Urol* 1997; **79**: 958–963.

30. Boolell M, Allen MJ, Ballard SA *et al.* Sildenafil: an orally active type 5 cyclic GMP specific phosphadiesterase inhibitor for the treatment of penile erectile dysfunction. *Int J Impot Res* 1996; **8**: 47–52.

31. Ryder RE, Close CF, Moriarty KT *et al.* Impotence in diabetes: aetiology, implications for treatment and preferred vacuum device. *Diabet Med* 1992; **9**: 893–898.

32. Price DE, Cooksey G, Jehu D *et al.* The management of impotence in diabetic men by vacuum tumescence therapy. *Diabet Med* 1991; **8**: 964–967.

33. Vale JA, Feneley MR, Lees WR, Kirby RS. Venous leak surgery: long term follow up of patients undergoing excision and ligation of the deep dorsal vein of the penis. *Br J Urol* 1995; **76**: 192–195.

34. Wilson SK, Delk JR II. Inflatable penile implant infection: predisposing factors and treatment suggestions. *J Urol* 1995; **153**: 659–661.

35. Wilson SK, Carson CC, Cleves MA, Delk JR II. Quantifying risk of penile prosthesis infection with elevated glycosylated hemoglobin. *J Urol* 1998; **159**: 1537–1539; discussion 1539–1540.

36. Bejany DE, Perito PE, Lustgarten M, Rhamy RK. Gangrene of the penis after implantation of penile prosthesis: case reports treatments and recommendations and review of the literature. *J Urol* 1993; **150**: 190–191.

37. Bishop JR, Moul JW, Sihelnik SA *et al.* Use of glycosylated haemaoglobin to identify diabetics at high risk for penile periprosthetic infections. *J Urol* 1992; **147**: 386–388.

13

Acute coronary syndromes: impact of diabetes on pathophysiology, outcome, and management

Laura Benzaquen and Richard Nesto

Coronary heart disease (CHD) is a major cause of morbidity and mortality among patients with diabetes mellitus. The Framingham Study found that diabetes doubled the risk for cardiovascular disease in men and tripled it in women.[1,2] Those with diabetes mellitus Type 1 had a cumulative mortality due to coronary artery disease of 35% by age 55 years, compared with 4–8% for non-diabetics.[3] Another study found that sudden cardiac death occurred 50% more often than average in diabetic men and 300% more than average in diabetic women.[4] Furthermore, diabetics had a greater incidence of multivessel disease and a greater number of diseased vessels.[5,6] Even when adjusting for advancing age, hypertension, smoking, hypercholesterolemia, and left ventricular hypertrophy, diabetes remains a major independent cardiovascular risk factor. In fact, the contribution of these risk factors taken together accounts for less than 25% of the increased coronary heart disease in diabetic patients.[7] The reasons for this disparity are multifactorial, reflecting the widespread effects of diabetes on multiple physiological processes. In this chapter, we will discuss many of the pathophysiological changes related to diabetes that together impact so significantly upon the incidence of CHD and sudden cardiac death. In addition, we will review current therapies, management issues, and outcomes in diabetics with CHD.

A brief introduction to both normal vascular anatomy and the pathogenesis of coronary artery disease and sudden cardiac death is necessary prior to exploring some of the changes that occur in diabetic patients. The coronary artery consists of three major layers: the intima, the media, and the adventitia. The intima is a continuous layer of endothelial cells which regulates the transport of substances through the arterial wall. These cells resist thrombogenesis, produce growth factors and vasoactive substances such as nitric oxide and prostacyclin PGI2, and contribute to a connective tissue matrix. The middle layer, the media, consists of smooth muscle cells which are surrounded by a proteoglycan matrix, collagen, and elastic fibers. The outermost layer of the arterial wall, the adventitia, is largely composed of connective tissue, though it also contains the autonomic nerve endings that help to regulate vascular tone.

Coronary artery disease is caused by atherosclerosis, a multifactorial process which leads to the extensive accumulation of smooth muscle cells within the intima of the affected artery. The advanced lesion of atherosclerosis is the atherosclerotic plaque, and the prevailing theory in plaque formation is the 'response-to-injury' hypothesis. This postulates that several forms of injury to the endothelium can lead to endothelial cell dysfunction, resulting in increased adherence of monocytes/macro-phages and T-lymphocytes, and contributing to smooth muscle cell proliferation and migration through the release of growth factors. The inflammatory cells migrate between the endothelial cells and accumulate subendothe-lially, releasing metalloproteinases capable of degrading the major constituents of the extra-cellular matrix. At the same time, low-density lipoprotein (LDL, which normally binds to specific endothelial cell receptors and mediates the transport of cholesterol) begins to accumu-late subendothelially. Macrophages act as scavenger cells to take up this lipid. LDL can also become modified by oxidation, which renders it cytotoxic, immunogenic, and chemo-tactic. Moreover, it is taken up by macrophages 10 times more readily than unmodified LDL. These macrophages become 'foam cells' which, together with the T-lymphocytes and smooth muscle cells, form the 'fatty streak', the initial lesion of atherosclerosis. As the lesion progresses, an increasing number of macro-phages scavenge still more lipid. At the same time, dysfunction of the endothelial cells impairs their ability to resist thrombogenesis, leading to the formation of platelet thrombi and the subsequent release of additional growth-regulatory proteins. Ultimately, the release of such growth factors and cytokines from cells within the lesion (including activated macrophages, T-lymphocytes, smooth muscle cells, and endothelial cells) leads to the evolu-tion of the 'fatty streak' into a 'fibrofatty lesion', and ultimately to a fibrous plaque – the advanced atherosclerotic plaque.[8]

Disruption of the atherosclerotic plaque plays a crucial role in the pathophysiology of acute coronary syndromes. Thrombi that become incorporated into existing atheroscler-otic lesions increase plaque size and worsen lumenal narrowing. When an advanced plaque forms cracks and fissures, the exposure of plaque contents to circulating blood products leads to further thrombus formation. Ultimately, this may lead to vessel occlusion, resulting in the acute coronary syndromes – unstable angina, myocardial infarction, and sudden death.[9]

In diabetic individuals, each stage of athero-genesis is accentuated. There is an increased propensity to vascular injury due to multiple causes, including enhanced vasoconstriction and hyperglycemia. Vasoconstriction reduces vessel caliber, resulting in increased turbulent flow, wall stress, and platelet aggregation – all of which facilitate endothelial damage. Several mechanisms are operative: inactivation of nitric oxide by either oxygen-free radicals or advanced glycation end-products, as well as an impaired vasodilatory response to both endoge-nous and exogenous nitric oxide; decreased prostacyclin production, which normally stimulates vasodilation and inhibits platelet aggregation; increased endothelin-1, a power-ful vasoconstrictor as well as a mitogen for smooth muscle cells; and increased relative sympathetic activation secondary to parasym-pathetic-related autonomic dysfunction.[10-13] Hyperglycemia is another factor favoring vascular injury and endothelial dysfunction; elevated serum glucose results in the nonenzy-matic 'glycation' of several proteins, leading to the generation of advanced glycated end-products. These glycated end-products accumu-late on extracellular matrix proteins and have been found in large amounts within the atherosclerotic plaque of diabetics, resulting in increased vessel stiffness, lipoprotein accumu-lation, and cytokine release. They also increase recruitment of monoctyes/macrophages, which release matrix metalloproteinases, weakening the fibrous cap and rendering the plaque more vulnerable to disruption.[14]

The next stage of atherosclerosis, the prolif-eration of smooth muscle cells, is exaggerated in diabetic patients through several different mechanisms. In addition to the proliferative actions of insulin-like growth factor and insulin, factors favoring muscle cell proliferation include increased production of platelet-derived growth factor (PDGF), increased endothelin, and decreased nitric oxide production.[13,15,16] As previously mentioned, advanced glycated end-products are chemotactic for monocytes/macrophages, inducing them to produce cytokines such as cachectin/tumor necrosis factor and interleukin 1 (IL-1), which have strong proliferative properties as well.[17]

In diabetes, changes in the lipid profile affecting several different lipoproteins, including LDL, very-low-density lipoprotein (VLDL), lipoprotein (a), and high-density lipoprotein (HDL), contribute to the progression of atherosclerosis. Although total LDL may not be elevated in patients with diabetes, modifications of LDL such as oxidation and glycation render it more atherogenic. Oxidized LDL is cytotoxic and chemotactic, and is taken up by macrophages more readily than unmodified LDL.[18,19] Glycation of LDL decreases its clearance by LDL receptors by up to 25%, favoring clearance through the scavenger pathway,[20,21] and also predisposes it to oxidative modification.[22,23] Diabetic patients with microalbuminuria or overt diabetic nephropathy may also have elevated total LDL levels secondary to renal dysfunction.[24,25] High levels of another lipoprotein, VLDL, are independently associated with the development of coronary artery disease in the diabetic patient, possibly by increasing intermediate density lipoprotein concentration.[26]

Lipoprotein (a) has been found to be elevated in Type 1 diabetics with poor metabolic control and microalbuminuria, and is an independent risk factor for coronary artery disease.[27] Although its atherogenic properties have been extensively studied, its functional role in vascular complications in Type 1 diabetes is not completely clear.[28-30] Curiously, lipoprotein (a) in not elevated in patients with Type 2 diabetes. Finally, the beneficial functions of HDL in coronary disease appear to be related to mobilization of cholesterol from the atherosclerotic plaque and its transport back to the liver.[31,32] However, in diabetic patients, HDL production is reduced and its catabolism is increased. Glycation of HDL also appears to interfere with its interaction with the HDL_3 receptor, impairing its ability to remove cholesterol from cells.[33] All of the above processes enhance the formation of lipid and cholesterol deposits, together resulting in a larger, softer, and more vulnerable plaque.

Even when correcting for the number of coronary plaques, diabetics still have more acute coronary events than non-diabetic individuals. In addition to more widespread atherosclerosis and the particular pathobiology of the plaques described previously, factors extrinsic to the plaque itself can lead to disruption and superimposed thrombosis. These include increased platelet aggregation, impaired fibrinolysis, and enhanced coagulability, all of which increase the likelihood of thrombosis in the setting of vascular injury. Platelet aggregation is a particularly important factor in occlusive thrombus formation. Platelets in diabetic patients appear to synthesize thromboxane A_2 in higher amounts, particularly in those with poor glycemic control or with vascular complications.[34] Also, platelet consumption is increased in diabetic patients, and the platelet-specific proteins β-thrombomodulin and platelet factor 4, thought to indicate platelet activation, are both elevated.[35]

In diabetic patients, the balance between the coagulation and fibrinolytic systems is impaired as well. They have higher levels of several coagulation factors, including Factors

VII, IX, X, and XII, as well as fibrinogen. An elevation in plasma fibrinogen is an independent risk factor for the development of coronary artery disease and myocardial infarction, and elevated fibrinogen in diabetic men correlates with myocardial ischemia and sudden death.[36-39] Similarly, elevations in Factor VII increase the risk of coronary events. The von Willebrand factor serves as the plasma carrier for Factor VIII and facilitates platelet adhesion; increased levels predispose to sudden death and myocardial infarction. Elevations of Factor VIII itself and thrombin–antithrombin complexes, both of which are thrombogenic, have been reported in diabetics as well.[40] In addition to increased levels of coagulants, an impairment in anticoagulants would predispose to thrombogenesis. In fact, the anticoagulants antithrombin III and activated protein C are decreased in patients with poorly controlled Type 1 diabetes.[41] Finally, impaired endogenous fibrinolysis as a result of increased plaminogen activator inhibitor-1 (PAI-1) is a risk factor for premature coronary disease and myocardial infarction.[42] High levels of PAI-1, which predispose to thrombus formation in the event of endothelial injury, appear to be associated with elevated levels of insulin and triglycerides, as well as glycated lipoproteins.[43]

Another factor possibly contributing to plaque disruption and thrombosis is autonomic nervous system dysfunction. This is a common complication, occurring in up to 50% of patients with Type 2 diabetes of more than 10 years' duration. Increased sympathetic activity may cause a hypercoagulable state as the release of catecholamines promotes platelet and thrombin activation.[44] Cardiac parasympathetic fibers are affected before sympathetic fibers, leading initially to a relative increase in sympathetic tone that results in resting tachycardia and hypertension, increasing myocardial oxygen demand. A decrease in parasympathetic

tone may be responsible for inappropriate coronary vasoconstriction, with its potentially destabilizing effect on the atherosclerotic plaque. Diabetic patients with autonomic neuropathy may fail to experience angina symptoms that may cause critical delays in presenting for medical evaluation. Furthermore, the lack of symptoms often slows physician recognition of the event, further delaying appropriate diagnostic and therapeutic intervention.[45]

With these multiple pathophysiogical changes, it is not surprising that the outcomes of diabetic patients differ considerably from those of non-diabetics. Mortality is particularly high in the immediate peri-myocardial infarction period in the diabetic population. Subgroup analyses of several large thrombolytic trials have yielded interesting data regarding the outcomes of diabetic patients with acute myocardial infarction. In the Thrombolysis and Angioplasty in Myocardial Infarction Study Group (TAMI), over 1,000 patients with acute myocardial infarction underwent coronary angiography within 90 minutes of the administration of tissue-plaminogen activator (t-PA). Diabetics (148 patients) and non-diabetics (923 patients) had similar infarct-related artery patency rates (71 vs 70%, respectively) after thrombolysis, although the in-hospital mortality was higher among diabetics (11 vs 6%, respectively; $p < 0.02$), and particularly high in diabetic women (21%). Coronary angiography in this setting showed that patients with diabetes had more severe anatomic disease (66 vs 46% had multivessel disease; $p < 0.0001$), and a higher incidence of pulmonary edema (11 vs 4%; $p = 0.001$), often despite similar infarct sizes and left ventricular ejection fractions.[46]

In the Global Utilization of Streptokinase and Tissue Plasminogen Activator for Occluded Coronary Arteries (GUSTO-I) trial, over 40,000 patients with evolving MI (approximately 15% of whom were diabetic) were randomized to four different thrombolytic strategies. Despite similarities among diabetics and non-diabetics in the infarct-related arterial patency rates in response to therapy, reocclusion rates, and left ventricular systolic function, diabetic patients had a higher mortality rate at 30 days (11.3% in diabetic patients compared with 5.9% in non-diabetic patients; $p < 0.0001$) and at 1 year (14.5 vs 8.9%; $p < 0.001$). After adjusting for the extent of coronary artery disease and other clinical variables, diabetes remained an independent determinant of short- and long-term mortality.[47]

Using data from the Gruppo Italiano per lo studio della Stretochinasi nell'Infarto miocardico 2 (GISSI-2) trial, the effects of diabetes on the outcome of patients with myocardial infarction who received thrombolytics was examined. Among the 11,667 patients with myocardial infarction in this study, the prevalence of diabetes was higher in women than in men (8.75 vs 1.85% for Type 1 diabetes; $p < 0.01$; 23.7 vs 13.8% for Type 2 diabetes; $p < 0.01$). The in-hospital mortality was moderately increased in diabetic men (8.7 and 10.1% for those with Types 1 and 2 diabetes, respectively, vs 5.8% for non-diabetic patients) and was markedly increased in Type 1 diabetic women (24 vs 15.8% in Type 2 and 13.9% in non-diabetic women). Similar differences in outcomes were found at 1 year follow-up (14.5 vs 8.9%; $p < 0.001$). The increased mortality rate seen in women has been attributed to the higher incidence of congestive heart failure and cardiogenic shock, though the reasons for the increased frequency of heart failure and shock among women are not known.[48]

The presence of congestive heart failure in diabetic patients has been evaluated in several studies. The Thrombolysis in Myocardial Infarction II (TIMI-II) trial found that during long-term follow-up after post-myocardial infarction, congestive heart failure developed more commonly in diabetic patients.[49] The Multicenter Investigation of the Limitation of Infarct Size (MILIS) Study included 500 patients with acute myocardial infarction (85 of whom were diabetic) who underwent serial assessments of left ventricular function. There was a higher incidence of congestive heart failure and death in diabetic patients when compared with non-diabetics at 3 and 6 months follow-up, despite smaller infarct size and similar levels of left ventricular systolic function at the time of presentation with heart failure.[50] There are several possible explanations for this. Metabolic factors related to diabetes place the left ventricle at a higher risk for maladaptive remodeling. In addition, previous silent infarction is often noted at the time of the first clinically recognized myocardial infarction, and cardiac autonomic neuropathy can cause systolic and diastolic dysfunction. Finally, left ventricular dysfunction may result from a subclinical diabetic and/or hypertensive cardiomyopathy.

In spite of significant differences in outcomes, the management of CHD in patients with diabetes remains similar to that of non-diabetics. In general, the therapy of patients with coronary artery disease is multipronged, comprising antithrombotic therapy (with antiplatelet agents, anticoagulants, and thrombolytic agents), beta-blockers, lipid-lowering drugs, ACE-inhibitors, and revascularization procedures (both percutaneous and surgical). In addition, optimization of glycemic control at the time of myocardial infarction can be considered another important strategy to decrease morbidity and mortality in the diabetic population.

Antithrombotic therapy with antiplatelet agents plays a crucial role in the treatment of acute coronary syndromes. The three major classes of antiplatelet agents include cyclooxygenase inhibitors, ADP receptor antagonists, and platelet glycoprotein IIb/IIIa receptor inhibitors. Cyclooxygenase inhibitors and ADP receptor antagonists are effective in secondary prevention of acute coronary syndromes, and the glycoprotein IIb/IIIa antagonists, which inhibit the binding of fibrinogen to glycoprotein IIb/IIIa on platelets, are more suitable for acute vascular thrombosis. The meta-analysis of randomized trials of antiplatelet therapy by the Antiplatelet Trialists' Collaboration found aspirin beneficial in the treatment of diabetic patients with cardiovascular disease or with a high risk for vascular disease; there was a reduction from 22.3 to 18.5% in the combined end-point of vascular death, myocardial infarction, or stroke in the aspirin group when compared with the control group. The benefit in the diabetic group was comparable to that observed in the non-diabetic population.[51] However, in the Second International Study of Infarct Survival (ISIS-2) trial, no additional reduction in mortality was shown in the diabetic group, although there was an overall absolute reduction of 2.4% in the 35-day vascular mortality rate in those treated with aspirin (160 mg of aspirin started at diagnosis of myocardial infarction).[52] Interpretation of results of this latter study are limited by the low dose of aspirin used. It is generally agreed that treatment with aspirin should be considered for all patients with diabetes and coronary disease. The ADP antagonists include ticlopidine and clopidogrel, both of them irreversibly inhibit the ADP platelet receptor. Ticlopidine has been shown to be effective in secondary prevention of acute coronary events in the general population, but no subgroup analysis in diabetics has been reported.[53] Finally, glycoprotein IIb/IIIa receptor antago-

nist therapy decreases acute coronary events and the requirement for additional revascularization procedures in patients who present with unstable angina and non-Q-wave myocardial infarction. In fact, treatment with heparin plus tirofiban, a specific inhibitor of glycoprotein IIb/IIIa receptor, resulted in a significant sustained reduction in ischemic complications in diabetic patients presenting with unstable angina or non-Q-wave myocardial infarction.[54]

Beta-blockers are a mainstay of therapy in patients with acute coronary syndromes and chronic stable angina. Treatment with beta-blockers after myocardial infarction reduces infarct size, infarct extension, recurrent ischemia, reinfarction, and cardiac sudden death.[55] Several large trials have shown that the long-term administration of beta-blockers to patients after myocardial infarction improves survival, and the diabetic population seems to benefit even more from beta-blockade than non-diabetics.[56] In the Bezafibrate Infarction Prevention (BIP) Study Group, which involved 14,417 patients with chronic coronary artery disease, 2,723 (19%) had non-insulin-dependent diabetes. Total mortality at 3 years in diabetics was 7.8% in those receiving beta-blockers, compared with 14% in those who were not (a 44% reduction in total mortality).[57] In the Miami trial, early treatment of MI with beta-blockers reduced mortality at 15 days by fourfold in diabetic patients compared with non-diabetics.[58] Additional data supporting the benefit of beta-blockers came from a recent randomized, placebo-controlled study of atenolol in patients with (or at risk for) cardiovascular events during non-cardiac surgery. That study found that diabetic patients treated with atenolol before and after surgery had no increase in mortality compared with non-diabetics for the 2-year study period, whereas the placebo group had a fourfold increase.[59]

Despite their clear benefit, however, beta-blockers are still underused, although the percentage of patients receiving this therapy has recently increased.[60] Though impaired glucose tolerance and a blunted response to hypoglycemia can occur with beta-blocker therapy, these events are rare when cardioselective agents (β_1-blockers) are used.

Thrombolytic therapy has dramatically changed the course of acute myocardial infarction, and diabetic patients appear to benefit from thrombolysis as much as do non-diabetics. This was demonstrated in the International Study of Infarct Survival-II (ISIS-II) trial, which found that diabetic patients receiving streptokinase had a 31% improvement in survival when compared with placebo; there was 23% improvement in survival in the non-diabetic population.[61] The Fibrinolytic Therapy Trialists' Collaborative Group confirmed the benefit of thrombolytics in diabetic patients; there was a 3.7% absolute reduction in mortality in diabetic patients when compared with a 2.1% reduction in the control group.[62] In those trials, no additional increase in serious bleeding or hemorrhagic stroke was seen in patients with diabetes. Although diabetic people respond to thrombolytic therapy, overall outcome is worse. Subgroup analyses of the TAMI trials, GUSTO-1, GISSI-2, and other trials have shown that the short- and long-term mortality rates remain 1.5–2 times higher in the diabetic population. As mentioned previously, the worse outcome in diabetic patients relates to the severity and extent of coronary artery disease, the higher frequency of non-infarct zone ventricular dysfunction and congestive heart failure, and the altered thrombotic–thrombolytic equilibrium at the time of the plaque rupture.

Treatment with angiotensin-converting enzyme inhibitors (ACE-I) in patients after an acute myocardial infarction reduces infarct size, limits ventricular remodeling, and reduces mortality. ACE-I have been shown to decrease mortality even more dramatically in diabetic individuals when compared with non-diabetics.[63] In the Gruppo Italiano per lo studio della Sopravvivenza nell'Infarto Miocardico-3 (GISSI-3) trial, which included 2,790 diabetic patients, early administration of the ACE-I lisinopril significantly reduced both 6-week and 6-month mortality in diabetics versus non-diabetics (6 weeks, 30 *vs* 5% reduction in mortality, respectively; 6 months, 20 *vs* 0%, respectively). The GISSI-3 trial also suggested that diabetic patients derive more benefit than non-diabetics when an ACE-I is administered within the first day of an acute myocardial infarction.[64] In addition to their effects on limiting ventricular remodeling and reducing infarct size, ACE-I may improve outcomes by decreasing further ischemic events. In the Survival and Ventricular Enlargement (SAVE) trial, recurrent myocardial infarctions were 25% less frequent in those treated with ACE-I.[65] Similarly, in the Captopril and Thrombolysis Study (CATS) trial, the use of ACE-I was associated with 37% fewer ischemic events.[66]

These beneficial effects of ACE-I in diabetic patients are probably multifactorial (for review see ref. 63). ACE-I may augment ischemic preconditioning by potentiating a bradykinin-dependent mechanism. Bradykinin is a potent vasodilator and inhibitor of vascular smooth muscle cell proliferation; however, it also stimulates the release of several endothelially derived vasodilators, including nitric oxide. ACE-I may also decrease insulin resistence, improve glycemic control, and restore fibrinolytic capacity. These studies strongly support administration of ACE-I as part of the regimen for the diabetic patient with an acute myocardial infarction and with left ventricular dysfunction.

Since plasma cholesterol level is a strong predictor of the risk of cardiovascular events both in patients with diabetes and in patients with coronary heart disease, the potential benefits of aggressive lipid-lowering therapy have been evaluated in several studies.[67,68] The subgroup analyses of the Scandanavian Simvastatin Survival Study (4S) examined 202 diabetic patients with previous angina or myocardial infarction.[69–71] Although there was no difference in total mortality, simvastatin therapy was more effective at decreasing coronary events in diabetic patients than in non-diabetics (55 vs 32%). However, in the Cholesterol and Recurrent Events (CARE) study there were similar reductions in major coronary events in diabetic and non-diabetic patients with pre-existing coronary heart disease when treated with pravastatin (25 and 23%, respectively).[72] Based on these and other studies, it is clear that the relative risk-reduction achieved with statins in the diabetic population is similar or slightly greater than in the non-diabetic population. Therefore, statins are indicated for the treatment of patients with diabetes plus hypercholesterolemia and/or mild-to-moderate hypertriglyceridemia. Finally, data from the subset analysis of the Helsinki Heart Study compared the effects of gemfibrozil and placebo on coronary events in diabetic patients.[73] Diabetic patients who received gemfibrozil had a lower incidence of coronary heart disease compared with those who received the placebo (3.4 vs 10.5%, respectively). It found the greatest benefit in those with baseline hypertriglyceridemia and low HDL cholesterol. Ultimately, combination therapy with statins and fibrates may be the optimum management of the dyslipidemia in diabetics with coronary heart disease.

In addition to the medical therapies discussed previously, surgical and percutaneous revascularization procedures have important roles in the management of patients with CHD. Indications for revascularization procedures are similar in diabetic and non-diabetic patients, and diabetic patients do well in the initial period after percutaneous revascularization with angioplasty, whether performed electively or after acute myocardial infarction. However, several studies have shown that diabetic patients have an increased rate of restenosis. The restenosis rate of single native vessel angioplasty was greater in 57 diabetics when compared with 243 non-diabetic patients (63 vs 36 %, respectively; p = 0.0002).[74] It is felt that restenosis in diabetic individuals is increased because of exuberant intimal hyperplasia rather than increased vessel remodeling.[75] Given these long-term results with percutaneous revascularization, surgical revascularization with coronary artery bypass grafting (CABG) is often performed in diabetic patients with angina and multivessel disease. As with CHD in general, short- and long-term survival after CABG is significantly reduced by the presence of diabetes.[76,77] This difference is mostly associated with more progressive disease in both the non-bypassed and bypassed vessels in diabetic individuals.

Most trials have shown similar outcomes comparing angioplasty to bypass surgery in non-diabetics with the two methods of revascularization. However, the Bypass Angioplasty Revascularization Investigation (BARI) trial has shown that diabetic patients with multivessel disease had an 81% survival rate at 5 years if the initial strategy was bypass surgery, compared with a 66% survival when the initial treatment strategy was angioplasty.[78] Increased rates of restenosis and more extensive disease in diabetic patients reduces the likelihood of complete revascularization with percutaneous techniques. Thus, surgery remains the preferred treatment in those diabetic individuals with multivessel disease.

All of the above management issues are relevant for both diabetic and non-diabetic individuals. However, an additional factor critical in the treatment of diabetic patients is glycemic control, as poor long-term glycemic control is associated with increased cardiac mortality and morbidity. Indeed, elevated glycosylated hemoglobin levels have been associated with a higher mortality rate after infarction.[79] The Diabetes Control and Complications Trial (DCCT) examined the effect of intensive insulin treatment in patients with Type 1 diabetes on the development and progression of microvascular disease. Intensive treatment delayed the onset and slowed the progression of microvascular disease by 35–74% and decreased the development of hypercholesterolemia by 43%. It also decreased the risk of major macrovascular events by 41%, although this reduction did not reach statistical significance.[80] The United Kingdom Prospective Diabetes Study (UKPDS) investigated the impact of glycemic control on the incidence and severity of vascular complications in Type 2 diabetic patients. This study included nearly 4,000 newly diagnosed patients with Type 2 diabetes who were randomized either to conventional therapy or to intensive treatment – the latter employing sulphonylureas, metformin, and/or insulin with a target hemoglobin A1c of less than 7.0%. Those in the intensive treatment arm had a 25% reduction ($p = 0.0099$) in the risk of microvascular disease, as well as a 16% risk reduction ($p = 0.052$) in myocardial infarction and sudden death.[81] Since the UKPDS enrolled patients with no known vascular disease, this degree of reduction in macrovascular events may not be experienced by diabetic patients with established CHD. It is also possible possible that Type 2 diabetic patients with CHD might derive further benefit from tight glycemic control; further clinical trials will be necessary to address this important issue.

Strict glycemic control during the hospital phase of acute myocardial infarction may protect ischemic myocardial cells. The heart typically utilizes free fatty acids as its major source of energy. However, the ischemic myocardium utilizes glucose as its major source of ATP production. The most important glucose transporter in cardiac myocytes is GLUT4; insulin as well as other factors such as ischemia and acidosis stimulate the translocation of this transporter to the cell surface increasing glucose uptake by myocytes.[82] In diabetic patients with ischemia, relative insulinopenia decreases translocation of GLUT4 resulting in decreased intracellular glucose. This results in depressed ATP production, generation of oxygen-free radicals, increased myocardial oxygen consumption, and myocardial contractile dysfunction, thereby reducing the compensatory capacity of the non-infarcted myocardium.[83] The DIGAMI study evaluated outcomes in 620 diabetic patients with an acute myocardial infarction randomized to either intensive insulin therapy (insulin–glucose infusion for 24 hours followed by subcutaneous insulin therapy four times daily for >3 months) or standard treatment. Those receiving the intense insulin regimen were found to have a significant reduction of mortality at 1 year when compared with those receiving conventional care (19 vs 26%). The greatest reduction in mortality was seen in patients who were not receiving insulin prior to the infarction.[84] If other studies support the findings of the DIGAMI trial, strict glycemic control may become standard therapy in diabetic patients with acute myocardial infarction.

Sulfonylurea drugs, the most widely used agents for achieving glycemic control in patients with non-insulin-dependent diabetes, have been associated with increased morbidity and mortality in patients with coronary artery disease.[85] This is probably a result of their inhibition of ATP-sensitive potassium channels (K^+_{ATP}). In the pancreas this inhibition ultimately increases the secretion of insulin, accounting for the hypoglycemic effects of the sulfonylureas. However, in the heart, the opening of K^+_{ATP} channels is believed to facilitate ischemic preconditioning, a cardioprotective mechanism. Sulfonylureas affecting this cardiac K^+_{ATP} channel may impair the myocardial preconditioning in the setting of ischemia, resulting in more extensive myocardial injury at the time of myocardial infarction. Finally, sulfonylureas may be both proarrhythmic and antiarrhythmic due to the role of the K^+_{ATP} channel in regulating the duration of the cardiac action potential.[86,87]

Conclusion

Diabetes mellitus is associated with an increased morbidity and mortality from coronary artery disease. In addition to the accelerated atherosclerosis seen in the diabetic population, there are other factors associated with diabetes that significantly impact in the pathophysiology of acute coronary syndromes. In this chapter, we have reviewed the similarities and differences between diabetic and non-diabetic people in the pathophysiology, outcomes, and management of coronary artery disease and acute coronary syndromes. Further understanding of these issues should lead to more specialized treatment modalities for this high-risk subset of patients.

It is also clear that several issues in diabetes and coronary heart disease require more intensive investigation. Most notably, the reasons for the far-worse outcomes of diabetic women with CHD compared with diabetic men need to be studied, with the goal of improving care for this large group of patients.

References

1. Kannel WB, McGee DL. Diabetes and cardiovascular risk factors: the Framingham Study. *Circulation* 1979; **59**: 8–13.
2. Kannel WB, McGee DL. Diabetes and cardiovascular disease: The Framingham Study. *JAMA* 1979; **241**: 2035–2038.
3. Krolewski AS, Kosinski EJ, Warran JH *et al*. Magnitude and determinants of coronary artery disease in juvenile-onset, insulin-dependent diabetes mellitus. *Am J Cardiol* 1987; **59**: 750–755.
4. Barrett-Connor E, Orchard TJ. Insulin-dependent diabetes mellitus and ischemic heart disease. *Diabetes Care* 1985; **8**: 65–70.
5. Robertson W, Strong J. Atherosclerosis in persons with hypertension and diabetes mellitus. *Lab Invest* 1968; **18**: 538.
6. Waller BF, Palumbo PJ, Lie JT, Roberts WC. Status of the coronary arteries at necropsy in diabetes mellitus with onset after age 30 years. Analysis of 229 diabetic patients with and without clinical evidence of coronary heart disease and comparison to 183 control subjects. *Am J Med* 1980; **69**: 498–506.
7. Pyörälä K, Laakso M, Uusitupa M. Diabetes and atherosclerosis: an epidemiologic view. *Diabetes Metab Rev* 1987; **3**: 463–524.
8. Ross R. The pathogenesis of atherosclerosis: a perspective for the 1990s. *Nature* **362**: 801–808.
9. Fuster V, Badimon L, Badimon JJ *et al*. The pathogenesis of coronary artery disease and the acute coronary syndromes (1). *N Engl J Med* 1992; **326**: 242–250.
10. Williams SB, Cusco JA, Roddy MA *et al*. Impaired nitric oxide-mediated vasodilation in patients with non-insulin-dependent diabetes mellitus. *J Am Coll Cardiol* 1996; **27**: 567–574.
11. Bucala R, Tracey KJ, Cerami A. Advanced glycosilation products quench nitric oxide and mediate defective endothelium-dependent vasodilatation in experimental diabetes. *J Clin Invest* 1991; **87**: 432–438.
12. Ferri C, Pittoni V, Piccoli A *et al*. Insulin stimulates endothelin-1 secretion from human endothelial cells and modulates its circulating levels *in vivo*. *J Clin Endocrinol Metab* 1995; **80**: 829–835.
13. Takahashi K, Ghatei MA, Lam HC *et al*.

Elevated plasma endothelin in patients with diabetes mellitus. *Diabetologia* 1990; **33**: 306–310.

14. Bucala R, Makita Z, Koschinsky T *et al*. Lipid advanced glycosylation induces transendothelial human monocyte chemotaxis and secretion of platelet-derived growth factor: role in vascular disease of diabetes and aging. *Proc Natl Acad Sci USA* 1990; **87**: 9010–9014.

15. Kawano M, Koshikawa T, Kanzaki T *et al*. Diabetes mellitus induces accelerated growth of aortic smooth muscle cells: association with overexpression of PDGF beta-receptors. *Eur J Clin Invest* 1993; **23**: 84–90.

16. Scherrer U, Randin D, Vollenweider P *et al*. Nitric oxide release accounts for insulin's vascular effects in humans. *J Clin Invest* 1994; **94**: 2511–2515.

17. Vlassara H, Brownlee M, Manogue KR *et al*. Cachectin/TNF and IL-1 induced by glucose-modified proteins: role in normal tissue remodeling. *Science* 1988; **240**: 1546–1548.

18. Henriksen T, Majoney EM, Steinberg D. Enhanced macrophage degradation of biologically modified low density lipoprotein. *Atherosclerosis* 1983; **3**: 149–159.

19. Steinberg D, Parthasarathy S, Carew TE *et al*. Beyond cholesterol. Modifications of low-density lipoprotein that increases its atherogenicity. *N Engl J Med* 1989; **320**: 915–924.

20. Kissebah AH. Low density lipoprotein metabolism in non-insulin-dependent diabetes mellitus. *Diabetes Metab Rev* 1987; **3**: 619–651.

21. Steinbrecher UP, Witztum JL. Glycosylation of low-density lipoproteins to an extent comparable to that seen in diabetes slows their catabolism. *Diabetes* 1984; **33**: 130–134.

22. Bowie A, Owens D, Collins P *et al*. Glycosylated low density lipoprotein is more sensitive to oxidation: implications for the diabetic patient? *Atherosclerosis* 1993; **102**: 63–67.

23. Hunt JV, Smith CC, Wolff SP. Autooxidative glycosylation and possible involvement of peroxides and free radicals in LDL modification by glucose. *Diabetes* 1990; **39**: 1420–1424.

24. The DCCT Research Group. Lipid and lipoprotein levels in patients with IDDM diabetes control and complication. Trial experience. *Diabetes Care* 1992; **15**: 886–894.

25. Winocour PH, Durrington PN, Bhatnagar D *et al*. Influence of early diabetic nephropathy on very low density lipoprotein (VLDL), intermediate density lipoprotein (IDL), and low density lipoprotein (LDL) composition. *Atherosclerosis* 1991; **89**: 49–57.

26. Goldschmid MG, Barrett-Conor E, Eldestein SL *et al*. Dyslipidemia and ischemic heart disease mortality among men and women with diabetes. *Circulation* 1994; **89**: 991–997.

27. Bottalico LA, Keesler GA, Fless GM *et al*. Cholesterol loading of macrophages leads to marked enhancement of native lipoprotein(a) and apoprotein(a) internalization and degradation. *J Biol Chem* 1993; **268**: 8569–8573.

28. Lawn RM. Lipoprotein (a) in heart disease. *Sci Am* 1992; **266**: 54–60.

29. Haffner SM. Lipoprotein (a) and diabetes. An update. *Diabetes Care* 1993; **16**: 835–840.

30. Maser RE, Usher D, Becker DJ *et al*. Lipoprotein(a) concentration shows little relationship to IDDM complications in the Pittsburgh Epidemiology of Diabetes Complications Study cohort. *Diabetes Care* 1993; **16**: 755–758.

31. Breslow JL. Transgenic mouse models of lipoprotein metabolism and atherosclerosis. *Proc Natl Acad Sci USA* 1993; **90**: 8314–8318.

32. Eisenberg S. High density lipoprotein metabolism. *J Lipid Res* 1984; **25**: 1017–1058.

33. Duell PB, Oram JF, Bierman EL. Non-enzymatic glycosilation of HDL and impaired HDL-receptor-mediated cholesterol efflux. *Diabetes* 1991; **40**: 377–384.

34. Davi G, Catalano I, Averna M *et al*. Thromboxane biosynthesis and platelet function in type II diabetes mellitus. *N Engl J Med* 1990; **322**: 1769–1774.

35. Rosove M, Harrison F, Harwig M. Plasma β-thromboglobulin, platelet factor 4, fibrinopeptide A, and other hemostatic functions during improved short-term glycemic control in diabetes mellitus. *Diabetes Care* 1984; **7**: 174–179.

36. Meade TW, North WR, Chakrabarti R *et al*. Haemostatic function and cardiovascular death: Early results of a prospective study. *Lancet* 1980; **1**: 1050–1054.

37. Kannel WB, D'Agostino RB, Belanger AJ. Fibrinogen, cigarette smoking, and risk of

cardiovascular disaese: Insights from the Framingham Study. *Am Heart J* 1987; **113**: 1006–1010.

38. Thompson SG, Kienast J, Pyke SD *et al*. Hemostatic factors and the risk of myocardial infarction or sudden death in patients with angina pectoris. European Concerted Action on Thrombosis and Disabilities Angina Pectoris Angina Group. *N Engl J Med* 1995; **332**: 635–641.

39. Wilhemsen L, Svardsudd K, Korsan-Bengten K *et al*. Fibrinogen as a risk factor for stroke and myocardial infarction. *N Engl J Med* 1984; **311**: 501–505.

40. Jones RL, Peterson CM. Hematologic alterations in diabetes mellitus. *Am J Med* 1981; **70**: 339–352.

41. Ceriello A, Quatraro A, Dello Russo P *et al*. Protein C deficiency in insulin-dependent diabetes: a hyperglycemia-related phenomenon. *Thromb Haemost* 1990; **64**: 104–107.

42. Aznar J, Estelles A, Tormo G *et al*. Plasminogen activator inhibitor activity and other fibrinolytic variables in patients with coronary artery disease. *Br Heart J* 1988; **59**: 535–541.

43. Nordt TK, Sawa H, Fujii S *et al*. Induction of plasminogen activator inhibitor type-1 (PAI-1) by proinsulin and insulin *in vivo*. *Circulation* 1995; **91**: 764–770.

44. Kaikita K, Ogawa H, Yasue H *et al*. Soluble P-selectin is released into the coronary circulation after coronary spasm. *Circulation* 1995; **92**: 1726–1730.

45. Jacoby RM, Nesto RW. Acute myocardial in the diabetic patient: pathophysiology, clinical course and prognosis. *J Am Coll Cardiol* 1992; **20**: 736–744.

46. Granger CB, Califf RM, Young S *et al*. Outcome of patients with diabetes mellitus and acute myocardial infarction treated with thrombolytic agents. *J Am Coll Cardiol* 1993; **21**: 920–925.

47. Woodfield SL, Lundergan CF, Reiner JS *et al*. Angiographic findings and outcome in diabetic patients treated with thrombolytic therapy for acute myocardial infarction: the GUSTO-I experience. *J Am Coll Cardiol* 1996; **28**: 1661–1669.

48. Zuanetti G, Latini R, Maggioni AP *et al*. Influence of diabetes on mortality in acute myocardial infarction: data from the GISSI-2 study. *J Am Coll Cardiol* 1993; **22**: 1788–1794.

49. Mueller HS, Braunwald E, and the TIMI investigators. Predictors of early morbidity and mortality after thrombolytic therapy of acute myocardial infarction. Analysis of patient subgroups in the thrombolysis in myocardial infarction (TIMI) trial, phase II. *Circulation* 1992; **85**: 1254–1264.

50. Stone PH, Mueller J, Hartwall T *et al*. The effect of diabetes mellitus on prognosis and serial left ventricular function after acute myocardial infarction: Contribution of both coronary disease and left ventricular dysfunction to the adverse prognosis, The MILIS Study Group. *J Am Coll Cardiol* 1989; **14**: 49–57.

51. Antiplatelet Trialists' Collaboration. Collaborative overview of randomized trials of antiplatelet therapy – I: Prevention of death, myocardial infarction, and stroke by prolonged antiplatelet therapy in various categories of patients. *Br Med J* 1994; **308**: 81–106.

52. ISIS-2 (Second International Study of Infarct Survival) Collaborative Group. Randomized trial of intravenous streptokinase, oral aspirin, both, or neither among 17,187 cases of suspected acute myocardial infarction: ISIS-2. *Lancet* 1988; **ii**: 349–360.

53. Balsano F, Rizzon P, Violi F *et al*. Antiplatelet treatment with ticlopidine in unstable angina, a controlled multicenter clinical trial. *Circulation* 1990; **82**: 17–26.

54. Theroux P, Ghannam A, Nasmith J *et al*. Improved cardiac outcomes in diabetic unstable angina/non-Q-wave myocardial infarction patients treated with tirofiban and heparin (Abstr). *Circulation* 1998; **98**: 1359.

55. Kendall MJ, Lynch KP, Hjalmarson Å, Kjekshus J. β-blockers and sudden cardiac death. *Ann Intern Med* 1995; **123**: 358–367.

56. Malmberg K, Herlitz J, Hjalmarson A, Ryden L. Effects of metoprolol on mortality and late infarction in diabetics with suspected acute myocardial infarction: Retrospective data from two large studies. *Eur Heart J* 1989; **10**: 423–428.

57. Jonas M, Reicher-Reiss H, Boyko V *et al*. Usefulness of beta-blocker therapy in patients with non-insulin-dependent diabetes mellitus and coronary artery disease. Bezafibrate

Infarctio Prevention (BIP) Study Group. *Am J Cardiol* 1996; **77**: 1273–1277.

58. Malmberg K, Herlitz J, Hjalmarson A, Ryden L. Effects of metoprolol on mortality and late infarction in diabetics with suspected acute myocardial infarction: Retrospective data from two large studies. *Eur Heart J* 1989; **10**: 423–428.

59. Mangano DT, Layug EL, Wallace A, Tateo I. Effect of atenolol on mortality and non-cardiovascular morbidity after non-cardiac surgery. *N Engl J Med* 1996; **335**: 1713–1720.

60. Gotlieb SS, McCarter RJ, Vogel RA. Effect of beta-blockade on mortality among high-risk and low-risk patients after myocardial infarction. *N Engl J Med* 1998; **339**: 489–497.

61. ISIS-2 Collaborative Group. Randomized trial of intravenous streptokinase, oral aspirin, both, or neither among 17,187 cases of suspected myocardial infarction: ISIS-2. *Lancet* 1988; **ii**: 349–360.

62. Fibrinolytic Therapy Trialists' (FTT) Collaborative Group. Indications for fibrinolytic therapy in suspected acute myocardial infarction: collaborative overview of early mortality and major morbidity results from all randomised trials of more than 1000 patients. *Lancet* 1994; **11**: 162–165.

63. Nesto RW, Zarich S. Acute myocardial infarction in diabetes mellitus. Lessons learned from ACE inhibition. *Circulation* 1998; **97**: 12–15.

64. Zuanetti G, Latini R, Maggioni AP *et al.* on behalf of the GISSI-3 Investigators. Effect of ACE inhibitor lisinopril on mortality in diabetic patients with acute myocardial infarction: Data from the GISSI-3 study. *Circulation* 1997; **96**: 4239–4245.

65. Moye LA, Pfeffer MA, Wun CC *et al.*, for the SAVE Investigators. Uniformity of captopril benefit in the SAVE study: subgroup analysis. *Eur Heart J* 1994; **15**: 2–8.

66. Van Den Heuvale AD, van Gilst WH, van Veldhuisen DJ *et al.* Long-term anti-ischemic effects of angiotensin-converting enzyme inhibition in patients after myocardial infarction. *J Am Coll Cardiol* 1997; **30**: 400–405.

67. Kannel WB, McGee DL. Diabetes and glucose tolerance as risk factors for cardiovascular disease: the Framingham Study. *Diabetes Care* 1979; **2**: 120–126.

68. Stamler J, Vaccaro O, Neaton JD, Wentworth D. Diabetes, other risk factors, and 12-yr cardiovascular mortality for men screened in the Multiple Risk Factor Intervention Trial. *Diabetes Care* 1993; **16**: 434–444.

69. Scandinavian Simvastatin Survival Study Group. Randomized trial of cholesterol lowering in 4444 patients with coronary heart disease: the Scandinavian Simvastatin Survival Study (4S). *Lancet* 1994; **344**: 1383–1389.

70. Pyörälä K, Pedersen TR, Kjekshus J *et al.* The Scandinavian Simvastatin Survival Study (4S) group: cholesterol lowering with simvastatin improves prognosis of diabetic patients with coronary heart disease: a subgroup analysis of the Scandinavian Simvastatin Survival study (4S). *Diabetes Care* 1997; **20**: 614–620.

71. Haffner SM. The Scandinavian Simvastatin Survival Study (4S) subgroup analysis of diabetic subjects: implications for the prevention of coronary artery disease. *Diabetes Care* 1997; **20**: 469–471.

72. Sacks FM, Pfeffer MA, Moye LA *et al.* The effect of pravastatin on coronary events after myocardial infarction in patients with average cholestarol level. *N Engl J Med* 1996; **335**: 1001–1009.

73. Koskinen P, Manttari M, Manninen V *et al.* Coronary heart disease incidence in NIDDM patients in the Helsinki heart study. *Diabetes Care* 1992; **15**: 820–825.

74. Van Belle E, Bauters C, Hubert E *et al.* Restenosis rate in diabetic patients: A comparison of coronary stenting and ballon angioplasty in native coronary arteries. *Circulation* 1997; **96**: 1454–1459.

75. Kornowski R, Mintz GS, Kent KM *et al.* Increased restenosis in diabetes mellitus after coronary interventions is due to exaggerated intimal hyperplasia. *Circulation* 1995; **91**: 979–989.

76. Barzilay JI, Kronmal RA, Bittner V *et al.* Coronary artery disease and coronary artery grafting in diabetic patients aged ≥65 years (report from the Coronary Artery Study [CASS] registry). *Am J Cardiol* 1994; **74**: 334–339.

77. Smith L, Harrell F, Rankin J *et al.* Determinants of early versus late cardiac death in patients undergoing coronary artery bypass graft surgery. *Circulation* 1991; **84 (Suppl 3)**: 422.

78. The Bypass Angioplasty Revascularization Investigation (BARI) Investigators. Comparison of coronary bypass surgery with angioplasty in patients with multivessel disease. *N Engl J Med* 1996; **335**: 217–225.

79. Oswald G, Corcoran S, Yudkin J. Prevalence and risks of hyperglycaemia and undiagnosed diabetes in patients with acute myocardial infarction. *Lancet* 1984; **9**: 1264–1267.

80. Diabetes Control and Complications Trial Research Group. The effect of intensive treatment of diabetes on the development and progression of long-term complications in insulin-dependent diabetes mellitus. *N Engl J Med* 1993, **329**: 977–986.

81. UK Prospective Diabetes Study Group. Intensive blood-glucose control with sulphonylureas or insulin compared with conventional treatment and risk of complications in patients with Type 2 diabetes (UKPDS 33). *Lancet* 1998; **352**: 837–853.

82. Sun D, Nguyen N, Degrado T *et al*. Ischemia induces translocation of the insulin-responsive glucose transporter GLUT4 to the plasma membrane of cardiac myocites. *Circulation* 1995; **91**: 635–640.

83. Rodrigues B, Vam MC, McNeill JH. Myocardial substrate metabolism: implications for diabetic cardiomyopathy. *J Molec Cell Cardiol* 1995; **27**: 169–179.

84. Malmberg K, Ryden L, Efendic S *et al*. Randomized trial of insulin–glucose infusion followed by subcutaneous insulin treatment in diabetic patients with acute myocardial infarction (DIGAMI Study): effects on mortality at 1 year. *J Am Coll Cardiol* 1995; **26**: 57–65.

85. University Group Diabetes Program. Effects of hypoglucemic agents on vascular complications in patients with adult-onset diabetes. *Diabetes* 1976; **25**: 1129–1153.

86. Cole W, McPherson CD, Sontag D. ATP regulated K channel protect the myocardium againt ischemia/reperfusion damage. *Circ Res* 1991; **69**: 571–581.

87. Kubota I, Yamaki M, Shibata T *et al*. Role of ATP-sensitive K channel on ECG ST elevation during a bout of myocardial ischemia: a study on epicardial mapping in dogs. *Circulation* 1993; **88**: 1845–1851.

14

Designer insulins: have they revolutionized insulin therapy?

David Owens and Anthony Barnett

Introduction

The isolation of insulin from pancreatic extracts by Banting and Best in 1921 ended the desperate search for the active principle from the islets of Langerhans.[1] This miracle of twentieth century medicine heralded major advances in the development of insulin preparations (*Table 14.1*), saving countless millions of lives. During the first 50 years, the evolutionary milestones encompassed the production and formulation of insulin to alter its time–action characteristics, and purification of animal insulin (bovine and porcine) preparations. More recently, the advent of recombinant DNA technology has made biosynthetic human insulin available for clinical use since 1982.[2–4] Modifications of the human insulin molecule quickly followed, with the production of many insulin analogues ('designer insulins') with altered physico-chemical and biological properties in an attempt to simulate better both meal-related and basal insulin requirements.[5,6]

The need to achieve near-normal blood glucose levels was recommended by Joslin in the 1930s, and since re-affirmed by others and supported by the more recent and conclusive findings of the Diabetes Control and Complications Trial (DCCT)[7] in patients with Type 1 diabetes and the United Kingdom Prospective Diabetes Study (UKPDS)[8,9] for patients with Type 2 diabetes. Therefore,

Table 14.1
Insulin preparations: milestones.

Year	Researchers	Milestone
1922	Banting, Best[244]	Isolation of insulin
1934	Scott[245]	Crystallization
1936	Hagedorn *et al.*[202]	Protamine insulin
1946	Krayenbühl, Rosenberg[203]	Isophane insulin
1952	Hallas-Møller *et al.*[246]	Lente insulins
1972	Schlichtkrull *et al.*[247]	Monocomponent insulin
1979	Goeddel *et al.*[2]	Recombinant human insulin
1987	Brange *et al.*[29]	'Monomeric' insulin analogues
1987	Markussen *et al.*[212]	Soluble prolonged-acting analogues
1996	Markussen *et al.*[218]	Acylated insulins

good glycaemic control in all patients with Type 1 and Type 2 diabetes translates into clinical benefit in the form of primary and secondary prevention of long-term diabetes-specific microvascular complications. In an update on their study, the DCCT Research Group also expressed an opinion that the risk of complications may be more dependent on the extent of post-prandial excursions than any summary measures of glycaemic control such as HbA_{1c}.[10]

Currently available conventional short-, intermediate- and long-acting insulin preparations, when given by bolus subcutaneous injection according to a variety of regimens and sites of injection, still fail to replicate a non-diabetic day-long circulating insulin profile. An initial 'lag-phase' in the absorption of human soluble (regular) insulin used for meal-related requirements results in peak concentrations in the blood within 1.5–3 hours, which necessitates injecting the insulin at least 15–30 minutes before eating. Insulin is still present in the blood 6–8 hours after administration, with between-meal snacks needed to counter the inappropriately prolonged hyperinsulinaemia, and thus avoid hypoglycaemia.

The intermediate- and long-acting insulins are suspensions of insulin in crystalline and/or amorphous forms (NPH or Lente type) necessitating thorough mixing to ensure homogeneity prior to injection in order to minimize the within- and between-patient variation in absorption, which has been estimated to account for up to 80% of the day-to-day variation in blood glucose concentration.[11] These insulin preparations fail to simulate basal insulin supply, resulting instead in peaks of circulating insulin and a relatively short duration of action, predisposing the patient to nocturnal hypoglycaemia and/or fasting hyperglycaemia when given before bed as part of a 'basal bolus' insulin regimen.

Considerable progress is being made in the quest to achieve more physiological replacement of insulin, with the introduction of the 'rapid-acting' insulin analogues to provide meal-related insulin requirements. To date, progress has been much slower in arriving at a suitable long-acting preparation for basal requirements. This hitherto 'elusive goal'[12] will undoubtedly remain a target into the next millennium, recognizing that pancreatic insulin was not evolved for exogenous administration and that, to date, subcutaneous insulin therapy has not succeeded in normalizing glycaemic control. Several reviews are now available on this subject.[13–20]

Rapid-acting insulin analogues
Concept and strategies

At physiological concentration, insulin circulates and binds to its receptor as a monomeric unit.[21] At higher concentrations, insulin dimerizes, and in neutral solution in the presence of zinc, three dimers associate into hexamers, which is the main association state found in U-100 (~0.6 mM) neutral soluble insulin.[22] The amino acid residues involved in the association of two insulin molecules into dimers are A21, B8, 9, 12, 16, 20, 21 and 23–29 (*Fig. 14.1a*). The insulin molecules in the dimer are held together predominantly by non-polar forces (hydrophobic surfaces), reinforced by four hydrogen bonds between B24 and B26 arranged as an antiparallel β-sheet structure between the two carboxy-terminal strands of the β-chain (*Fig. 14.1b*). Packing of the three dimers around two zinc ions, which results in the burial of the remaining non-polar surface, involves amino acid residues A13, 14 and 17, and B1, 2, 4, 10, 13, 14 and 17–20. The assembly between dimers in the hexamer is much

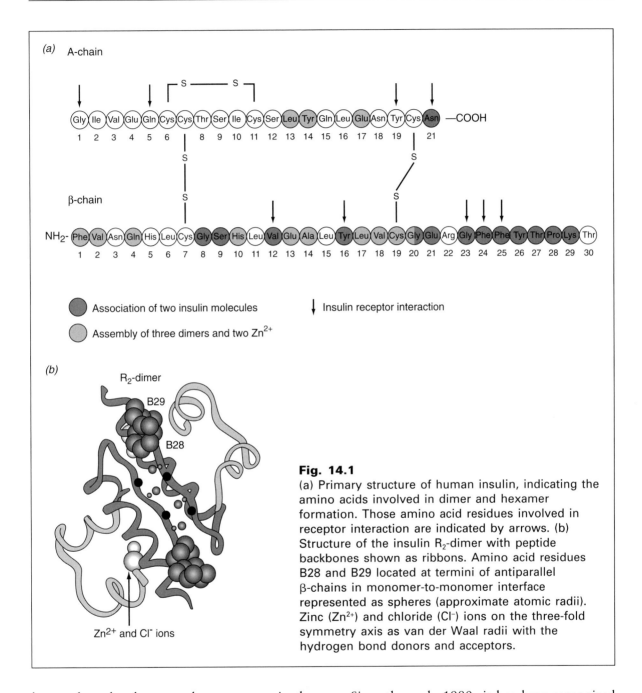

Fig. 14.1

(a) Primary structure of human insulin, indicating the amino acids involved in dimer and hexamer formation. Those amino acid residues involved in receptor interaction are indicated by arrows. (b) Structure of the insulin R_2-dimer with peptide backbones shown as ribbons. Amino acid residues B28 and B29 located at termini of antiparallel β-chains in monomer-to-monomer interface represented as spheres (approximate atomic radii). Zinc (Zn^{2+}) and chloride (Cl^-) ions on the three-fold symmetry axis as van der Waal radii with the hydrogen bond donors and acceptors.

looser than that between the monomers in the dimers. Putative amino acid residues interacting with the insulin receptor site include A1, 5, 19 and 21, and B12, 16 and 23–25[23,24] which, therefore, should remain unaltered.

Since the early 1980s it has been recognized that factors known to influence insulin absorption, such as the species and concentration of insulin, and especially subcutaneous blood flow, have an influence on the association state

Table 14.2
Insulin analogues.

Strategy		Examples
Charge repulsion		
• with pre-existing charge		Asp^{B9}, Glu^{B27}; Asp^{B25}, Asp^{B28}; Asp^{B28}
• introducing charge counterparts		Asp^{A21}, Glu^{B27}; Asp^{B25}
• Removal of metal-binding sites		Asp^{B10}, Thr^{B10}
• Hydrophobic into hydrophilic residues		Glu^{B16}, Glu^{B27}; Glu^{B26}
Stearic manipulation		
Type 1		Ile^{B12}
Type 2	β-sheet residue	
	Deletion	desB27
	Reversal	Lys^{B28}, Pro^{B29} (Lispro)

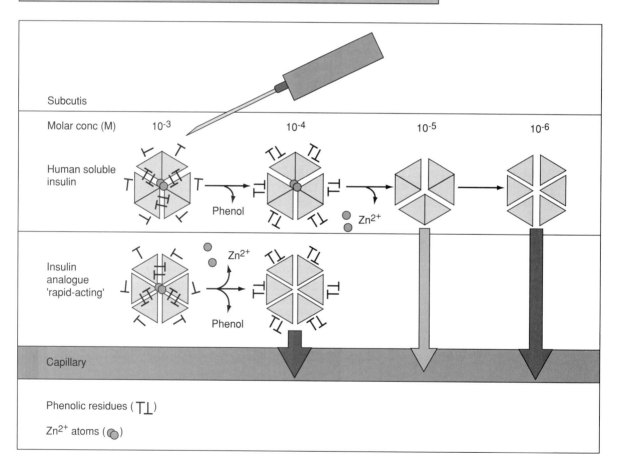

Fig. 14.2
Schematic representation of the dissociation process and subsequent absorption of insulin from the subcutaneous tissue for both human soluble insulin and the rapid-acting human insulin analogues following subcutaneous injection.

of insulin and its propensity to dissociate.[13,16] Many insulin analogues with a reduced tendency to self-associate have been made utilizing a variety of different strategies to include charge repulsion, removal of metal-binding sites, exchanging hydrophobic with highly hydrophilic residues thus decreasing interface hydrophobicity, and stearic manipulation of the C-terminal part of the B-chain to interfere with both hydrophobic interactions and β-sheet formation (*Table 14.2*).

The association state and the increased tendency to dissociate of the many rapid-acting insulin analogues have been demonstrated in the laboratory using a variety of methods to include osmometry, ultracentrifugation, circular dichronism spectroscopy, and size-exclusion chromatography. In pharmaceutical formulations it is important for both chemical and physical stability that the insulin is associated as hexameric units, which is promoted by the presence of zinc ions and phenol or cresole molecules. In the subcutaneous tissue, the initial step in the dissociation process is likely to be that phenol is released from the hexomeric complex, which then rapidly dissociates into dimers and monomers, with zinc diffusing into the subcutaneous tissue (*Fig. 14.2*). The potential clinical relevance of the rate of dissociation of the hexamer to subcutaneous insulin absorption was quickly realized when the first three insulin analogues, Asp^{B9}, Glu^{B27} and Asp^{B10}, and then Asp^{B28}-human insulins were studied in healthy subjects following a single bolus subcutaneous injection.[25–28] The initial 'lag-phase' observed in the absorption of human soluble insulin is abolished with these 'monomeric' insulin analogues (*Fig. 14.3*),[27,29] resulting in an earlier hypoglycaemic response compared with human soluble insulin when given by bolus subcutaneous injection in both normal and diabetic subjects.[25,26,28] Interestingly, despite marked differences in *in vitro* potency (free fat cell bioassay) between these analogues the hypoglycaemic effect seen was nevertheless equivalent.[27] This is due to reciprocal differences in receptor binding and receptor-mediated insulin clearance,[30] meaning that a low-affinity

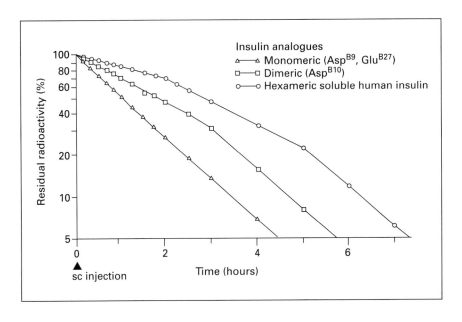

Fig. 14.3
Disappearance curves of ^{125}I-labelled human soluble insulin (○) and the human insulin analogues Asp^{B9}, Glu^{B27} (△), and Asp^{B10} (□) following bolus subcutaneous injection into the anterior abdominal wall. Means ± SE.

analogue with consequently high plasma concentrations is equivalent to a high-affinity analogue accompanied by low plasma concentrations.[31]

Pharmacokinetic and pharmacodynamic studies

The first proof of concept study in insulin-treated diabetic patients was carried out with the Asp[B9], Glu[B27]-HI analogue, which was compared with soluble human insulin (Actrapid HM), with both being given by bolus subcutaneous injection immediately before a meal.[32] The insulin analogue resulted in a much higher and earlier insulin peak, with a markedly reduced post-prandial glucose excursion. Further studies in insulin-treated diabetics, when comparing soluble insulin injected 30 minutes before eating versus three 'monomeric' human insulin analogues given immediately before the meal (basal insulin provided by a low-dose constant-rate insulin infusion), revealed that the post-prandial incremental glucose excursions were 21–57% lower with the series of rapid-acting insulin analogues (*Fig. 14.4*).[26]

The rapid-acting insulin analogue Asp[B10]-human insulin was the first to be tested in a clinical setting over a 2-month treatment period in insulin-treated diabetics against human soluble insulin (Actrapid HM), both given as the mealtime insulin with NPH insulin at bedtime as part of a basal/bolus insulin regimen.[33] Despite improved post-prandial plasma insulin/analogue and glucose concentrations seen predominantly after breakfast with the insulin analogue, the overnight glucose profile was worse than with human soluble insulin. Consequently, no overall improvement in HbA_{lc} was achieved. The unadjusted night-time dose of NPH was, therefore, clearly inadequate in support of the

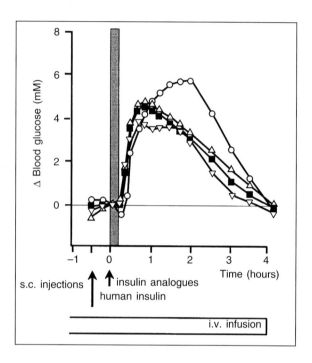

Fig. 14.4

Post-prandial incremental plasma glucose excursions in Type 1 patients on a constant low-dose intravenous infusion of insulin, given human soluble insulin (○) 30 minutes before the meal, compared with the three insulin analogues Asp[B9], Glu[B27] (■), Asp[B10] (△) and Asp[B28] (▽), all given by bolus subcutaneous injection into the anterior abdominal wall.

shorter-acting Asp[B10] analogue. This analogue was later discontinued due to its carcinogenic effect in female rats (mammary tumours) during long-term studies in the Sprague–Dawley strain of rats,[30] later to be confirmed with human breast epithelial cells.[34] As a consequence, there is now a greater understanding of the molecular basis of the mitogenic effects of insulin analogues, which is due primarily to the differential residence times on the insulin receptor.[35,36] A slow insulin receptor dissociation rate is associated with a sustained activation of the insulin receptor tyrosine kinase and phosphorylation of the Shc protein,[35] a likely cause of the increased mitogenicity of some insulin analogues such as the Asp^{B10}-human insulin analogue. In human breast cells, Asp^{B10} has been shown to possess enhanced mitogenic effects due to the activation of both insulin and IGF-1 receptors.[34]

Insulin Lispro

Recognition of the existence of the insulin homologue insulin-like growth-factor 1 (IGF-1) molecule as a monomer, with inversion of the Pro^{B28}, Lys^{B29} sequence seen in insulin, led to the development of Lys^{B28}, Pro^{B29}-human insulin (insulin Lispro).[37] This structural change removed two hydrophobic interactions involving Pro^{B28} and also caused a weakening of the two β-pleated sheet hydrogen bonds essential for the stability of the dimer subunits within the hexamer.[38] The combination of removing proline from B28 and its introduction to B29 resulted in a marked decrease in self-association. In solution, in the presence of zinc, this analogue is a stable hexamer with a much faster rate of dissociation than human soluble insulin when in the subcutaneous tissue resulting in a more rapid absorption profile.[6,39,40] *In vitro* properties of the analogue were found to be comparable to those of human insulin, with only slightly greater binding to the IGF-1 receptor, due to the presence of the basic amino acid at B29, but with no enhanced mitogenicity relative to human insulin.[41,42] In a functional type of mitogenic assay, measuring growth of human mammary epithelial cells in culture, the mitogenic potencies of insulin Lispro and human insulin were comparable,[37] reflecting similar insulin receptor dissociation kinetics in the presence of only marginally enhanced IGF-1 receptor affinity.[42] With insulin Lispro, no adverse toxicological effects were seen in year-long studies in dogs and rats, and no

mutagenicity or mammary gland tumours, no adverse effects on reproduction or development, nor significant immunogenicity in a rhesus monkey study.[43–45] The Fischer 344 strain of rats was used, known to have a lower spontaneous tumour rate compared with the Sprague–Dawley strain used in the toxicology study with the Asp^{B10}-human insulin analogue.[30] The potency of insulin Lispro has been shown to be equivalent to that of soluble human insulin in a number of assay systems.[46,47]

The pharmacokinetic properties of insulin Lispro have been extensively assessed and compared with human soluble insulin following subcutaneous administration in both healthy subjects[39] and patients with Type 1 diabetes mellitus.[48–52] When given by bolus subcutaneous injection, insulin Lispro is rapidly absorbed, reaching peak plasma concentration approximately 1 hour after administration and being cleared within 4–5 hours, in marked contrast to soluble human insulin (*Fig. 14.5*). Dose-ranging studies with insulin Lispro revealed dose-related increases in peak action with little or no change in duration of effect, in contrast to human soluble insulin, where both the peak and especially the duration of action are increased.[53] The faster rate of absorption with insulin Lispro also minimizes the difference between sites of injection such as the anterior abdominal wall, thigh or upper arm regions.[54]

Asp^{B28}-human insulin analogue (insulin aspart)

The Asp^{B28}-human insulin analogue (insulin aspart) represents another strategy for reducing self-association by the introduction of a negative charge counterpart to an existing negative charge on Glu^{B21} on the aggregating surface of the other insulin molecule (*Table 14.2*). This is not, however, as previously

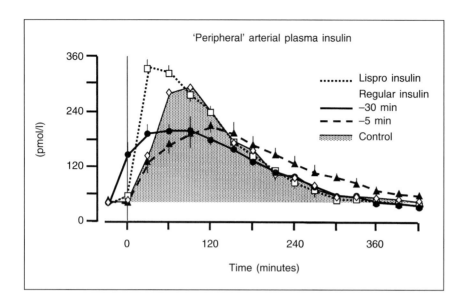

Fig. 14.5
Peripheral 'arterial' plasma insulin profiles following bolus subcutaneous injection of human soluble insulin at −30 minutes (●) or −5 minutes (▲) and insulin Lispro (□) immediately before food in patients with Type 1 diabetes. Non-diabetic subjects were given the same meal (◇). Adapted from Pampanelli et al.[181]

proposed, the main mechanism for inhibiting dimer formation, but rather the removal of the contact between Pro^{B28} and Gly^{B23} at the monomer to monomer interface.[19] The substitution of aspartic acid for proline at position B28 leads to a small conformational change at the C-terminus, but has little effect on the overall conformation. The binding affinity of Asp^{B28}-human insulin analogue to the insulin receptor is 80% relative to human insulin.[30,55] The insulin receptor binding characteristics, internalization, degradation, and kinase activation are indistinguishable from human insulin. Also, binding to the IGF-1 receptor is similar for the analogue and human insulin. The *in vivo* potencies of Asp^{B28}-human insulin and human insulin are identical.[56] Long-term toxicological studies revealed similar mutagenicity and immunogenicity of the analogue and human insulin.[57]

Following bolus subcutaneous administration in healthy subjects, Asp^{B28}-human insulin analogue is more rapidly absorbed than human soluble insulin, with peak concentrations in plasma occurring within 1 hour and returning to basal values within 4–5 hours. This is in contrast to a more protracted peak (plateau) with human insulin from 1–3 hours, with a much slower return towards pre-injection insulin concentration remaining above basal levels for up to 6 hours post-injection.[28,58,59,60] Using the euglycaemic clamp technique in healthy subjects, the glucose infusion rate confirmed the much earlier action of the Asp^{B10}-human insulin analogue, with less variability in the pharmacokinetic parameters compared with human soluble insulin.[59] Within the first hour, the glucose infusion rate was 80% higher with the insulin analogue compared with human soluble insulin. The intra- and inter-individual variability in time to maximum concentrations was lower for insulin aspart than for human soluble insulin, but with comparable variability of action following subcutaneous administration into the anterior abdominal wall.[61] In Type 1 diabetics given Asp^{B28}-human insulin analogue subcutaneously immediately before a meal, the prandial glycaemic excursion was 43% of that observed with human soluble insulin when given 30 minutes before the meal.[26] In a double-blind study in subjects with Type 1 diabetes, insulin aspart given immediately before a standard meal achieved post-prandial glucose excursions 68 and 84% that of human insulin when given 30 minutes or immediately before the meal, respectively.[62] Insulin aspart revealed peak concentrations twice that of soluble insulin in half the time. Similar results were evident between human soluble insulin and insulin aspart in another double-blind study involving Type 1 diabetic subjects where the test preparations were given before each of the three meals during the day and where the biggest difference between the insulins occurred following the first meal of the day, consistent with the pharmacokinetic differences.[63] A study in healthy subjects comparing the main sites of injection (abdomen, deltoid, thigh) demonstrated no difference in bioavailability over the 10 hour post-injection period or in the time to maximum plasma concentration, although a higher maximum plasma concentration was achieved from the abdomen compared with the thigh. The pharmacokinetics of Asp^{B10}-human insulin analogue following subcutaneous administration is similar in children, adolescents, and adult patients with Type 1 diabetes.

Clinical studies with fast-acting insulin analogues

The currently available conventional insulin preparations fail to achieve the necessary quality of glycaemic control required to minimize the onset and progression of the specific microvascular complications of diabetes without considerable disruption to lifestyle.[7] The availability of recombinant DNA technology offers the opportunity to 'design' insulins better suited to replicate the basal and meal-related insulin requirements necessary for maintaining normoglycaemia when using the subcutaneous route of administration.[64] The relatively slow absorption of human soluble insulin compounded by a relatively prolonged clearance from the circulation allows the development of excessive prandial hyperglycaemia, followed by a susceptibility to late hypoglycaemia. The recommendation to inject the human soluble insulin 30 minutes before a meal to restrain better the post-prandial glucose excursions[65,66] is, however, rarely followed in practice.[67] The problem of insulin replacement therapy is further compounded by inadequacies in the current 'intermediate-' and 'long'-acting preparations which result in discernible peak concentrations in the blood, with poor intra- and inter-subject variability in the rate of absorption from the subcutaneous tissue.[68–71]

The first clinical trial to be carried out with a rapid-acting insulin analogue involved a comparison of the ill-fated Asp^{B10}-human insulin analogue versus human soluble insulin in a double-blind crossover design.[33] Each treatment period lasted for 2 months, during which the rapid-acting analogue was given immediately, and soluble insulin 30 minutes before meals, respectively, and NPH administered before bed as the basal insulin. Despite the marked reduction in the post-prandial glucose excursion after breakfast and a more physiological insulin profile with the rapid-acting analogue, the ensuing pre-meal and overnight glucose concentrations were higher during the insulin analogue arm of the study. This accounts for the lack of difference in the overall glycaemic control, as represented by the glycosylated haemoglobin (HbA_{1c}), between the two treatment regimens. There was also no change in the frequency of hypoglycaemia.

A summary of the single-dose studies with the rapid-acting insulin analogues in subjects with diabetes is represented in *Table 14.3*.

Table 14.3
Summary of single-dose studies in diabetic subjects.

Authors	Analogue	Patient type (No.)	Basal insulin	Change in 2 hours post-prandial glucose* (%)
Kang *et al.* 1990[32]	Asp[B9], Glu[B27]	Type 1 (6)	i.v. infusion discontinued	−43[†]
Kang *et al.* 1991[26]	Asp[B10]	Type 1 (6)	i.v. infusion constant	−46[‡]
	Asp[B9], Glu[B27], Asp[B28]			−49[‡] −61[‡]
Lutterman *et al.* 1993[63]	Asp[B28]	Type 1 (14)	NPH − bedtime	−19[†]
Pampanelli *et al.* 1995[181]	Insulin Lispro	Type 1 (6)	i.v. infusion constant	−21[‡], −38[†]
Torlone *et al.* 1996[50]	Insulin Lispro	Type 1 (10)	i.v. infusion constant	−25[†,‡]
Wiefels *et al.* 1995[139]	Asp[B28]	Type 1 (6)	i.v. infusion constant	−34[†]
Lindholm *et al.* 1998[62]	Asp[B28]	Type 1 (24)	i.v. infusion constant	−16[†], −32[‡]

* Relative to human soluble insulin injected (s.c.) at [†] −30 minutes or [‡] −50 minutes pre-prandially.

Insulin Lispro

An extensive array of both single- and repeat-dose studies in several thousands of patients with Type 1 and Type 2 diabetes have consistently demonstrated improved prandial glucose concentrations with insulin Lispro, when injected 0–5 minutes before breakfast, compared with human soluble insulin given at various times up to three-quarters of an hour pre-prandially (*Tables 14.3 and 14.4*). The findings are well represented in a few large, multinational, randomized controlled studies in patients with Type 1 and Type 2 diabetes,[72,73] comparing human soluble insulin given 30–45 minutes pre-breakfast, with insulin Lispro immediately before eating, following injection into the anterior abdominal wall. Basal insulin was provided by NPH or ultralente on a once- or twice-daily basis according to the patient's need. The increments in prandial glucose at 1 and 2 hours post-prandial were 36 and 64% lower, respectively, in Type 1 patients, and 19 and 48% lower, respectively, in Type 2 patients. Essentially, similar differences were observed when using a twice-a-day regimen of soluble or insulin Lispro admixed with NPH insulin in both Type 1 and Type 2 patients.[74]

Meta-analysis of all identifiable long-term randomized controlled trials up to 1997 comparing insulin Lispro with human soluble insulin in Type 1 or 2 patients revealed significant differences in favour of the rapid-acting insulin analogue with respect to post-prandial glycaemic excursions.[75] There were no significant differences in long-term glycaemic control (HbA$_{1c}$), fasting glucose, or frequency of hypoglycaemia between the insulin Lispro and human soluble insulin treatment groups. However, a reduction in night-time hypoglycaemia was observed in Type 1 patients.[72] All studies acknowledge the improved patient convenience with insulin Lispro, a better post-prandial glycaemic control with no increase in hypoglycaemia.

Table 14.4
Summary of clinical studies with rapid-acting insulin analogues in diabetic subjects.

Authors	Analogue	Study design	Patient type (No.)	Treatment duration (minutes)	Basal insulin	% change (Δ) ΔHbA$_{1c}$	ΔHypo freq (total)
Neilsen et al. 1995[33]	Asp[B10]	DB, crossover	Type 1 (21)	2	NPH*	none	-14
Garg et al. 1996[105]	Insulin Lispro	Parallel	Type 1 (39)	12	NPH/Ultralente	+0.2	-54
Pfützner et al. 1996[97]	"	Crossover	Type 1 (104)	3	NPH*,†	none	-11
Rowe et al. 1996[76]	"	DB, crossover	Type 1 (93)	3	NPH*	none	-4
Anderson et al. 1997a[72]	"	Crossover	Type 1 (1,008)	3	NPH/Ultralente*,†,‡	none	-12
Anderson et al. 1997b[73]	"	Parallel	Type 1 (336)	12	NPH/Ultralente*,†,‡	-0.2	-34
			Type 2 (295)			none	-33
Anderson et al. 1997c[86]	"	Crossover	Type 2 (722)	3	NPH/Ultralente*,†,‡	none	-38
Ebeling et al. 1997[184]	"	Sequential	Type 1 (66)	5	NPH	-0.8	-11
Holleman, Hoekstra 1997[18]	"	Crossover	Type 1 (199)	3	NPH*	none	-38
Jacobs et al. 1997[110]	"	Crossover	Type 1 (12)	1	NPH*	none	-3
Zinman et al. 1997[78]	"	DB, crossover	Type 1 (30)	3	CSII	-0.3	-19
Vignati et al. 1997[74]	"	Crossover	Type 1 (379)	2	NPH†,‡	-0.2	none
			Type 2 (328)				
Home et al. 1998[91]	Asp[B28]	DB, crossover	Type 1 (90)	1	NPH bedtime	none	≥20%

NPH given at * bedtime, † before evening meal and ‡ during the daytime.

Amongst the large volume of clinical studies, only two double-blind studies were conducted with insulin Lispro (*Table 14.4*), the reason being to retain the optimum timing of administration of the human soluble insulin. A large proportion of patients (approximately 80%) inject their meal-related soluble insulin within 20 minutes of taking the meal, being easier to remember and more convenient.[67] In one multicentre, double-blind, randomized crossover study the rapid-acting insulin analogue insulin Lispro was compared with human soluble insulin, with both being given pre-prandially within 15 minutes of meals, with NPH given before bed as the basal insulin for overnight control.[76] Glucose control was determined using self-monitored profiles. The study confirmed the earlier observations of significantly lower post-breakfast glucose levels with insulin Lispro, but with higher pre-prandial and fasting glucose values, due to its shorter action.[76] There was no difference in the frequency of symptomatic hypoglycaemia or overall glycaemic control with almost 60% of patients expressing a preference for insulin Lispro.

Most of these early studies either did not allow or, due to time constraints, achieved little or no dosage adjustment of the basal insulin in an attempt to restrain the development of nocturnal hyperglycaemia.[77] The results from these studies reaffirmed what was seen earlier during 24-hour glucose profiling with the first rapid-acting insulin analogue Asp[B10], despite more physiologically normal meal-related insulin profiles during the early part of the day.[33] Both highlight the obvious need to increase the basal insulin supplement to accommodate the relatively shorter duration of action of the 'rapid'-acting insulin analogues compared with human soluble insulin which has a much longer clinically relevant hypoglycaemic effect than has previously been recognized. It was later observed that during the use of continuous subcutaneous infusion (CSII) of insulin Lispro, or soluble human insulin, with basal delivery rates between meals and overnight and bolus delivery immediately before meals in a double-blind study over a 3-month period a significant reduction in the HbA_{1c} was achieved without increasing the risk of hypoglycaemia.[78] This pivotal study confirmed the need for adequate basal insulin supply in order to be able to convert or translate the pharmacokinetic differences between insulin Lispro and human soluble insulin into potential clinical benefit.

When given post-prandially (+15 minutes), insulin Lispro has been shown to obtain similar prandial glucose excursions to that achieved with human soluble insulin injected up to 20 minutes before a meal.[79] The control of incidental hyperglycaemia also seems easier with insulin Lispro than human soluble insulin.[80]

Type 2 diabetes

Whereas insulin is now widely used in the management of patients with Type 2 diabetes to improve control when oral agents have failed, there is little consensus regarding the optimal insulin regimen,[81] although intermediate-acting insulin or premixed preparations administered on a once- or twice-daily basis is most commonly used. The recent results from the UKPDS supports the use of insulin in this group of patients, highlighting the importance of achieving good control to avoid diabetes-related complications.[8]

There is a substantial defect in the early insulin response to a carbohydrate challenge in patients with Type 2 diabetes resulting in excessive prandial hyperglycaemia.[82,83] The early prandial delivery of insulin to patients with Type 2 diabetes underlines the physiological importance of timely prandial insulin supply.[84,85]

Mealtime treatment with insulin Lispro in a 6-month multinational, randomized crossover clinical trial when given immediately before a meal reduced post-prandial glycaemia compared with soluble human insulin injected 30–45 minutes before eating.[86] Basal insulin was given by NPH or ultralente insulin. The difference in the 1 and 2 hour post-prandial glucose levels was 30%, and 53% lower with insulin Lispro. The rate of hypoglycaemia, especially overnight, was also reduced with insulin Lispro. No difference in HbA_{lc} was evident between the two mealtime insulin regimens. Similar results were obtained in a 12-month parallel design study comparing insulin Lispro and human soluble insulin given before meals with an intermediate- (NPH) or long-acting (ultralente) insulin as the basal supplement.[72] Again there was no difference between the insulins in overall glycaemic control (HbA_{lc}) or hypoglycaemia rates. Other studies imply insulin Lispro's suitability in combination with oral agents,[87,88] and its ability to induce a prompt inhibition in hepatic glucose production[89] with change toward normalization of circadian plasma glucose and insulin levels in Type 2 patients with secondary failure.[90]

In the light of the results from the UKPDS,[8] further careful consideration needs now to be given to the pharmacological management of patients with Type 2 diabetes mellitus in the era of new oral agents and insulin analogues.

Asp^{B28}-human insulin analogue (insulin aspart)

The initial single-dose studies in patients with Type 1 diabetes demonstrated the greater reduction in post-prandial glycaemia with the Asp^{B28}-human insulin analogue given immediately before eating compared with human soluble insulin given 30 minutes before.[26] Relative to human soluble insulin, the incre-

mental area under the glucose curve over a 4 hour period was approximately 43%. The daytime glucose profile in a small number of subjects with the same insulin regimen confirmed the reduction in post-prandial glycaemia following breakfast, with no difference at lunch-time, but with improvement in post-prandial glycaemia reappearing again after the evening meal.[63] Insulin aspart was compared with human soluble insulin in a multicentre randomized double-blind cross-over study involving 90 Type 1 diabetics.[91] Insulin aspart or human soluble insulin (Actrapid HM) was given pre-prandially thrice daily with NPH insulin as the basal supply administered before bed; 24-hour profiles were carried out at the beginning of the study and at the end of the two 4-week treatment periods (*Fig. 14.6*). The insulin analogue was consistently absorbed more rapidly than human soluble insulin, with improved post-prandial glucose concentrations following the three meals, and without any deterioration in pre-prandial glycaemic control during the day, in contrast to what was found earlier with insulin Lispro.[76] During the night-time, however, the mean plasma glucose concentration was higher on the Asp^{B28}-human insulin analogue, thus negating the benefit of reduced daytime prandial glucose excursions, which was reflected in the lack of difference in fructosamine levels at the end of each of the two treatment periods. The duration of the study restricted the opportunity to adjust the night-time insulin dose sufficiently in an attempt to optimize glycaemic control. The number of severe hypoglycaemic episodes requiring third-party intervention was significantly lower on the rapid-acting insulin analogue.

The findings, to date, indicate that Asp^{B28}-human insulin analogue (insulin aspart), as part of a basal bolus regimen, is superior to the

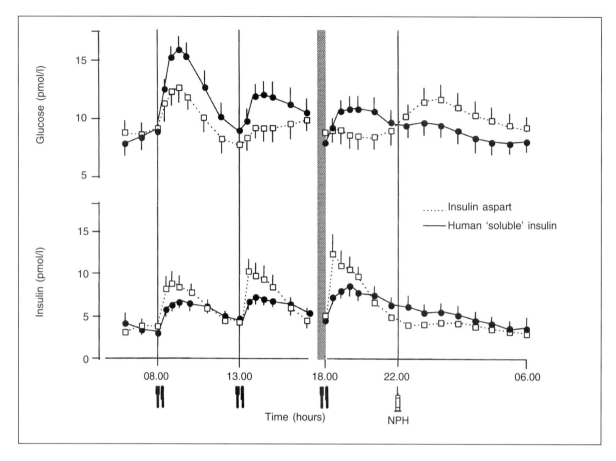

Fig. 14.6

Plasma glucose and serum insulin profiles in patients with Type 1 diabetes with pre-meal subcutaneous injections of human soluble insulin (●) or the human insulin analogue, insulin aspart (□). Basal insulin supplementation was human NPH insulin given before bed. Adapted from Home et al.[91]

reference human soluble insulin for meal-related glycaemic control, but with little or no change in basal insulin supply overnight there is no overall improvement in HbA$_{1c}$. These findings are consistent with earlier observations with both the Asp^{B10} and insulin Lispro human insulin analogues,[33,72,76] pointing to the need to increase the basal insulin supply either by increasing the dose and/or frequency of the NPH insulin, currently used as the basal supply in the majority of patients, so as to realize the

full potential of the rapid-acting insulin analogues.

Preliminary results from a large study involving almost 2,000 patients with Type 1 diabetes in a multinational, parallel, open study comparing the Asp^{B28}-human insulin analogue with human soluble insulin as meal-related insulin over a 6-month period showed better overall control (HbA$_{1c}$) with the rapid-acting analogue. Based on the findings of the DCCT,[7] the difference of 0.12–0.15% in HbA$_{1c}$

observed could potentially reduce microvascular complications by 5–7%.

There is, however, only very limited data in patients with Type 2 diabetes, from single-dose studies showing a similar post-prandial glucose profile with Asp[B28]-human insulin analogue injected immediately before eating compared with human soluble insulin injected 30 minutes pre-prandially.

Hypoglycaemia

Hypoglycaemia is amongst the most feared consequence of insulin therapy, with associated morbidity and some mortality.[92–94] In the DCCT, the frequency of hypoglycaemia was up to threefold higher in the intensive insulin treatment group compared with the conventional treatment group.[7,95,96]

The initial short-term multicentre clinical studies with insulin Lispro as the meal-related insulin did not reveal a consistent change (reduction) in the overall frequency of hypoglycaemia when compared with human soluble insulin in Type 1 diabetic patients.[75] In a randomized, open-label, controlled, crossover trial in 107 patients with Type 1 diabetes, over a 3-month treatment period, insulin Lispro improved post-prandial glycaemic control and also reduced the frequency of hypoglycaemia.[97] Subsequently, a much larger multicentre study in 1,008 Type 1 patients demonstrated a 12% reduction in the rate of hypoglycaemia with insulin Lispro over a 3-month treatment period, the largest relative improvement occurring overnight.[72,98] Similarly, in Type 2 patients, mealtime treatment with insulin Lispro, compared with human soluble insulin, reduced both the post-prandial hyperglycaemia and overall rate of asymptomatic hypoglycaemia by 8%, with a 36% reduction in night-time episodes, i.e. from midnight to 0600 hours.[73] In contrast, another multicentre trial in both Type 1 and Type 2 patients, when conducted

over a longer period of 12 months, demonstrated a similar reduction in the rate of hypoglycaemia for both insulin Lispro and human soluble insulin, 34 and 33%, respectively, during the course of the study.[86] Similarly, in a double-blind study comparing insulin Lispro with human soluble insulin over a relatively short-term treatment period of 3 months, no difference in the frequency of symptomatic hypoglycaemia was recorded.[76]

A cumulative meta-analysis was carried out on the incidence of severe hypoglycaemia (resulting in coma and/or requiring intravenous glucose or intramuscular glucagon) from a series of eight large clinical studies involving approximately 2,000 patients with Type 1 diabetes, comparing insulin Lispro and human soluble insulin treatment over 6–12 months duration.[99] Whilst there was no difference in overall glycaemic control (HbA$_{1c}$) between the treatment groups, a 30% reduction in the incidence of severe hypoglycaemia (3.1 *vs* 4.4%) was seen with insulin Lispro compared with human soluble insulin. Other studies in well-controlled Type 1 diabetic patients demonstrated that, whilst there was no difference between the overall rates of hypoglycaemia, the incidence of severe hypoglycaemic events, including hypoglycaemic coma, was lower with insulin Lispro than with human soluble insulin.[100–104] Also, the frequency of nocturnal hypoglycaemia with insulin Lispro was decreased, whereas episodes of morning hypoglycaemia increased. A reduction in nocturnal hypoglycaemia with insulin Lispro compared with human soluble insulin is important in adolescents with Type 1 diabetes.[105,106] Early pre-prandial hypoglycaemia has also been reported in a few well-controlled patients,[107] emphasizing the need to be aware of this possibility. Meal composition[108] and the timing of exercise[109] need special consideration to avoid hypoglycaemia. Studies demonstrate that the symptomatic and hormonal counterregulatory responses to hypoglycaemia are similar for human soluble insulin and insulin Lispro.[48,94,110]

In contrast to the findings of the DCCT, where hypoglycaemic episodes are increased with decreasing levels of HbA$_{1c}$ with human soluble insulin,[7] this relation was not observed with insulin Lispro.[97,99,111,112] Essentially similar findings have been observed with the rapid-acting Asp^{B28}-human insulin analogue, in a double-blind study over a 4-week treatment period, with a reduction by half of the episodes of hypoglycaemia requiring third-party intervention with equivalent overall glycaemic control.[91]

Any reduction in the incidence of severe hypoglycaemia without having to compromise glycaemic control offers considerable benefits to the insulin-treated diabetic patient. A reduced risk of hypoglycaemia can facilitate the quest for better glycaemic control with intensive insulin therapy, and prevent the damaging influence of recurrent severe hypoglycaemia on cognitive function and hypoglycaemia unawareness.[113,114]

Lipid metabolism

Little detailed published information is available relating to the impact on lipid metabolism of insulin Lispro in comparison to human soluble insulin in patients with Type 1 diabetes.[105,115] In one open, randomized, crossover study involving a small number of well-controlled patients on intensive insulin therapy, the fasting and 2-hour post-prandial total cholesterol, triglyceride levels, and LDL/HDL-C were lower on human soluble insulin than insulin Lispro, without there being any change in overall glycaemic control between the two 3-month treatment periods, which involved NPH as the basal insulin.[115] The LDL, HDL, HDL$_2$ and HDL$_3$ composition remained equally abnormal in both treatment groups, with the 2-hour post-prandial VLDL composition improved with human soluble

insulin, becoming normal on insulin Lispro. The full clinical significance of these observations is unclear. There was no change in serum lipid and lipoprotein levels between insulin Lispro and human soluble insulin in a 6-month, randomized, crossover study in patients with Type 2 diabetes.[86] In view of the extensive nature of the clinical trials, there must be a large body of information on lipids which needs to be made available, especially as cardiovascular disease is a major concern in this patient population.

Pre-mixed formulations of insulin analogues

A large proportion of patients with insulin-requiring diabetes (approximately 40%) are treated with pre-mixed preparations comprising different ratios of soluble to NPH insulin, according to needs. The use of pre-mixed insulins has been shown to reduce errors in dosage, along with improving convenience.[116-118]

Initial problems in admixing the rapid-acting analogue insulin Lispro with NPH insulin[49] have been overcome with the introduction of NPL, where insulin Lispro is co-crystallized with protamine.[119] However, a detailed study in healthy subjects did not reveal a blunting of the action profile of insulin Lispro by mixing with NPH.[120] Clinical practice demonstrates that insulin Lispro is suitable as part of a variety of intensive insulin regimens when admixed with NPH and ultralente.[108,121-123]

Admixing insulin Lispro and isophane insulin as part of a twice-a-day regimen given just before meals lowers the 2 hour post-prandial glucose concentration compared with a 30-minute pre-prandial separate injection of human soluble and isophane insulin.[124] The rapid absorption of insulin Lispro is not adversely affected when mixed with ultralente insulin in Type 1 patients,[121] although some delay in absorption was evident from studies in healthy subjects using the glucose clamp technique.[50] Others, in an open-label study over a 2–3-month period showed no difference in glycosylated haemoglobin (HbA$_{1c}$) between admixtures of insulin Lispro with NPH or ultralente as the basal insulin in patients with Type 1[122] or Type 2 diabetes.[74]

A study of three pre-mixed formulations of insulin Lispro and NPL (75:25; 50:50, and 25:75, respectively) in healthy subjects did not reveal any alteration in the absorption profile of insulin Lispro during glucose clamp studies (*Fig. 14.7*).[125] A clinical study in patients with Type 2 diabetes comparing pre-mixed insulin Lispro/NPL (25:75) with human soluble insulin/NPH (30:70) and NPH demonstrated a reduced post-prandial (breakfast) glucose excursion relative to NPH with the insulin Lispro combination of 36% compared with 56% with the human soluble/NPH pre-mixed formulation.[126] The peak increment in serum insulin was higher with the insulin Lispro/NPH than the soluble/NPH pre-mixed preparation or NPH. The difference between the two pre-mixed formulations was evident only in the first 2–3 hours after administration. The overall glucose excursion, however, remained higher on all the insulins compared with the control group of healthy subjects.

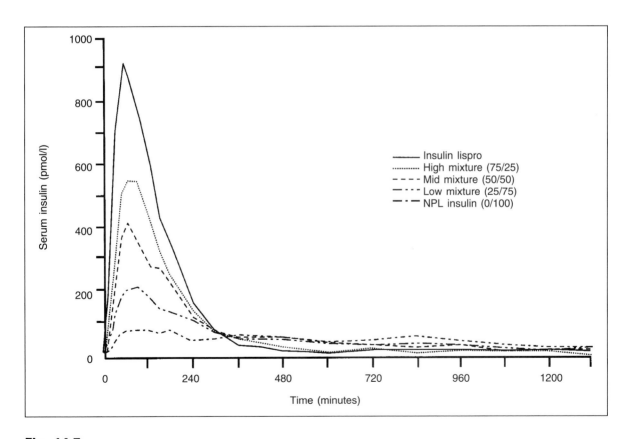

Fig. 14.7
Serum insulin concentrations following bolus subcutaneous administration of insulin Lispro, NPL insulin, and the pre-mixtures 75:25, 50:50 and 25:75, respectively. Adapted from Meise et al.[125]

Clinical experience is rapidly increasing with the pre-mixed formulations of insulin Lispro, and preliminary results indicate a lower rate of nocturnal hypoglycaemia with the 25:75 (insulin Lispro:NPH-MIX25) preparation given before bed.[127,128]

Similarly, a 30/70 pre-mixed formulation of Asp[B28]-human insulin analogue and NPH insulin evaluated in a double-blind, euglycaemic glucose clamp study in healthy subjects indicated that the rapid absorption of the insulin analogue fraction was unaffected, and that it retained its pharmacokinetic and pharmacodynamic properties.[129]

Physical exercise

Physical exercise enhances the affinity of insulin for its receptor, resulting in both an increase in peripheral glucose utilization and inhibition of hepatic glucose output. The risk of hypoglycaemia during exercise in insulin-treated diabetics is well recognized,[130,131] necessitating a reduction in subcutaneously administered short- and/or intermediate-acting insulin, or additional more rapidly absorbable carbohydrate intake prior to exercise in order to avoid hypoglycaemia. In comparison to human soluble insulin, the rapid-acting insulin analogue insulin Lispro, when given immediately prior to a meal, has been shown to be twice as likely to cause exercise-induced hypoglycaemia in the early post-prandial period, but was only half as likely when exercise was performed later than 2–3 h after the meal.[109] Moderate exercise, within 1½–2 hours after a standard meal, in patients on insulin Lispro or human soluble insulin pre-prandially with ultralente twice daily as the basal insulin, resulted in lower post-exercise glucose levels with insulin Lispro, accompanied by a higher frequency of mild hypoglycaemia, but no moderate or severe hypoglycaemia.[132]

Accepting the importance of exercise in diabetes care, serious consideration needs to be given to these findings, so as to reduce the potential for exercise-induced hypoglycaemia, necessitating a reduction in the dose of insulin Lispro or any other rapid-acting insulin analogues, such as the Asp[B28]-human insulin analogue in patients intent on exercising soon after a meal.

Meal consumption and snacks

Meal composition and/or size of meals is a major determinant of prandial glucose concentration, with the general recommendation given to patients to take between-meal snacks in order to avoid hypoglycaemia as a result of the delayed absorption and relatively prolonged action of pre-prandial subcutaneous soluble insulin.[133] When using insulin Lispro in association with low carbohydrate meals there is a tendency for early post-prandial hypoglycaemia compared with soluble insulin[134,135] (*Fig. 14.8*). Others have suggested that post-prandial administration of Lispro insulin may be preferable in certain dietary circumstances.[94,136] With a high carbohydrate meal, giving insulin Lispro pre-prandially, as opposed to 20 minutes post-prandially, achieves a greater reduction in prandial glucose excursions. However, with a high-fat-content meal, accompanied by delayed absorption, post-prandial administration of insulin Lispro is preferable, to avoid the risk of early hypoglycaemia. These findings re-emphasize the need to consider meal composition and also the option of transferring calories from snacks to the preceding main meal when switching from soluble insulin to the rapid-acting insulin analogues.[137] When 50% or more of the carbohydrate content of a snack was incorporated in the main meals, in association with the introduction of insulin Lispro, a small improvement in overall glycaemic control of 0.25% HbA_{1c} was seen only in those patients deemed compliant with the dietary instructions.[80] There was a slightly

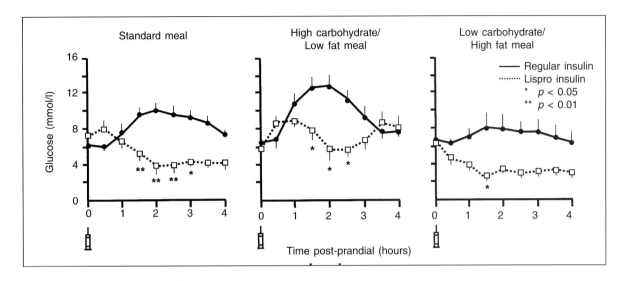

Fig. 14.8

The influence of meal composition on post-prandial glucose profiles following the subcutaneous injection of insulin Lispro immediately before eating. Adapted from Burge et al.[108]

greater fall in those patients with poorer glycaemic control before conversion. The number of hypoglycaemic episodes was also lower with this modification in the dietary habits of the patients. Lispro, when given before a meal combined with a snack, is equivalent to soluble insulin injected 30 minutes before the same meal followed by a snack 2½ hours later.[138] Therefore, reducing between-meal snacks, when switching from soluble insulin to insulin Lispro, is not only safe, but can achieve some improvement in glycaemic control in those dietary compliant patients. However, insulin Lispro given with traditional meal patterns without dosage reduction risks early post-prandial hypoglycaemia.[108,138]

CSII: insulin Lispro in external pump systems

In view of the lack of benefit in overall glycaemic control (HbA$_{1c}$) with the use of insulin Lispro over human soluble insulin in the majority of the early clinical studies,[71–75] due to the inadequacy of the basal insulin supplement, the potential for continuous subcutaneous insulin infusion (CSII) was explored in a small number of studies.[139–142] The first experience was with the insulin analogue Asp^{B28}, administered by CSII over a 6-day period.[139] Improved 1-hour post-prandial glucose concentrations with a small, but nevertheless important, reduction in overall glycaemic control (HbA$_{1c}$) of 0.34% was achieved with insulin Lispro compared with human soluble insulin in the only double-blind crossover CSII study, with the meal-related boluses given immediately prior to the meals for both human soluble and insulin Lispro preparations.[140] Further improvement might be expected if the basal insulin requirement had been better optimized during the night. The hypoglycaemia rate fell during the study with both insulin preparations, but no significant difference in the overall frequency of hypogly-caemia between insulin Lispro and human soluble insulin was noted.

This CSII study was followed by other open-label, randomized, crossover studies where the bolus meal-related human soluble insulin was commenced 20–30 minutes before the meal.[141–144] Improved overall glycaemic control (HbA$_{1c}$) with insulin Lispro was observed over the 3-month treatment periods in some of these studies.[141,143,145,146] Despite improved glycaemic control on insulin Lispro, there has been either no change or very little change,[140,141,143,145] in the frequency of hypoglycaemia. The counter-regulatory hormone response to hypoglycaemia was not adversely affected by CSII with insulin Lispro or human soluble insulin over a 3-month period.[145] In a few patients, cannula occlusion has been observed with insulin Lispro,[140,147] but the consensus is that it is as suitable as any other insulin for external pumps, although not regarded as stable enough in implantable devices.[148] The stability of insulin Lispro in different infusion systems (Disetronic, MiniMed pumps) is suitable for prolonged infusion when the syringes and catheters are replaced at 18-hour intervals.[149] There is, however, concern that due to its rapid clearance from the circulation, patients with pump malfunction would be at a greater risk of developing ketoacidosis. Monitoring the deterioration in metabolic control after inter-ruption of CSII in patients on regular pump therapy revealed a similar increase in mean plasma glucose and β-hydroxybutyrate over the first 6 hours post-cessation observation period for both soluble insulin and insulin Lispro.[150] Only two out of the nine patients on insulin Lispro, and three out of nine patients treated with human soluble insulin treatment group, continued to 8 hours before developing ketonuria, as depicted by the β-hydroxybu-tyrate concentration. There was no apparent

difference in the rate or extent of metabolic decompensation between human soluble and insulin Lispro. The deterioration in metabolic control after interruption of the insulin is considered to be delayed enough for both human and insulin Lispro to be safely used by CSII.[151] More recent studies suggest improved reproducibility of insulin absorption with insulin Lispro by CSII,[152] and less variability in the blood glucose response,[153] when compared with human soluble insulin. However, whatever the insulin employed during CSII, particular attention needs to be given to pump function and catheter maintenance in order to avoid a potentially lethal situation.

Special populations/situations

Young patients

There is a consistent and significant improve-ment in post-prandial glucose excursions with pre-prandial insulin Lispro over human soluble insulin in studies involving young patients with Type 1 diabetes who use multiple pre-prandial insulin injection therapy.[97,105,106,154,155] However, little or no change in HbA$_{1c}$ was evident in these studies. The frequency of mild hypogly-caemia was reduced by up to 50% in subjects receiving pre-meal insulin Lispro,[154,156] with a marked reduction seen in nocturnal hypogly-caemia in a large multinational, crossover, randomized, open-labelled study involving 481 pubertal children.[157] The lack of change in HbA$_{1c}$ may be due to increasing nocturnal hyperglycaemia, compounded by hormonal and psychosocial factors in addition to the non-compliance characteristic of puberty and adolescence.[158]

Post-prandial (+15 minutes) injection of insulin Lispro is equally as effective as human soluble insulin injected 20 minutes before eating in controlling prandial hyperglycaemia in adolescent patients, and could therefore be of benefit in a number of clinical situations such as illness, eating difficulties, and unpredictability of mealtimes and/or content.[155] Both pre- and post-prandial administration of insulin Lispro has also been seen to be equally safe and efficacious in very young children below the age of 5 years.[154] Also, the pharmacokinetics of the Asp[B28]-human insulin analogue in children and adolescents is similar to that in adults.

Consistently, the greatest perceived advantage of insulin Lispro in the young person (children and adolescents) with Type 1 diabetes is the convenience of administration either within 5 minutes before a meal,[97,152,156,159] or post-prandially.[154,155] The rapid-acting insulin analogues offer considerable advantages to the young Type 1 diabetic subject with respect to hypoglycaemia, as most severe events occur at night, with the majority related to missed meals and/or increased activity, although nearly 40% still remain unexplained.[160] Long-term studies are required to ascertain whether improvement in overall glycaemic control can be achieved with the rapid-acting insulin analogues compared with human soluble insulin in the young diabetic during early childhood, puberty, and adolescence.

Elderly diabetic patients

An increasing proportion (approximately 20–30%) of elderly patients with Type 2 diabetes are being treated with insulin.[161] There is little or no meaningful efficacy or safety data on the use of insulin analogues such as insulin Lispro in this ever-increasing population of diabetic patients. The perceived advantages could be the reduced risk of late post-prandial hypoglycaemia, with more flexibility in relation to often very variable eating habits,[162] with the added option of post-prandial administration,[79,136] especially in patients with autonomic neuropathy resulting in delayed gastric emptying.[161]

Pregnancy

Concern has recently been expressed relating to the use of insulin Lispro during pregnancy.[163] Reference was made to congenital abnormalities in the offspring of two well-controlled Type 1 primiparous women treated with insulin Lispro during pregnancy. Subsequently, a limited study involving five women (four Type 1 and one Type 2) well controlled prior to pregnancy and treated with insulin Lispro throughout the first trimester resulted at 38 weeks of gestation in four normal babies and one with septal hypertrophy,[164] suggesting that the insulin analogue did not induce any adverse foetal effect during pregnancy. Similarly, unplanned pregnancies during controlled clinical trials involving several thousands of female patients treated with insulin Lispro resulted in 19 live births, with only one neonate having any abnormality (one dysplastic kidney).[165]

One recent study which compared insulin Lispro and human soluble insulin injected 5 and 30 minutes, respectively, before a test meal in 35 subjects with gestational diabetes mellitus (GDM) demonstrated lower post-prandial glucose at 3 hours with insulin Lispro.[166] The rapid action of insulin Lispro to control post-prandial glucose excursions makes it particularly suitable for patients with GDM. Surveillance of all pregnancies in patients with Type 1 or GDM using insulin Lispro pre-conceptually and/or during pregnancy is required to better elicit the relative safety of insulin Lispro to human soluble insulin in human pregnancy. Studies in pregnant CD rats and rabbits treated prior to and throughout pregnancy with insulin Lispro revealed no developmental toxicity or impaired reproductive performance at doses up to 10 times higher than the expected human dose.[167] There are even fewer data relating to the used of Asp[B28]-human soluble insulin during pregnancy. However, until more comprehensive data are available, insulin Lispro and the Asp[B28]-human insulin analogues should be restricted according to clinical need in the insulin-requiring patient both prior to and throughout pregnancy.

Insulin resistance

There are no immunological differences between insulin Lispro and human soluble insulin in insulin-naïve Type 1 and Type 2 diabetic patients.[168] Neither has insulin Lispro been shown in insulin-treated patients with Type 1 or Type 2 diabetes over a 1-year period to display any differences in immunogenicity from human soluble insulin, with no change in antibody status over the study period.[169] However, a small number of patients with severe insulin antibody-mediated insulin resistance have benefited from the substitution of insulin Lispro for human soluble insulin, resulting in a reduction in insulin requirements and a more stable glycaemic status.[170–174]

Other clinical situations

Insulin Lispro has certain advantages over human soluble insulin in different situations, such as incidental hyperglycaemia due to inappropriate insulin dosage adjustments relation to diet, exercise, or even insulin withdrawal.[80] Exposure to a hot environment such as a Finnish sauna enhances the absorption of insulin Lispro, but with little or no change in glycaemia, due possibly to an increased counterregulatory response.[175] Patients with cystic fibrosis-related diabetes also benefit from insulin Lispro's rapid- and short-lived effect, which is eminently suitable for controlling the prominent post-prandial hyperglycaemia (personal communication) seen in this condition.

Lipohypertrophy at injection sites remains a well-recognized local complication of insulin therapy[176] which results in delayed insulin absorption.[177] It has been suggested that the shorter residence time of the short-acting insulin analogue insulin Lispro in the subcutaneous tissue may lead to less stimulation of subcutaneous adipocytes than human soluble insulin.[178]

Optimization strategies

The importance of timing of pre-prandial subcutaneous soluble insulin with respect to post-prandial glycaemic excursions is well recognized.[65,66] Both rapid-acting insulin analogues, insulin Lispro and Asp[B28]-human insulin, when given just before a meal, in either Type 1 or Type 2 patients, control the post-prandial glucose concentrations better than pre-prandial human soluble insulin for at least the first 2–3 hours of the post-prandial period.[26,28,39,50,72,73,77]

In those well-controlled Type 1 diabetic patients, insulin Lispro, when given immediately before a meal, is more effective in reducing post-prandial hyperglycaemia than human soluble insulin injected up to 40 minutes pre-prandially.[79] However, in patients who are markedly hyperglycaemic before mealtimes, it is necessary to give insulin Lispro 15–30 minutes before, to improve both pre- and post-prandial hyperglycaemia.[179] However, extending the interval between injection of insulin Lispro and the meal to 30 minutes in some patients results in loss of late post-prandial glucose control due to the short duration of action of the insulin Lispro itself. Even injecting insulin Lispro 15 minutes after the commencement of a meal is still better than pre-prandial human soluble insulin.[79]

Based on the findings from the initial large-scale series of randomized control studies comparing insulin Lispro and human soluble insulin, despite the favourable outcome on post-prandial glycaemia by insulin Lispro, there was little or no improvement in overall long-term glycaemic control (HbA$_{1c}$).[72,75–77] These studies were designed essentially to examine post-prandial glycaemia and hypoglycaemia, and not necessarily the optimization of insulin therapy. Those studies which have determined day-long or overnight glucose profiles clearly illustrate the pronounced lack of overnight glycaemic control when little or no adjustment is made to the night-time basal insulin supplement, in support of the rapid-acting, but short duration of action, human insulin analogues.[33,91,102,103,180]

These findings emphasize the need to implement new strategies of basal insulin supplementation utilizing currently available intermediate- and long-acting insulin preparations to derive the full advantage of the rapid-acting insulin analogues whilst awaiting the availability of pharmacokinetically more suitable basal insulin preparations. This requirement is supported by the observation in newly diagnosed Type 1 diabetics where insulin Lispro controlled the post-prandial glucose for longer due to the presence of residual pancreatic β-cell function,[181] in contrast to C-peptide-negative patients who require additional basal insulin supplementation to maintain near-normal glycaemia.[50] Therefore, in order for insulin Lispro to maintain improved glycaemic control beyond 4 hours, in C-peptide-negative patients, basal insulin in between meal times and overnight must be optimally replaced to avoid progressive insulin deficiency and ketosis.[49,103,180]

Increasing the bedtime dose of NPH by 25%, whilst reducing the evening insulin Lispro dose by 20%, compared with standard pre-meal human soluble insulin and evening NPH in an open-label, randomized study, achieved an improvement in the post-evening meal blood glucose control without deteriorating overnight glucose levels.[104] The earlier administration of NPH before the evening meal does not, however,

always ameliorate the night-time hyperglycaemia associated with current regimens involving the rapid-acting insulin analogues.

The addition of daytime NPH extends the post-prandial efficacy of insulin Lispro with improved overall glycaemic control.[50,180,182,183] One study compared soluble insulin and insulin Lispro given pre-prandially (lunch, dinner) plus NPH given at night versus insulin Lispro at a 30% reduced dose with NPH before each meal.[182] The reduced dose Lispro plus NPH at lunch-time was able to maintain the improvement in post-prandial blood glucose for 6 hours before the next meal, in contrast to insulin Lispro without NPH, where the blood glucose and 3-hydroxybutyrate concentration started to escape 3 hours after the lunch. These results supported earlier findings.[50,180] Therefore, adjustment of both the dose and number of injections (2–4) of the basal NPH insulin according to home blood glucose monitoring can achieve an improvement in overall glycaemic control.[184] In this 5-month open study, an increase in the proportion of basal insulin from approximately 40–60% of the daily dose was observed, with improvement in HbA$_{1c}$ of 0.8% achieved but with no change (increase) in the frequency of hypoglycaemia or body-weight. The total daily insulin dose increased only marginally, with a 43% rise in basal insulin and a reduction in the pre-meal dosage of 20%.

Similarly, improved overall glycaemic control (HbA$_{1c}$ reduced by 0.4%) was also achieved with a 26% reduction in the daily dosage of the meal-related insulin of insulin Lispro, and a 34% increase in the dose of NPH when compared with human soluble and NPH as part of an intensive multiple insulin regimen.[185] There was no change in the total daily insulin dosage, with NPH given at a low dose 2–3 times during the day, in addition to the night-time administration.[185] Combining insulin

Lispro with NPH at each meal over a 1-year period maintained a decrease in the HbA_{lc} and frequency of mild hypoglycaemia when compared with human soluble insulin.[112]

Admixing ultralente with insulin Lispro also improves between-meal glycaemia for up to 8 hours.[135] Both open-label[135,122] and double-blind[123] studies demonstrate that NPH and ultralente are equally effective in providing basal insulin replacement with insulin Lispro.

Pre-mixtures of the fast-acting analogues with NPH offer a real alternative to separate injections, as demonstrated from the use of the insulin Lispro/NPL 25:75 preparation,[126] and extrapolated insulin profiles of a fixed combination (30:70) of the Asp^{B28}-human insulin analogue with NPH.[19] The lower individual pre-prandial doses of such admixtures given two or three times daily may also reduce the within and day-to-day variation in absorption.

For a small number of patients, the CSII of the rapid-acting analogue with the use of an external pump is another alternative.[139,140] Awareness of possible consequences of pump malfunction is essential in such patients. Improved post-prandial and overall glycaemic control (HbA_{lc}) was consistently achieved with insulin Lispro compared with human soluble insulin via external pumps.

Therefore, newer strategies for basal insulin supplementation need to be considered in clinical practice to realize better the full potential of the rapid-acting insulin analogues in both C-peptide-negative and newly diagnosed patients with Type 1 diabetes.

In any optimization schedule, serious consideration also needs to be given to other major factors such as diet and exercise. The current convention with human soluble insulin is to recommend between-meal snacks, the necessity for which may be less with the use of pre-prandial fast-acting insulin analogues.[137]

Transference of approximately 50% of the between-meal snacks to the main meals with insulin Lispro has also been shown to be safe in a prospective study, resulting in improved glycaemic control accompanied by a significant reduction in hypoglycaemic events.[18] However, if daytime NPH is concomitantly used, this dietary change need not apply. Physical exercise and many other situations which affect insulin absorption will also have an impact on short-term glycaemic control.

Therefore, recommendations as to the most appropriate regimen need to be made on an individual patient basis so as to capitalize on the advantages offered by the newer insulins. (Differences are not only evident between patients, but also between countries, which is predominantly due to differences in eating habits.)

Quality of life issues

There are many studies which have assessed quality of life measures, relating predominantly to patient preferences, treatment satisfaction, flexibility in lifestyle, hypoglycaemic episodes, and well-being whilst comparing human soluble insulin with the rapid-acting insulin analogues.[186] The most frequently perceived quality of life benefit of insulin Lispro appears to be flexibility in lifestyle, as it relates to timing of meals and planning of physical and social activities as a consequence of being able to inject their insulin either immediately before mealtimes, or post-prandially in young subjects with Type 1 diabetes and adults with either Type 1 or Type 2 diabetes.[72,86,101,105,187,188] This is not surprising, as it is well known that compliance is low with injection instructions for human soluble insulin requiring administration 15–30 minutes before meals.[66,67] A recognized lower risk of severe hypoglycaemia and coma during the night has also contributed to treatment satisfaction,[91,97,101] although, unfortunately, this is due to deteriorating glycaemic control. Therefore, unsurprising higher pre-bed and fasting glucose levels are associated with lower hypoglycaemic rates.[189] In an open, randomized crossover study involving 481 adolescents with diabetes and their parents, comparing insulin Lispro and human soluble insulin over a 4-month period with NPH insulin given 1–3 times daily as the basal insulin, more than 85% of patients indicated their preference to continue on insulin Lispro, and 82% of patients and parents agreed that insulin Lispro made their life easier.[187]

Health-related quality of life (HRQoL) measures from two randomized, multinational, comparative studies over 3-month periods found higher treatment satisfaction and treatment flexibility scores for insulin Lispro compared with human soluble insulin.[186] Similar findings were obtained using a diabetes quality of life (DQoL) questionnaire in a Spanish population,[190] and other patient groups in Europe,[191–193] and the USA.[194] Although a small proportion of patients, (<10%), mention difficulties with insulin Lispro,[192] the vast majority have expressed that insulin Lispro provides more flexibility in their lifestyle, both in general and specifically related to timing of meals, physical and social activities.[101] Using a validated Diabetes Treatment Satisfaction Questionnaire (DTSQ) and a Well-Being Questionnaire (WBQ), in Type 1 diabetics on a multiple injection regimen, significant differences in favour of insulin Lispro was seen in the DTSQ total and convenience scores, as well as the total WBQ score, and three out of four subscales (depression, anxiety, energy, but not positive well-being).[195] Whereas in most open studies, upwards of 70% expressed a preference to continue on insulin Lispro in the one double-blind study with Lispro insulin as part of a basal bolus regimen with night-time NPH,

only half of the patients identified their insulin correctly and 59% expressed a preference for insulin Lispro.[76]

With respect to the rapid-acting Asp[B28]-human insulin analogue, overall satisfaction with treatment measured using the DTSQ was significantly higher than in the human soluble insulin group after 6 months of treatment. The main differences betweeen the treatments were related to convenience and flexibility.

The opportunity to administer the rapid-acting analogues post-prandially[79,154,155] and the reduced reliance on site of injection[54] further adds to the flexibility of treatment. Less-frequent hypoglycaemia,[72,73,101,187] together with improved quantity of life,[195] offers real opportunity for achieving improved compliance with intensive insulin therapy regimens in an attempt to improve the long-term outcome for the patients.

Safety

There was no difference in cardiovascular events, including sudden death, between insulin Lispro and soluble insulin in a large multicentre study involving 3,634 patients (>2,000 patient years).[196]

Treatment with insulin Lispro or human soluble insulin, together with human NPH or ultralente, has little immunological impact in Type 1 or Type 2 patients.[169] Forty to sixty per cent of patients treated with either human insulin or insulin Lispro developed insulin antibodies which did not relate to clinically meaningful increases in insulin dosage requirements.[197]

In long-term multinational safety studies in both Type 1 and Type 2, no clinically relevant differences in adverse events have been observed between insulin Lispro and human soluble insulin.[198]

There is no difference in glucose counter-regulation following s.c. administration between insulin Lispro and human soluble insulin.[48,110]

Long-acting insulin analogues

A continuous low secretion of insulin is required to inhibit hepatic glucose production in the post-absorptive state, especially during the night, which is complicated by increased requirements during the waking hours ('dawn phenomenon').[199,200] Delaying the absorption of insulin from the subcutaneous tissue has been a goal ever since the availability of insulin. The initial attempts to reduce the number of daily injections, involving mixing insulin with gum arabic, oil suspensions, lecithin emulsions, or vasoconstrictor substances, were unsuccessful due to poor stability, pain on injection, and unreliable absorption (*Table 14.5*).[201] Attempts at reducing insulin's solubility, thereby delaying its absorption, by the addition of strong basic proteins and metal ions, was rewarded with the introduction of various protamine insulins[202,203] and zinc-stabilized (Lente) insulin preparations,[204] which have remained the mainstay of 'basal' insulin therapy over the last 40–50 years (*Table 14.5*). Accepting the obvious benefits, the limitations of injecting NPH and Lente insulins for basal insulin supplementation are also well recognized.[71] After subcutaneous administration, these 'intermediate-acting insulin preparations' all result in 'peaks' in plasma insulin concentrations and considerable intra- and inter-patient variation,[205] and therefore are not ideal as a once-daily injection.[11,58,68,205] Attempts to increase the night-time dose, so as to reduce fasting hyperglycaemia, merely increases the risk of night-time hypoglycaemia. Beef ultralente insulin had most of the desired features of a 'basal' insulin,[205–207] but its immunogenicity was deemed disadvantageous and it was therefore discontinued. The advent of human insulin formulated as NPH, Lente, and Ultralente insulins compounded the problem due to more pronounced and earlier peak insulin concentrations and shorter duration of action compared with their forerunner animal-insulin-derived preparations,[58,205] resulting in a propensity to early nocturnal hypoglycaemia and fasting hyperglycaemia, respectively.

Table 14.5
Insulin preparations with prolonged effect.

- 1922–1936: First generation – mixing insulin with:

1923	Gum arabic
1929	Oil suspensions
1930	Lecithin emulsions
1933–34	Vasoconstrictor substances

- 1936–1980: Second generation – mixing insulin with:

Protamine	1936	Protamine, Protamine Zinc Insulin (PZI)
	1946	Isophane insulin (NPH)
Zinc	1951	Lente insulins
Others	1938	Surfen insulins
	1939	Globin insulins
	1940	Iso insulins

In 1982, human proinsulin (hPI) was produced by recombinant DNA technology[208] and was shown to have pharmacokinetic characteristics of an 'intermediate-acting' insulin, but development was discontinued due to excess cardiovascular events in clinical studies as compared with human insulin.[209] Consequently, the metabolite of hPI, the des (64, 65) hPI, was produced,[210] which had the full potency of human insulin, but as duration of action in diabetic patients was shorter than NPH,[211] it was also discontinued.

Different strategies were then adopted to evolve the next generations of insulin analogues (*Table 14.6*), which included altering the isoelectric point of human insulin from 5.4 towards neutral pH, which meant that the insulin analogue would be soluble in an acidic solution and precipitate at the neutral pH of the subcutaneous tissue.[212–216] Other attempts have included producing a cobalt–insulin complex which is essentially non-dissociable, but even this strategy did not result in significant retardation of insulin absorption, as seen with NPH insulin.[217] The latest technique has been to modify the insulin to enhance its binding to albumin, thereby also reducing its absorption from the subcutaneous tissue (*Table 14.6*).[218,219]

At present, continuous subcutaneous insulin infusion (CSII) is currently the best method available of simulating basal insulin secretion. This method of insulin delivery is limited to a relatively small number of patients due to 'pump' and people-related costs.

Insulin analogues with increased isoelectric pH

A series of soluble, prolonged-acting, insulin analogues have been produced by substitution at the β-chain terminus, with basic amino acids accompanied by blocking the C-terminal carboxyl group of the β-chain which crystallizes instantly when the pH is adjusted from 5.4 to 7.0.[213] The analogue Gly^{A21}, Arg^{B27}, Thr^{B30}–NH_2 HI (NovoSol Basal) formed microcrystals in the subcutaneous tissue and its absorption was seen to be much slower than human ultralente, with a $T_{50\%}$ (time to 50% disappearance of radioactivity from site of injection) of 35 hours compared with 26 hours, respectively.[214] The prolonged absorption rate of NovoSol Basal was also associated with a much reduced intra- and inter-patient variability in absorption. However, in clinical studies this analogue failed to control adequately the blood glucose, despite substantial dose increments,[220] which could possibly be related to a local inflammatory reaction.

- 1982: Third generation – rDNA derived:

  1982 Human proinsulin
  1988 Gly^{A21}, Asp^{B27}, Thr^{B30}–NH_2 (NovoSol Basal)
  1990 Arg^{B31}, Arg^{B32}–insulin
  1992 Gly^{A21}, Arg^{B31}, Arg^{B22}–insulin (HOE901)

- 1996: Fourth generation – rDNA derived:

  1996 Lys^{B29}-tetradecanoyl des-(B30)-insulin(NN304)
  1996 *N*-palmitoyl, Lys^{B29}-human insulin

Table 14.6
Insulin preparations with prolonged effect.

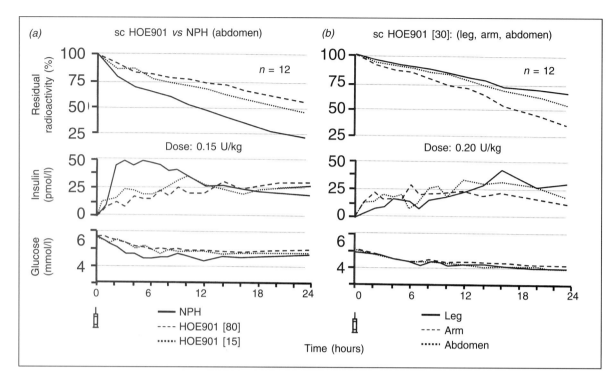

Fig. 14.9
(a) Disappearance curves of ^{125}*I-labelled di-arginyl insulin (HOE901 [15], HOE901 [80]), and NPH insulin, with plasma glucose and estimated exogenuous insulin profiles following bolus subcutaneous injection into the anterior abdominal wall. (b) Disappearance curves of* ^{125}*I-labelled di-arginal insulin (HOE901 [30]) following bolus subcutaneous injection into the anterior abdominal wall, upper arm, and thigh region.*

Based on the same concept, the analogue di-arginyl human insulin (Arg^{B31}, Arg^{B32}) an intermediate in the metabolism of proinsulin, was developed,[215] but when tested was found to have a shorter blood-glucose-lowering effect than NPH insulin.[211] However, the additional substitution of asparagine by glycine at position A21 to improve stability also resulted in a much slower onset and prolonged hypoglycaemic effect compared with NPH insulin, as reflected indirectly in the glucose infusion rates following subcutaneous administration in a clamp study in normal humans.[216] The Gly^{A21}, Arg^{B31}, Arg^{B32}-human insulin analogue (HOE901) was then further

tested in healthy subjects comparing two ^{125}I-labelled formulations varying only in zinc content (15 and 80 µg/ml) versus NPH.[221] The disappearance rate from the site of injection revealed a much delayed absorption of the HOE901 [15] and HOE901 [80] preparations compared with NPH, following subcutaneous absorption into the anterior abdominal wall, with a $T_{75\%}$ of 8.8, 11.0, and 3.2 hours, respectively. This was associated with a slow appearance in plasma of the HOE901 analogues, with a peakless concentration profile over 24 hours, in marked contrast to NPH's exhibiting peak plasma concentrations 4–6 hours after administration (*Fig. 14.9a*). A further study with HOE901 [30] revealed little or no difference in the disappearance rate from the subcutis and the appearance in plasma when HOE901 [30] was injected subcutaneously either into the anterior abdominal wall, thigh, or upper arm regions with a $T_{75\%}$ of 13.2–15.3 hours (*Fig. 14.9b*).[222] There was no clinically discernible local irritation at the site of injection with HOE901 [30].

In vitro studies using rat fibroblast cells revealed similar binding characteristics with human soluble insulin, HOE901, and the Asp^{B10}-human insulin analogue, but the insulin receptor dissociation kinetics were very different, with only the Asp^{B10} insulin analogue causing prolonged phosphorylation and post-receptor events, and thereby possessing increased mitogenicity.[223] The IGF binding affinity of HOE901 using cardiac myocytes was intermediate between human soluble insulin and Asp^{B10}.[224] The growth promoting effect of the Asp^{B10}-human insulin analogue is much greater than HOE901, which was essentially equipotent to human insulin.[224,225] The addition of arginine residues at B31 or B32 increases marginally the affinity for the IGF-1 receptor, with no enhanced mitogenicity relative to human insulin.[226]

To date, relatively few clinical studies have been conducted with HOE901 using a variety of formulations differing only in their zinc content, either 15, 30, or 80 µg/ml.[227–230] An initial 4-day study, with once a day HOE901 given at night-time, achieved a blood glucose profile equivalent to that of NPH, when administered up to four times a day, at the same total daily dosage.[227] This was followed by longer-term multicentre studies involving a four-week treatment period comparing HOE901 given at night with NPH once or twice daily.[229,230] In both studies, the fasting plasma at the end of 4 weeks was lower with HOE901 with one of the studies reporting, in addition, a reduction in HbA_{1c} and nocturnal hypoglycaemia.[229] Similarly, in a large multi-centre 4-week study, overall glycaemic control was similar with HOE901, 15 and 30 mg/ml, and NPH in patients with Type 2 diabetes on concomitant oral hypoglycaemic agents.[228] Significantly fewer hypoglycaemic episodes were recorded on HOE901 compared with NPH or ultralente insulin as the basal insulin supply. These initial findings are encouraging and now await the outcome of longer-term studies.[231]

Acylated insulin analogues binding to albumin

A series of insulin analogues have been produced by acylation of the ϵ-amino group in the side-chain of Lys^{B29}, with deletion of Thr^{B30} thereby placing the acylated Lys^{B29} residue in the C-terminal position of the β-chain (*Fig. 14.10a*).[232,233] Of the saturated fatty acids, maximal binding affinity to human serum albumin was observed with Lys^{B29}-tetradecanoyl des-B30) insulin (NN304) (*Fig. 14.10a,b*). The $T_{50\%}$ for NN304, when studied in pigs, was significantly longer at 14.3 hours, compared with 10.5 hours with NPH insulin with maximum glucose disposal rates in a eugly-caemic clamp study of 6.6 and 9.9 mg kg^{-1} min^{-1} at 6.4 and 3.4 hours, respectively (*Fig. 14.10c*). A reduced coefficient of variation of the $T_{50\%}$ was observed with NN304 at 15%, compared with 41% with NPH. Further clamp studies in dogs demonstrated similar steady-state glucose disposal rates for NN304 and human insulin, but at concentrations of 10–12-fold higher with NN304 (due to the albumin binding).[234,235] *In vitro* competitive binding studies with human serum albumin have been carried out with a variety of drugs (sulphonylureas, valproate, diazepam), varying concentrations of FFA and drugs known to increase FFA concentration

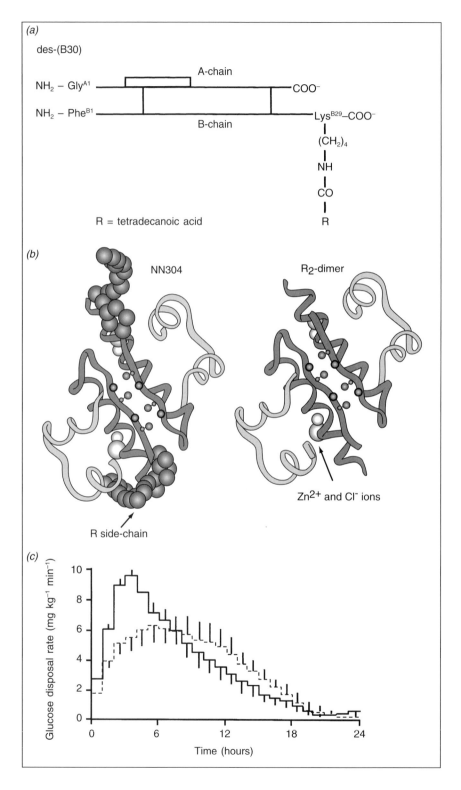

Fig. 14.10

(a) Schematic representation of human insulin and des-(B30) human insulin acylated in the ε-amino group of the side-chain of Lys^{B29}. (b) Structure of the acylated insulin analogue NN304-dimer, with the myristoyl side-chains as well as the hydrogen bond donors and acceptors. The zinc (Zn^{2+}) and chloride (Cl^{-}) ions are included on the three–fold symmetry axis as van der Waal spheres (in the background). (c) Time–action profiles (glucose disposal rate during euglycaemic clamp) following bolus subcutaneous injection of human NPH (—) and the fatty acid acylated insulin analogue Lys^{B29}-tetradecanoyl des-(B30) insulin: NN304 (----) in pigs. Means ± SE. Adapted from Markussen et al.[218]

(heparin, β-agonists), with little or no influence on NN304 albumin binding.[236] Marked elevation in free fatty acids can cause displacement of NN304 due to competition for binding sites on albumin, but with little or no metabolic consequences.[237,238] Pharmacokinetic studies in healthy subjects at three dose levels of NN304 in an isoglycaemic clamp study demonstrated a dose-related increase in the area under the plasma insulin profile for NN304, with a much reduced peak concentration compared with NPH insulin.[239] NN304 achieved a more even metabolic effect than NPH insulin; however, no clear-cut dose-response relationship was observed. Long-term studies in humans are awaited.

A second insulin acylated at Lys^{B29}, but with palmitic acid (N-ε-palmitoyl Lys^{B29})-human insulin has also been demonstrated to have a longer hypoglycaemic effect than NPH insulin in diabetic dogs, and associated with both a lower variability in absorption and a flatter plasma insulin concentration profile compared with NPH insulin after subcutaneous administration.[240] The duration of the hypoglycaemic action of Lys^{B29}-palmitoyl insulin following subcutaneous injection was 16 hours, compared with 8 hours with NPH. The plasma concentration was 20 to 30 times higher and the dose approximately 80% higher than NPH insulin due to the very significant albumin binding. The T_{50} following bolus intravenous administration was 27 minutes compared with 4 minutes for native human insulin, and the hypoglycaemic potency of Lys^{B29}-palmitoyl insulin in healthy subjects was 20–25% that of human insulin.[241] Studies in Type 1 diabetic patients using the euglycaemic clamp confirmed the more prolonged action of the Lys^{B29}-palmitoyl human insulin, with similar metabolic effects and reduced potency compared with NPH insulin.[242]

These two acylated human insulin analogues demonstrate that binding of insulin to albumin in the subcutaneous tissue and vascular compartment can lead to extended time–action characteristics with potential as basal insulin supplementation. Studies will be necessary to confirm efficacy and safety of these new and exciting analogues in various clinical situations, especially in relation to conditions associated with very high or low serum albumin concentrations.

Summary

The full impact of major advances that have occurred in the understanding of the molecular assembly, biological activity, and therapeutic properties of insulin, and the ensuing modifications in its amino acid structure resulting in novel designer insulins are yet to be fully realized. These important evolutionary steps are an inherent part of a long-term revolution aimed to achieve more physiological insulin replacement.

The recent arrival of the rapid-acting and short-lived insulin analogues, insulin Lispro and the Asp^{B28} human insulin analogue, when compared with human soluble insulin, offer improved post-prandial glucose control, a reduction in the frequency of hypoglycaemia, and a more flexible lifestyle with improved quality of life. The site of injection is seemingly less critical, and post-prandial administration is an additional option. Meal composition, need for snacks, and the interval between meals and timing of exercise all necessitate special consideration when introducing the rapid-acting insulin analogues. The clinical use of these analogues must therefore reflect the pharmacokinetic differences with human soluble insulin.

The potential of the rapid-acting insulin analogues may well not be realized until the availability of better basal insulin supplementation. In the meantime, optimization of therapy requires both a reduction in dose of the rapid-acting insulin analogues compared with human soluble insulin when given before meals, and an equivalent increase in the dose of the presently available 'basal' insulin preparations, in order to compensate for the shorter duration of action of the rapid-acting insulin analogues compared with their forerunners. The need for different strategies (frequency of administration) of basal insulin supplementation has been recognized in an attempt both to achieve better overall glycaemic control and to accommodate the many different lifestyles and nutritional habits of the insulin-requiring diabetic patients worldwide. In this respect, therefore, the issue of co-administration of the rapid-acting insulin analogues with insulin preparations having a more protracted action is very important, especially as the majority of patients with both Type 1 and Type 2 diabetes are currently managed with pre-mixed insulin preparations comprising different ratios of conventional short- and intermediate-acting insulin.

Expectations now reside with the new generation of long-acting insulin analogues to provide a near-constant basal insulin supply in marked contrast to the currently available insulin preparations with protracted action. Earlier protamine zinc insulin and bovine ultralente insulin preparations met in part the pharmacokinetic requirements of a basal insulin, but both had perceived drawbacks including high immunogenic potencies and pharmaceutical incompatabilities, which led to their discontinuation. However, HOE901 appears to be the first long-acting insulin analogue on the clinical horizon, followed possibly by the acylated human insulin analogues. Whilst we await the availability of these new basal insulins, greater clinical experience is still needed with the rapid-acting insulin analogues to answer the many remaining questions, which include how to optimize their use and achieve the short- and long-term clinical benefits whilst also establishing the safety of these new chemical entities.[243]

It is prudent to slowly improve blood glucose control with the introduction of new insulin analogues, especially during pregnancy and in all patients previously poorly controlled, in an attempt to avoid the appearance and/or progression of microvascular complications of diabetes, especially diabetic retinopathy.

These latest developments in insulin chemistry have also served as a potent stimulus to the clinician to re-examine in more depth current practices in insulin therapy and their limitations. The findings of both the DCCT and UKPDS will ensure a continuing commitment, by both scientists and clinicians, to achieve a more physiological insulin replacement based both on insulin analogues ('designer' insulins) and/or different methods of insulin delivery.

The complexity of the subject of insulin replacement therapy to achieve normoglycaemia without incurring unwanted hypoglycaemic events using the subcutaneous route of administration cannot be overestimated. However, the availability of insulin analogues represents a significant evolutionary milestone in this continuing challenge.

Acknowledgements

We acknowledge the secretarial support of Catherine Murray, Angela White and Jane Spickett, and Adrian Shaw for the illustrations, and Helle Birk Olsen for Figs 14.1b and 14.10b.

References

1. Bliss M. *The Discovery of Insulin*. Toronto: McClelland and Stewart, 1982.
2. Goeddel DV, Kleid DG, Bolivar F *et al.* Expression in Escherichia coli of chemically synthesized genes for human insulin. *Proc Natl Acad Sci USA* 1979; **76**: 106–110.
3. Markussen J, Damgaard U, Diers I *et al.* Biosynthesis of human insulin in yeast via

single-chain precursors. In: Theodoropoulos D, ed. *Peptides* Berlin: de Gruyter & Co's, 1986: 189–194.

4. Brogden RN, Heel RC. Human insulin. A review of its biological activity, pharmacokinetics and therapeutic use. *Drugs* 1987; **34**: 350–371.

5. Brange J, Ribel U, Hansen JF *et al.* Monomeric insulins obtained by protein engineering and their medical implications. *Nature* 1988; **333**: 679–682.

6. DiMarchi RD, Mayer JP, Fan L *et al.* Synthesis of a fast-acting insulin based on structural homology with insulin-like growth factor 1. 1992. Smith JA, Rivier JE, eds. *Peptides XII (Proceedings of the 12th American Peptide Symposium)*. Leiden: Escom, 1992: 26–28.

7. DCCT. The effect of intensive treatment of diabetes on the development and progression of long-term complications in insulin-dependent diabetes mellitus. *N Engl J Med* 1993; **329**: 977–986.

8. UKPDS33. Intensive blood glucose control with sulphonylureas or insulin compared with conventional treatment and risk of complications in patients with Type 2 diabetes. *The Lancet* 1998; **352**: 837–853.

9. UKPDS34. Effect of intensive blood-glucose control with metformin on complications in overweight patients with type 2 diabetes. *Lancet* 1998; **352**: 854–865.

10. DCCT. The relationship of glycemic exposure (HbA$_{1c}$) to the risk of development and progression of retinopathy in the Diabetes Control and Complications Trial. *Diabetes* 1995; **44**: 968–983.

11. Lauritzen T, Faber OK, Binder C. Variation in ^{125}I-insulin absorption and blood glucose concentration. *Diabetologia* 1979; **17**: 291–295.

12. Zinman B. The physiological replacement of insulin: an elusive goal. *N Engl J Med* 1989; **321**: 363–370.

13. Brange J, Owens DR, Kang S, Vølund A. Monomeric insulins and their experimental and clinical implications. *Diabetes Care* 1990; **13**: 923–954.

14. Galloway JA, Chance RE. *Approaches to Insulin Analogues. The Diabetes Annual/8.* Amsterdam: Elsevier, 1994: 277–279.

15. Barnett AH, Owens DR. Insulin analogues. *Lancet* 1997; **349**: 47–51.

16. Burge MR, Schade DS. Insulins. *Curr Therap Diabetes* 1997; **26**: 575–598.

17. Hoffman A, Ziv E. Pharmacokinetic considerations of new insulin formulations and routes of administration. *Clin Pharmacokinet* 1997; **33**: 285–301.

18. Holleman F, Hoekstra JBL. Insulin Lispro. *N Engl J Med* 1997; **337**: 176–183.

19. Brange J, Vølund A. Insulin analogues with improved pharmacokinetic profiles. In: Baudys M, Kim SW, eds. *Insulin Delivery. Advanced Drug Delivery Reviews* 1999; **35**: 307–335.

20. Bolli GB, DiMarchi R, Park G *et al.* Insulin analogues and their potential in the management of Type 1 Diabetes Mellitus. *Diabetologia* 1998; in press.

21. Blundell T, Dodson G, Hodgkin D, Mercola D. Insulin: The structure in the crystal and its reflection in chemistry and biology. *Adv Protein Chem* 1972; **26**: 279–402.

22. Cunningham LW, Fischer RL, Vestling CS. A study of the binding of zinc and cobalt by insulin. *J Am Chem Soc* 1955; **77**: 5703–5707.

23. Pullen RA, Lindsay DG, Wood SP *et al.* Receptor-binding region of insulin. *Nature* 1976; **259**: 369–373.

24. Gammeltoft S. Insulin receptors: binding kinetics and structure–function relationship of insulin. *Physiolog Rev* 1984; **64**: 1321–1378.

25. Vora JP, Owens DR, Dolben J *et al.* Recombinant DNA derived monomeric insulin analogue: comparison with soluble human insulin in normal subjects. *Br Med J* 1988; **297**: 1236–1239.

26. Kang S, Creagh FM, Peters JR *et al.* Comparison of subcutaneous soluble human insulin and insulin analogues (Asp^{B9}; Glu^{B27}; Asp^{B10}; Asp^{B28}) on meal-related plasma glucose excursions in Type 1 diabetic subjects. *Diabetes Care* 1991; **14**: 571–577.

27. Kang S, Brange J, Burch A *et al.* Subcutaneous insulin absorption explained by insulin's physicochemical properties: evidence from absorption studies of soluble human insulin and insulin analogues in humans. *Diabetes Care* 1991; **14**: 942–948.

28. Kang S, Brange J, Burch A *et al.* Absorption

kinetics and action profiles of subcutaneously administered insulin analogues (Asp^{B9}; Glu^{B27}; Asp^{B10}; Asp^{B28}) in healthy subjects. *Diabetes Care* 1991; **14**: 1057–1065.

29. Brange J, Diers I, Hansen MT *et al.* Monomeric insulin are absorbed three times faster from subcutis than human insulin. *Diabetes* 1987; **36** (**Suppl 1**): 77A.

30. Drejer K. The bioactivity of insulin analogues from *in vitro* receptor binding to *in vivo* glucose uptake. *Diabetes Metab Rev* 1992; **8**: 259–286.

31. Ribel U, Hougaard P, Dreger K, Sørensen AR. Insulin analogues and human insulin: equivalent *in vivo* biological activity of insulin analogues and human insulin different *in vivo* potenices. *Diabetes* 1990; **39**: 1033–1039.

32. Kang S, Owens DR, Vora JP, Brange J. Comparison of insulin analogue Asp^{B9} Glu^{B27} and soluble human insulin in insulin-treated diabetes. *Lancet* 1990; **335**: 303–306.

33. Neilsen FS, Jørgensen LN, Ipsen M *et al.* Long-term comparison of human insulin analogue B10Asp and soluble human insulin in IDDM patients on a basal/bolus insulin regimen. *Diabetologia* 1995; **38**: 592–598.

34. Milazzo G, Sciacca L, Papa V *et al.* Asp^{B10} insulin induction of increased mitogenic responses and phenotypic changes in human breast epithelial cells: Evidence for enhanced interactions with the insulin-like growth factor-1 receptor. *Molec Carcino* 1997; **18**: 19–25.

35. Hansen BF, Danielsen GM, Drejer K *et al.* Sustained signalling from the insulin receptor after stimulation with insulin analogues exhibiting increased mitogenic potency. *Biochem J* 1996; **315**: 271–279.

36. Ish-Shalom D, Christoffersen CT, Vorwerk P *et al.* Mitogenic properties of insulin and insulin analogues mediated by the insulin receptor. *Diabetologia* 1997; **40**: S25–S31.

37. Slieker LJ, Brooke GS, Chance RE *et al.* Insulin and IGF-I analogs: Novel approaches to improved insulin pharmacokinetics. In: LeRoith D, Raizada MK, eds. *Current Directions in Insulin-Like Growth Factor Research.* New York: Plenum Press, 1994: 25–32.

38. Ciszak E, Beals JM, Frank BH *et al.* Role of C-terminal B-chain residues in insulin assembly: the structure of hexameric $Lys^{B28}Pro^{B29}$-human insulin. *Structure* 1995; **3**: 615–622.

39. Howey DC, Bowsher RR, Brunelle RL, Woodworth JR. [Lys(B28), Pro(B29)]-human insulin: a rapidly absorbed analogue of human insulin. *Diabetes* 1994; **43**: 396–402.

40. DiMarchi RD, Chance RE, Long HB *et al.* Preparation of an insulin with improved pharmacokinetics relative to human insulin through consideration of structural homology with insulin-like growth factor-I. *Horm Res* 1994; **41** (**Suppl 2**): 93–96.

41. Slieker LJ, Sundell K. Modifications in the 28–29 position of the insulin B-chain after binding to the IGF-I receptor with minimal effect on insulin receptor binding. *Diabetes* 1991; **40** (**Suppl 1**): 168A.

42. Slieker LJ, Brooke GS, DiMarchi RD *et al.* Modifications in the B10 and B26-30 regions of the B-chain of human insulin alter affinity for the human IGF-1 receptor more than for the insulin receptor. *Diabetologia* 1997; **40**: S54–S61.

43. Zimmerman J. A 12-month chronic toxicity study of LY275585 (human insulin analog) administered subcutaneously to Fischer 344 Rats. *Diabetes* 1994; **4** (**Suppl 1**): 166A.

44. Buelke-Sam J, Byrd RA, Holt JA, Zimmerman JL. A reproductive and developmental toxicity study in CD rats of LY275585 [Lys(B28), Pro (B29)]-human insulin. *J Am Coll Toxicity* 1994; **13**: 247–260.

45. Zwickl CM, Smith HW, Zimmerman JL, Weirda D. Immunogenicity of biosynthetic human LysPro insulin compared to native-sequence human and purified porcine insulins in rhesus monkeys immunized over a 6-week period. *Arzneimittel-Forschung* 1995; **45**: 524–528.

46. Shaw WN, Su KSE. Viological aspects of a new human insulin analogue: [Lys (B^{28}), Pro (B^{29})]-human insulin. *Diabetes* 1991; **40** (**Suppl 1**): 464A.

47. Radziuk J, Candas B, Davies J *et al.* The absorption kinetics of subcutaneously injected insulin and two monomeric analogs. *Diabetes* 1991; **40** (**Suppl 1**): 465A.

48. Torlone E, Fanelli C, Rambotti AM *et al.* Pharmacokinetics, pharmacodynamics and glucose counterregulation following subcutaneous injection of the monomeric insulin analogue [Lys(B28), Pro(B29)] in IDDM. *Diabetologia* 1994; **37**: 713–720.

49. Torlone E, Pampanelli S, Lalli C *et al*. Postprandial glycemic control in IDDM after sc. LysPro insulin analogue or human regular insulin, alone or mixed with NPH. *Diabetologia* 1995; **38** (**Suppl 1**): A190.

50. Torlone E, Pampanelli S, Lalli C *et al*. Effects of short-acting insulin analog [Lys(B28), Pro(B29)] on post-prandial blood glucose control in IDDM. *Diabetes Care* 1996; **19**: 945–952.

51. Howey DC, Bowsher RR, Brunelle RL *et al*. [Lys(B28), Pro(B29)]-human insulin: Effect of injection time in post-prandial glycaemia. *Clin Pharmcol Therap* 1995; **58**: 459–469.

52. Heinemann L, Heise T, Wahl LC *et al*. Prandial glycaemia after a carbohydrate-rich meal in Type 1 diabetic patients: Using the rapid-acting insulin analogue [Lys(B28), Pro(B29)] human insulin. *Diabet Med* 1996; **13**: 625–629.

53. Woodworth JR, Howey DC, Bowsher RR *et al*. [Lys (B28), Pro (B29)] human insulin: dose ranging versus Humulin R. *Diabetes* 1993; **42** (**Suppl 1**): 170A.

54. Ter Braak EW, Erkelens DW, Woodworth JR *et al*. Injection site effects on the pharmacokinetics and glucodynamics of insulin Lispro and regular insulin. *Diabetes Care* 1996; **19**: 1437–1440.

55. Drejer K, Kruse V, Larsen UD *et al*. Receptor binding and tyrosine kinase activation by insulin analogues with extreme affinities studied in human heptoma HepG2 cells. *Diabetes* 1991; **40**: 1488–1495.

56. Vølund A, Brange J, Drejer K *et al*. *In vitro* and *in vivo* potency of insulin analogues designed for clinical use. *Diabet Med* 1991; **8**: 839–847.

57. Ottersen JL, Nilsson P, Jami J *et al*. The potential immogenicity of human insulin and insulin analogues evaluated in a transgenic mouse model. *Diabetologia* 1994; **37**: 1178–1185.

58. Owens DR. *Human Insulin. Clinical Pharmacological Studies in Normal Man*. Lancaster: MTP Press, 1986.

59. Heinemann L, Heise T, Jørgensen LN *et al*. Action profile of the rapid acting insulin analogue: Human insulin [B28]Asp. *Diabet Med* 1993; **10**: 535–539.

60. Home PD, Barriocanal L, Lindholm A. Comparative pharmacokinetics and pharmacodynamics of the novel rapid-acting insulin analogue, insulin aspart, in healthy volunteers. *Eur J Clin Pharmacol* 1999; **55**: 199–203.

61. Heinemann L, Weyer C, Rauhaus M *et al*. Variability of the metabolic effect of soluble insulin and the rapid-acting insulin analogue insulin aspart. *Diabetes Care* 1998; **21**: 1910–1914.

62. Lindholm A, McEwen J, Riis A. Significantly improved postprandial glycaemic control with the novel rapid-acting insulin aspart. *Diabetologia* 1998; **41** (**Suppl 1**): A49.

63. Lutterman JA, Pijpers E, Netten PM, Jørgensen LN. Glycaemic control in IDDM patients during one day with injection of human insulin or the insulin analogues insulin X14 and insulin X14 (+Zn). In: Berger M, Gries FA, eds. *Frontiers in Pharmacology*. Stuttgart: Thieme, 1993: 102–109.

64. Brange J. The new era of biotech insulin analogues. *Diabetologia* 1997; **40**: S48–S53.

65. Dimitriadis GD, Gerich JE. Importance of timing of pre-prandial subcutaneous insulin administration in the management of diabetes mellitus. *Diabetes Care* 1983; **6**: 374–377.

66. Lean ME, Ng LL, Tennison BR. Interval between insulin injection and eating in relation to blood glucose control in adult diabetics. *Br Med J* 1985; **290**: 105–108.

67. Jørgensen LN, Nielsen FS. Timing of pre-meal insulins in diabetic patients on a multiple daily injection regimen. A questionnaire study. *Diabetologia* 1990; **33**: A116.

68. Binder C. Absorption of injected insulin. *Actual Pharmacolog Toxicological* 1969; (**Suppl 2**): 1–87.

69. Galloway TA, Spradlin CT, Nelson RL *et al*. Factors influencing the absorption, versus insulin concentration and blood glucose responses after injections of regular insulin an various insulin mixtures. *Diabetes Care* 1981; **4**: 366–376.

70. Lauritzen T, Pramming S, Deckert T, Binder C. Pharmacokinetics of continuous subcutaneous insulin infusion. *Diabetologia* 1983; **24**: 326–329.

71. Binder C, Lauritzen T, Faber O, Pramming S. Insulin pharmacokinetics. *Diabetes Care* 1984; **7**: 188–199.

72. Anderson JH Jr, Brunelle RL, Koivisto VA *et al*. Multicenter Insulin Lispro Study Group.

Reduction of postprandial hyperglycemia and frequency of hypoglycemia in IDDM patients on insulin-analog treatment. *Diabetes* 1997a; **46**: 265–270.

73. Anderson JH, Brunelle RL, Koivisto VA *et al.* Improved mealtime treatment of diabetes mellitus using an insulin analogue. *Clin Therap* 1997b; **19**: 62–72.

74. Vignati L, Anderson JH, Iversen PW. Efficacy of insulin lispro in combination with NPH human insulin twice per day in patients with insulin-dependent or non-insulin-dependent diabetes mellitus. *Clin Therapeutics* 1997; **19**: 1408–1421.

75. Davey P, Grainger D, MacMillan J *et al.* Clinical outcomes with insulin lispro compared with human regular insulin: A meta-analysis. *Clin Therapeutics* 1997; **19**: 656–674.

76. Rowe R, James H, Anderson JR, Gale E. A double-blind comparison of insulin Lispro and regular insulin in patients on a multiple injection regimen. *Diabetes* 1996; **45 (Suppl 2)**: 71A.

77. Wilde MI, McTavish D. Insulin Lispro: a review of its pharmacological properties and therapeutic use in the management of diabetes mellitus. *Drugs* 1997; **54**: 597–614.

78. Zinman B. Tildesley H, Chiasson JL *et al.* Insulin Lispro in CSII: Results of a double-blind cross-over study. *Diabetes* 1997; **46**: 440–443.

79. Schernthaner G, Wein W, Sandholzer K *et al.* Post-prandial insulin Lispro: a new therapeutic option for Type 1 diabetic patients. *Diabetes Care* 1998; **21**: 570–573.

80. Holleman F, DerTweel I, van der Brand JJG *et al.* Comparison of LysB28, ProB29-human insulin analog and regular human insulin in the correction of incidental hyperglycaemia. *Diabetes Care* 1996; **19**: 1426–1429.

81. Yki-Jarvinen H, Kauppila M, Kujansuu E *et al.* Comparison of insulin regimens in patients with non-insulin-dependant diabetes mellitus. *N Engl J Med* 1992; **327**: 1426–1433.

82. Colwell JA, Lean A. Diminished insulin response to hyperglycaemia – prediabetes and diabetes. *Diabetes* 1967; **16**: 560–565.

83. Owens DR, Luzio SD, Coates PA. Insulin secretion and sensitivity in newly diagnosed NIDDM caucasions in the UK. *Diabetic Med* 1996; **13**: S19–S24.

84. Bruce DG, Chrisholm DJ, Storlien LH, Kraegen EW. The physiological importance of the deficiency in early prandial insulin secretion in non-insulin dependant diabetes. *Diabetes* 1998; **37**: 736–744.

85. Coates PA, Ollerton RL, Luzio SD *et al.* A glimpse of the 'natural history' of established Type 2 (non-insulin dependent) diabetes mellitus from the spectrum of metabolic and hormonal responses to a mixed meal at the time of diagnosis. *Diabetes Res Clin Pract* 1994; **26**: 139–153.

86. Anderson JH, Brunelle RL, Keohane P *et al.* Mealtime treatment with insulin analog improves postprandial hyperglycemia and hypoglycemia in patients with non-insulin-dependent diabetes mellitus. *Arch Intern Med* 1997c; **157**: 1249–1255.

87. Feinglos MN, Lane JD, Thacker CH, English JS. Pre-prandial insulin Lispro improves glucose control in patients with secondary sulfonylurea failure. *Diabetes* 1996; **45 (Suppl 2)**: 286A.

88. Gudat U, Trautmann M, Pfützner A *et al.* Combination therapies with insulin Lispro in NIDDM patients at oral agent failure. *Diabetologia* 1997; **40 (Suppl 1)**: A363.

89. Bruttomesso D, Pianta A, Mari A *et al.* Restoration of early rise in plasma insulin levels improves the glucose tolerance of Type 2 diabetic patients. *Diabetes* 1999; **48**: 99–105.

90. Brabant G, Braun D, Ellermann A *et al.* Normalization of circadian plasma glucose and insulin levels by prandial s.c. short-acting insulin in NIDDM with secondary failure to sulphonylureas. *Diabetes* 1996; **45 (Suppl 2)**: 218A.

91. Home PD, Lindholm A, Hylleberg B, Round P, for the UK Insulin Aspart Study Group. Improved glycaemic control with insulin aspart – a multicentre randomized double-blind cross-over trial in type 1 diabetes mellitus. *Diabetes Care* 1998; **21**: 1904–1909.

92. The DCCT Research Group. Epidemiology of severe hypoglycaemia in the Diabetes Control and Complications Trial. *Am J Med* 1991; **90**: 450–459.

93. Macleod KM, Hepburn DA, Frier BM. Frequency and morbidity of severe hypoglycaemia in insulin-treated diabetic patients. *Diabetic Med* 1993; **10**: 238–245.

94. McCrimmon RJ, Frier BM. Symptomatic and physiological responses to hypoglycaemia induced by human soluble insulin and the analogue lispro human insulin. *Diabetic Med* 1997; **14**: 929–936.

95. The Diabetes Control and Complications Trial Research Group. Hypoglycaemia in the Diabetes Control and Complications Trial. *Diabetes* 1997; **46**: 271–286.

96. Egger M, Smith GD, Stettler C, Diem P. Risk of adverse effects of intensified treatment in insulin-dependent diabetes mellitus: a meta-analysis. *Diabetic Med* 1997; **14**: 919–928.

97. Pfützner A, Küstner E, Forst T *et al*. Intensive insulin therapy with insulin Lispro in patients with type 1 diabetes reduces the frequency of hypoglycaemia episodes. *Exp Clin Endocrinol Diabetes* 1996; **104**: 25–30.

98. Anderson JH, Brunelle RL, Arora V *et al*. Effect of basal insulin on reduced frequency of nocturnal hypoglycaemia in patient treated with insulin lispro (Abstr). *Diabetologia* 1996; **39 (Suppl 1)**: A221.

99. Brunelle RL, Llewelyn J, Anderson JH *et al*. Meta-analysis of the effect of insulin lispro on severe hypoglycaemia patients with type 1 diabetes. *Diabetes Care* 1998; **21**: 1726–1731.

100. Heller SR, Amiel SA, James J. Hypoglycaemia during intensive insulin therapy: a comparison of lispro and regular insulin. *Diabetes* 1997; **46 (Suppl 1)**: 151A.

101. Holleman F, Schmitt H, Rottiers R *et al*. Reduced frequency of severe hypoglycaemia and coma in well-controlled IDDM patients treated with insulin Lispro. *Diabetes Care* 1997; **20**: 1827–1832.

102. Ahmed ABE, Home PD. Reduced nocturnal hypoglycaemia with insulin analogue Lispro in Type 1 diabetic patients. *Diabetologia* 1997; **40 (Suppl 1)**: A10.

103. Ahmed ABE, Home PD. The effect of insulin analog lispro on nighttime blood glucose control in type 1 diabetic patients. *Diabetes Care* 1998; **21**: 32–37.

104. Ahmed ABE, Mallias J, Home PD. Optimisation of evening insulin dose in patients using the short-acting insulin analog lispro. *Diabetes Care* 1998; **21**: 1162–1166.

105. Garg SK, Carmain JA, Braddy KC *et al*. Pre-meal insulin analogue insulin Lispro vs. Humulin® R

106. Holcombe J, Zalani S, Arora V *et al*. Insulin lispro (LP) results in less nocturnal hypoglycaemia compared with regular human insulin in adolescents with Type 1 diabetes. *Diabetes* 1997; **46 (Suppl 1)**: 103A.

107. Iafusco D, Angius E, Prisco F. Early pre-prandial hypoglycaemia after administration of insulin lispro. *Diabetes Care* 1998; **21**: 1777–1778.

108. Burge MR, Castillo KR, Schade DS. Meal composition is a determinant of Lispro-induced hypoglycemia in IDDM. *Diabetes Care* 1997; **20**: 152–155.

109. Tuominen JA, Karonen SL, Melamies L *et al*. Exercise-induced hypoglycaemia in IDDM patients treated with a short-acting insulin analogue. *Diabetologia* 1995; **38**: 106–111.

110. Jacobs MAJM, Salobir P, Pop-Snijders C *et al*. Counterregularly hormone response and symptoms during hypoglycaemia induced by porcine, human regular insulin, and Lys (B28), Bro (B29) human insulin analogue (insulin lispro) in healthy male volunteers. *Diabetic Med* 1997; **14**: 248–257.

111. Del Sindaco P, Ciofetta M, Lalli C *et al*. Use of short acting insulin analogue lispro in intensive treatment of Type I diabetes mellitus: Importance of appropriate replacement of basal insulin and time-interval injection-meal. *Diabetic Med* 1998; **15**: 592–600.

112. Lalli C, Ciofetta C, del Sindaco P *et al*. Long-term intensive treatment of Type 1 diabetes with the short-acting insulin analog Lispro in variable combination with NPH insulin at mealtime. *Diabetes Care* 1999; **22**: 468–477.

113. Langan SJ, Deary IJ, Hepburn DA, Frier BM. Cumulative cognitive impairment following recurrent severe hypoglycaemia in adult patient with insulin-treated diabetes mellitus. *Diabetologia* 1991; **34**: 337–344.

114. Fanelli CG, Epifano L, Rambotti AM *et al*. Meliculous prevention of hypoglycaemia normalises the glycaemic thresholds and magnitude of most neuroendocrine responses to, symptoms of and cognitive function during hypoglycaemia in intensively treated patients with short-term IDDM. *Diabetes* 1993; **42**: 1683–1689.

115. Caixàs A, Pérez A, Payés A *et al*. Effects of a short-acting insulin analog (insulin Lispro)

versus regular insulin on lipid metabolism in insulin-dependent diabetes mellitus. *Metabolism* 1998; **47**: 371–376.

116. Bell DSH, Clements RS Jr, Perentesis SG *et al.* Dosage accuracy of self-mixing versus premixed insulin. *Arch Intern Med* 1991; **155**: 2265–2269.

117. Coscelli C, Calabrese G, Fedele D *et al.* Use of pre-mixed insulin among the elderly. Reduction of errors in patient preparation of mixtures. *Diabetes Care* 1992; **15**: 1628–1630.

118. Arunoff S, Goldberg R, Kumar D *et al.* Use of pre-mixed insulin regimen (Novolin 70/30) to replace self-mixed insulin regimens. *Clin Therapeutics* 1994; **16**: 41–49.

119. DeFelippis MR, Bakaysa DL, Youngman KM *et al.* Preparation and characterization of neutral protamine lispro (NPL) suspension. *Diabetes* 1996; **45** (**Suppl 2**): 74A.

120. Joseph SE, Hopkins D, Korzon-Burakowska A *et al.* The action profile of lispro is not blunted by mixing in the syringe with NPH insulin. *Diabetes Care* 1998; 21; **12**: 2098–2102.

121. Bastyr EJ, Holcombe JH, Anderson JH, Clove JN. Mixing insulin Lispro and Ultralente insulin (Letter). *Diabetes Care* 1997; **20**: 1047–1048.

122. Llewelyn J, Birkett M, Boggs B *et al.* Comparison of the effect of using insulin Lispro with Ultralente and NPH basal regimens in IDDM patients. *Diabetologia* 1997; **40** (**Suppl 1**): A352.

123. Zinman B, Ross S, Campos R, Strack T. Effectiveness of human Ultralente versus NPH insulin in providing basal insulin replacement for an insulin Lispro multiple daily injection regimen. *Diabetes Care* 1999; **22**: 603–608.

124. Burden AC, Janes J, Collier A *et al.* P24. The metabolic effects of twice daily Lispro and isophane compared to soluble and isophane. *Diabetic Med* 1996; **14** (**Suppl 3**): 521.

125. Heise T, Weyer C, Serwas A *et al.* Time-action profiles of novel premixed preparations of insulin Lispro and NPL insulin. *Diabetes Care* 1998; **21**: 800–803.

126. Koivisto VA, Tuominen JA, Ebeling P. Lispro MIX25 insulin as pretrial therapy in Type 2 diabetic patients. *Diabetes Care* 1999; **22**: 459–462.

127. Roach P, Trautmann M, Anderson J. Lower incidence of nocturnal hypoglycaemia during treatment with a novel protamine-base formulation of insulin lispro. *Diabetes* 1998; **47** (**Suppl 1**): A92.

128. Malone J, Roach P, Anderson J. Less nocturnal hypoglycaemia during treatment with evening administration of lispro mixture 25, a lispro/intermediate insulin mixture. *Diabetic Med* 1999; in press.

129. Weyer C, Heise T, Heinemann L. Insulin aspart in a 30/70 premixed formulation: Pharmacodynamic properties of a rapid-acting insulin analog in stable mixture. *Diabetes Care* 1997; **20**:1612–1614.

130. Lawrence RD. The effect of exercise on insulin action in diabetics. *Br Med J* 1926; **1**: 648–650.

131. Vranic M, Berger M. Exercise and diabetes mellitus. *Diabetes* 1979; **28**: 147–163.

132. Robinson-Pleadwell M, Morrical L, Hills S *et al.* Comparison of glucose and insulin excursions after insulin Lispro or Humulin R followed by moderate exercise. *Diabetologia* 1998; **41** (**Suppl 1**): A16.

133. Franz MJ, Horton ES, Bantle JP *et al.* Nutritional principles for the management of diabetes and related complications. *Diabetes Care* 1994; **17**: 490–518.

134. Bergis K, Schimers S, Kuhn-Röpke A *et al.* Meal composition at breakfast and treatment with insulin Lispro. *Diabetologia* 1996; **39** (**Suppl 1**): A223.

135. Burge MR, Waters DL, Holcombe JH, Schade DS. Prolonged efficacy of short-acting insulin Lispro in combination with human ultralente in insulin-dependent diabetes mellitus. *J Clin Endocrinol Metab* 1997; **82**: 920–924.

136. Strachan M, Frier B. Efficacy of insulin Lispro administered before and after food: Influence of meal composition. *Diabetes* 1997; **46** (**Suppl 1**): 150A.

137. Rönnemaa T, Viikari J. Reducing snacks when switching from conventional soluble to Lispro insulin treatment: effects on glycaemic control and hypoglycaemia. *Diabetic Med* 1998; **15**: 601–607.

138. Kong N, Ryder REJ. What is the role of between meal snacks with intensive basal bolus regimens using preprandial Lispro? *Diabetic Medicine* 1999; **16**: 325–331.

139. Wiefels K, Hübinger A, Dannehi K, Gries FA. Insulin kinetic and dynamic in diabetic patients under insulin pump therapy after injection of human insulin or the insulin analogue (Asp^{B28}). *Horm Metab Res* 1995; **27**: 421–424.

140. Zinman B, Tildesley H, Chiasson J-L *et al*. Insulin Lispro in CSII: results of a double-blind cross-over study. *Diabetes* 1997; **46**: 440–443.

141. Melki V, Renard E, Lassmann-Vague V *et al*. Improvement of HbA1c and blood glucose stability in IDDM patients treated with Lispro insulin analog in external pumps. *Diabetes Care* 1998; **21**: 977–982.

142. Schmauß S, König A, Landgraf R. Human insulin analogue [LYS(B28)], PRO(B29)]: The ideal pump insulin? *Diabetic Med* 1998; **15**: 247–249.

143. Hanaire H, Bringer J, Lassmann-Vague V *et al*. Improvement of HbA1c without increasing hypoglycemia risk in diabetic patients treated with insulin Lispro in external pumps. *Diabetologia* 1997; **40** (**Suppl 1**): A10.

144. Hoss U, Salgado M, Sternberg F *et al*. Insulin Lispro improves glycemic control in IDDM patients under continuous subcutaneous insulin infusion (CSII). *Diabetologia* 1997; **40** (**Suppl 1**): A335.

145. Tsui EYL, Chiasson J-L, Tildesley H *et al*. Counterregulatory hormone responses after long-term continuous subcutaneous insulin infusion with Lispro insulin. *Diabetes Care* 1998; **21**: 93–96.

146. Holcombe J, Zalan S, Hoen H, Harris C. Comparison of insulin Lispro and regular insulin in continuous insulin infusion pump therapy. *Diabetologia* 1998; **41** (**Suppl 1**): A227.

147. Wright AWD, Little JA. Cannula occlusion with use of insulin Lispro and insulin infusion system. *Diabetes Care* 1998; **21**: 874.

148. Demirdjian S, Bardin C, Savin S *et al*. Lispro insulin is suitable for external pumps but not for implantable pumps. *Diabetes Care* 1998; **21**: 867–868.

149. Lougheed WD, Zinman B, Strack TR *et al*. Stability of insulin Lispro in insulin infusion systems. *Diabetes Care* 1997; **20**: 1061–1065.

150. Attia N, Jones TW, Holcombe J, Tamborlane WV. Comparison of human regular and Lispro insulins after interruption of continu-ous subcutaneous insulin infusion and in the treatment of acutely decompensated IDDM. *Diabetes Care* 1998; **21**: 817–821.

151. Pein M, Hinselmann C, Pfützner A, Dreyer M. Catheter disconnection in Type 1 diabetic patients treated with CSII: comparison of insulin Lispro and human regular insulin. *Diabetologia* 1996; **39** (**Suppl 1**): A223.

152. Johansson U, Wredling R, Lins P, Adamson U. Reproducibility of insulin absorption with insulin Lispro and regular insulin during CSII. *Diabetes* 1998; **47** (**Suppl 1**).

153. Lins P, Johansson U, Wredling R, Adamson U. Blood glucose variability and well-being during CSII using insulin Lispro and regular insulin. *Diabetes* 1998; **47** (**Suppl 1**): A10.

154. Rutledge KS, Chase HP, Klingensmith GJ *et al*. Effectiveness of postprandial humalog in toddlers with diabetes. *Pediatrics* 1997; **100**: 968–972.

155. Rami B, Schober E. Postprandial glycaemia after regular and Lispro in children and adolescents with diabetes. *Eur J Pediatr* 1997; **15**: 838–840.

156. Garg SK, Carmain JA, Braddy KC *et al*. Pre-meal insulin analog (Lys-Pro) vs: human regular insulin treatment in young subjects with Type 1 Diabetes. *Diabetes* 1994; **93** (**Suppl 1**): A162.

157. Holcombe J, Zalani S, Arona V. Comparative study of insulin Lispro and regular insulin in 481 adolescents with type 1 diabetes. *Diabetologia* 1997; **40** (**Suppl 1**): A344.

158. Mortensen HB, Robertson KJ, Aanstoot HJ *et al*. for the Hvidøre Study Group. Insulin management and metabolic control of Type I diabetes mellitus in childhood and adolescence in 18 countries. *Diabetic Med* 1998; **15**: 752–759.

159. Holcombe J, Zalani S, Arora V *et al*. Patient preference for insulin Lispro versus Humulin R in adolescents with type 1 diabetes. *Diabetologia* 1996; **40** (**Supp 1**): A343.

160. Davis EA, Russell M, Keating B *et al*. Hypoglycaemia: Incidence and clinical predic-tors in a large population-based sample of children and adolescents with IDDM. *Diabetes Care* 1997; **20**: 22–25.

161. Benbarka MM, Prescott PT, Aoki TT. Practical guidelines on the use of insulin Lispro in elderly diabetic patients. *Drugs Ageing* 1998; **12**: 103–113.

162. Hoogwerf BJ, Mehta A, Reddy S. Advances in the treatment of diabetes mellitus in the elderly: development of insulin analogues. *Drugs Ageing* 1996; **9**: 438–448.

163. Diamond T, Kormas N. Possible adverse fetal effect of insulin Lispro. *N Engl J Med* 1997; **37**: 1009–1010.

164. Rosen SG, Engel SS. Use of insulin Lispro in pregnant women with diabetes mellitus. *Diabetes* 1998; **47** (**Suppl 1**): A437.

165. Anderson JH, Bastyr EJ, Wishner KL. Possible adverse fatal effect of insulin lispro. *N Engl J Med* 1997; **37**: 1010.

166. Jovanovic L, Ilic S, Pettitt D *et al.* Insulin Lispro and regular insulin: postprandial glucose and insulin in gestational diabetes mellitus (GDM). *Diabetologia* 1998; **41** (**Suppl 1**): A245.

167. Beulke-Sam J, Byrd RA, Hoyt JA, Zimmermann JL. A reproductive and developmental toxicity study in CD Rats of LY275585, {Lys(B28), Pro(B29)}-Human Insulin. *J Am Coll Toxicol* 1994; **13**: 247–260.

168. Fineberg SE, Fineberg NS, Anderson JH, Birkett M. Does the use of short-acting (LysPro) human insulin in insulin naive patients augment the insulin immune response or differ between type 1 and type 2 patients? *Diabetes* 1995; **44** (**Suppl 1**): 231A.

169. Fineberg NS, Fineberg SE, Anderson JH *et al.* Immunologic effects of insulin Lispro [Lys(B28), Pro(B29) Human insulin] in IDDM and NIDDM patients previously treated with insulin. *Diabetes* 1996; **45**: 1750–1754.

170. Braimon J, O'Brien M, Kaulbach H, Moses A. The insulin analog lispro effectively treats anti-insulin antibody mediated insulin resistance. *Diabetes* 1996; **45** (**Suppl 2**): 185A.

171. Henrichs HR, Unger H, Trautmann ME, Pfützer A. Severe insulin resistance treated with insulin Lispro. *Lancet* 1996; **348**: 1248.

172. Hermoso F, Vázquez M, Chaves G *et al.* Generalised allergy to human insulin treated with insulin Lispro. *Diabetologia* 1997; **40** (**Suppl 1**): A349.

173. Lahtela JT, Knip M, Paul R *et al.* Severe insulin antibody-mediated human insulin resistance: successful treatment with insulin analog Lispro. *Diabetes Care* 1997; **20**: 71–73.

174. Kumar D. Lispro analog for treatment of generalized allergy to human insulin. *Diabetes Care* 1997; **20**: 1357–1359.

175. Pöyry K, Kostano E, Karonen S-L. The effect of Finnish sauna on the absorption of short-acting insulin analogue. *Diabetes* 1995; **44** (**Suppl 1**): 106A.

176. Hauner H, Stockamp B, Haastet B. Prevalence of lipohypertrophy in insulin treated diabetic patients and predisposing factors. *Exper Clin Endocrinol Diabetes* 1996; **104**: 106–110.

177. Young RJ, Hannan WJ, Frier BM *et al.* Diabetic lipohypertrophy delays insulin treated diabetic patients and predisposing factors. *Diabetes Care* 1984; **7**: 479–480.

178. Roper NA, Bilous RW. Resolution of lipohypertrophy following change of short-acting insulin to insulin (Humalog). *Diabetic Med* 1998; **15**: 1063–1064.

179. Rassam AG, Zeise TM, Burge MR, Schade DS. Optimal administration of Lispro insulin in hyperglycaemic Type 1 diabetes. *Diabetes Care* 1999; **22**: 133–136.

180. Torlone E. Recombinant human insulin analogues. *Bio Drugs* 1998; **9**: 363–374.

181. Pampanelli S, Torlone E, Lalli C *et al.* Improved postprandial metabolic control after subcutaneous injection of a short-acting insulin analog in IDDM of short duration with residual pancreatic beta-cell function. *Diabetes Care* 1995; **18**: 1452–1459.

182. Ahmed ABE, Home PD. Optimal provision of daytime NPH insulin in patients using the insulin analogue lispro. *Diabetes Care* 1998; **21**: 1707–1713.

183. Colombel A, Murat A, Krempf M *et al.* Improvement of blood glucose control in Type 1 diabetic patients treated with Lispro and multiple NPH injections. *Diabetic Medicine* 1999; **16**: 319–324.

184. Ebeling P, Jansson P-A, Smith U *et al.* Strategies toward improved control during insulin Lispro therapy in IDDM. *Diabetes Care* 1997; **20**: 1287–1289.

185. Del Sindaco P, Ciofetta M, Lalli C *et al.* Importance of basal insulin to improve control without increasing hypoglycaemia in intensively treated IDDM using a short-acting insulin analog at meals. *Diabetologia* 1997; **40** (**Suppl 1**): A352.

186. Kotsanos JG, Vignati L, Huster W *et al.* Health-related quality-of-life results from multinational clinical trials of insulin Lispro. *Diabetes Care* 1997; **20**: 948-958.

187. Holcombe J, Zalani S, Arora V *et al.* Patient preference for insulin Lispro versus Humulin R in adolescents with Type 1 diabetes. *Diabetologia* 1997; **40** (**Suppl 1**): A343.

188. Pfützner A, Linder U, Trautmann M *et al.* Insulin Lispro and quality of life – results from the German QoL study. *Diabetes* 1998; **47** (**Suppl 1**): A354.

189. Pramming S, Thorsteinsson B, Bendtson I *et al.* Nocturnal hypoglycaemia in patients receiving conventional treatment. *Br Med J* 1985; **291**: 376–379.

190. Reviriego J, Millan M. Health-related quality of life and insulin Lispro (Letter). *Diabetes Care* 1998; **21**: 1203–1204.

191. Letiexhe MR, Rutters A, Schmitt H. [LYS(B28), PRO(B29)] Human insulin: patients treated with Lyspro vs. human regular insulin: Quality of life assessment. *Diabetologia* 1994; **37** (**Suppl 1**): A648.

192. De Leeuw I, Rutters A, Schmitt H, de Roeck K. [Lys (B28), Pro (B29)] Human insulin (LysPro): patients treated with LysPro vs human regular insulin: quality of life assessment (QoL). 15th International Diabetes Federation Congress, Kobe. November 6–11, 1994. 07A5PP0395.

193. Hovorka K, Pumprla J, Schlusche D *et al.* Insulin Lispro changes treatment satisfaction under flexible functional insulin treatment. *Diabetologia* 1997; **40** (**Suppl 1**): A353.

194. Desmet M, Rutters A, Schmitt H, Satter E. [Lys (B28), Pro (B29)] Human insulin (LysPro): Patients treated with LysPro vs human regular insulin – quality of life assessment (QoL). *Diabetes* 1994; **43** (**Suppl 1**): 167A.

195. Janes JM, Bradley C, Rees A. Preferences for, and improvements in aspects of quality of life (QoL) with, insulin Lispro in a multiple injection regimen. *Diabetologia* 1997; **40** (**Suppl 1**): A353.

196. Glazer B, Zalani S, Symanowski SM *et al.* The cardiovascular safety profile of insulin Lispro (LP). *Diabetologia* 1997; **40** (**Suppl 1**): A351.

197. Roach P, Varshavsky JA, Gatner K, Anderson JH. Immune antibody formation during treatment with human insulin or insulin Lispro does not affect insulin dose requirements. *Diabetes* 1996; **45** (**Suppl 2**): 261A.

198. Symanowski SM, Brunelle RI, Anderson JH. A new technique of population subgroup analysis to evaluate the safety of insulin Lispro. Abstract of 15th International Diabetes Federation Congress, Kobe. 1994; p. 120.

199. Bolli GB, Gerich JE. The 'dawn phenomenon' a common occurrence in both non-insulin-dependant and insulin-dependant diabetes mellitus. *N Engl J Med* 1984; **310**: 746–750.

200. Perriello G, De Feo P, Torlone E *et al.* The dawn phenomenon in Type 1 (insulin dependent) diabetes mellitus: magnitude, frequency, variability, and dependency on glucose counterregulation and insulin sensitivity. *Diabetologia* 1991; **34**: 21–28.

201. Best CH. The prolongation of insulin action symposium on hormones (Sigma XI Lecture). 1937; 362–377.

202. Hagedorn HC, Hensen BN, Krarup NB, Woodstrup I. Protamine insulinate. *J Am Med Assoc* 1936; **106**: 177–180.

203. Krayenbühl C, Rosenberg T. Crystalline protamine insulin. *Rep Steno Hosp* (Copenhagen) 1946; **1**: 60–73.

204. Hallas-Møller K, Petersen K, Schlichtkrull J. Crystalline and amorphous insulin-zinc compounds with prolonged action. *Ugeskr Laeg* 1951; **113**: 1761–1767.

205. Owens DR, Vora JP, Heding LG *et al.* Human, porcine and bovine ultralente insulin: subcutaneous administration in normal man. *Diabetic Med* 1986; **3**: 326–329.

206. Francis AJ, Hanning I, Alberti KGGM. Human ultralente insulin: a comparison with provine lente insuolin as a twice-daily insulin in insulin dependant diabetic patients with fasting hyperglycaemia. *Diabetes Res* 1986; **3**: 263–268.

207. Seigler DE, Olsson GM, Agramonte RF *et al.* Pharmacokinetics of long-acting (ultralente) insulin preparations. *Diabetes Nutr Metab* 1991; **4**: 267–273.

208. Frank BH, Pettee JM, Zimmerman RE, Burek PJ. The production of human proinsulin and its transformation to human insulin and C-peptide. In: Rich DH, Gross E, eds. *Peptides: Synthesis–Structure–Function.* Rockford, IL: Pierce Chemical Co., 1981: 729–738.

209. Galloway JA, Hooper SA, Spradlin CT *et al.* Biosynthetic human proinsulin: review of chemistry, *in vitro* and *in vivo* receptor binding, animal and human pharmacology studies, and clinical trial experience. *Diabetes Care* 1992; **15**: 661–692.

210. Howey DC, Bowsher RR, Brunelle R *et al.* des(64, 65) human proinsulin: a potent insulin agonist with intermediate action. *Diabetes* 1992; **41** (**Suppl 1**): 191A.

211. Heinemann L, Heise T, Klepper A *et al.* Time action profiles of the intermediate-acting insulin analogue des(64, 65)-human proinsulin. *Diabetes Metab* 1995; **21**: 415–419.

212. Markussen J, Hougaard P, Ribel U *et al.* Soluble, prolonged-acting insulin derivatives. I. Degree of protraction and crystallizability of insulins substituted in the termini of the B-chain. *Prot Eng* 1987; **1**: 205–213.

213. Markussen J. Engineering novel, prolonged-acting insulins. In: Hook JB, Post G, eds. *Protein Design and the Development of New Therapeutics and Vaccines*, Vol. 19. Plenum Publishing Co., 1990: 397–422.

214. Jørgensen S, Vaag A, Lang-kjaer L *et al.* NovoSol Basal: pharmacokinetics of a novel soluble long-acting soluble insulin analogue. *Br Med J* 1989; **299**: 415–419.

215. Zeuzem S, Stahl E, Jungmann E *et al.* *In vitro* activity of biosynthetic human diarginyl insulin. *Diabetologia* 1990; **33**: 65–71.

216. Dreyer M, Pein M, Schmidt C *et al.* Comparison of the pharmacokinetics/dynamics of Gly(A21)-Arg(B31,B32)-human insulin (HOE71GT) with NPH-insulin following subcutaneous injection by using euglycaemic clamp technique. *Diabetologia* 1994; **37** (**Suppl 1**): A78.

217. Kurtzhals P, Ribel U. Action profile of cobalt(III)-insulin. A novel principle of protraction of potential use for basal insulin delivery. *Diabetes* 1995; **44**: 1381–1385.

218. Markussen J, Havelund S, Kurtzhals P *et al.* Soluble, fatty acid acylated insulins bind to albumin and show protracted action in pigs. *Diabetologia* 1996; **39**: 281–288.

219. Myers SR, Yakubu-Madus FE, Johnson WT *et al.* Acylated of human insulin with palmitic acid extends the time action of human insulin in diabetic dogs. *Diabetes* 1997; **46**: 637–642.

220. Holman RR, Steenson J. OPID 194: a novel long-acting insulin preparation. *Diabetic Med* 1989; **6** (**Suppl 1**): A41.

221. Coates PA, Mukherjee S, Luzio S *et al.* Pharmacokinetics of a 'long-acting' human insulin analogue (HOE901) in healthy subjects. *Diabetes* 1995; **44** (**Suppl 1**): 130A.

222. Owens D, Luzio S, Tinbergen J, Kurzhals R. The absorption of HOE 901 in healthy subjects. *Diabetologia* 1998; **41** (**Suppl 1**): A245.

223. Berti L, Bossenmeier B, Kellerer M *et al.* Comparison of the human insulin analogue HOE901 and Asp(B10): Characteristics of receptor binding, activation and tyrosine phosphorylatioin of different substrate proteins. *Diabetologia* 1995; **38** (**Suppl 1**): A191.

224. Liu L, Koenen M, Seipke G, Eckel J. IGF-I Receptor-mediated signalling of the human insulin analogue HOE 901. *Diabetologia* 1997; **40** (**Suppl 1**): A355.

225. Bähr M, Kolter T, Seipke G, Eckel J. Growth promoting and metabolic activity of the human insulin analogue [Gly^{A21}, Arg^{B31}, Arg^{B32}] insulin (HOE901) in muscle cells. *Eur J Pharmacol* 1997; **320**: 259–265.

226. Slieker LJ, Brooke GS, DiMarchi RD *et al.* Modifications in the B10 and B26-30 regions of the B-chain of human insulin alter affinity for the human IGF-1 receptor more than for the insulin receptor. *Diabetologia* 1997; **40**: 554–561.

227. Talaulicar M, Willms B, Roßkamp. HOE 901, Ein Neues Insulinanalogon, zur Substitution des Basalen Insulin-beddarfs bei Typ-1-Diabetes. *Diabetes Stoffwechsel* 1996; **5**: 3–6.

228. Matthews DR, Pfeiffer C. A new long-acting insulin (HOE901) demonstrates less nocturnal hypoglycaemia when compared with protamine insulin in a clinical trial. *Diabetologia* 1998; **41** (**Suppl 1**): A245.

229. Pieber T, Eugene-Jolchine I, Derobert E. Efficacy and safety of HOE 901 in patients with Type 1 diabetes mellitus: a four-week randomized NPH insulin-controlled trial. *Diabetes* 1998; **47** (**Suppl 1**): A62.

230. Rosenstock J, Park G, Zimmermann J. Efficacy and safety of HOE 901 in patients with Type 1 diabetes mellitus: a four-week

randomized NPH insulin-controlled trial. *Diabetes* 1998; **47** (**Suppl 1**): A92.

231. Home PD. Insulin glargine: the first clinically useful extended-acting insulin in half a century? *Exp Opin Invest Drugs* 1999; **8**: 307–314.

232. Markussen J, Havelund S, Kurtzhals P *et al.* Soluble, fatty acid acylated insulins bind to albumin and show protracted action in pigs. *Diabetologia* 1996; **39**: 281–288.

233. Kurtzhals P, Havelund S, Jonassen I *et al.* Albumin binding of insulins acylated with fatty acids: characterization of the ligand–protein interaction and correlations between binding affinity and timing of insulin effect *in vivo. Biochem J* 1997; **312**: 725–731.

234. Hamilton-Wessler M, Adam M, Getty L *et al.* Glucose turnover profiles during continuous intravenous infusion of long-acting NN304. *Diabetologia* 1996; **39** (**Suppl 1**): A24.

235. Hamilton-Wessler M, Ader M, Dea M *et al.* Dose response with long-acting insulin analog NN304 follows analog dynamics in hind limb lymph in dogs. *Diabetologia* 1997; **40** (**Suppl 1**): A10.

236. Kurtzhals P, Havelund S, Jonassen I, Markussen J. Effect of fatty acids and selected drugs on the albumin binding of long-acting, acylated insulin analogue. *J Pharm Sci* 1997; **86**: 1365–1368.

237. Ribel U, Jensen-Holm HB, Havelund S, Jonassen I. Effect of circulating free fatty acids on the *in vivo* kinetics of NN304. *Diabetologia* 1997; **40** (**Suppl 1**): A353.

238. Hamilton-Wessler M, Markussen J. Elevation in free fatty acids influences albumin-binding but not metabolic effects of fatty acid acylated insulin, NN304, in dogs. *Diabetes* 1998; **47** (**Suppl 1**): A296.

239. Sinha K, Weyer C, Heinemann L *et al.* Time-action profile of the soluble, fatty acid acylated long-acting insulin analogue NN304. *Diabetic Med* 1999; **16**: 332–338.

240. Myers SR, Yakubu-Madus FE, Johnson WT *et al.* Acylated of human insulin with palmitic acid extends the time action of human insulin in diabetic dogs. *Diabetes* 1997; **46**: 637–642.

241. Howey DC, Woodworth JR, Bowsher RR, Reviergo J. Pharmacokinetic and pharmacodynamic assessments of N-palmitoyl, Lys(B29) human insulin in healthy volunteers. *Diabetologia* 1997; **40** (**Suppl 1**): A354.

242. Radziuk J, Pye S, Bradley B *et al.* Basal activity of NPH and [N-palmitoyl Lys(B29)] human insulin in subjects with IDDM. *Diabetologia* 1998; **41**: 116–120.

243. Berger M, Heinemann L. Are presently available insulin analogues clinically beneficial? *Diabetologia* 1997; **40**: 591–596.

244. Banting FG, Best CH. The internal secretion of the pancreas. *J Lab Clin Med* 1922; **7**: 251–256.

245. Scott DA. Crystalline insulin. *Biochem J* 1934; **28**: 1592–1602.

246. Hallas-Møller K, Jersild M, Petersen K, Schlichtkrull J. Zinc insulin preparations for single preparations for single daily injections. *JAMA* 1952; **150**: 1667–1671.

247. Schlichtkrull J, Brange J, Christiansen AH *et al.* Clinical aspects of insulin – antigenicity. *Diabetes* 1972; **21**: 649–656.

15

Insulin sensitizers: a new era in the management of Type 2 diabetes

John J Nolan

Background

The insulin sensitizers are a new class of oral antidiabetic agents. Although developed originally for the treatment of Type 2 diabetes, this class of drugs has significant potential for the treatment of other clinical syndromes. The insulin sensitizers share a common thiazolidinedione chemical structure, and are often referred to by the alternative term 'glitazones'. The glitazones act primarily as insulin sensitizers, that is they enhance the effects of endogenously secreted insulin in target tissues, primarily skeletal muscle, liver, and fat. The insulin sensitizers are the first major new class of drugs for diabetes in almost 40 years. They are completely unrelated structurally and in their mode of action to any of the older oral hypoglycaemic drugs. Their arrival has promoted a new therapeutic approach to Type 2 diabetes, targeting insulin resistance rather than insulin secretion. The glitazones are effective in non-diabetic animal models of insulin resistance as well as in several important prediabetic human syndromes of insulin resistance. Unlike any of the previously available oral agents for the treatment of diabetes, the glitazones act through nuclear receptors and have effects primarily on gene expression. Recent research on their mechanism of action is making an important contribution to basic research on insulin action *per se* and on the fundamental cellular events leading to insulin resistance.

Since the discovery of insulin more than 75 years ago, clinical research has gradually led to an understanding of the heterogeneity of human diabetes. After insulin was introduced, oral medications were developed which were variably effective in some forms of diabetes, mostly in overweight subjects with a later onset of the disease. Only in the last 20 years has there been a clear distinction between the two most common types of diabetes. Type 1 diabetes is an autoimmune disease leading to absolute loss of endogenous insulin secretion. Type 2 diabetes is a complex disease of altered homeostasis in both carbohydrate and fat metabolism. Type 2 diabetes is ultimately a genetically determined syndrome of progressive failure of the pancreatic islets to maintain sustained hyperinsulinaemia in the face of peripheral insulin resistance.[1] Subjects with Type 2 diabetes are typically obese, and hypertension, dyslipidaemia, and early cardiovascular disease are frequent in this population. In Type 1 diabetes, treatments and improvements have focused on the challenge of insulin replacement therapy. In Type 2 diabetes, treatment has traditionally followed a stepwise approach through diet and exercise with weight reduction, followed by the oral agents

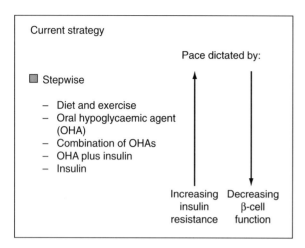

Fig. 15.1
Stepwise therapy in Type 2 diabetes prior to the availability of the thiazolidinedione insulin sensitizers.

alone or in combination, and eventually insulin (see *Fig. 15.1*). This treatment approach suffers from several limitations which may account for the disappointing long-term success of current treatments for Type 2 diabetes. Firstly, significant long-term improvements in diet, exercise, and body-weight are extremely difficult to achieve in anything more than a minority of overweight subjects. This may be explained by both behavioural and biological factors relating to obesity and by the modes of action of currently available antidiabetic drugs. The current status of Type 2 diabetes treatments has been well represented in the findings of the recently published United Kingdom Prospective Diabetes Study (UKPDS).[2,3] Despite close clinical follow-up during that study over a 20-year period, glycaemic control in all groups showed a gradual and definite upward drift, following a U-shaped curve after diagnosis and initial treatment. The important microvascular benefits from better control of glucose and

blood pressure were not clearly associated with better macrovascular outcomes, which are more closely associated with insulin resistance.

The thiazolidinedione insulin sensitizers have now been clearly shown to be as effective in terms of glucose lowering as the older oral hypoglycaemic agents. This glycaemic lowering occurs without additional demands on depleted islet cell insulin reserves. On the contrary, there is evidence that insulin secretion probably improves on using these agents. Furthermore, there is abundant evidence from both pre-clinical and clinical studies that these new agents lead to additional indirect benefits on blood pressure, albuminuria, and lipid metabolism, all of these parameters being directly related to insulin resistance itself. Given the historical development of diabetes treatments, it is likely that the insulin sensitizers will fulfil expectations as the next major advance in the treatment of diabetes and the prevention of its long-term complications.

Introduction

Type 2 diabetes is increasing in prevalence worldwide and is currently estimated to affect 200 million people.[4] The main complications of diabetes include retinopathy, nephropathy, neuropathy, and early cardiovascular disease due to accelerated atherosclerosis. Thus Type 2 diabetes is a leading cause of blindness, renal failure, amputation, and death from cardiovascular disease. The total health expenditure for diabetes and its complications is considerable, and has been estimated at between 10 (UK) and 15% (US) of the total national health budget.

Three principal metabolic abnormalities characterize the typical subject with Type 2 diabetes: increased hepatic glucose production, impaired insulin secretion, and insulin resistance in skeletal muscle, liver and adipose tissue.[5,6]

Treatments of Type 2 diabetes until recently have been based on three mechanistic approaches: increasing the circulating concentrations of insulin (by sulphonylureas, other insulin secretagogues, or insulin itself), suppressing elevated hepatic glucose production (metformin), and reducing carbohydrate absorption from the small intestine (alphaglucosidase inhibitors). Treatment failure with the oral agents is common, and none of these drug categories has proven effective at restoring near-normal glucose homeostasis in the long-term treatment of the disease. The recently published findings of the UKPDS illustrate this problem very clearly.[2,3] The thiazolidinediones or glitazones act through a new mechanism, by directly improving peripheral insulin resistance in the target tissues for insulin. Because insulin resistance is closely associated with the dyslipidaemia, hypertension, endothelial abnormalities, and early cardiovascular disease,[7] the insulin sensitizer drugs may have a much greater effect than the currently available drugs on the long-term complications of Type 2 diabetes.

Ciglitazone was the first glitazone to be synthesized, in 1982, and was shown to reduce insulin resistance in obese and diabetic animals.[8] Several similar compounds were later developed, all sharing a thiazolidine-2,4-dione moiety and having different pharmacological and side-effect profiles. Currently, the three leading members of the thiazolidinedione or glitazones are troglitazone, rosiglitazone, and pioglitazone. Their chemical structures are shown in *Fig. 15.2*. Troglitazone incorporates an alpha-tocopherol (vitamin E) side-chain which adds an important and potent anti-oxidant function to the molecule. Troglitazone has been licensed for use in the US and Japan since early 1997. Rosiglitazone and pioglitazone are in the late stages of clinical development. At the time of writing there is only limited published clinical trial data from

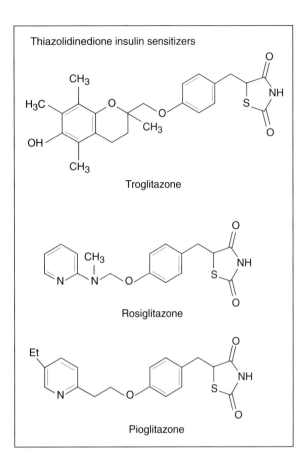

Fig. 15.2
Chemical structures of the thiazolidinedione insulin sensitizers.

human subjects on either rosiglitazone or pioglitazone, whereas the clinical portfolio of troglitazone is already extensive.[9–11] Hence, these troglitazone clinical data will be the main focus of this chapter. Other thiazolidinediones are at earlier stages in the development process. A further potentially important class of drugs in development is the non-thiazolidinediones, which can bind to DNA through the retinoid X receptor (RXR) and act as nuclear transcription factors in a similar manner to the glitazones.[12]

Mechanism of action

The insulin sensitizers have their primary effect on peripheral insulin action.[9–11] They lower blood glucose and insulin concentrations simultaneously. This is an important distinguishing point between these and other antidiabetic agents. The glitazones have the potential to preserve endogenous insulin secretory reserve. In addition to effects on glucose and insulin, the glitazones have favourable effects on lipid metabolism, blood pressure, endothelial and fibrinolytic activity, and ovarian steroid synthesis.[9–11] These non-glucose effects can be explained indirectly by effects on peripheral insulin sensitivity, but the exact mechanisms require further elucidation.

The glitazones are now known to be ligands which bind to and activate a specific nuclear receptor, formerly considered an 'orphan' receptor, known as peroxisome proliferator-activated receptor (PPAR).[10,13] The PPARs are a family of nuclear receptors including three subtypes, PPAR alpha, PPAR gamma, and PPAR delta. The normal biological function of the PPARs has not been fully elucidated, but it appears that they play a regulatory role in the expression of genes involved in carbohydrate and lipid metabolism, as well as in adipocyte differentiation.[9–11,13] In support of their role in the cellular effects of the glitazones, a close correlation has been demonstrated between the antidiabetic actions of the various glitazones and their ability to activate PPAR gamma.[14] The closely related PPAR alpha receptor is the ligand for the fibric acid hypolipidaemic agents,[10] with which some of the glitazones share biological effects *in vivo*. The glitazones have been shown to increase the expression of GLUT1 and GLUT4 and to reduce leptin, tumor necrosis factor alpha (TNF-α), and hepatic glucokinase, through effects on PPAR gamma.[14,15] The exact sequence of effects of the

glitazones on adipose tissue is incompletely understood, and while PPAR gamma appears to promote adipocyte differentiation, smaller adipocytes are favoured over larger cells, and lower circulating free fatty acid and triglyceride concentrations observed in many studies reflect improved sensitivity of adipose tissue to insulin.[16,17]

Since over 80% of *in vivo* insulin-mediated glucose disposal occurs in skeletal muscle, considerable attention has been focused on the effects of the glitazones in muscle, both in pre-clinical and clinical studies. A recent study in cultured human skeletal muscle has shown that troglitazone treatment leads to a marked increase in PPAR gamma expression as well as the expression of several other genes concerned with glucose and lipid metabolism.[18] In cultured muscle, troglitazone had both acute and chronic effects on glucose uptake and on the activity of the enzyme glycogen synthase. GLUT1 mRNA and protein were increased, in contrast to GLUT4 and GS which did not change. Research on the transcriptional effects of the glitazones (through their interaction with the PPAR system) is still at an early stage. It is likely that a wide range of gene expression is altered by these agents, and it remains to be clarified how this nuclear transcription system participates in the pathogenesis of insulin resistance and Type 2 diabetes independent of any pharmacological agents. In order to influence gene transcription, the PPAR receptor must first form a heterodimer with the RXR; this complex then binds to DNA. A recent paper has reported the exact three-dimensional structure of the ligand-binding domain of PPAR gamma, by X-ray crystallography.[19] This domain is large, and supports the finding that a wide variety of ligands can bind to it. Ongoing and future research will certainly focus on the differences between the various glitazone agents in terms of their agonist or partial agonist status and the effect of these binding interactions on downstream regulation of glucose and lipid metabolism.

Pre-clinical studies

Effects on liver

Troglitazone has been shown in a variety of animal models to reduce hepatic glucose production, probably by inhibition of fatty acid oxidation.[20–23] Hepatic glycogen synthesis is increased in cultured Hep G2 cells.[24]

Effects on pancreatic insulin secretion

Since the glitazones appear to act primarily on peripheral insulin resistance, direct effects on pancreatic islets seemed less likely. From many of the models studied, as well as human subjects with insulin resistance, improvements in glucose metabolism were accompanied by reductions in circulating insulin concentrations. There is interesting evidence that troglitazone treatment increases insulin synthesis and the insulin content of islet cells as well as improving the secretory response of islets.[25] In isolated rat pancreatic cells and in hamster β-cell lines, there is evidence that the glucose-stimulated insulin secretory response is enhanced at low concentrations of troglitazone and inhibited at high concentrations.[26] Rosiglitazone has been studied in the Zucker fatty rat to assess its effects on the prevention or treatment of features of the insulin resistance syndrome, including hyperinsulinaemia, insulin resistance, hypertension, and dyslipidaemia.[27] In this study, pancreatic islet hyperplasia, along with other ultrastructural abnormalities, could be prevented or ameliorated by treatment with rosiglitazone.

Effects on insulin action

The glitazones have been studied in a wide range of settings from tissue culture to animal models and ultimately to human subjects. Both acute and chronic increases in insulin sensitivity have been demonstrated in culture and animal model systems.[11,18,22] Both troglitazone[28,29] and pioglitazone[30] can prevent and reverse the cellular insulin resistance due to hyperglycaemia and troglitazone can increase the expression of glucose transporters (GLUT1 and GLUT4) and their translocation to the cell membrane. Another possible mechanism of the glitazones' action is through effects on TNF-α. Both troglitazone and pioglitazone have been shown to block the inhibitory effects of TNF-α on the insulin-signalling cascade.[31] This could be an important mechanism both in obesity and in Type 2 diabetes. There is evidence that pioglitazone can reduce the production of TNF-α in Wistar fatty rats, while glucose and insulin concentrations are improved.[32] Rosiglitazone has recently been shown to block the lipolytic effects of TNF-α in cultured adipocytes.[33] It is likely that each of these postulated mechanisms of improving insulin action plays some role in the *in vivo* actions of the glitazones. Further mechanistic studies in human subjects will be required in order to understand which of these mechanisms is most relevant in the treatment of diabetic subjects.

Effects on vascular smooth muscle

In an obese hypertensive rat model, troglitazone has been shown to lower systolic blood pressure as well as increase creatinine clearance and sodium excretion.[34] Pioglitazone has also been shown to lower blood pressure in a rat model system.[35] There is evidence that pioglitazone acts as a calcium channel blocker in vascular smooth muscle. A recent study has compared the effects of the glitazones on vascular smooth muscle in human adipose tissue. Troglitazone, but not rosiglitazone, was shown to vasodilate small arteries.[36] This effect could be inhibited by treatment with indomethacin, and was shown not to be due to the vitamin E moiety of troglitazone. A further study in arteries from the Wistar rat has shown that the vasodilatory effect of troglitazone is mediated through effects on calcium conduction, but not through the nitric oxide pathway.[37]

Effects on endothelium and platelets

Insulin resistance is associated with a number of abnormalities in endothelial function. These are considered to be an important component of the insulin-resistance syndrome and to account for at least some of the increased risk for early atherosclerotic disease in diabetes. Proliferation of vascular smooth muscle and intimal hyperplasia are important features of early atherosclerosis. Both have been shown to be inhibited by troglitazone in a rodent model.[38] Abnormalities of platelet function are also characteristic of the insulin-resistance syndrome. In a study of the effects of the glitazones on various aspects of platelet activity, it was found that troglitazone, but not pioglitazone, was a potent inhibitor of thrombin-induced activation of phophoinositide signalling in platelets.[39] The authors concluded that this inhibitory effect on platelet aggregation was due to the vitamin E component of troglitazone.

Effects on lipoproteins

Troglitazone has been shown in many studies to reduce triglycerides and free fatty acids while increasing HDL-cholesterol.[9–11,20] Furthermore, it has been shown to be a potent antioxidant both *in vitro* and *in vivo*, a unique feature, due

to its alpha-tocopherol side-chain.[40] Early studies in the Zucker fatty rat showed reductions in free fatty acids, triglycerides, and very-low density lipoproteins (VLDLs) after treatment with troglitazone.[20] Total cholesterol concentrations were unchanged. Various mechanisms could account for these changes, including both increased clearance and decreased synthesis. Troglitazone is a partial agonist at the PPAR alpha, which is the main receptor for the fibric acid hypolipidaemic drugs. This may explain the observed effects on lipid metabolism, and may also explain differences between the various glitazones with regard to their effects on lipids, although data on this question are still limited for the other glitazones.

Effects on myocardium

During the early development of the thiazolidinediones, it was noted that high doses of troglitazone could lead to reversible increases in heart weight in Wistar rats. The mechanism for this change was not clear. Owing to this, long-term studies were later carried out in both primates and human subjects (see below), specifically to test the effects on myocardial structure and function. In these studies, no myocardial hypertrophy has been found, and in contrast to initial concerns, improvements in cardiac function including reduction in blood pressure have been confirmed.[41] A cardioprotective effect has also been shown in the streptozotocin-induced diabetic rat after treatment with troglitazone.[42]

Clinical studies

This section will review the available clinical data on the thiazolidinedione insulin sensitizers. The majority of the available data concern troglitazone, while data on the other agents in the class are accumulating and can be expected in published form in the near future. In reviewing the clinical data, the various mechanistic studies will first be discussed, dealing with the separate effects on liver, muscle, pancreas, and so on, and the effects in different subject groups. Then the large-scale efficacy studies will be reviewed, along with current data on side-effects and safety.

Effects on liver

The thiazolidinediones have now been shown to be effective glucose-lowering agents, equal in efficacy to sulphonylureas and metformin. The mechanism of this glucose-lowering effect is less clearly understood. Fasting and post-prandial glucose are reduced, while plasma insulin concentrations are also reduced, to a lesser degree, in various studies of subjects with poorly controlled diabetes.[9-11] The relative contribution of the effects on liver and peripheral insulin action required tracer studies in combination with the glucose clamp technique. The first such study by Suter and co-workers reported on 11 subjects with Type 2 diabetes who underwent clamp studies with tritiated glucose tracer before and after 6–12 weeks treatment with troglitazone 200 mg b.d.[43] Eight of 11 subjects responded to treatment, with a reduction in fasting glucose from 12.7 to 8.3 mM. Basal hepatic glucose output was reduced significantly in the responder group, to almost normal levels (see *Fig. 15.3*). There was a good correlation between the reduction in hepatic glucose output and the reduction in fasting plasma glucose. In a subsequent, much larger, multicentre study, 93 patients with mean fasting glucose at 11.2 mM underwent glucose clamp studies, with stable isotope as tracer, before and after 6 months' treatment with either placebo or 100, 200, 400, or 600 mg of

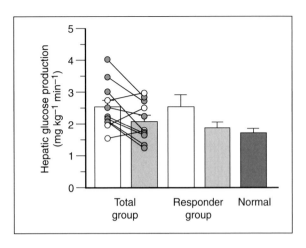

Fig. 15.3
*Hepatic glucose production rates. Bars represent mean ± SE hepatic glucose production rates before (open bars) and during (cross-hatched bars) troglitazone treatment in total group and responders. Solid bar: mean ± SE basal hepatic glucose production rate in 17 weight-matched non-diabetic control subjects for comparison. Differences between pre-treatment and during treatment were p < 0.01 (responders) and p < 0.05 (total). Non-responders are indicated by open circles. (From Suter SL, Nolan JJ, Wallace P et al. Metabolic effects of new oral hypoglycemia agent CS-045 in NIDDM subjects. Diabetes Care 1992; **15**: 193–203.)*

troglitazone.[44] The effects on hepatic glucose production were much more modest in this study, although fasting plasma glucose was reduced by 20%. A significant reduction in hepatic glucose production was observed only at the 600 mg dose of troglitazone. A further study in 13 obese, poorly controlled (fasting glucose 15.3 mM) subjects with diabetes confirmed these findings after 3 months' treatment with 400 mg troglitazone daily.[45] Using stable isotopes, this study compared the effects of troglitazone with those of metformin. In the metformin group, hepatic glucose production was reduced by 19%, consistent with its mechanism of action. Troglitazone and metformin led to similar reductions in fasting plasma glucose (20%), although clearly by different mechanisms (see below). A further study has shown no effect of troglitazone on hepatic glucose production. When obese, non-diabetic subjects were treated with troglitazone and studied with the glucose clamp technique and tritiated glucose tracer, significant improvements in glucose tolerance and insulin resistance were confirmed in the absence of any effect on basal hepatic glucose production.[46] These subjects included some with impaired glucose tolerance, but fasting plasma glucose and basal hepatic glucose production were normal prior to treatment with troglitazone. In summary, troglitazone has modest effects on net hepatic glucose production, particularly at high doses and only in those diabetic subjects with clearly elevated basal hepatic glucose production. The effects of troglitazone on fasting glucose must therefore derive mainly from its effects on peripheral insulin resistance.

Effects on peripheral insulin resistance

A number of studies have focused on the effects of the glitazones on insulin resistance. The glucose clamp technique has been used in some studies, and less-direct techniques such as the intravenous glucose tolerance test (IVGTT) have been used in others. These are the most important studies of these new agents, since their principal mechanism of action is on peripheral insulin resistance. The studies to be discussed below include those in subjects with typical Type 2 diabetes, both obese and lean, and also pre-diabetic groups well recognized for their increased potential for subsequent development of diabetes. These include subjects with impaired glucose tolerance, women with the polycystic ovary syndrome, and women with a prior history of gestational diabetes, the latter group having a very high rate of later conversion to established diabetes.

Insulin resistance in Type 2 diabetes

Two early studies employed the glucose clamp to assess insulin sensitivity before and after treatment with troglitazone. The first study,[43] in the US, was conducted in 11 obese subjects (mean body-mass index (BMI) 32.3 kg/m^2) with a mean fasting plasma glucose of 12.5 mM. The mean reduction in fasting plasma glucose was 1.8 mM after 6–12 weeks. Three of the 11 subjects did not show a reduction in plasma glucose, and were deemed to be non-responders (see *Fig. 15.4*). Glucose clamp studies were conducted at two insulin infusion rates, 120 mU m^{-2} min^{-1} and 300 mU m^{-2} min^{-1} at euglycaemia. The overall improvement in glucose disposal was impressive, at 59% in the 120 mU study and 31% in the 300 mU study (see *Fig. 15.5*). Even those subjects who did not show a reduction in fasting glucose (the non-responders) showed a 25 and 18% increase, respectively, in glucose disposal in the two clamp studies. If the non-responders were excluded from the analysis, the eight responders showed 76 and 38% increases, respectively. Consistent with these findings, the glucose and insulin responses in a 7-hour meal tolerance test were significantly reduced, as were the basal and post-meal concentrations of free fatty acids.

A second study was carried out in Japan[47] on much leaner subjects (BMI 22 kg/m^2), comparing the effects of 400 mg/day troglitazone with placebo in a total of 14 subjects. These subjects were better controlled at baseline, with fasting glucose at less than 10 mM, and less hyperinsulinaemic than those in the US study. In a three-step hyperinsulinaemic euglycaemic clamp study, the increases in glucose disposal in the

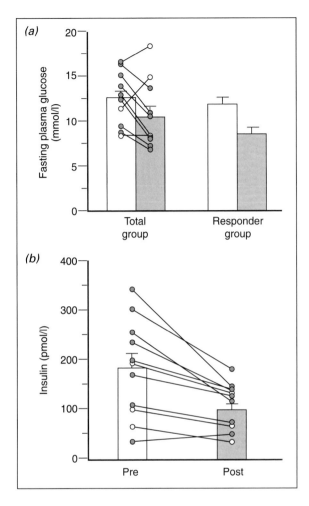

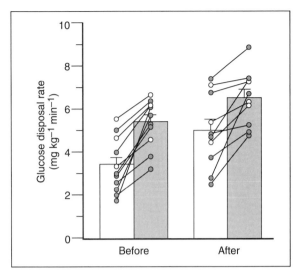

Fig. 15.5

Glucose clamp studies. Glucose disposal rates before (open bars) and during (hatched bars) troglitazone treatment during 120 mU min⁻¹ m⁻² insulin infusion (left side) and 300 mU min⁻¹ m⁻² insulin infusion studies (right side). (From Suter SL, Nolan JJ, Wallace P et al. Metabolic effects of new oral hypoglycemic agent CS-045 in NIDDM subjects. Diabetes Care *1992;* **15:** *193–203.)*

Fig. 15.4

(a) Fasting plasma glucose values before (open bars) and during (hatched bars) troglitazone treatment in total group and responder group. Non-responders are indicated by open circles. (b) Fasting plasma insulin values before and during troglitazone treatment. (From Suter SL, Nolan JJ, Wallace P et al. Metabolic effects of new oral hypoglycemic agent CS-045 in NIDDM subjects. Diabetes Care *1992;* **15:** *193–203.)*

troglitazone-treated group were 51, 34, and 20%. Fasting glucose decreased by 15% in the treated group after 12 weeks. These findings confirmed the impressive insulin-sensitizing effects of troglitazone in the Japanese subjects, even though they were much leaner and less hyperglycaemic than their American counterparts. Further studies in lean Japanese subjects, using the IVGTT to assess insulin resistance, have shown more modest but similar effects on both glucose and insulin responses after a glucose load.

Two Japanese studies have reported on the effects on pioglitazone on insulin sensitivity using the glucose clamp approach. In the first study,[48] 20 relatively lean (BMI 24 kg/m²) subjects were studied, 17 of whom had been on sulphonylureas prior to the investigation. After 3 months' oral administration of

30 mg/day pioglitazone, fasting glucose decreased from 11.0 mM to 8.9 mM and HbA$_{1C}$ decreased from 9.2 to 8.3%. Glucose disposal increased by 51%. Consistent with these findings, fasting serum insulin and C-peptide were also reduced by 20 and 7%, respectively. Levels of fasting triglycerides and free fatty acids decreased, and HDL increased. In the second study from the same Japanese group,[49] the effects of 3 months' treatment with pioglitazone (30 mg/day) were compared with placebo, in a double-blind study. A total of 30 subjects were studied. The glucose clamp study was combined with an oral glucose load, to measure whole body and splanchnic glucose uptake. Glucose disposal increased by 12% in the group treated with pioglitazone, and splanchnic glucose uptake was more than doubled.

With the aim of obtaining a better quantitative assessment of the effects of troglitazone on insulin sensitivity, two larger, multicentre clamp studies were carried out in the US. In both studies, a 120 mU m^{-2} min^{-1} euglycaemic clamp was used in conjunction with stable isotope to measure glucose turnover. Maggs et al.[44] studied 93 Type 2 diabetic subjects (BMI 32 kg/m^2 and fasting glucose 11.2 mM) before and after 6 months' treatment with either placebo or various doses of troglitazone (from 100 to 600 mg). Fasting and post-prandial glucose was reduced in the troglitazone treated groups. Increases in glucose disposal were found at all troglitazone doses and reached approximately 45% at the two higher doses (see Fig. 15.6). Further evidence of improved insulin sensitivity were reductions in fasting and post-prandial triglycerides and fasting C-peptide. Fasting hepatic glucose production was reduced only at the 600 mg dose. Using stepwise regression, the authors showed that fasting C-peptide was the strongest predictor of the glucose-lowering effect of troglitazone. This

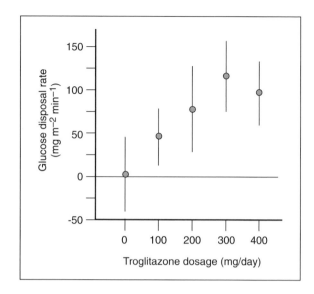

Fig. 15.6
Mean changes in glucose disposal rates measured during a hyperinsulinaemic euglycaemic clamp procedure. Changes are given as the rate after treatment minus the rate before treatment. Steady-state glucose disposal increased in all troglitazone-treated groups compared with placebo (p < 0.005). Vertical bars represent 95% confidence intervals. (From Maggs DG, Buchanan TA, Burant CF et al. Metabolic effects of troglitazone monotherapy in type 2 diabetes mellitus: a randomized, double-blind, placebo-controlled trial. Ann Int Med *1998;* **128:** *176–185.)*

is consistent with the concept that the most insulin-resistant subjects benefit the most from a treatment which works through insulin resistance primarily.

Inzucchi et al.[45] directly compared the effects of 400 mg/day troglitazone with 1 g b.d. metformin during 3 months' treatment in a group of 29 obese poorly controlled diabetic subjects (BMI 34 kg/m^2, fasting glucose 15.5 mM). After 3 months' treatment, the glucose-lowering effects of troglitazone and

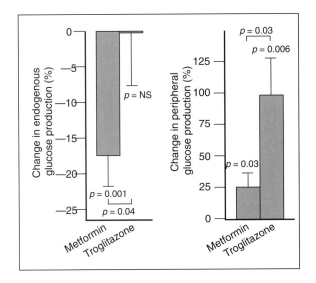

Fig. 15.7
*Mean ± SE changes within subjects in hepatic glucose production and glucose disposal rate under hyperinsulinaemic clamp conditions after 3 months' therapy with metformin 1 g b.d. or troglitazone 400 mg daily. (From Inzucchi SE, Maggs DG, Spollett GR et al. Efficacy and metabolic effects of metformin and troglitazone in type 2 diabetes mellitus. N Engl J Med 1998; **338**: 867–872.)*

metformin were similar, at 20–25%. During the glucose clamp studies, troglitazone led to a much greater increase in glucose disposal, at 54% compared with 13% with metformin (*Fig. 15.7*). Metformin was more potent at suppressing basal hepatic glucose production, at −19% compared with −3% with troglitazone. This is a critically important study, which distinguishes between the complementary effects of the glitazones and metformin. After the initial treatment phase with either troglitazone or metformin, subjects were treated for a further 3 months on both agents together, and re-studied using the clamp technique. Somewhat surprisingly, metformin-treated subjects were

shown to have a further 24% increase in glucose disposal when troglitazone was added for 3 months. When metformin was added to those already treated with troglitazone, the increment in glucose disposal was a more modest 15%.

Prigeon and colleagues[50] have used IVGTT to measure changes in insulin sensitivity in somewhat leaner subjects (BMI 27.7 kg/m², fasting glucose 11.1 mM) treated with troglitazone for 3 months. Fasting glucose was reduced by 1.7 mM in these subjects, while the insulin sensitivity index (Si) increased by 75 ± 35%. One European study, by Sironi et al.,[51] has used the insulin suppression test to assess insulin action in diabetic subjects (BMI 28.8 kg/m², fasting glucose 12.2 mM) treated for 2 months with 200 mg/day troglitazone. Fasting glucose was reduced by about 1 mM, and insulin sensitivity improved, with a reduction in the steady-state plasma glucose from 13.8 to 10.0 mM during the insulin suppression test.

In summary, in a variety of studies in both lean and obese subjects, from various continents, both troglitazone and pioglitazone have been shown to be potent insulin sensitizers. This mechanism appears to be the main mode of glucose lowering for the glitazones, which is equal to that of metformin, although, when directly compared, troglitazone is clearly a much more powerful insulin sensitizer.

Insulin resistance in pre-diabetic conditions

Impaired glucose tolerance (IGT) is the commonest and therefore the most important easily classifiable pre-diabetic condition. Progression from IGT to Type 2 diabetes occurs at varying rates depending primarily on ethnicity, degree of obesity and other factors.[52] Groups at particularly high risk include those from ethnic minorities such as native Americans, Latinos, and certain immigrant

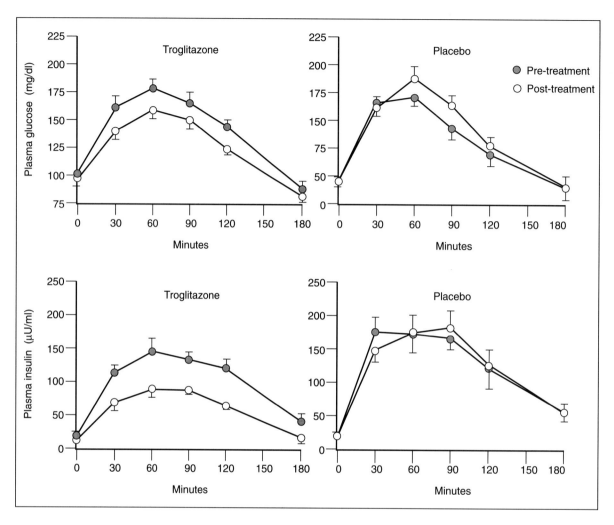

Fig. 15.8
Results of oral glucose tolerance tests before and after the administration of troglitazone or placebo for 12 weeks in obese subjects without diabetes. (From Nolan JJ, Ludvik B, Beerdsen P et al. Improvement in glucose tolerance and insulin resistance in obese subjects treated with troglitazone. N Engl J Med *1994; **331**: 1188–1193.)*

Asian populations. Troglitazone has been studied in several of these high-risk groups.

The first in-depth metabolic study of troglitazone in non-diabetic subjects examined the effects of 12 weeks' treatment with 200 mg b.d. troglitazone in 18 obese subjects, nine of whom had IGT.[46] These were randomized to receive placebo (*n* = 6) or troglitazone (*n* = 12). After troglitazone treatment, the glycaemic response to glucose or mixed meals was significantly decreased. In fact, glucose tolerance was normalized in six of seven subjects who previously had had IGT (*Fig. 15.8*). Fasting insulin was reduced by 48%,

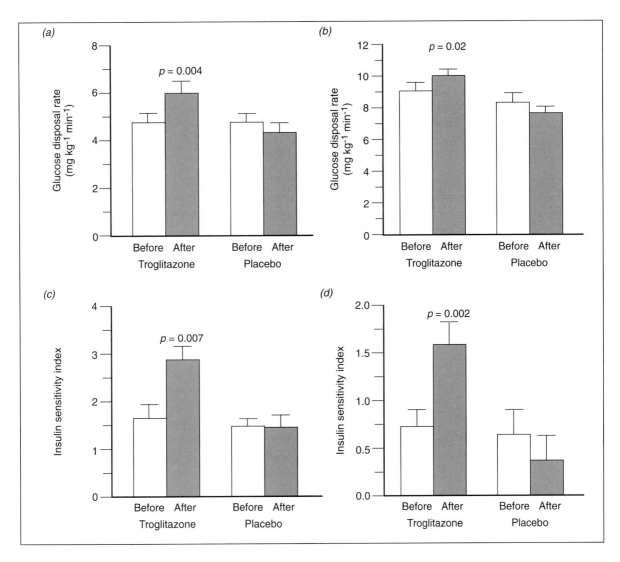

Fig. 15.9

*Measurements of insulin resistance before and after the administration of troglitazone or placebo for 12 weeks in obese subjects without diabetes. (a) 40 mU clamp study; (b) 300 mU clamp study; (c) clamp-derived insulin sensitivity index; (d) minimal model-derived insulin sensitivity index, from the IVGTT. (From Nolan JJ, Ludvik B, Beerdsen P et al. Improvement in glucose tolerance and insulin resistance in obese subjects treated with troglitazone. N Engl J Med 1994; **331:** 1188–1193.)*

and the insulin response to glucose and mixed meals was reduced by 40% (see *Fig. 15.8*) . Peripheral glucose disposal increased by 22% during clamp studies at 40 mU m⁻² min⁻¹. The clamp-derived insulin sensitivity index increased by 75%, and the IVGTT-derived Si was more than doubled after troglitazone (*Fig. 15.9*).

A later study by Berkowitz *et al.* studied the effects of troglitazone treatment in 42 Latino women with IGT and a history of gestational diabetes.[53] This is one of the highest risk groups for progression from IGT to Type 2 diabetes, with an estimated 5-year risk of 80%. An IVGTT and oral glucose tolerance test were performed before and after 3 months' treatment. The IVGTT-derived Si increased by 40% after 200 mg troglitazone and by 88% after 400 mg. Despite these impressive effects on peripheral insulin action, oral glucose tolerance had not improved after treatment. The most plausible explanation for these findings is the well-documented defect in pancreatic insulin secretion which characterizes women with gestational diabetes,[54] which accelerates their later progression to Type 2 diabetes if they become more insulin resistant, either through weight gain or through subsequent pregnancies, or both.[55]

Subjects with IGT were again studied by Antonucci *et al.* in a randomized, double-blind, placebo-controlled design.[56] A total of 51 subjects were included; 25 received 400 mg once-daily troglitazone and 26 received placebo. After 6 weeks, 75% of those taking troglitazone had improved to normal glucose tolerance, compared with 38% of those on placebo ($p = 0.008$). After 12 weeks, 80% of the treated group had normal glucose tolerance, compared with 48% of those on placebo ($p = 0.016$). Along with the improvements in glucose tolerance, troglitazone led to reductions in insulin and C-peptide responses in the oral glucose tolerance test. Fasting triglycerides were decreased by −0.45 mM in the treatment group by 12 weeks.

In a later study in IGT, Cavaghan *et al.* randomized 14 subjects to treatment with troglitazone 400 mg/day and seven subjects to placebo for 3 months.[57] Using the IVGTT, these authors demonstrated a doubling of the insulin Si.

Consistent with earlier studies, the glucose response in the OGTT was reduced by 10% and the insulin response was reduced by 39%. An important additional finding by this group was an improvement in the β-cell response to glucose. This was the first evidence in human subjects that the insulin sensitizers may actually improve pancreatic insulin secretion *per se*.

Troglitazone has been studied in women with polycystic ovarian syndrome (PCOS), a classic insulin-resistant syndrome with an increased risk of conversion to diabetes.[58] Women with PCOS are typically obese and hyperinsulinaemic with hyperandrogenaemia and associated menstrual disturbances. In one study of PCOS, troglitazone at 400 mg/day in 13 obese women resulted in a 60% increase in the insulin Si, as well as reductions in fasting and post-load insulin concentrations.[58] Furthermore, these changes were accompanied by reduction in androgens and the return of ovulatory menses in some subjects. Ehrmann and colleagues subsequently studied 13 obese women who had both PCOS and IGT, and who thus represented a particularly insulin-resistant subgroup.[59] Treatment with troglitazone 400 mg/day for 12 weeks led to marked improvements in glucose tolerance, reduction in glycosylated haemoglobin, and a 63% increase in the insulin Si, studied by the IVGTT. Most importantly, the β-cell responsiveness to an oscillatory glucose infusion improved significantly after troglitazone treatment. Consistent with the earlier study in PCOS, androgen levels were reduced, as were the concentrations of plasminogen activator inhibitor (PAI-1), a marker of fibrinolytic capacity.

In summary, troglitazone has been studied in a variety of pre-diabetic insulin-resistant conditions. Treatment has consistently demonstrated the possibility of restoring glucose tolerance towards normal, in addition to improving β-cell function and reducing hyperinsuli-naemia. In all the common non-diabetic forms of human insulin resistance, troglitazone leads to substantial increases in glucose disposal.

Effects on pancreatic insulin secretion

As has been described above, various studies in pre-diabetic insulin-resistant states such as IGT and PCOS have shown that islet cell insulin responsiveness can be improved by troglitazone treatment. The technique of the oscillatory glucose infusion has been employed in these settings to test the capacity of the β-cell to detect and respond to increases in circulating glucose.[59] Some authors have measured the proportion of proinsulin to insulin, which reflects β-cell health. There have been two reports of a decreased proinsulin to insulin ratio after troglitazone therapy.[50,60] This is consistent with the theory that the insulin sensitizers may directly improve islet cell signalling or physiology.

Effects on lipids, and lipid oxidation

The classical dyslipidaemia associated with Type 2 diabetes, and with its pre-diabetic insulin-resistant precursor states, is elevation of VLDLs and reduction of HDLs.[7,61] Although LDL concentrations are typically normal in diabetic subjects, the LDL particle is smaller and denser, and is glycated and more prone to oxidation.[61] Taken together, these lipid disturbances are thought to account for at least some of the increased risk of macrovascular disease in Type 2 diabetes. Troglitazone treatment has been consistently shown to be associated with reductions in trigly-cerides and an increase in HDL-cholesterol.[9–11] LDL-cholesterol has been shown to increase slightly (by up to 10%), while apolipoprotein B

levels remain unchanged. In more detailed studies, it has been shown that the LDL particles are qualitatively changed to the larger, less-dense, less-oxidizable form, which is thought to be less atherogenic.[62,63] The anti-oxidant property of troglitazone has been studied both *in vitro* and *in vivo*.[40] Troglitazone is, in fact, a potent anti-oxidant molecule, and the combination of its effects on lipoprotein concentrations combined with its effects on oxidation suggest that its long-term effects on atherogenesis could be considerable. Pioglitazone has been shown to have similar effects on lipids to those of troglitazone, although it is not an anti-oxidant.[48]

Effects on blood pressure

Hypertension is an important component of the insulin-resistance syndrome, and occurs with greater frequency in subjects with diabetes.[64] Insulin may affect blood pressure in several ways, potentially raising blood pressure through increased renal sodium retention and increased peripheral sympathetic activity, and potentially lowering blood pressure through a vasodilator effect on arteries and arterioles. The insulin-sensitizer agents could be expected to have some effect on blood pressure, depending on the net balance between these various mechanisms in any particular group of subjects.

The effects of troglitazone on blood pressure were studied in obese non-diabetic subjects (some with IGT) before and after 12 weeks' treatment with 200 mg b.d. troglitazone.[46] Twenty-four-hour ambulatory blood pressure recording was performed pre- and post-treatment. These subjects were not hypertensive at the outset, but troglitazone treatment led to a significant reduction in both systolic (–6 mmHg) and diastolic (–4 mmHg) blood pressure. In a study of Japanese diabetic subjects with mild hypertension, a similar dose of troglitazone for 8 weeks led to much greater improvements in systolic (–18 mmHg) and diastolic (–12 mmHg) blood pressure, which was correlated to the reduction in plasma insulin concentration.[65] A longer-term study, by Ghazzi and colleagues,[41] has followed the effects of troglitazone at 800 mg/day in 154 obese subjects with Type 2 diabetes. These subjects have been followed for up to 96 weeks in the majority of cases. Modest but significant improvements in diastolic blood pressure and mean arterial pressure have been shown to persist at the 96-week-time point. Blood pressure did not change in the comparison arm of this study, in which subjects received gliben-clamide. Importantly, plasma insulin concentrations were reduced by 25% in the troglitazone group, compared with no change in those treated with glibenclamide. This study was originally designed to address concerns about the possibility of cardiac hypertrophy developing during glitazone therapy, as had been observed in rodents (see above). Echocardiography was carried out, along with pulse Doppler, at regular intervals in all subjects to assess the effects on the myocardium. After 2 years, left-ventricular-mass index was unchanged in the troglitazone-treated group of patients. Furthermore, an increase in stroke volume and cardiac index were noted, in addition to the reduction in mean arterial pressure and peripheral vascular resistance mentioned above.

Effects on endothelium

Abnormalities in endothelial function are thought to be an important component of the insulin-resistance syndrome.[66] Studies with the insulin-sensitizer drugs indicate that they have favourable effects on platelet function, on vascular smooth muscle, and on the intima. A Japanese group has studied the effects of 6 months' 400 mg daily troglitazone treatment in 135 subjects with Type 2 diabetes.[67] A B-mode ultrasound was used to measure carotid artery intimal and medial thickness (IMT). After 3 months, a significant reduction in IMT was noted, which was sustained at 6 months.

A recent study has shown that troglitazone can markedly inhibit platelet aggregation through suppression of thrombin-induced signalling within the platelets.[39] This effect was not seen with pioglitazone, an observation that might be explained by the vitamin E moiety on troglitazone.

Insulin resistance has been shown to be associated with impaired fibrinolysis and increased PAI-1 levels. In diabetic subjects, troglitazone treatment has been shown to decrease levels of PAI-1, either during monotherapy or in combination with insulin.[68] Similarly, in women with PCOS and IGT, troglitazone treatment led to reduction in PAI-1.[59]

The effects of troglitazone on insulin-mediated vasodilation have also been studied. Tack and colleagues performed whole-body and forearm glucose uptake studies in a group of obese insulin-resistant subjects before and after 8 weeks' treatment with troglitazone at 400 mg/day.[69] Glucose disposal was increased in the clamp study by 23%, consistent with earlier similar studies. No change was noted in insulin-induced vasodilation in these subjects, and the endothelium-dependent and endothelium-independent vascular responses were normal and unchanged.

Effects on body-weight

A most important long-term issue is the effect, if any, of the insulin-sensitizer drugs on body-weight. This is a very complex issue, and can only be addressed in a satisfactory way by long-term prospective studies. In theory, the improvements in insulin sensitivity seen with these agents could be expected to result in an increase in weight. What is more difficult to calculate is the combined effect of improved insulin sensitivity together with an overall reduction in circulating insulin concentrations, which has been observed in most clinical studies to date. At the molecular level, the thiazolidinediones decrease the expression of leptin in adipocytes.[70] In a recently reported study in Japanese diabetic subjects, 12 weeks' treatment with 200 mg b.d. troglitazone led to reduced glucose and insulin levels, as well as reduction in leptin.[71] Interestingly, more than half of these patients reported increased hunger after troglitazone administration. In contrast to these findings, leptin levels did not change in 13 non-diabetic obese subjects (eight with IGT) who were treated with the same dose of troglitazone (200 mg b.d.) for 12 weeks, despite substantial improvements in insulin sensitivity and reductions in insulin levels.[72] It is clear that a wide variety of biological and behavioural factors interact in the long-term determination of body mass, and only long-term studies will indicate whether these new agents have any net effect on this process.

Large-scale trials

Among the three leading thiazolidinediones, troglitazone is still the only member of the class for which substantial clinical trial data are available. For the other glitazones, trials are in progress or being analysed and prepared for publication at the time of writing.

The traditional treatment strategy for Type 2 diabetes has been a stepwise process through education, diet and exercise, oral agents combination therapy, and then insulin. The timing of these steps in treatment follows algorithms based on glycaemic goals, but is largely determined by both the degree of insulin resistance, which increases as diabetes progresses, and the reserves of endogenous insulin, which continue to decrease (see *Fig. 15.1*). One of the most important broad questions relating to the new insulin sensitizers is whether they can actually spare insulin reserves and delay progression to the final step of insulin treatment. There is a growing body of evidence that the glitazones are safe and effective antidiabetic drugs when used as monotherapy or in combination with either sulphonylureas or insulin.

Monotherapy

Troglitazone monotherapy has been studied in Europe, Japan, and the US. In the multicentre European Troglitazone Study, 330 Type 2 diabetic subjects who were moderately obese (BMI 28–29 kg/m^2) were treated with 200, 400, 600, or 800 mg troglitazone once daily, or 200 or 400 mg b.d. for 12 weeks.[73] Troglitazone treatment lowered HbA$_{1C}$ by 0.6–1.0% and fasting glucose by 2 mM, as well as lowering fasting insulin by 12–26%. Higher doses of troglitazone led to reduction in triglycerides and free fatty acids, and an increase in HDL-cholesterol. LDL-cholesterol increased by 10–15% at the 400 and 600 mg doses. The drug was well tolerated. In a subsequent Japanese study of troglitazone, also of 12 weeks' duration, 262 lean subjects with Type 2 diabetes were treated with 400 mg daily.[74] Glycaemic lowering was less in this group, at 1.25 mM, with HbA$_{1C}$ reduction of 0.5%. The responder group in this study (more than 50% of the participants) achieved >20% reduction in fasting glucose or >1% reduction in HbA$_{1C}$. This subgroup was more obese, with a higher baseline HbA$_{1C}$. Lipids and blood pressure did not change, and a slight weight gain of 0.5 kg was reported.

Two multicentre US trials of troglitazone monotherapy have recently been published. In the first these studies, mentioned above, 93 obese Type 2 diabetic subjects were treated with placebo or troglitazone in doses from 100 to 600 mg daily for 6 months.[44] This study was conducted in six centres capable of performing the glucose clamp technique, which was part of the investigations. After 6 months, troglitazone significantly reduced fasting and post-prandial glucose, triglycerides, and serum C-peptide. Fasting free fatty acids were also reduced and serum insulin was reduced in the 200 mg and 600 mg groups. At 400 mg and 600 mg, the reduction in fasting glucose was 20%. Among baseline characteristics, the fasting C-peptide concentrations were the strongest predictor of a response in fasting and post-prandial glucose. The glucose clamp data demonstrated that improvement in peripheral insulin resistance was the main mechanism for the glycaemic response to troglitazone (*Fig. 15.6*). Only the 600 mg dose was associated with modest reduction in hepatic glucose output. In a second large US multicentre study, 402 obese (mean BMI 32.4 kg/m²) Type 2 diabetic subjects were treated for 6 months with either placebo, or 200, 400, or 600 mg troglitazone.[75] Prior to the study, one-fifth of subjects had been on a special diet alone (and had a shorter duration of diabetes) and four-fifths had been on oral agents. Oral agents were withdrawn in a wash-out phase prior to baseline study. Fasting glucose was reduced by 2.2, 2.9, and 3.2 mM at the 200, 400, and 600 mg doses, respectively. The 100 mg dose was ineffective at glycaemic lowering. HbA_{1C} was reduced by −0.7 and −1.1% at the 400 and 600 mg doses, respectively. An HbA_{1C} of <8% was achieved in 40% subjects at the 400 mg dose and in 42% at 600 mg. Consistent with earlier studies, fasting insulin was reduced by 20–25% and C-peptide by 36%. It is interesting to compare the treatment response in the two groups studied. Those whose prior treatment was diet alone (22% of subjects) had a much better glycaemic response (−2.7 mM) to troglitazone than those who had been on oral agents (78% of the group), which were first withdrawn in a wash-out period prior to the study. In this group, insulin levels fell during wash-out, and glycaemic response was much less (−1.9 mM).

To date, results have been published for one of the multicentre studies of rosiglitazone in Type 2 diabetes. Lebovitz and colleagues randomized 493 subjects with Type 2 diabetes to treatment with either placebo, or 4 mg or 8 mg of rosiglitazone daily, for 6 months.[76] On average, these subjects were poorly controlled at baseline, with a mean HbA_{1C} of 8.9%. After 6 months, compared with placebo-treated patients (in whom fasting glucose rose), there was an overall difference in fasting glucose of 3.2 mM at 4 mg and 4.2 mM at 8 mg of rosiglitazone. The net reduction in HbA_{1C} was 1.21 and 1.54 %, respectively. When the subset of subjects who were naïve to drug therapy was analysed, the glycaemic lowering was significantly greater with rosiglitazone.

All of these monotherapy studies were conducted in poorly controlled patients mainly treated with sulphonylureas prior to study. The withdrawal of the oral agent prior to the introduction of the glitazone caused a further deterioration in control. From what is known about the mechanism of action of the glitazones, a more logical approach would be to test their efficacy in combination with sulphonylureas. These combination studies are now discussed.

Combination with sulphonylureas

Combining the effects of an insulin secretagogue with an insulin sensitizer is a logical approach to the treatment of Type 2 diabetes, given the fact that in most patients both impaired insulin secretion and peripheral insulin resistance contribute to the elevated glucose levels. This has been studied in one large multicentre trial in the US, where a total of 542 patients were treated for 1 year in a randomized, double-blind protocol.[77] Seven treatment arms were included as follows: 12 mg micronized glyburide, 200 mg troglitazone, 400 mg or 600 mg once daily (all monotherapy), and the same three doses in combination with glyburide. At baseline, all these subjects had failed maximal doses of sulphonylureas, and had a mean fasting glucose of 12.3 mM, a mean HbA$_{1C}$ of 9.6% and a mean fasting C-peptide >1.5 ng/ml. After 1 year, the addition of troglitazone to glyburide reduced fasting glucose by −3.0, −3.3, and 4.3 mM in the 200, 400, and 600 mg groups, respectively, and reduced HbA$_{1C}$ by −1.61, −1.81, and −2.65%, respectively. Consistent with earlier studies, fasting insulin was also reduced. The proportion of patients achieving the target of HbA$_{1C}$ <7% was 32% in the 200 and 400 mg combination groups and 58% in the 600 mg combination group. Maximal glyburide alone allowed this goal to be reached in only 6% of subjects. There was no increase in adverse events in any of the treatment groups. Clearly, the addition of troglitazone to maximal sulphonylurea therapy offered very significant benefits to those subjects who were failing the sulphonylurea approach and who would normally have been under consideration for insulin therapy.

Combination with metformin

Only one study to date has reported the effects of troglitazone in combination with metformin in diabetic patients. Inzucchi and colleagues[45] recruited 29 subjects who had failed diet or sulphonylureas (basal fasting glucose prior to starting therapy was 15.4 mM), and treated them with either 400 mg daily troglitazone or 1 g b.d. metformin. After 3 months, each group was then given the second drug for a further 3-month period. After the first 3 months on parallel treatment, troglitazone and metformin led to similar reductions in fasting (−20%) and post-prandial (−25%) glucose. At the end of the second 3-month period, during which subjects were on combination therapy, there was a further decrease in fasting (−2.3 mM) and post-prandial (−3.0 mM) glucose. Glucose clamp studies showed clearly that metformin's effect was primarily through suppression of elevated hepatic glucose production (*Fig. 15.7*). Troglitazone's effect was almost entirely due to stimulation of peripheral glucose uptake. There was no significant change in plasma insulin or body-weight during the 6-month study. Thus, troglitazone and metformin have complementary effects in patients with Type 2 diabetes, and can act synergistically to improve abnormalities in glucose metabolism.

Combination with insulin

Troglitazone was first licensed for use in the US only as add-on treatment for those Type 2 diabetic subjects already treated with insulin. Prior to licensing, two large multicentre studies were carried out to investigate this combination therapy. Both studies lasted 6 months and were conducted in the US. In the first study, 350 poorly controlled (mean HbA$_{1C}$ 9.5%) patients who were already insulin treated were randomized to receive troglitazone 200 mg or 600 mg daily.[78] The insulin dose was reduced if two consecutive fasting glucose levels were <5.5 mM. At 6 months, HbA$_{1C}$ was reduced by 0.8% in the 200 mg group, by 1.41% in the 600 mg group, and by 0.1% in those on placebo. Exogenous insulin doses were reduced by 11% in those on 200 mg troglitazone and by 42% in those on the 600 mg dose. The study was continued for an open-label extension for nearly 2 years, and the improvements in glycaemic control and insulin requirements persisted.

In a second study, 222 obese subjects with Type 2 diabetes were recruited for a trial of combination therapy.[79] At baseline, insulin doses ranged from 30 to 150 units per day. After 6 months, subjects receiving 200 mg troglitazone (with insulin) required a reduction in daily insulin of 41%. In the 400 mg group, the insulin dose was reduced by 58%, and with the placebo group, the dose reduced by 14%. At the 200 mg dose, 51% of subjects had their dose reduced to half or less of baseline, and at the 400 mg dose 70% reached this target. Insulin could actually be discontinued in 7% of those on 200 mg and in 15% of those on 400 mg troglitazone, compared with just 1.5% of those on placebo. Insulin could be given less frequently when in combination with troglitazone. Glycaemic control improved, despite the major reduction in exogenous insulin. This study was also extended for 18 months, during which the reduced insulin dose was sustained while glycaemic parameters continued to improve, with a further 1% reduction in HbA_{1C}. Patients gained 4.7 kg and 3.0 kg in the 200 mg and 400 mg combination groups, respectively, during the extension phase of this study. These two studies illustrate most directly the insulin-sensitizing, and therefore insulin-sparing, effects of troglitazone. The glitazones would appear to be most effective when used in combination with either insulin or with the sulphonylurea insulin secretagogues.

In the majority of the clinical studies summarized above, patients were poorly controlled at entry and had already reached a late stage in the diabetic syndrome, with marked insulin resistance and depleted reserves of endogenous insulin. At this stage of diabetes, a combination therapy approach is most effective since it targets each of the major metabolic defects which lead to hyperglycaemia, namely, impaired insulin secretion (insulin or secretagogues), elevated hepatic glucose production (metformin), and insulin resistance (glitazones). In the insulin combination studies, troglitazone was generally well tolerated. Small reductions in red cell indices were found (previously noted in earlier studies of troglitazone), but within the normal reference range. Hypoglycaemia was increased slightly in the troglitazone combination groups. Because of its effects of promoting insulin sensitivity, troglitazone can lead to hypoglycaemia when used in combination with either sulphonylureas or insulin. This is a key point, as thiazolidinediones when used as monotherapy do not cause hypoglycaemia.

Combination with sulphonylurea and metformin

Only one study to date has reported the use of a triple combination of troglitazone, metformin, and sulphonylurea. Ovalle and colleagues performed a retrospective analysis of the response in 35 obese subjects of the addition of 600 mg daily troglitazone to the combination of metformin and glimepiride.[80] These subjects had been very poorly controlled at baseline, with HbA_{1C} >10%. HbA_{1C} improved to <8% after 6 months on triple therapy. Patients gained approximately 4 kg during the first 3 months, but had returned to baseline weight by the end of 6 months. This study suggests an important potential role for the glitazones in the subgroup of patients failing the current maximal oral combination therapy. Provided the glycaemic benefits could be sustained in the long term, such a combination therapy could postpone the need for exogenous insulin.

Safety

Side-effects

The glitazones in general are well-tolerated, once-daily oral agents without serious adverse effects. During the clinical development stage, the incidence of adverse events has been similar to that in placebo-treated subjects. Withdrawal from trials has been similar to placebo at about 5%. Minor side-effects noted for the class include a very slight reduction (within normal limits) in plasma haemoglobin, haematocrit, and neutrophils. These minor changes in the peripheral haematologic profile can occur within weeks of starting therapy, but have been shown to remain stable for up to 2 years without progression.

Licensing of troglitazone in Europe was postponed in 1997 because of concerns about rare but serious adverse effects on liver function. During the clinical development of troglitazone, it was noted that reversible elevations in AST and ALT to greater than three times the upper limit of 'normal' occurred at 2% in troglitazone-treated subjects, compared with 0.6% of those treated with placebo. These changes were reversible and no serious sequelae were noted. However, more serious hepatic side-effects were first noted during the post-marketing phase after initial licensing in the US and Japan.[81,82] There have been a series of reported cases of fulminant liver damage necessitating liver transplant or causing death. To date, the incidence of serious liver damage is still rare and estimated at 1:60,000 treated patients.[83] The hepatic side-effects appear to be idiosyncratic and can develop over a short time. As a result, the Food and Drug Administration (FDA) has introduced new product-labelling measures requiring regular monitoring of liver function prior to and during therapy. Serum transaminases should be checked prior to therapy, monthly for the first 8 months, then every 2 months for the first year, and periodically thereafter. Troglitazone should not be given if the subject has liver disease or has elevated transaminases (greater than two times the upper limit of normal). If a patient treated with troglitazone develops symptoms suggestive of liver disease, liver function tests should be checked. For moderate elevation of transaminases (alanine aminotransferase (ALT) $>1.5 \times N$), the liver enzymes should be checked within a week and weekly until they normalize. If the patient becomes jaundiced, or if the ALT is elevated to greater than three times the normal level, troglitazone should be discontinued.

Hepatic adverse effects have not been noted to date during the clinical development of either rosiglitazone or pioglitazone.

Research in rodents has led to concerns that troglitazone could lead to cardiac enlargement, albeit at much higher doses of the drug than would be used in human subjects. On account of this, a 2-year prospective study was carried out in diabetic subjects who were treated with 600–800 mg troglitazone daily.[41] This study conclusively showed no adverse effects on myocardial structure or function. In fact, improvement in cardiac contractility was demonstrated, along with improvement in peripheral vascular resistance.

The glitazones do not cause hypoglycaemia when used as monotherapy. However, when used in combination with sulphonylureas or insulin, hypoglycaemia can occur. It is necessary to reduce the dose of other antidiabetic treatments when a glitazone is introduced, because of the insulin-sensitizing effect. Even with combination therapy, severe hypoglycaemia is still extremely rare. In the US insulin/troglitazone combination trials, only one case of serious hypoglycaemia was reported.

Contraindications

The glitazones have not been studied in pregnant or breast-feeding women, and so, these agents should not be administered to either of these groups. Similarly, the treatment of children is contraindicated until these drugs have been formally studied in the paediatric age group. Troglitazone has been shown to improve the metabolic defects in PCOS and can lead to resumption of ovulation. Therefore, such subjects should be counselled in relation to the increased risk of becoming pregnant during treatment for insulin resistance.

Drug interactions

Troglitazone (but not rosiglitazone) may inhibit enzymes from the hepatic cytochrome P_{450} class, and may alter the circulating concentrations of various drugs. No major drug interaction has been reported. These drugs should not be given with cholestyramine, which reduces their absorption. Troglitazone can cause a reduction in the plasma concentrations of oral contraceptives.

Clinical indications

The findings of the wide range of clinical studies of the thiazolidinediones are consistent and confirm the hypothesis that these agents primarily reduce insulin resistance. They are effective agents in the treatment of Type 2 diabetes. For troglitazone in particular, these beneficial effects are also seen in impaired glucose tolerance, in women with prior gestational diabetes, and in women with the PCOS. The glitazones are effective when administered once daily, orally. The FDA has approved the use of troglitazone as monotherapy in Type 2 diabetic subjects whose glycaemic control is unsatisfactory with diet and exercise alone. The effective dose range is from 200–600 mg daily, the usual starting dose being 400 mg. In a recent Position Statement,[84] the American Diabetes Association has recommended a target fasting glucose of 4.3–6.6 mM and an HbA_{1C} of <7%. When introducing troglitazone as combination therapy (in patients already failing maximal doses of sulphonylurea or metformin), troglitazone should be started at 200 mg daily and titrated, with the knowledge that hypoglycaemia may occur on such a combination. Substitution of troglitazone for one of the other agents makes no sense, given that the glitazones have a similar glycaemic lowering effect as the older agents. When adding troglitazone to insulin therapy, the starting dose should also be 200 mg. This dose may be titrated every 2–4 weeks, with careful instruction to the patient to monitor their capillary glucose more frequently. Once the fasting glucose is below 6.6 mM, the insulin dose should then be reduced by 10–25% (as was done in the large clinical trial). The ideal therapeutic model would be to achieve near-normal glycaemia at the lowest exogenous insulin dose.

Because troglitazone can lead to serious hepatic dysfunction, the FDA's guidelines on testing of liver function should be followed strictly, both prior to commencement of therapy and during the first year, as outlined above. The hepatic toxicity is idiosyncratic, and can develop quickly. Rosiglitazone and pioglitazone have not been reported to lead to any hepatotoxicity. Clinical selection of those patients most likely to benefit from the thiazolidinediones is not completely straightforward. In theory, those patients who are most insulin resistant stand to benefit the most from these drugs. When all the clinical trial data are integrated, the more obese individuals tend to show a better response. In addition to insulin resistance, the degree of residual pancreatic insulin secretory reserve is also an important determinant of response to the insulin sensitizers. In one of the multicentre studies, fasting C-peptide was an independent predictor of response to troglitazone. As a result of our increasingly better understanding of the heterogeneity of Type 2 diabetes (or, non-Type 1 diabetes), it is likely that in the future, more attention will be focused on the evaluation of the degree of insulin resistance and insulin secretion at baseline. Variables such as BMI, waist/hip ratio, blood pressure, fasting lipids, and fasting C-peptide, and possibly other parameters, can be used to predict response and to tailor therapy to each individual's insulin-replacement and insulin-resistance requirements. Patients with primarily insulin secretory failure and no insulin resistance are unlikely to benefit from these agents. The arrival of this new class of antidiabetic drugs will eventually lead to important changes in clinical practice. A revised stepwise strategy, which represents the future potential uses of the glitazones is summarized in *Fig. 15.10.*

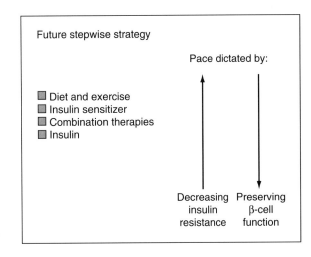

Fig. 15.10

Proposed stepwise therapy in Type 2 diabetes and pre-diabetic conditions based on the proven efficacy of the thiazolidinedione insulin sensitizers.

Conclusion

The thiazolidinedione/glitazone group of insulin sensitizer agents are an exciting new family of antidiabetic drugs which work by a completely novel mechanism involving the regulation of gene transcription. They are at least as effective as other antidiabetic drugs in terms of glucose lowering, but achieve this with concomitant reduction in circulating insulin levels, because of very substantial effects on skeletal muscle insulin resistance. Other consequences of insulin resistance are improved, including a wide range of vascular and endothelial risk factors. The insulin-sensitizer drugs are particularly effective in combination with the current antidiabetic drugs, including sulphonylureas, metformin, and insulin. Troglitazone is the most extensively studied agent, whereas the published clinical data on the other agents are still limited. Troglitazone

ameliorates several of the pre-diabetic syndromes through its effects in improving insulin sensitivity. The only important side-effect is a rare hepatotoxicity, which to date has only been observed with troglitazone. The exact mechanism of this adverse effect has not been explained, but this has led to a cautious regulatory stance on these agents until more is understood. The most important future perspective on these agents is as preventive therapy in the earliest stages of the diabetic syndrome, with a real potential to prevent or delay the more serious cardiovascular complications of diabetes.

References

1. Polonsky KS, Sturis J, Bell GI. Non-insulin dependent diabetes mellitus – a genetically programmed failure of the beta cell to compensate for insulin resistance. *N Engl J Med* 1996; **334**: 777–783.

2. UK Prospective Diabetes Study Group. Effect of intensive blood glucose control with metformin on complications in overweight patients with type 2 diabetes (UKPDS 34). *Lancet* 1998; **352**: 854–865.

3. UK Prospective Diabetes Study Group. Intensive blood glucose control with sulphonylureas or insulin compared with conventional treatment and risk of complications in patients with type 2 diabetes (UKPDS 33). *Lancet* 1998; **352**: 837–853.

4. Zimmet P, McCarthy D. The NIDDM epidemic: Global estimates and projection: a look into the crystal ball. *IDF Bulletin* 1995; **40**: 8–16.

5. Nolan JJ, Olefsky JM. Insulin action and insulin resistance in NIDDM. In: Draznin B, Rizza R, eds. *Clinical Research in Diabetes and Obesity: Volume II: Diabetes and Obesity.* Totawa, NJ: The Humana Press, 1997: 137–158.

6. DeFronzo RA, Bonadonna RC, Ferrannini E. Pathogenesis of NIDDM: a balanced overview. *Diabetologia* 1992; **35**: 389–397.

7. Reaven GM. Role of insulin resistance in human disease. *Diabetes* 1998; **37**: 1595–1607.

8. Fujita T, Sugiyama Y, Taketomi S *et al.* Reduction of insulin resistance in obese and/or diabetic animals by 3[-4-(1-methyl-cyclohexyl-methoxy)benzyl]-Thiazolidine-2,4-dione (ADD-3870, U-63,287, ciglitazone), a new antidiabetic agent. *Diabetes* 1983; **32**: 804–810.

9. Henry RR. Thiazolidinediones. *Endocrinol Met Clinics North Am* 1997; **26**: 553–573.

10. Saltiel A, Olefsky J. Thiazolidinediones in the treatment of insulin resistance and Type 2 diabetes. *Diabetes* 1996; **45**: 1661–1669.

11. Henry RR. Type 2 diabetes care: the role of insulin-sensitizing agents and practical implications for cardiovascular disease prevention. *Am J Med* 1998; **105(1A)**: 20S-26S.

12. Mukherjee K, Davis PJ, Crombie DL *et al* Sensitization of diabetic and obese mice to insulin by RXR agonists. *Nature* 1997; **386**: 407–410.

13. Lemberger T, Desvergne B, Wahli W. Peroxisome proliferator-active receptors: a nuclear receptor signaling pathway in lipid physiology. *Ann Rev Cell Dev Biol* 1996; **12**: 335–363.

14. Willson TM, Cobb JE, Cowan DJ *et al.* The structure–activity relationship between peroxisome-proliferator-activated receptor agonism and the antihyperglycemic activity of thiazolidinediones. *J Med Chem* 1996; **39**: 665–668.

15. Bahr M, Spelleken M, Bock M *et al.* Acute and chronic effects of troglitazone (CS-045) on isolated rat ventricular cardiomyocytes. *Diabetologia* 1996; **39**: 766–774.

16. Olefsky JM. The effects of spontaneous obesity of insulin binding, glucose transport and glucose oxidation of isolated rat adipocytes. *J Clin Invest* 1976; **57**: 842–851.

17. Abbott WG, Foley JE. Comparison of body composition, adipocyte size and glucose and insulin concentration in Pima Indians and Caucasian children. *Metabolism* 1987; **36**: 576–579.

18. Park KS, Ciaraldi TP, Carter LA *et al.* Troglitazone regulation of glucose metabolism in human skeletal muscle cultures from obese type 2 diabetic subjects. *J Clin Endocrinol Metab* 1998; **83**: 1636–1643.

19. Nolte RT, Wisely GB, Westin S *et al.* Ligand binding and co-activator assembly of the peroxisome proliferator-activated receptor gamma. *Nature* 1998; **395**: 137–143.

20. Fujiwara T, Okuno A, Yoshioka S *et al.* Suppression of hepatic gluconeogenesis in long term troglitazone treated diabetic KK and CS7BL/KSJ-db/db mice. *Metabolism* 1995; **44**: 486–490.

21. Fulgencio JP, Kohl C, Girard J *et al.* Troglitazone inhibits free fatty acid oxidation and esterification, and gluconeogenesis in isolated hepatocytes from starved rats. *Diabetes* 1996; **45**: 1556–1562.

22. Horikoshi H, Fujiwara T, Shimada M *et al.* Suppression of hepatic gluconeogenesis by CS-045 in KK mice and in perfused liver (abstr). *Diabetes* 1990; **39 (Suppl 1)**: 111A.

23. Tominaga M, Igarashi M, Daimon M *et al.* Thiazolidinediones (AD-4833 and CS-045) improve hepatic insulin resistance in streptozotocin-induced diabetic rats. *Endocrine J* 1993; **40**: 343–349.

24. Ciaraldi TP, Gilmore A, Olefsky JM *et al. In vitro* studies on the action of CS-045, a new antidiabetic agent. *Metabolism* 1990; **39**: 1056–1062.

25. Inoue Y, Tanigawa K, Nakamura S *et al.* Lack

of effect of CS-045, a new antidiabetic agent, on insulin secretion in the remnant pancreas after 90% pancreatectomy in rats. *Diabetes Res Clin Pract* 1995; **27**: 19–26.

26. Masuda K, Okamoto Y, Tsuura Y *et al.* Effects of troglitazone (CS-045) on insulin secretion in isolated rat pancreatic islets and HIT cells: an insulinotropic mechanism distinct from glibenclamide. *Diabetologia* 1995; **38**: 24–30.

27. Buckingham RE, Al-Barazanji K, Toseland CD *et al.* Peroxisome proliferator-activated receptor gamma agonist, rosiglitazone, protects against nephropathy and pancreatic islet abnormalities in Zucker fatty rats. *Diabetes* 1998; **47**: 1326–1334.

28. Kellerer M, Kroder G, Tippmer S *et al.* Troglitazone prevents glucose-induced insulin resistance of insulin receptor in rat-1 fibroblasts. *Diabetes* 1994; **43**: 447–453.

29. Kroder G, Bossenmaizer B, Kellerer M *et al.* Tumor necrosis factor alpha and hyperglycemia-induced insulin resistance: evidence for different mechanisms and different effects on insulin signaling. *J Clin Invest* 1996; **97**: 1471–1477.

30. Maegawa H, Ide R, Hasegawa M *et al.* Thiazolidine derivatives ameliorate high glucose-induced insulin resistance via the normalization of protein-tyrosine phosphatase activities. *J Biol Chem* 1995; **270**: 7724–7730.

31. Peraldi P, Xu M, Spiegelman BM. Thiazolidinediones block tumor necrosis factor-alpha-induced inhibition of insulin signalling. *J Clin Invest* 1997; **100**: 1863–1869.

32. Murase K, Odaka H, Suzuki M *et al.* Pioglitazone time-dependently reduces tumour necrosis factor-alpha level in muscle and improves metabolic abnormalities in Wistar fatty rats. *Diabetologia* 1998; **41**: 257–264.

33. Souza SC, Yamamoto M, Franciosa M *et al.* BRL 49653 blocks the lipolytic actions of tumour necrosis factor-alpha: a potential new insulin-sensitizing mechanism for thiazolidinediones. *Diabetes* 1998; **47**: 691–695.

34. Yoshioka T, Nishino H, Shiraki T *et al.* Antihypertensive effects of CS-045 treatment in obese Zucker rats. *Metabolism* 1993; **42**: 75–80.

35. Yoshimoto T, Naruse M, Nishikawa M *et al.* Antihypertensive and vasculo- and renoprotec-

tive effects of pioglitazone in genetically obese diabetic rats. *Am J Physiol* 1993; **272**: E989–E996.

36. Walker AB, Naderali EK, Chattington PD *et al.* Differential vasoactive effects of the insulin sensitizers Rosiglitazone (BRL 49653) and Troglitazone on human small arteries *in vitro*. *Diabetes* 1998; **47**: 810–814.

37. Song J, Walsh MF, Igwe R *et al.* Troglitazone reduces contraction by inhibition of vascular smooth muscle cell Ca^{2+} currents and not endothelial nitric oxide production. *Diabetes* 1997; **46**: 659–664.

38. Law RE, Meehan WP, Xi X-P *et al.* Troglitazone inhibits vascular smooth muscle cell growth and intimal hyperplasia. *J Clin Invest* 1996; **98**: 1897–1905.

39. Ishizuka T, Itaya S, Wada H *et al.* Differential effect of the antidiabetic thiazolidinediones troglitazone and pioglitazone on human platelet aggregation mechanism. *Diabetes* 1998; **47**: 1494–1500.

40. Cominacini L, Garbin U, Pastorino AM *et al.* Effects of troglitazone on *in vitro* oxidation of LDL and HDL induced by copper ions and endothelial cells. *Diabetologia* 1997; **40**: 165–172.

41. Ghazzi M, Perez J, Antonucci T *et al.* The Troglitazone Study Group and Whitcomb R: cardiac and glycemic benefits of troglitazone treatment in NIDDM. *Diabetes* 1997; **46**: 433–439.

42. Shimabukuro M, Higa S, Shinzato T *et al.* Cardioprotective effects of troglitazone in streptozotocin-induced diabetic rats. *Metabolism* 1993; **45**: 1168–1169.

43. Suter S, Nolan JJ, Wallace P *et al.* Metabolic effects of new oral hypoglycemic agent CS-045 in NIDDM subjects. *Diabetes Care* 1992; **15**: 193–203.

44. Maggs DG, Buchanan TA, Burant CF *et al.* Metabolic effects of Troglitazone Monotherapy in Type 2 Diabetes Mellitus: a randomized, double-blind, placebo-controlled trial. *Ann Int Med* 1998; **128**: 176–185.

45. Inzucchi SE, Maggs DG, Spollett GR *et al.* Efficacy and metabolic effects of metformin and troglitazone in type 2 diabetes mellitus. *N Engl J Med* 1998; **338**: 867–872.

46. Nolan JJ, Ludvik B, Beerdsen P *et al.* Improvement in glucose tolerance and insulin

resistance in obese subjects treated with troglitazone. *N Engl J Med* 1994; **331**: 1188–1193.

47. Mimura K, Umeda F, Hiramatsu S *et al*. Effects of new oral hypoglycemic agent (CS-045) on metabolic abnormalities and insulin resistance in type 2 diabetes. *Diabet Med* 1994; **11**: 685–691.

48. Yamasaki Y, Kawamori R, Wasada T *et al*. Pioglitazone (AD-4833) ameliorates insulin resistance in patients with NIDDM. AD-4833 Glucose Clamp Study Group, Japan. *Tohoku J Exp Med* 1997; **183**: 173–183.

49. Kawamori R, Matsuhisa M, Kinoshita J *et al*. Pioglitazone enhances splanchnic glucose uptake as well as peripheral glucose uptake in non-insulin-dependent diabetes mellitus. AD-4833 Clamp-IGL Study Group. *Diabetes Res Clin Pract* 1998; **41**: 35–43.

50. Prigeon RL, Kahn SE, Porte D. Effect of troglitazone on B cell function, insulin sensitivity and glycemic control in subjects with type 2 diabetes mellitus. *J Clin Endo Metab* 1998; **83**: 819–823.

51. Sironi AM, Vichi S, Gastaldelli *et al*. Effects of troglitazone on insulin action and cardiovascular risk factors in patients with non-insulin dependent diabetes. *Clin Pharmacol Therapeut* 1997; **62**: 194–202.

52. Harris MI. Impaired glucose tolerance in the US population. *Diabetes Care* 1989; **12**: 464–474.

53. Berkowitz K, Peters R, Kjos S *et al*. Effect of troglitazone on insulin sensitivity and pancreatic beta-cell function in women at high risk for NIDDM. *Diabetes* 1996; **45**: 1572–1579.

54. Metzger BE, Cho NH, Roston SM, Radvany R. Prepregnancy weight and antepartum insulin secretion predict glucose tolerance five years after gestational diabetes mellitus. *Diabetes Care* 1995; **16**: 1598–1605.

55. Peters RK, Kjos SL, Xiang A, Buchanan TA. Long-term diabetogenic effect of single pregnancy in women with previous gestational diabetes mellitus *Lancet* 1996; **347**: 227–230.

56. Antonucci T, Whitcomb R, McLain R, Lockwood D. Impaired glucose tolerance is normalized by treatment with the thiazolidinedione troglitazone. *Diabetes Care* 1997; **20**: 188–193.

57. Cavaghan M, Ehrmann D, Byrne M, Polonsky K. Treatment with the oral antidiabetic agent

Troglitazone improves beta-cell responses to glucose in subjects with impaired glucose tolerance. *J Clin Invest* 1997; **100**: 530–537.

58. Dunaif A, Scott D, Finegood D *et al*. The insulin sensitizing agent troglitazone improves metabolic and reproductive abnormalities in the polycystic ovary syndrome. *J Clin Endocrinol Metab* 1996; **81**: 3299–3306.

59. Ehrmann DA, Schneider DJ, Sobel BE *et al*. Troglitazone improves defects in insulin action, insulin secretion, ovarian steroidogenesis, and fibrinolysis in women with polycystic ovary syndrome. *J Clin Endocrinol Metab* 1997; **82**: 2108–2116.

60. Iwamoto Y, Shiraishi I, Kuzuya T *et al*. Effect of CS-045 treatment on serum proinsulin level in NIDDM patients. *Diabetes* 1993; **42 (Suppl 1)**: 57A.

61. Garg A. Dyslipoproteinemia and diabetes. *Endocrine Metab Clin N Am* 1998; **27**: 613–626.

62. Tack CJ, Demacker PN, Smits P, Stalenhoef AF. Troglitazone decreases the proportion of small, dense LDL and increases the resistance of LDL to oxidation in obese subjects. *Diabetes Care* 1998; **21**: 796–799.

63. Hirano T, Yoshino G, Kazumi T. Troglitazone and small low-density lipoprotein in type 2 diabetes. *Ann Int Med* 1998; **129**: 162–163.

64. Simonson DC. Etiology and prevalence of hypertension in diabetic patients. *Am J Hypertension* 1995; **8**: 316–320.

65. Ogihara T, Rakugi H, Ikegami H *et al*. Enhancement of insulin sensitivity by troglitazone lowers blood pressure in diabetic hypertensives. *Am J Hypertens* 1995; **8**: 316–320.

66. Hseuh WA, Law RE. Cardiovascular risk continuum: Implications of insulin resistance and diabetes. *Am J Med* 1998; **105(1A)**: 4S-14S.

67. Minamikawa J, Tanaka S, Yamauchi M *et al*. Potent inhibitory effect of troglitazone on carotic arterial thickness in type 2 diabetes. *J Clin Endocrinol Metab* 1998; **83**: 1818–1820.

68. Fonseca V, Reynolds T, Hemphill H *et al*. Effect of troglitazone on fibrinolysis and coagulation. *Diabetes* 1997; **46 (Suppl 1)**: 336.

69. Tack CJJ, Ong MKE, Lutterman JA *et al*. Insulin-induced vasodilation and endothelial function in obesity/insulin resistance. Effects of

troglitazone. *Diabetologia* 1998; **41**: 569–576.

70. Kallen CB, Lazar MA. Antidiabetic thiazolidinediones inhibit leptin (ob) gene expression in 3Te-L1 adipocytes. *Proc Natl Acad Sci USA* 1996; **93**: 5793–5796.

71. Shimizu H, Tsuchiya T, Sato N. Troglitazone reduces plasma leptin concentration, but increases hunger in NIDDM patients. *Diabetes Care* 1998; **21**: 1470–1474.

72. Nolan JJ, Olefsky JM, Nyce MR *et al*. Effect of troglitazone on leptin production. *Diabetes* 1996; **45**: 1276–1278.

73. Kumar S, Boulton AJM, Beck-Nielsen H *et al*. Troglitazone, an insulin action enhancer, improves metabolic control in NIDDM patients. *Diabetologia* 1996; **39**: 701–709.

74. Iwamoto Y, Kosaka K, Kuzuya T *et al*. Effects of troglitazone, a new hypoglycemic agent in patients with NIDDM poorly controlled by diet therapy. *Diabetes Care* 1996; **19**: 151–156.

75. Fonseca VA, Valiquett TR, Huang SM *et al*. Troglitazone monotherapy improves glycemic control in patients with Type 2 diabetes mellitus: a randomized, controlled study. *J Clin Endocrinol Metab* 1998; **83**: 3169–3175.

76. Lebowitz HE, Patel J, Dole J, Patwardhan R. Rosiglitazone monotherapy has significant glucose effect in Type 2 diabetic patients. *Diabetologia* 1998; **41** (**Suppl 1**): 922, A238.

77. Horton ES, Whitehouse F, Ghazzi MN *et al*. and the Troglitazone Study Group. Troglitazone in combination with sulfonylurea restores glycemic control in patients with type 2 diabetes. *Diabetes Care* 1998; **21**: 1462–1469.

78. Schwartz S, Raskin P, Fonseca V, Graveline JF, for the Troglitazone and Exogenous Insulin Study Group. Effect of troglitazonein insulin-treated patients with type 2 diabetes. *N Engl J Med* 1998; **338**: 861–866.

79. Buse JB, Gumbiner B, Mathias NP *et al*. Troglitazone use in insulin-treated type 2 diabetic patients. The Troglitazone Insulin Study Group. *Diabetes Care* 1998; **21**: 1455–1461.

80. Ovalle F, Bell DSH. Triple oral antidiabetic therapy in type 2 diabetes mellitus. *Endocrine Pract* 1998; **4**: 146–147.

81. Gitlin N, Neil J, Spurr CL *et al*. Two cases of severe clinical and histologic hepatotoxicity associated with troglitazone. *Ann Int Med* 1998; **129**: 36–38.

82. Neuschwander-Tetri BA, Isley WL, Oki JC *et al*. Troglitazone-induced hepatic failure leading to liver transplantation. *Ann Int Med* 1998; **129**: 38–41.

83. Watkins PB, Whitcomb RW. Hepatic dysfunction associated with troglitazone. *N Engl J Med* 1998; **338**: 916–917.

84. American Diabetes Association. Standards of medical care for patients with diabetes mellitus (Position Statement). *Diabetes Care* 1998; **21** (**Suppl 1**): S23–S31.

16

Optimal control of Type 2 diabetes: current and future prospects

Robert J Heine, Jeroen JJ de Sonnaville and Stephan JL Bakker

Introduction

Type 2 diabetes is a very common disease that is asscoiated with microvascular and macrovascular complications.[1,2] These complications largely explain the severely enhanced mortality (three- to sixfold) in this population.[3,4]

The obvious and well-known objective of treatment in Type 2 diabetes is lowering of the burden caused by these complications. A major hindrance in accomplishing this objective is that Type 2 diabetes is usually diagnosed late; this has been estimated to be approximately 7–10 years following the actual occurrence of hyperglycaemia. This delay in diagnosis allows the hyperglycaemia to cause the tissue damage: for example, already at the time of diagnosis about 30% of these patients have demonstrable diabetic retinopathy.[5,6] Probably for even longer than that, i.e. at the stage of impaired glucose tolerance or impaired fasting glucose, patients have been exposed to a cluster of cardiovascular risk factors.[7,8] This probably explains the frequent presence of macrovascular complications and the high rate of coronary events in newly diagnosed Type 2 diabetic patients.[4,9] In some studies an enhanced risk of cardiovascular disease has been observed in subjects with impaired glucose tolerance.[10,11] Several epidemiological surveys have shown high rates of obesity, dyslipidaemia, and hypertension in this high-risk group, risk factors which are known to be associated with insulin resistance.[7,8,12]

During the past few years more risk factors have been identified, some of which are also related to insulin resistance. The emergence of these other 'new' cardiovascular risk factors, as for example von Willebrand factor, PAI-1, and qualitative changes in some lipoproteins, is of great interest, as they may assist the clinician to identify patients at particular risk of developing ischaemic heart disease.[13–15]

The availability of potent, but expensive, lipid-lowering drugs has stimulated a fierce debate on the pros and cons of lipid-lowering drugs in clinical practice,[16–20] and whether the reported results are also applicable for persons with abnormal glucose tolerance.[21–24] Several relevant questions have been raised in this context: does the benefit outweigh the risk to the patient?[20] How effective is the drug in reducing the risk in the diabetic population as compared with the general population?[20,22–24] Which clinical and laboratory data are needed to make a therapeutic decision? In this chapter we will not provide an answer to all these relevant questions. The focus of our attention will be directed on the practical issues concerning the identification and treatment of the patient at risk. We will suggest a practical approach; this is to try to identify the patient who has a low risk due to the absence of the various risk factors, except hyperglycaemia.

These patients obviously still require adequate treatment to normalize glycaemia. The prevailing evidence strongly suggests that microvascular disease can be prevented by sustaining normoglycaemia. This treatment target is supported by several observational and intervention studies in Type 1, but now also in Type 2 diabetes. In our minds, normoglycaemia should be emphasized more strongly in the guidelines for clinicians.[25] A relevant question still is: does it matter how we attain and maintain normoglycaemia? On the one hand, the growing arsenal of blood-glucose-lowering agents provides us with the opportunity to achieve the normoglycaemic treatment target via several mechanisms, but on the other hand, it leaves us with the difficult question of whether we should give preference to one drug above another?[26]

For example, is there a drug to which we should give preference in newly diagnosed Type 2 diabetic patients? These considerations readily illustrate the complexity of the treatment of Type 2 diabetes. As we all know, it is a heterogeneous disease, involving insulin resistance and β-cell dysfunction.[27] Insulin resistance is a putative risk factor for cardiovascular disease, whereas β-cell dysfunction is considered to be the main cause of hyperglycaemia, caused by the inability of the β-cell to compensate for the enhanced insulin requirements. This latter abnormality may be regarded as justification for the use of insulin secretagogues and/or of insulin to supplement for the (relative) insulin deficiency. An alternative approach would be to enhance insulin sensitivity, by which one lowers the insulin requirements to a level which can be sustained, at least transiently, by the compromised β-cells.[26,28] The potential consequences of these

widely different approaches, for the cardiovascular risk in particular, have to be discussed. The ongoing United Kingdom Prospective Diabetes Study (UKPDS) provides us with information with which we can rationalize our treatment.[26]

Finally, what do we know about the efficacy of the different interventions for lowering the incidence rate of cardiovascular disease in Type 2 diabetes? As we only, at present, have data from major studies in non-diabetic populations, we have to rely on *post-hoc* analyses in the small subgroups of diabetic patients in these major studies. In this chapter we will discuss the therapeutic options in Type 2 diabetes, including those which are required to lower the burden of cardiovascular disease.

Treatment objectives

The primary objectives for the treatment of patients with diabetes mellitus are summarized in *Table 16.1*. To achieve these objectives in daily practice, treatment targets for the prevention of micro- and macroangiopathic complications were defined by the European NIDDM Policy Group in 1993[29] (*Table 16.2*); these are currently under revision.

Table 16.1
Treatment objectives.

- Relief of symptoms
- Improvement of quality of life
- Prevention of acute and chronic complications
- Reduction of morbidity and mortality
- Reduction of burden and side-effects of treatment

	Good	*Poor*
• Blood glucose (mmol/l)		
Fasting	4.4–6.1	>7.8
Post-prandial	4.4–8.0	>10.0
• Glycated haemoglobin		
HbA$_{1c}$ (%)	<6.5	>7.5
• Lipids (mmol/l)		
Total cholesterol	<5.2	>6.5
HDL-cholesterol	>1.1	<0.9
Fasting triglycerides	<1.7	>2.2
• Body-mass index (kg/m^2)		
Men	20–25	>27
Women	19–24	>26
• Blood pressure (mmHg)	<140/90	>160/95
• Smoking (cigarettes)	No	Yes

Table 16.2
Targets for control (European NIDDM Policy Group 1993).

The great importance to strive not only for normoglycaemia, but also for normalization of other risk factors for both micro- and macroangiopathy, has now been widely recognized. However, Table 16.2 ignores the fact that the risk for developing cardiovascular complications may vary greatly between individuals. The clinical question then is: is it reasonable to attain these stringent values at all costs and for any associated treatment burden in all our patients? Or should we try to focus our attention and scarce resources to those who are at high risk? For this it is essential that we understand the factors which contribute to the elevated risk, and know how to assess this risk in the individual patient.

Cardiovascular risk assessment and risk stratification in Type 2 diabetes: when and how to treat?

Risk stratification and the use of statins

Since the 1960s, attention has been focused primarily on serum cholesterol concentrations, blood pressure, and relative risks. Now a different approach seems to emerge, one in which initiation of treatment of an individual subject is based upon multiple rather than single factors and on absolute rather than relative risk. For a similar relative risk reduction, those with the highest absolute risk gain the greatest benefit of treatment.[30] Also, one has to take into consideration the balance between the obtained reduction in cardiovascular events and the incidence of adverse effects. A meta-analysis of cholesterol-lowering interventions performed prior to the statin (3-hydroxy-3-methylglutaryl-coenzyme A reductase inhibitor) era illustrates this well.[31] A great number of trials (35), with a wide range of absolute risks (1.2–127.5 coronary heart disease (CHD) deaths per 1,000 person years) were included. There was net benefit, in terms of reduction in total mortality, when the mortality from CHD was over 30 events per 1,000 person years. In the subjects with a risk below this level, an increase of total mortality

was observed in the treatment group. Based on these calculations and observations, an annual event rate of 3% per year – 30 events/1,000 person years – was accepted as a threshold of absolute risk above which cholesterol-lowering treatment should be initiated. However, statins are more potent and have been shown to have less adverse effects than the old cholesterol-lowering drugs. It has been clearly established that statins lower total mortality in populations with CHD death rates below 30 per 1,000 person years. These rates ranged from 3.9 in the WOSCOPS to 16.7 in the 4S (Table 16.3).[16,17,32] From these trials, no important side-effects were reported.

Despite their unchallenged potency, the benefits of statins in the trials are small if expressed in calculated average life extension.

Table 16.3 Efficacy of statins, aspirin and antihypertensives in the prevention of coronary heart disease (CHD) death, with absolute risks expressed in event rate per 1,000 person years (ER).

		ER_c	ER_t	$ER_c–ER_t$	RRR	NNT
Statin trials	WOSCOPS	3.9	2.6	1.3	33	156
	4S	16.7	9.7	7.1	42	28
	Care	12.0	9.6	2.4	20	84
Aspirin trials	PHS	0.5	0.2	0.3	62	690
	TPT	3.3	3.7	–0.4	–12	–
	HOT*	3.9	3.7	0.2	5	1,026
	Post-MI meta*	44.1	37.6	6.5	15	31
Hypertension trials		4.0	3.5	0.5	12	417

ER = number of subjects who died from the event × 1,000/(mean follow-up (years) × ((number of subjects – total number of subjects who died during study) + 0.5 × total number of subjects who died during study)); AR = absolute risk; ER_c = AR placebo group; ER_t = AR treatment group; $ER_c–ER_t$ = Reduction of AR; RRR = Reduction of RR (%) = 100× $(ER_c–ER_t)/ER_c$; NNT: number needed to treat to prevent one event during 5 years of trial = 1,000/(5 × $(ER_c–ER_t)$); * = total cardiovascular mortality instead of death from CHD; WOSCOPS = West of Scotland Coronary Prevention Study; 4S = Scandinavian Simvastatin Survival Study; CARE = Cholesterol and Recurrent Events Study; PHS = Physicians Health Study; TPT = Thrombosis Prevention Trial; HOT = High blood pressure Optimal Treatment trial; post-MI meta = post-MI meta-analysis.

This value was 24 days for 5.4 years of treatment in the 4S (high risk) and about 1 week for 5 years of treatment in the WOSCOPS (low risk).[33] Few will take the burden of taking a tablet every day, irrespective of costs and potential adverse events, if the benefit is expressed in this way. However, these gains are not so futile as they may seem, as they are averaged over all people receiving treatment.[34] For example, if all cancer were to be eradicated, the average gain in life expectancy would be only 1 year, although for the people who would otherwise have developed cancer the gain would be measured in decades.[35] In the field of cardiovascular risk prevention, a gain in quality-adjusted life expectancy of 2 or more months is considered important.[34] It is difficult to appreciate and more so to define what constitutes a large or small gain.[36] However, statins, just like antihypertensive drugs and aspirin, not only save lives, they also prevent non-fatal cardiovascular events such as coronary events and strokes.[37] Moreover, they may reduce morbidity of heart failure,[38] angina

pectoris, and peripheral vascular disease.[39]

Rather than using life extensions as outcomes, it is more justifiable and persuasive to express the benefits in numbers needed to treat (NNT) to prevent one cardiovascular event during 5 years of treatment.[40] The NNT resulting from the trials can be seen in *Tables 16.3–16.6* for different outcome variables. A separate table (*Table 16.7*) shows the NNTs calculated from these trials for Type 2 diabetic subjects who had already suffered a myocardial infarction. In this latter setting, the numbers are very small for any intervention. Mainly for reasons of cost-effectiveness, current guidelines recommend statin treatment when the estimated total (fatal + non-fatal) CHD event rate is 3% per year or above. This is in accordance with current recommendations for secondary prevention following a non-fatal myocardial infarction in almost all subjects. In Finland, for instance, these subjects have a rate of new events of approximately 3% per year.[41] Type 2 diabetics with no history of myocardial infarction have a cardiovascular event rate

Table 16.4 *Efficacy of statins, aspirin and antihypertensives in the prevention of non-fatal myocardial infarction, with absolute risks expressed in event rate per 1,000 person years (ER).*

		ER_c	ER_t	ER_c–ER_t	RRR	NNT
Statin trials	WOSCOPS	15.6	11.4	4.1	27	48
	4S	4.4	30.7	13.7	31	15
	Care	17.5	13.6	3.9	22	51
Aspirin trials	PHS	3.9	2.4	1.5	39	132
	TPT	8.5	5.8	2.7	32	74
	HOT	12.2	11.1	1.1	9	182
	Post-MI meta	30.5	21.7	8.8	29	23
Hypertension trials		4.6	3.9	0.7	15	282

For key, please refer to the footnote to Table 16.3.

Table 16.5 *Efficacy of statins, aspirin and antihypertensives in the prevention of fatal or non-fatal stroke, with absolute risks expressed in event rate per 1,000 person years (ER).*

		ER_c	ER_t	ER_c–ER_t	RRR	NNT
Statin trials	WOSCOPS	3.2	2.9	0.3	11	588
	4S	9.6	6.5	3.1	32	64
	Care	7.9	5.4	2.5	31	81
Aspirin trials	PHS	1.8	2.2	−0.4	−22	–
	TPT	3.0	2.9	0.0	3	5,000
	HOT	4.2	4.1	0.1	2	2,500
	Post-MI meta*	6.1	3.9	2.2	36	91
Hypertension trials		5.4	3.2	2.2	41	90

* Only non-fatal stroke included.
For key, please refer to the footnote to Table 16.3.

Table 16.6 *Efficacy of statins, aspirin and antihypertensives in the prevention of overall mortality, with absolute risks expressed in event rate per 1,000 person years (ER).*

		ER_c	ER_t	ER_c–ER_t	RRR	NNT
Statin trials	WOSCOPS	8.5	6.7	1.9	22	106
	4S	22.6	15.8	6.8	30	29
	Care	19.8	18.1	1.7	9	116
Aspirin trials	PHS	4.1	4.0	0.2	4	1,176
	TPT	12.2	13.0	−0.7	−6	–
	HOT	8.6	8.0	0.6	7	332
	Post-MI meta	48.7	42.9	5.8	12	34
Hypertension trials		11.3	9.8	1.5	13	132

For key, please refer to the footnote to Table 16.3.

which is at least as high (*Table 16.8*).[41] Given this fact, one could argue for primary and secondary prevention in every person with Type 2 diabetes. However, this would be an oversimplification, since the cardiovascular risk inevitably will vary greatly between subjects and populations.[42] The increased incidence of cardiovascular disease in Type 2 diabetes can, at least for the greater part, be explained by the presence of insulin resistance. Many 'classic' and other cardiovascular risk factors have been identified which cluster with each

Table 16.7 *Numbers needed to treat (NNT) for different outcome variables standardized for the risk in Type 2 diabetic subjects who have suffered a myocardial infarction.*

		CHD death	Non-fatal MI	Stroke	Total mortality
Statin trials	WOSCOPS	8	9	53	12
	4S	7	8	18	9
	Care	14	12	19	28
Aspirin trials	PHS	4	7	–	64
	TPT	–	8	196	–
	HOT	55	28	294	37
	Post-MI meta	18	9	16	23
Hypertension trials		23	17	14	20

For key, please refer to the footnote to Table 16.3.

Table 16.8 *Incidence of cardiovascular events in relation to history of myocardial infarction in subjects with Type 2 diabetes and in non-diabetic subjects in events per 1,000 person years.*

	Non-diabetic subjects		Subjects with Type 2 diabetes	
	Prior MI	No prior MI	Prior MI	No prior MI
Death from CVD	26	3	73	25
Fatal or non-fatal MI	30	5	78	32
Fatal or non-fatal stroke	12	3	34	16

other. Examples of these 'new' risk factors are von Willebrand factor, PAI-1, apolipoprotein B, and hypertriglyceridaemia.[12–14,43] This phenomenon is now often referred to as the insulin-resistance syndrome. General guidelines indicating primary prevention through cholesterol lowering with statins in every Type 2 diabetic patient will consequently result in overtreatment among those with a low risk. Also, one has to assume that the results of

statin trials in non-diabetic subjects are applicable to diabetic subjects. This seems to be the case. The 4S and the CARE study accidentally include some Type 2 diabetic subjects. *Post-hoc* analyses of these data revealed at least a comparable efficacy.[32,44] This should not come as a surprise. The insulin-resistance-associated cardiovascular risk factors are also common in non-diabetic subjects with established cardiovascular disease.[45] Therefore, the pathogenesis of cardiovascular disease in Type 2 diabetics seems not to differ widely from that in the glucose-tolerant population. The apparent importance of the insulin-resistance-associated risk factors may also allow us to identify a subgroup of Type 2 diabetics with a relatively low cardiovascular risk in whom statin treatment may not confer a marked benefit. These are likely to be the persons with no cardiovascular risk factors apart from hyperglycaemia. Not included in the Framingham risk tables, but very important for risk assessment in Type 2 diabetic subjects, is hypertriglyceridaemia.[43] If hypertriglyceridaemia is present, a diabetic subject should be considered to be at high risk.

Aspirin

Aspirin is an effective and safe drug in high-risk patients.[46] In these patients it lowers the rate of CHD death, non-fatal myocardial infarction, stroke, and total mortality (*Tables 16.3–16.6*). If we extrapolate the results obtained in a subgroup with a CHD death event rate of 44.1 per 1,000 person years (*Table 16.3*, post MI meta-analysis) to Type 2 diabetic subjects that have suffered a myocardial infarction, it can be seen that efficacy of aspirin is comparable to that of statins (*Table 16.7*). Aspirin trials with low event rates, ranging from 0.5 CHD deaths per 1,000 person years in the Physicians Health Study (PHS) to 3.9 in the Hypertension Optimal Treatment (HOT),[47–49] only show a consistent reduction in incidence of non-fatal myocardial infarction (*Tables 16.3–16.6*), but not of total mortality. This may be due to aspirin-related gastrointestinal bleeding and haemorrhagic stroke. The NNT to prevent one non-fatal myocardial infarction is very high in these low-risk subjects (*Table 16.4*). In this scenario, the benefit is outweighed by treatment-associated adverse events.

Again, no trials in Type 2 diabetic subjects have been performed, but subanalyses of those included in the studies teach us that Type 2 diabetics benefit to a degree comparable to non-diabetic subjects.[49,50] This is again consistent with the central role of insulin resistance in the pathophysiology of Type 2 diabetes mellitus and cardiovascular disease. An increased tendency to clot formation and an impaired fibrinolysis have been identified as components of the insulin-resistance syndrome.[51–53] As acute thrombus formation on pre-existent atherosclerotic lesions is now considered the major cause of most acute cardiovascular events, it is scarcely astonishing that aspirin has been demonstrated to consistently reduce cardiovascular event rates and total mortality in high-risk populations.

Blood-pressure-lowering agents

Approximately 40% of Type 2 diabetic patients are hypertensive (blood pressure above 140/90 mmHg) at diagnosis.[54] In albuminuric (>300 mg/24 hours) patients, the prevalence of hypertension is even as high as 60%.[54] Insulin resistance seems to play a major role in the association between Type 2 diabetes and hypertension. In patients with diabetes, hypertension has been shown to enhance the risk of coronary events, strokes, congestive heart failure, and peripheral vascular disease. Also, progression of retinopathy and renal failure is accelerated with elevated blood pressure.[55,56] Recently a large randomized trial has investigated the efficacy of treatment of hypertension in patients with Type 2 diabetes mellitus.[57] The recently published HOT study also investigated the association between target blood pressures and major cardiovascular events during antihypertensive treatment in 1,501 patients with diabetes mellitus (probably mostly Type 2).[49] The results of both studies showed a clear benefit in major cardiovascular events and cardiovascular mortality when the diastolic blood pressure was lowered to 80–85 mmHg or below. The total mortality showed the same tendency. It is of great interest that in the HOT study these results were achieved while 78% of the patients were receiving felodipine, one of the calcium channel blockers, a class of drugs that has been suggested to increase the incidence of coronary events in both non-diabetic and diabetic hypertensive subjects.[58,59] In two recent trials in diabetic subjects, calcium channel blockers were compared with angiotensin-converting enzyme (ACE) inhibitors.[58,59] The only conclusion that can be drawn from these studies, due to the lower rate of cardiovascular events, is that ACE inhibitors should be preferred above calcium channel blockers. The data of the HOT study suggest that calcium channel blockers can safely be added if blood pressure cannot be adequately managed by ACE inhibitors.

Diuretics and beta-blockers are the only antihypertensive drugs that have unequivocally been proven to lower cardiovascular and total mortality. In meta-analyses including low- and high-risk populations, these drugs decreased CHD death, non-fatal MI, strokes, and overall mortality.[60] If the risk reduction achieved in a relatively low-risk population (CHD death event rate of 4.0 per 1,000 person years, *Table 16.3*) is extrapolated to high-risk Type 2 diabetic subjects, their efficacy expressed in NNT is even comparable to those with statins and aspirin (*Table 16.7*). Diuretics and beta-blockers have the potential disadvantage of enhancing pre-existing insulin resistance. Therefore, it has been suggested that these drugs should be avoided in diabetics.[61,62] This suggestion is not justified. As already mentioned, subjects at high risk are almost always insulin resistant. Also, when these drugs are used at a low dose, the effect on insulin

sensitivity is negligible.[63] Thus, the disadvantage is the same for high-risk groups and Type 2 diabetics. This is in good agreement with recent results, which show that diuretics and beta-blockers have the same protective effect in Type 2 diabetics as in glucose-tolerant populations.[57,60]

Treatment goals and benefits

Currently, no studies are available that allow us to define precisely the indications for statins or blood-pressure-lowering drugs in Type 2 diabetes. In a largely non-diabetic population in the CARE study, it was suggested that no benefit was obtained in subjects with low-density lipid (LDL)-cholesterol concentrations below 3.2 mmol/l.[64] For the Type 2 diabetic population it is important that this study also found that the reduction of triglycerides with pravastatin contributed to the reduction of coronary events, independent of the effect on LDL-cholesterol. Triglycerides are an important risk factor in Type 2 diabetic subjects, probably also due to their association with small dense LDL particles.[43] On the grounds of their proven efficacy and low adverse event rate, we strongly support the recent recommendation that statins should be prescribed as secondary prevention to patients with diabetes whose total cholesterol is above 4.0 mmol/l,[65] or whose triglycerides are above 2.2 mmol/l.[24] The recommendation to treat residual hypertriglyceridaemia with a fibric acid or a nicotinic acid derivative[24] is not supported by evidence from randomized clinical trials. Primary prevention should be initiated at a lower estimated cardiovascular risk than the normally recommended 3% per year on the basis of the Framingham risk tables, because these tables do not include hypertriglyceridaemia and other additional risk factors that are frequently present in diabetic patients. An easier and more practical approach is to withhold statin treatment in those without additional risk factors. Blood pressure-lowering treatment, when initiated, should aim at a value of 150/85 mmHg or below.[49,57] Aspirin should, if there are no contraindications, be given to any diabetic person with one or more risk factors including hypertriglyceridaemia, and always in the case of secondary prevention.[50,65]

Treatment of hyperglycaemia

The majority of patients with Type 2 diabetes are relatively asymptomatic at diagnosis, i.e. they do not complain of the classic hyperglycaemic triad of thirst, polyuria, and weight loss. Vague symptoms such as dry mouth, lethargy, and poor concentration may be present, but are often attributed to age, not to diabetes. In general, these patients have fasting glucose levels below 15 mmol/l. The current therapeutic options in these patients include lifestyle adjustments, oral hypoglycaemic agents, and insulin treatment[29,66] (Table 16.9).

Primary insulin therapy

Primary insulin therapy should be considered in lean, symptomatic patients with high fasting glucose values (>15 mmol/l).[67] These patients are likely to have ordinary Type 1 diabetes or slow-onset Type 1 diabetes. This 'latent autoimmune diabetes in adults (LADA)' may mimic Type 2 diabetes.[68] The response to oral hypoglycaemic therapy is often poor and of short duration, as insulin deficiency develops with 1–3 years. The use of sulphonylurea in these patients may even enhance the rate at which insulin deficiency develops. Therefore it is of clinical relevance to recognize these patients at an early stage. Initial treatment with insulin, as in fact is the case in the honeymoon phase of Type 1 diabetes, allows the use of low dosages and facilitates the control of glycaemia.[69]

Lifestyle adjustments

Lifestyle adjustments (i.e. proper nutrition, physical exercise, and smoking cessation) are the first steps in the management of patients

Step 1	Lifestyle intervention: diet, physical activity and stop smoking
Step 2	Non-obese: sulphonylureas or acarbose Obese: metformin or acarbose
Step 3	Sulphonylureas; metformin; acarbose in combination (maximum of two agents)
Step 4	Self-monitoring of blood glucose
Step 5	Isophane insulin at bedtime, combined with oral hypoglycaemic agents (maximum of two)
Step 6	Isophane insulin twice daily
Step 7	Add short-acting insulin/start premix insulin

Table 16.9
Glycaemic treatment of Type 2 diabetes.

with only moderate hyperglycaemia. Attention is focused on lowering saturated fat intake to less than 10% of total calories in order to reduce the high risk of heart disease.[70] Restricting energy intake to realistic target levels may help the patient to lose weight. Although difficult to achieve, modest weight loss and exercise have beneficial effects on glycaemic control, serum lipid values, and blood pressure. When the fasting blood glucose target (in general, a fasting blood glucose value of <6.1 mmol/l or HbA_{1c} <6.5%) is not achieved within 3 months, treatment with oral hypoglycaemic agents should be considered. Cigarette smoking is an important modifiable risk factor for cardiovascular disease, and probably more so than in the general population. Moreover, it has been identified as an independent risk factor for retinopathy and nephropathy in Type 1 diabetes.[71] Therefore, especially in patients with diabetes, smoking habits deserve the attention of the diabetes team. In general, it appears difficult to persuade people to cessate this harmful habit, even when nicotine replacement (e.g. chewing gum, nicotine patches) is applied in order to minimize withdrawal effects.

Oral hypoglycaemic agents

Sulphonylureas, metformin, and acarbose are similarly effective in lowering blood glucose in patients with Type 2 diabetes mellitus[72] (*Table 16.10*). The clinician should be aware of side-effects and drug interactions, particularly in the elderly. Since β-cell function gradually decreases in the natural course of the disease, failure of oral agents should not primarily, as is often the case, be attributed to poor patient compliance.

Sulphonylureas (SUs) stimulate insulin secretion by promoting closure of the ATP-dependent potassium channels on the pancreatic β-cells. SUs are good first-choice agents in non-obese patients.[73] Due to their insulin-enhancing effect, weight gain is often a consequence of treatment. This is not observed with oral hypoglycaemic agents, which do not stimulate insulin secretion as do, for example, metformin and acarbose. The most serious side-effect of SUs is long-lasting hypoglycaemia, which can be avoided by using the lowest possible starting dose and by selecting short-acting SUs (e.g. glipizide or gliclazide), especially in the elderly.

	Initial dose (mg)	Maximum total daily dose (mg)
Sulphonylureas		
Tolbutamide	500	2,000
Glibenclamide	2.5	15
Glipizide	2.5	20
Gliclazide	80	240
Glimepiride	1	6
Metformin	500	3,000
Acarbose	50	600

Table 16.10
Oral agents used to lower blood glucose in Type 2 diabetes.

Short-acting non-SU insulin secretagogues (e.g. repaglinide and nateglinide) are being developed which probably bear a lower risk of serious hypoglycaemia.

The vascular system (heart and large vessels) also has SU receptors associated with ATP-dependent potassium channels. These channels play an important role in the protection of the myocardium against ischaemic reperfusion damage, and their closure by SUs could lead to amplified ischaemic damage. Theoretically, selective SU derivatives which act on β-cells, but not on the cardiac muscle (as has now been demonstrated for gliclazide and glimepiride), may for this reason be preferred above non-selective SU (glibenclamide, tolbutamide), especially in patients with cardiovascular disease.[74,75] However, so far there is no real evidence to support this preliminary recommendation. Further studies comparing selective and non-selective SU derivatives are warranted to elucidate this putative problem.

Weight loss, liver or renal impairment, alcohol, or co-medication (e.g. sulphonamides) may necessitate dose reduction in order to prevent hypoglycaemia. Flushing may sometimes occur when sulphonylureas are combined with use of alcohol. Plasma creatinine levels should be checked annually.

Metformin lowers blood glucose primarily by reducing hepatic glucose production. It is a good first-choice drug in obese, insulin-resistant patients, as it does not induce weight gain.[76,77] Gastrointestinal side-effects (e.g. nausea, diarrhoea) are usually transient and dose dependent; therefore a low dose is recommended initially (e.g. 500 mg once or twice a day). Less than 5% of patients do not tolerate metformin. Because of the risk of lactic acidosis, metformin should not be used in patients with severe renal or liver impairment, chronic hypoxaemia, or a history of alcohol misuse.

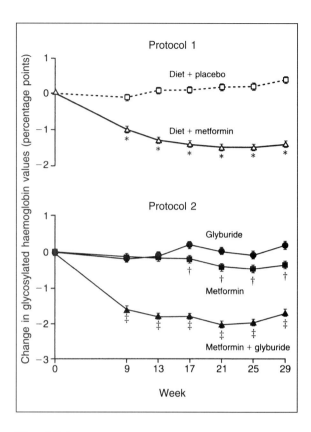

Fig. 16.1
*Mean (± SE) changes in glycosylated haemoglobin values in patients with NIDDM who were enrolled in Protocol 1 or 2; * indicates differences (p < 0.001) between the groups in Protocol 1, † indicates significant differences (p < 0.01) between the metformin and glyburide groups, and ‡ indicates significant differences (p < 0.001) between the combination therapy and glyburide groups. Reproduced with permission from DeFronzo RA, Goodman AM. N Eng J Med 1995; **333**: 541–549.*

Acarbose retards intestinal glucose absorption by inhibiting the hydrolysis of polysaccharides in the gut.[78] It can be given as a first-line or second-line drug in obese and non-obese patients, and particularly to those with post-prandial hyperglycaemia. Common gastrointestinal side-effects (e.g. flatulence, abdominal cramps and diarrhoea) are due to the fermentation of undigested sugars in the colon. Tolerance is improved by a low starting dose (50 mg/day), which is slowly increased at weekly intervals. Acarbose does not cause weight gain.

Combination therapy of two oral drugs is often required to achieve good blood glucose control. The various hypoglycaemic agents potentiate each other, as their mechanisms of action are different (*Fig. 16.1*). If the glycaemic targets cannot be achieved, insulin therapy is preferred to the addition of a third oral hypoglycaemic agent.

Secondary insulin therapy

Insulin therapy is indicated when the combination of two oral agents fails to establish glycaemic target values (secondary failure).

A simple, effective regimen combines 8 IU isophane insuline (neutral protamine Hagedorn; NPH) at bedtime with oral blood-glucose-lowering agents (sulphonylurea, metformin, or acarbose) during the day. The most experience exists with sulphonylurea and/or metformin.[79–81] Besides its safety, effectiveness, and feasibility, the main advantage of this combination therapy is the prevention of weight gain despite improvements in glycaemic control. When combining insulin with acarbose, patients must be aware that hypoglycaemia must be corrected by taking glucose and not complex carbohydrates or polysaccharides (e.g. sucrose). The insulin dose is adjusted with 2–4 IU twice weekly until the fasting glucose target (4.4–6.1 mmol/l) is reached.

If at this stage the HbA_{1c} target is not achieved, oral drugs are stopped and a twice-daily isophane insulin regimen (before breakfast and dinner) is started. The morning dose is adjusted according to glucose levels before dinner (4.4–6.1 mmol/l). Some advise to continue metformin in overweight persons to minimize further rise of body-weight.[79] Alternatively, the classic regimen comprises a twice-daily mixture of 30% short-acting insulin and 70% isophane insulin (e.g. 10 IU before breakfast and 5 IU before dinner). Although it may further encourage weight gain, snacks between main meals and at bedtime are mandatory, to prevent hypoglycaemia. The major disadvantage of this latter regimen as compared with the former are the necessity of two injections, the more complex education requirements, and the greater weight gain.

Therapeutic education

Diabetes education (e.g. home blood-glucose monitoring) is the main tool for achieving good glycaemic control with lowest risk of hypoglycaemia in patients treated with insulin. In patients treated with neutral protamine Hagedorn (NPH)-insulin once or twice daily, only fasting and pre-dinner glucose values are needed for adjustments of insulin doses. In patients treated with short-acting or premixture insulin, pre-lunch and evening glucose values are also requested, due to the increased risk of hypoglycaemia at these moments.

Diabetes education is a continuous process which is essential for successful self-care (*Table 16.11*). Diabetes education is not primarily aimed at making patients more knowledgeable about their disease, but to provide them with skills and tools to manage their treatment better. It may help them better adapt the diabetes control to the constant changes in daily life.[82] Especially in patients treated with insulin injections, self-monitoring of blood glucose is a prerequisite, as it may improve quality of glycaemic control, safety of treatment, patient compliance, and self-confidence.

- Aims of treatment
- Nutritional requirements and meal planning
- Benefits of physical activity
- Interaction of food intake, physical activity, and oral blood-glucose-lowering drugs/insulin
- Improvements in lifestyle (e.g. stop smoking, reduce excess alcohol intake)
- How to cope with emergencies and special activities (e.g. illness, hypoglycaemia, physical exercise)
- Signs, symptoms, and prevention of chronic complications (e.g. foot care)
- Self-monitoring of blood glucose, significance of values, and action to be taken
- Insulin injection technique, when required
- Practice must accompany knowledge

Table 16.11
What the patient with Type 2 diabetes should know.

Organization of care

Diabetes is a serious and chronic disorder and therefore requires a well-organized and targeted therapeutic approach. Ideally, the care structure needs to enhance a multidisciplinary team and a quality programme by which the quality of delivered care can be monitored.[83] The major objectives of diabetes care include the correction of the metabolic abnormalities in order to avoid the occurrence of complications, and to limit as much as possible the treatment-related adverse effects. For example, the benefit of attaining normoglycaemia should always, at an individual level, be balanced against the risks of severe hypoglycaemia.[79] Other possible adverse effects of therapy which have to be considered are (further) weight gain, often seen with drugs that enhance insulin levels, and gastrointestinal side-effects of the oral hypoglyaemic agents.[66,72]

Requirements of care

In order to accomplish the above-mentioned targets one has to keep in mind that:

- we are dealing with a large and growing population of elderly patients with frequent occurrence of co-morbidity;
- diabetes is a complex disease, with somatic and psychosocial aspects;
- persons with diabetes play an important role in their own care; in fact they should be enabled to share responsibility for accomplishing treatment targets;
- diabetes treatment encompasses both glycaemic control and monitoring/surveillance of complications.

The large number of patients and the complex treatment requirements make it necessary to utilize primary-care facilities for this purpose.

However, one has to realize that, at least in many countries, primary care has not been developed and designed for structured care of a chronic disease or for preventive medicine in general. On the contrary, the activities in primary care are patient driven, i.e. by symptoms and complaints; thus attention is focused on the major actual complaint of the patient. The great risk therefore is that time allocated for diabetes control always has to compete for complaints/symptoms of other ailments (e.g. arthrosis), during consultation.

In order to be able to accommodate diabetes care in the primary-care setting, the following requirements have to be fulfilled.

- Educational facilities need to be present. Only structured education will enable the patient to share the responsibility of achieving the pre-defined targets of therapy. Education has to be provided by trained educators, thus preferably by nurses and/or dieticians.
- Facilities to monitor metabolic control need to be present. These include measurements of blood glucose, serum lipids, and micro-albuminuria. Regular visits, mostly at 3-month intervals, have to be scheduled for glycaemic control. At these visits, well-being and symptoms suggestive for hyper- or hypoglycaemic episodes have to be assessed, and parameters of glycaemic control (fasting blood glucose/HbA$_{1c}$) be measured and discussed with the patient.
- Glycaemic control assessments have to be translated to clinical decision-making. How is the decision made to increase the dose of the blood-glucose-lowering drug or to transfer the patient from oral hypoglycaemic agents to insulin treatment?

These treatment steps, seemingly simple, are often not followed.[84,85] Several barriers have been identified and attributed to either patient-

or doctor-related factors or to the deficiencies in the care organization. Therefore, these barriers need to be addressed by implementing treatment guidelines which have been approved by the primary-care physician. In addition, the organization has to facilitate the required treatment steps by providing the opportunity for teaching home blood-glucose monitoring and to acquire the required skills for insulin treatment (e.g. insulin injection technique, coping with incipient hypoglycaemia).

The annual review

The annual review can be considered as the key visit to the diabetes team. During the visit the occurrence of complications is surveyed and the general well-being is assessed. Also the educational needs of the patients have to be estimated. Presence of complications can be assessed in several ways:

- diabetic eye complications, by ophthalmoscopy or fundus photography;
- kidney damage, by measuring albumin excretion rates;
- foot problems, by inspection of the feet and footwear;
- ischaemic heart disease, by asking for symptoms and smoking habits, and performance of physical and laboratory examination, including blood pressure, peripheral pulses, and serum lipids;
- neuropathy, by asking for the specific symptoms suggestive for sensory abnormalities and autonomic impairment, including sexual function.

These findings have to be recorded and discussed with the patient by the treating physician. These results should also be used to review the therapeutic and the educational needs. Taken together, the organizational requirements for diabetes care are very high.[29] The large number of patients does not allow centralized treatment in specialized clinics, and the therapeutic requirements as defined above make it very difficult to implement this care in general practice. To facilitate the implementation it is necessary to define exactly what the minimal requirements are, both in terms of facilities and in terms of personnel.

For individual patient care, the following care functions rather than professionals, should be made available.

- Medical care. This can be a general practitioner or diabetologist.
- Education: diabetes nurse/physician.
- Nutritional advice: dietician.
- Foot-care advice: nurse, podotherapist, or physician.
- The annual review of complications and risk factors require the additional support of an ophthalmologist and/or the possibility of fundus photography.

Obviously, when complications are present or psychological problems occur, other additional professional care providers need to be available. These include, amongst others, the ophthalmologist, having the facilities to treat diabetes-related eye complications, the psychologist, experienced in the treatment of persons with diabetes, the nephrologist, the cardiologist, and the vascular surgeon. The large variety of different professions involved in diabetes care makes it necessary to coordinate strictly these functions and to emphasize the importance of communication. In a primary-care setting, the responsibility has to be carried either by the general practitioner or by a diabetes clinic, facilitating the care for the general practitioner. This already illustrates how important it is to be very explicit about

how to organize the care for the diabetic patients in a particular region. This choice determines who is responsible, how to communicate, and how to allocate resources.

Quality monitoring

A quality development programme is mandatory for the assessment of whether the results of the provided care agrees with the set of predefined goals and criteria.

Various criteria may be considered for this purpose:

- Organization of care: A relevant question in this context is: do all patients benefit in a similar way from the diabetes care provided? This requires a proper registration of the diabetic patients in a region.
- Process of care: What is the proportion of patients undergoing the annual review process?
- Efficiency of care: Several parameters are required to answer this specific question. These may include metabolic and clinical outcome data, quality-of-life parameters, and costs.

How to implement diabetes care at a regional level?

The development and implementation of any care system should be guided by and is dependent on the available health-care system and resources. It is therefore important for a specific region, however defined, to make a choice for a certain diabetes-care system. This has to be explicit and all parties involved, thus both professionals and patients, have to be informed. This will avoid competing initiatives, confusing referrals of patients, and counterproductive resource allocation.

They key players at a regional level, the 'task force', should include representatives of the regional hospital, primary health care, diabetes educators, dieticians, podotherapists, and the patients' association. A well-known point of debate or controversy is whether the inclusion of one of the potential payers (government or health insurance company) is helpful at an early stage. Our view is that an early involvement of this important player in the field is a must. Early involvement of these representatives has stimulated rather than inhibited commitment and therefore the process of implementation of structured care in our region.[25]

Concomitantly, the introduction of a quality development programme is mandatory to enable monitoring of the number of patients undergoing the prescribed annual review examination. Taken together, all parties involved, thus payers, professionals, and patients alike, share responsibility for the development of the diabetes-care structure that is required to achieve an appropriate quality of diabetes care.

Future developments

New drugs will become available and insight into the pathophysiology should improve. Perhaps, more importantly, we should be able to estimate more reliably individual risks. The near future will probably bring us handheld computers which guide our estimation of the absolute risk of subjects, and help us to choose the appropriate therapy. Cardiovascular risk factors such as waist measurement, fasting, and post-prandial triglycerides, microalbuminuria, LDL size, and apolipoprotein B will probably be included. Currently, it seems unlikely that one unifying risk factor will replace all others. Several potentially interesting oral agents with different hypoglycaemic

and hypolipidaemic properties, and side-effects are currently under study. The most promising agents for the near future are mentioned below.

The mode of action of thiazolidinedione derivatives (troglitazone and rosiglitazone) is mediated by binding to the peroxisome proliferator-activated receptor gamma (PPAR-γ). This results in an improvement of insulin sensitivity (enhanced insulin-mediated glucose uptake), as reflected by lowering glucose and insulin levels.[86] The hypoglycaemic effect is comparable to that of SU or metformin, and additive in combination therapy.[87] A potentially important advantage of thiazolidinedione derivatives in comparison to other oral hypoglycaemic agents are the beneficial effects on serum lipids and other compounds of the insulin-resistance syndrome. Of interest also is the apparent low failure rates. The most important side-effect is hepatic toxicity. As a few patients died due to hepatic failure, studies with troglitazone were cancelled in Europe in 1998. In the USA and Japan, new guidelines have been issued, urging physicians to assess more frequently liver function during the first year of troglitazone use.

Pramlintide is a synthetic analogue of the human β-cell hormone amylin. Its hypoglycaemic effect is assumed to be due to modulation of the rate of gastric emptying and to inhibition of hepatic glucose output by suppressing glucagon secretion during physiologic conditions, but not during hypoglycaemia. Various studies in patients with Types 1 and 2 diabetes have shown reduction in HbA_{1c} associated with improvements in especially post-prandial glucose excursions, without weight gain. Nausea and vomiting are the most frequent reported side-effects.[72,87]

Repaglinide, a benzoic acid derivative, is a non-sulphonylurea insulin-releasing drug. It has a short hypoglycaemic effect and has therefore to be prescribed before every main meal, thus in general, three times a day. Owing to its short duration of action, the risk of hypoglycaemia is low. No information is yet available on cardiovascular effects, i.e. whether it is specifically targeted to the pancreatic β-cell sulphonylurea receptor.[72,88]

References

1. Harris MI, Hadden WC, Knowler WC, Bennett PH. Prevalence of diabetes and impaired glucose tolerance and plasma glucose levels in US population aged 20–74 years. *Diabetes* 1987; **36**: 523–534.

2. Klein R. Hyperglycaemia and microvascular and macrovascular disease in diabetes. *Diabetes Care* 1995; **18**: 258–268.

3. Garcia MJ, McNamara PM, Gordon T, Kannel WB. Morbidity and mortality in diabetics in the Framingham population. Sixteen year follow-up study. *Diabetes* 1974; **23**: 105–111.

4. Turner RC, Milns H, Neil HA *et al*. Risk factors for coronary artery disease in non-insulin dependent diabetes mellitus. *Br Med J* 1998; **316**: 823–828.

5. Harris MI, Klein R, Welborn TA, Knuiman MW. Onset of NIDDM occurs at least 4–7 years before clinical diagnosis. *Diabetes Care* 1992; **15**: 815–819.

6. Heine RJ, Mooy JM. Impaired glucose tolerance and unidentified diabetes. *Postgrad Med J* 1996; **72**: 67–71.

7. Haffner SM, Stern MP, Hazuda HP *et al*. Cardiovascular risk factors in confirmed prediabetic individuals. Does the clock of coronary heart disease start ticking before the onset of clinical diabetes? *JAMA* 1990; **263**: 2893–2898.

8. De Vegt F, Dekker JM, Stehouwer CDA *et al*. The 1997 ADA versus the 1985 WHO criteria for the diagnosis of abnormal glucose tolerance: poor agreement in the Hoorn Study. *Diabetes Care* 1998; **21**: 1686–1690.

9. Turner R, Cull C, Holman R. United Kingdom Prospective Diabetes Study 17: a 9-year update of a randomized, controlled trial on the effect of improved metabolic control on complications in non-insulin-dependent diabetes mellitus. *Ann Int Med* 1996; **124**: 136–145.

10. Fuller JH, Shipley MJ, Rose G *et al*. Coronary-heart-disease risk and impaired glucose tolerance. The Whitehall study. *Lancet* 1980; **1**: 1373–1376.

11. Alberti KG. The clinical implications of impaired glucose tolerance. *Diabetic Med* 1996; **13**: 927–937.

12. Reaven GM, Banting lecture 1988. Role of insulin resistance in human disease. *Diabetes* 1988; **37**: 1595–1607.

13. Stehouwer CD, Nauta JJ, Zeldenrust GC *et al*. Urinary albumin excretion, cardiovascular disease, and endothelial dysfunction in non-insulin-dependent diabetes mellitus. *Lancet* 1992; **340**: 319–323.

14. Gray RP, Yudkin JS, Patterson DL. Plasminogen activator inhibitor: a risk factor for myocardial infarction in diabetic patients. *Br Heart J* 1993; **69**: 228–232.

15. Austin MA, Breslow JL, Hennekens CH *et al*. Low-density lipoprotein subclass patterns and risk of myocardial infarction. *JAMA* 1988; **260**: 1917–1921.

16. Anonymous. Randomised trial of cholesterol lowering in 4444 patients with coronary heart disease: the Scandinavian Simvastatin Survival Study (4S). *Lancet* 1994; **344**: 1383–1389.

17. Shepherd J, Cobbe SM, Ford I *et al*. Prevention of coronary heart disease with pravastatin in men with hypercholesterolemia. West of Scotland Coronary Prevention Study Group. *N Engl J Med* 1995; **333**: 1301–1307.

18. Sacks FM, Pfeffer MA, Moye LA *et al*. The effect of pravastatin on coronary events after myocardial infarction in patients with average cholesterol levels. Cholesterol and Recurrent Events Trial investigators. *N Engl J Med* 1996; **335**: 1001–1009.

19. Frick MH, Elo O, Haapa K *et al*. Helsinki Heart Study: primary-prevention trial with gemfibrozil in middle-aged men with dyslipidemia. Safety of treatment, changes in risk factors, and incidence of coronary heart disease. *N Engl J Med* 1987; **317**: 1237–1245.

20. Huttunen JK, Heinonen OP, Manninen V *et al*. The Helsinki Heart Study: an 8.5-year safety and mortality follow-up. *J Int Med* 1994; **235**: 31–39.

21. Durrington P. Statins and fibrates in the management of diabetic dyslipidemia. *Diabetic Med* 1997; **14**: 513–516.
22. Pyörälä K, Pedersen TR, Kjekshus J *et al.* Cholesterol lowering with simvastatin improves prognosis of diabetic patients with coronary heart disease. A subgroup analysis of the Scandinavian Simvastatin Survival Study (4S). *Diabetes Care* 1997; **20**: 614–620.
23. Koskinen P, Manttari M, Manninen V *et al.* Coronary heart disease incidence in NIDDM patients in the Helsinki Heart Study. *Diabetes Care* 1992; **15**: 820–825.
24. Haffner SM. Management of dyslipidemia in adults with diabetes. *Diabetes Care* 1998; **21**: 160–178.
25. De Sonnaville JJJ, Bouma M, Colly LP *et al.* Sustained good glycaemic control in NIDDM patients by implementation of structured care in general practice: 2-year follow-up study. *Diabetologia* 1997; **40**: 1334–1340.
26. Anonymous. UK Prospective Diabetes Study (UKPDS) Group. Intensive blood-glucose control with sulphonylureas or insulin compred with conventional treatment and risk of complications in patients with Type 2 diabetes (UKPDS 33). *Lancet* 1998; **352**: 837–853.
27. Yki-Jarvinen H. Pathogenesis of non-insulin-dependent diabetes mellitus. *Lancet* 1994; **343**: 91–95.
28. Nolan JJ, Ludvik B, Beerdsen P *et al.* Improvement in glucose tolerance and insulin resistance in obese subjects treated with troglitazone. *N Engl J Med* 1994; **331**: 1188–1193.
29. Alberti KG, Gries FA, Jervell J, Krans HM. A desktop guide for the management of non-insulin-dependent diabetes mellitus (NIDDM): an update. European NIDDM Policy Group. *Diabetic Med* 1994; **11**: 899–909.
30. Smith GD, Egger M. Who benefits from medical interventions? *Br Med J* 1994; **308**: 72–74.
31. Smith GD, Song F, Sheldon TA. Cholesterol lowering and mortality: the importance of considering initial levels of risk. *Br Med J* 1993; **306**: 1367–1373.
32. Sacks FM, Pfeffer MA, Moye LA *et al.* The effect of pravastatin in coronary events after myocardial infarction in patients with average cholesterol levels. Cholesterol and Recurrent Events Trial investigators. *N Engl J Med* 1996; **335**: 1001–1009.
33. Krut LH. On the statins, correcting plasma lipid levels, and preventing the clinical sequelae of atherosclerotic coronary heart disease. *Am J Cardiol* 1998; **81**: 1045–1046.
34. Richardson WS, Detsky AS. Users' guides to the medical literature. VII. How to use a clinical decision analysis. B. What are the results and will they help me in caring for my patients? Evidence Based Medicine Working Group. *JAMA* 1995; **273**: 1610–1613.
35. Robson J. Information needed to decide about cardiovascular treatment in primary care. *Br Med J* 1997; **314**: 277–280.
36. Wright JC, Weinstein MC. Gains in life expectancy from medical interventions – standardizing data on outcomes. *N Engl J Med* 1998; **339**: 380–386.
37. Bucher HC, Griffith LE, Guyatt GH. Effect of HMGcoA reductase inhibitors on stroke. A meta-analysis of randomized, controlled trials. *Ann Int Med* 1998; **128**: 89–95.
38. Kjekshus J, Pedersen TR, Olsson AG *et al.* The effects of simvastatin on the incidence of heart failure in patients with coronary heart disease. *J Cardiac Fail* 1997; **3**: 249–254.
39. Pedersen TR, Kjekshus J, Pyorala K *et al.* Effect of simvastatin on ischemic signs and symptoms in the Scandinavian simvastatin survival study (4S). *Am J Cardiol* 1998; **81**: 333–335.
40. Cook RJ, Sackett DL. The number needed to treat: a clinically useful measure of treatment effect. *Br Med J* 1995; **310**: 452–454.
41. Haffner SM, Lehto S, Ronnemaa T *et al.* Mortality from coronary heart disease in subjects with type 2 diabetes and in nondiabetic subjects with and without prior myocardial infarction. *N Engl J Med* 1998; **339**: 229–234.
42. Zimmet PZ, Alberti KG. The changing face of macrovascular disease in non-insulin-dependent diabetes mellitus: an epidemic in progress. *Lancet* 1997; **350** (**Suppl 1**): 1–4.
43. Syvanne M, Taskinen MR. Lipids and lipoproteins as coronary risk factors in non-insulin-dependent diabetes mellitus. *Lancet* 1997; **350** (**Suppl 1**): S120–S123.
44. Pyörälä K, Pedersen TR, Kjekshus J *et al.* Cholesterol lowering in simvastatin improves prognosis of diabetic patients with coronary

heart disease. A subgroup analysis of the Scandinavian Simvastatin Survival Study (4S). *Diabetes Care* 1997; **20**: 614–620.

45. Bressler P, Bailey SR, Matsuda M, DeFronzo RA. Insulin resistance and coronary artery disease. *Diabetologia* 1996; **39**: 1345–1350.

46. Anonymous. Collaborative overview of randomised trials of antiplatelet therapy – I: Prevention of death, myocardial infarction, and stroke by prolonged antiplatelet therapy in various categories of patients. Antiplatelet Trialists' Collaboration. *Br Med J* 1994; **308**: 81–106.

47. Anonymous. Final report on the aspirin component of the ongoing Physicians' Heath Study. Steering Committee of the Physicians' Health Study Research Group. *N Engl J Med* 1989; **321**: 129–135.

48. Anonymous. Thrombosis prevention trial: randomised trial of low-intensity oral anticoagulation with warfarin and low-dose aspirin in the primary prevention of ischaemic heart disease in men at increased risk. The Medical Research Council's General Practice Research Framework. *Lancet* 1998; **351**: 233–241.

49. Hansson L, Zanchetti A, Carruthers SG *et al.* Effects of intensive blood-pressure lowering and low-dose aspirin in patients with hypertension – principal results of the hypertension optimal treatment (HOT) randomised trials. *Lancet* 1998; **351**: 1755–1762.

50. Colwell JA. Aspirin therapy in diabetes. *Diabetes Care* 1997; **20**: 1767–1771.

51. Panahloo A, Yudkin JS. Diminished fibrinolysis in diabetes mellitus and its implication for diabetic vascular disease. *J Cardiovasc Risk* 1997; **4**: 91–99.

52. Lindahl B, Asplund K, Eliasson M, Evrin P-E. Insulin resistance syndrome and fibrinolytic activity: the northern Sweden MONICA study. *Int J Epidemiol* 1996; **25**: 291–299.

53. Hamsten A, Eriksson P, Karpe F, Silveira A. Relationships of thrombosis and fibrinolysis to atherosclerosis. *Curr Opin Lipidol* 1994; **5**: 382–389.

54. Schrier RW. Antihypertensive treatment in type 2 diabetes. *Hospit Pract* 1998; **33**: 13–16.

55. Clark CM, Lee DA. Prevention and treatment of the complications of diabetes mellitus. *N Engl J Med* 1995; **332**: 1210–1217.

56. Webster MW, Scott RS. What cardiologists need to know about diabetes. *Lancet* 1997; **350** (**Suppl 1**): S123–S128.

57. Anonymous. Tight blood pressure control and risk of macrovascular and microvascular complications in Type 2 diabetes: UKPDS 38. UK Prospective Diabetes Study Group. *BMJ* 1998; **317**: 703–713.

58. Estacio RO, Jeffers BW, Hiatt WR *et al.* The effect of nisoldipine as compared with enalapril on cardiovascular outcomes in patients with non-insulin-dependent diabetes and hypertension. *N Eng J Med* 1998; **338**: 645–652.

59. Tatti P, Pahor M, Byington RP *et al.* Outcome results of the Fosinopril Versus Amlodipine Cardiovascular Events Randomized Trial (FACET) in patients with hypertension and NIDDM. *Diabetes Care* 1998; **21**: 597–603.

60. Collins R, Peto R, MacMahon S *et al.* Blood pressure, stroke, and coronary heart disease. Part 2, Short-term reductions in blood pressure: overview of randomised drug trials in their epidemiological context. *Lancet* 1990; **335**: 827–838.

61. Bonner G. Hyperinsulinemia, insulin resistance, and hypertension. *J Cardiovasc Pharmacol* 1994; **24** (**Suppl 2**): S39–S49.

62. Ramsay LE, Yeo WW, Jackson PR. Influence of diuretics, calcium antagonists, and alpha-blockers on insulin sensitivity and glucose tolerance in hypertensive patients. *J Cardiovasc Pharmacol* 1992; **20** (**Suppl 11**): S49–S53.

63. Moser M. Why are physicians not prescribing diuretics more frequently in the management of hypertension? *JAMA* 1998; **279**: 1813–1816.

64. Sacks FM, Moye LA, Davis BR *et al.* Relationship between plasma LDL concentrations during treatment with pravastatin and recurrent coronary events in the cholesterol and recurrent events trial. *Circulation* 1998; **97**: 1446–1452.

65. MacDonald TM, Butler R, Newton RW, Morris AD. Which drugs benefit diabetic patients for secondary prevention of myocardial infarction? DARTS/MEMO Collaboration. *Diabetic Med* 1998; **15**: 282–289.

66. De Sonnaville JJJ, Heine RJ. Non-insulin dependent diabetes mellitus: presentation and treatment. *Medicine* 1997; **25**: 23–26.

67. Heine RJ. Insulin treatment of non-insulin-

dependent diabetes mellitus. *Baillieres Clin Endocrinol Metab* 1988; **2**: 477–492.

68. Seissler J, de Sonnaville JJJ, Morgenthaler NG *et al.* Immunological heterogeneity in type 1 diabetes: presence of distinct autoantibody patterns in patients with acute onset and slowly progressive disease. *Diabetologia* 1998; **41**: 891–897.

69. Kobayashi T, Nakanishi K, Murase T, Kosaka K. Small doses of subcutaneous insulin as a strategy for preventing slowly progressive beta-cell failure in islet cell antibody-positive patients with clinical features of NIDDM. *Diabetes* 1996; **45**: 622–626.

70. Anonymous. Recommendations for the nutritional management of patients with diabetes mellitus. *Diab Nutr Metab* 1995; **8**: 1–4.

71. Chaturvedi N, Stephenson JM, Fuller JH. The relationship between smoking and microvascular complications in the EURODIAB IDDM Complications Study. *Diabetes Care* 1995; **18**: 785–792.

72. Melander A. Oral antidiabetic drugs: an overview. *Diabetic Med* 1996; **13**: S143–S147.

73. Groop LC. Sulphonylureas in NIDDM. *Diabetes Care* 1992; **15**: 737–754.

74. Bijlstra PJ, Lutterman JA, Russel FG *et al.* Interaction of sulphonylurea derivatives with vascular ATP-sensitive potassium channels in humans. *Diabetologia* 1996; **39**: 1083–1090.

75. Leibowitz G, Cerasi E. Sulphonylurea treatment of NIDDM patients with cardiovascular disease: a mixed blessing? *Diabetologia* 1996; **39**: 503–514.

76. DeFronzo RA, Goodman AM. Efficacy of metformin in patients with non-insulin-dependent diabetes mellitus. The Multicenter Metformin Study Group. *N Engl J Med* 1995; **333**: 541–549.

77. Stumvoll M, Nurjhan N, Perriello G *et al.* Metabolic effects of metformin in non-insulin-dependent diabetes mellitus. *N Engl J Med* 1995; **333**: 550–554.

78. Bayraktar M, van Thiel DH, Adalar N. A comparison of acarbose versus metformin as an adjuvant therapy in sulfonylurea-treated NIDDM patients. *Diabetes Care* 1996; **19**: 252–254.

79. Yki-Jarviven H, Kauppila M, Kujansuu E *et al.* Comparison of insulin regimens in patients with non-insulin-dependent diabetes mellitus. *N Engl J Med* 1992; **327**: 1426–1433.

80. Johnson JL, Wolf SL, Kabadi UM. Efficacy of insulin and sulfonylurea combination therapy in type 2 diabetes. A meta-analysis of the randomized placebo-controlled trials. *Arch Int Med* 1996; **156**: 259–264.

81. Pugh JA, Wagner ML, Sawyer J *et al.* Is combination sulfonylurea and insulin therapy useful in NIDDM patients? A metaanalysis. *Diabetes Care* 1992; **15**: 953–959.

82. Assal JP, Jacquemet S, Morel Y. The added value of therapy in diabetes: the education of patients for self-management of their disease. *Metabolism* 1997; **46**: 61–64.

83. Anonymous. Diabetes care and research in Europe: the Saint Vincent declaration. *Diabetic Med* 1990; **7**: 360.

84. Peters AL, Legorreta AP, Ossorio RC, Davidson MB. Quality of outpatient care provided to diabetic patients. A health maintenance organization experience. *Diabetes Care* 1996; **19**: 601–606.

85. Chesover D, Tudor-Miles P, Hilton S. Survey and audit of diabetes care in general practice in south London. *Br J Gen Pract* 1991; **41**: 282–285.

86. Saltiel AR, Olefsky JM. Thiazolidinediones in the treatment of insulin resistance and type 2 diabetes. *Diabetes* 1996; **45**: 1661–1669.

87. Inzucchi SE, Maggs DG, Spollett GR *et al.* Efficacy and metabolic effects of metformin and troglitazone in type 2 diabetes mellitus. *N Engl J Med* 1998; **338**: 867–872.

88. Wolffenbuttel BH, Nijst L, Sels JP *et al.* Effects of a new oral hypoglycaemic agent, repaglinide, on metabolic control in sulphonylurea-treated patients with NIDDM. *Eur J Clin Pharmacol* 1993; **45**: 113–116.

17

Optimum dietary approach in Type 2 diabetes
Joyce Barnett and Abhimanyu Garg

Introduction

The goals of dietary therapy for management of diabetes mellitus, as outlined by The American Diabetes Association (ADA), include normalization of blood glucose levels, optimization of blood lipoprotein levels, provision of adequate energy for attaining a desirable body-weight, and prevention of acute and chronic complications, in addition to improvement of overall health.[1,2] Specifically, for patients with Type 2 diabetes mellitus, there are two major considerations for achieving these goals: (a) diet composition and (b) reduction in total energy intake to achieve desirable body-weight. In this chapter we will review scientific data supporting dietary recommendations for patients with Type 2 diabetes, followed by discussion of practical aspects of implementing the diet.

Scientific rationale

Total energy intake

With 60–90% of patients with Type 2 diabetes in Western countries being overweight, energy control is an important part of dietary management. The threshold for insulin resistance in response to adiposity may vary in different ethnic groups as well as in different individuals belonging to the same ethnic group.[3–5] In addition to generalized excess of body fat, some patients with Type 2 diabetes are prone to truncal obesity.[3,6] Even patients not considered overweight by weight-for-height standards may have excess adiposity; therefore, all patients with Type 2 diabetes may benefit from weight loss. Weight loss of 5–10% has been shown to be beneficial in improving glycemic control and serum lipid levels in overweight individuals with Type 2 diabetes.[7–16] We strongly advocate reduction of body fat to lean levels for the obese and even the 'non-obese' patient with Type 2 diabetes.

Whether high-carbohydrate diets are more effective in causing weight loss than high-fat diets is quite controversial, as studies indicate that isoenergetic weight-reducing diets are equally effective in promoting weight loss. Metabolic studies under isoenergetic conditions report no change in energy balance when fat intake is increased, but with substantial increase in carbohydrate intake, a negative fat balance is reported. Substantial weight gain, however, can occur over time with overfeeding of either fat or carbohydrate. Spontaneous energy intake on an unrestricted high-fat diet tends to be higher when compared with a high-carbohydrate diet, but long-term effects have not been studied.[17] Therefore, for weight reduction, primary emphasis should be on restriction of total energy intake.

Two approaches for reducing total energy intake may be considered. A moderate reduction in energy intake of 250–500 kcal (1,050–2,100 kJ) per day will provide for gradual weight loss.[1] This approach is favoured by us in view of potential to induce and maintain weight loss, and will be discussed later. Another approach is to use a very low-calorie diet (VLCD) (less than 800 kcal or 3,350 kJ per day), which can lead to rapid weight loss and improvement in serum glucose and lipid levels, as well as decreases in blood pressure. Adequate medical supervision, however, is required to safely implement a VLCD, whether it is food-based or a liquid formula. Care must be exercised to include adequate protein (1.0–1.4 g/kg of ideal body weight per day), vitamins, electrolytes, and fluid. VLCDs may be employed in moderate to severely obese patients (body-mass index (BMI) >30 kg/m²), but not in mildly overweight individuals. Side-effects of VLCDs include rapid loss of lean body mass and electrolytes, cardiac arrhythmias, gout, and gallstones. Other less-serious side-effects include hair loss, cold intolerance, anemia, nervousness, constipation, fatigue, and menstrual irregularities.[18] Furthermore, these diets may not have long-term success in maintaining the reduced weight. In addition, there is some evidence that VLCDs may produce disordered binge eating in some people.[19]

Diet composition

Carbohydrate

The digestible carbohydrates are usually classified as simple (mono- and disaccharides) and complex carbohydrates. Historically, complex carbohydrates have been recommended and simple carbohydrates discouraged. However, when equal amounts of complex and naturally occurring simple carbohydrates are consumed, no significant differences in glycemic response are observed.[20] These findings have displaced the notion that simple sugars are more rapidly

absorbed and therefore should be avoided in order to limit wide fluctuations in blood glucose.[2] A number of studies have found no adverse effects on glycemia with sucrose as compared with starch; however, ingestion of sucrose or fructose can significantly increase the post-prandial concentration of serum triglycerides by impairing clearance of triglyceride-rich lipoproteins.[21-29] However, other investigators have reported no adverse effects from a high-fructose or high-sucrose diet on serum lipids.[30-32] Dietary fructose does produce a lower glycemic response than isoenergetic amounts of sucrose.[31,33-35] Nonetheless, while small amounts of simple carbohydrate can be incorporated into a healthy diet, large quantities of sucrose, fructose, or glucose are discouraged.[36] Simple sugars, especially sucrose, contribute to development of dental caries, and are often associated with high-energy containing foods and thus may interfere with weight reduction efforts. Simple sugars from fruits and vegetables are preferred because these foods also contain vitamins, minerals, and other essential nutrients.

Protein

Adequate protein intake is required to maintain lean body mass in adults. The ADA recommendation for protein intake is 10–20% of total energy intake.[1] The recommended dietary allowance (RDA) for protein is 0.8 g/kg, approximately 10% of total energy intake, while intake of protein in Western countries typically ranges from 15 to 20% of total energy intake.[37] Protein needs are increased during periods of rapid growth, pregnancy, catabolic illness or stress in the elderly, and during vigorous exercise. It is especially important to include adequate protein when using reduced-energy diets.[18] In patients with diabetic renal disease and chronic renal insufficiency, reduction of total protein to 0.8 g/kg is recommended, but protein malnutrition can occur at lower intakes.[38]

Studies suggest that decreasing protein intake in people with Type 1 diabetes may delay the progression of nephropathy; however, whether all patients with diabetes should reduce protein intake has not been determined.[39,40] Furthermore, whether different types of protein, e.g. from meat, vegetables, egg, or milk, have variable effects on renal function is not clear.[41–43]

Dietary fat

Dietary fats can be classified into three major categories: saturated fats (no double bonds), polyunsaturated fat (two or more double bonds) and monounsaturated fats (one double bond) (*Tables 17.1–17.3*).[44] Unsaturated fats, particularly monounsaturated fats, can be further classified by the geometric configuration of the bond, either *cis* or *trans*. A major consideration in diet planning is to reduce the intake of cholesterol-raising fatty acids (mainly saturated fats and *trans* fats) to achieve maximum reduction in serum low-density lipoprotein (LDL)-cholesterol levels.[45]

Saturated fat: Saturated fatty acids should be limited to <10% of total energy intake.[1,45] Saturated fatty acids with a carbon chain

Table 17.1
Common saturated fatty acids and their dietary sources.

Common name	Notation	Sources
Butyric	C4:0	Butterfat
Caproic	C6:0	Butterfat
Caprylic	C8:0	Palm kernel oil, coconut oil, butterfat
Capric	C10:0	Coconut oil, palm kernel oil, butterfat
Lauric	C12:0	Cinnamon oil, coconut oil, palm kernel oil, babassu fat
Myristic	C14:0	Coconut oil, palm kernel oil, nutmeg butter, ucuhuba butter
Palmitic	C16:0	Palm oil; cocoa butter; chinese vegetable tallow; fat of pigs, cattle, sheep, goats, and chickens; butterfat; cotton seed oil; fish oils (such as herring, menhaden and sardine); rice bran oil
*Stearic	C18:0	Cocoa butter; illipe or Borneo tallow; shea nut oil; sal fat; fat of sheep, goats, pigs, cattle, and chickens
Arachidic	C20:0	Ground nuts (peanuts), rambutan tallow, kusum
Behenic	C22:0	Ground nuts
Lignoceric	C24:0	Ground nuts

Source: Padley FB, Gunstone FD, Harwood JL, in *The Lipid Handbook*, 2nd edn, 1993.[44]
* Stearic acid does not raise serum LDL-cholesterol.

Table 17.2
Common polyunsaturated fatty acids and their dietary sources.

Common name	Notation	Sources
Linoleic	C18:2 (n-6)	Safflower oil, sunflower oil, corn oil, tobacco seed oil, grapeseed oil, wheat germ oil, soybean oil, cotton seed oil, buffalo gourd oil, sesame oil, ground nut oil, rice bran oil, candlenut oil, walnuts, pinenuts
α-Linolenic	C18:3 (n-3)	Linseed oil, chia oil, black sesame seeds, perilla, candlenut oil
γ-Linolenic	C18:3 (n-6)	Evening primrose oil, borage oil, blackcurrant seed oil
Arachidonic	C20:4 (n-6)	Animal fats, ground nut oil
Eicosapentaenoic	C20:5 (n-3)	Fish oils (such as menhaden, salmon, sardine, and herring) and marine fish such as anchovies, mackerel, and bluefin tuna
Docosahexaenoic	C22:6 (n-3)	Fish oils (such as salmon, sardine, menhaden, and herring) and marine fish such as anchovies, bluefin tuna, Atlantic salmon, blue fish, and mackerel

Source: Padley FB, Gunstone FD, Harwood JL, in *The Lipid Handbook*, 2nd edn, 1993.[44]

Table 17.3
Common monounsaturated fatty acids and their dietary sources.

Common name	Notation	Sources
Cis-monounsaturated		
Lauroleic	C12:1	Fish oils
Myristoleic	C14:1	Fish oils, beef fat
Palmitoleic	C16:1	Fish oils, beef and pork fat
Oleic	C18:1	Oils: olive; canola; high oleic safflower and sunflower; ground nut (peanuts); avocado; aceituno; shea nut; rice bran; sesame; *Jessenia bataua*; tea seed. Nuts: filberts, almonds, pistachios, pecans, macadamias, cashews. Others: mowrah butter; illipe butter; *fat of cattle, pigs, goats, chicken, and sheep; *cocoa butter
Gadoleic	C20:1	Fish oils (such as herring, sardines and mackerel), jojoba oil
Erucic	C22:1	Mustard seed oil, rape seed oil, nasturtium seed oil
Trans-monounsaturated		
Elaidic	C18:1	Margarine; cookies, crackers, cakes, and candies prepared with partially hydrogenated oils

Source: Padley FB, Gunstone FD, Harwood JL, in *The Lipid Handbook*, 2nd edn, 1993.[44]
* Although a source of oleic acid, these fats should be used sparingly because they are high in cholesterol-raising saturated fatty acids (Table 17.1).

length of 12 (lauric), 14 (myristic), and 16 (palmitic), have the most potent effect on raising serum LDL-cholesterol[46] (*Table 17.1*).[44] On the other hand, stearic acid does not raise serum LDL-cholesterol.[47,48] Interestingly, even medium-chain (caprylic, C8:0, capric, C10:0) and a long-chain (behenic, C22:0) saturated fatty acids have recently also been found to raise serum LDL-cholesterol concentrations.[49,50]

Polyunsaturated fat: Polyunsaturated fatty acids should be limited to 10% or less of total energy intake.[45] Polyunsaturated fatty acids are classified as n-6 (ω-6) or n-3 (ω-3), depending upon the position of the first double bond in the carbon chain, counting from the methyl end. Linoleic acid (C18:2) is the major n-6 polyunsaturated fatty acid in the diet and is essential for humans (*Table 17.2*).[44] The other essential fatty acid is α-linolenic acid (C18:3). Arachidonic and γ-linolenic acids can be formed from linoleic acid. The requirements for essential fatty acids can be easily met by consuming n-6 polyunsaturated fats equalling 2–3% of total energy intake. In addition to meeting demands for essential fatty acids, linoleic acid lowers LDL-cholesterol when substituted for saturated fats, but does not decrease triglycerides.

Eicosapentaenoic (EPA) and docosahexaenoic acid (DHA), n-3 fatty acids, have been shown to reduce serum triglycerides by inhibiting hepatic triglyceride synthesis. The major sources of EPA and DHA are fish oils (*Table 17.2*).[44] Although reduction of serum triglycerides would appear to be beneficial for the hypertriglyceridemic person with Type 2 diabetes, some studies have found a deterioration in glycemic control with high doses of fish oil supplements. A recent review concluded, however, that fish oil does not worsen glycemic control in Type 2 diabetes or impaired-glucose-tolerance patients with adequate control of

energy intake.[51] Another potentially beneficial effect of n-3 fatty acids is inhibition of platelet aggregation, which could possibly reduce risk of acute myocardial infarction. Routine use of fish oil supplementation, however, should not be recommended to patients with Type 2 diabetes.[52]

Monounsaturated fat: cis *and* trans *fatty acids*: Cis-monounsaturated fatty acids are the most abundant in nature and for many years were considered to have a neutral effect on serum cholesterol. Recent studies, however, have shown that oleic acid (C18:1), when substituted for saturated fatty acids, lowers serum LDL-cholesterol just as much as polyunsaturated fatty acids.[53–59] Although less is known about other monounsaturated fatty acids such as palmitoleic (C16:1), gadoleic (C20:1), and erucic acid (C22:1), a preliminary study showed that erucic acid may also have cholesterol-lowering properties similar to those of oleic acid.[60]

In a previous randomized, crossover trial, substitution of a diet high in *cis*-monounsaturated fatty acids for a diet high in carbohydrate content for patients with Type 2 diabetes, lowered plasma triglycerides and very-low-density lipoprotein (VLDL)-cholesterol levels, and increased high-density lipoprotein (HDL)-cholesterol and apolipoprotein A-I.[61] Plasma total cholesterol, LDL-cholesterol, and apolipoprotein B remained the same for both diets. Glycemic control improved, and daily insulin requirements were significantly lower on the high monounsaturated fat diet.[61] A recent meta-analysis of published studies shows that, compared with a high-carbohydrate diet, a high-monounsaturated-fat diet reduces fasting plasma triacylglycerol by 19% and VLDL-cholesterol concentrations by 22%, with a modest increase in HDL-cholesterol and no adverse effects on LDL-cholesterol concentrations (*Figs 17.1 and 17.2*).[61–70]

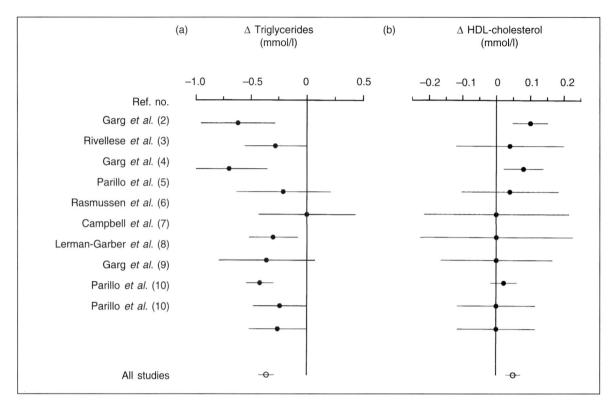

Fig. 17.1
*Net change in plasma triacylglycerol and HDL-cholesterol concentrations with consumption of a high-monounsaturated-fat diet compared with a high-carbohydrate diet in nine studies. The values shown are the mean changes (with 95% CIs) in triacylglycerol and HDL-cholesterol concentrations while patients consumed the high-monounsaturated diet minus values for the high-carbohydrate diet. The weighted mean of all studies with 95% CIs was calculated from the metaanalysis. Reprinted with permission from Garg A. Am J Clin Nutr 1998; **67 (Suppl):** 577S-582S.*

Trans fatty acids, either mono- or polyunsaturated, are formed during the process of partial hydrogenation of oils to increase physical characteristics such as firmness, and to enhance oxidative stability. The partially hydrogenated oils are thus suitable for use as shortenings, in spreads, or for frying, thus providing a dietary replacement for saturated fats. However, the *trans* fatty acids such as elaidic (C18:1) acid increase serum LDL-cholesterol and apolipoprotein B levels (*Table 17.3*).[44] In addition, they may lower serum HDL-cholesterol and apolipoprotein A-I levels, and therefore their intake should be limited as much as possible.[71,72]

Cholesterol
High intake of dietary cholesterol increases serum LDL- and total cholesterol, although

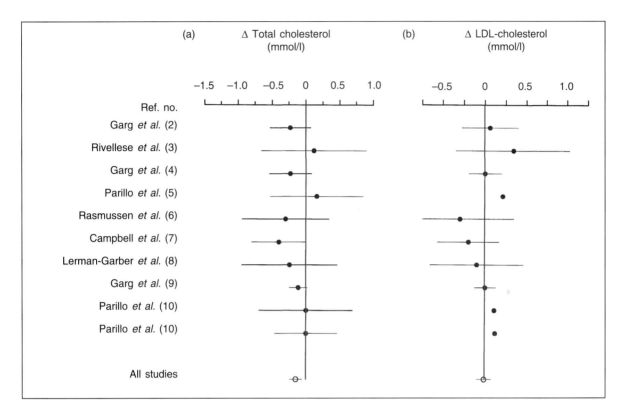

Fig. 17.2
Net change in plasma total cholesterol and LDL-cholesterol concentrations with consumption of a high-monounsaturated-fat diet compared with a high-carbohydrate diet in nine studies. The values shown are the mean changes (with 95% CIs) in total and LDL-cholesterol concentrations while patients consumed the high-monounsaturated diet minus values for the high-carbohydrate diet. The weighted mean of all studies with 95% CIs was calculated from the meta-analysis. Reprinted with permission from Garg A. Am J Clin Nutr 1998; **67 (Suppl):** *577S-582S.*

individual responsiveness may vary. Since dietary cholesterol is found solely in animal products, limiting total intake of animal products can help to lower overall dietary cholesterol intake. Limiting dietary cholesterol to 300 mg or less per day is recommended; further reductions to 200 mg or less per day may be needed for maximal lowering of LDL–cholesterol levels[1,45] (*Tables 17.4 and 17.5*).[73,74]

Sodium

Sodium intake is generally much greater than the minimum needed for normal body function. The role of sodium in management of hypertension is controversial, but some people appear to be more sensitive to sodium than others.[75] People with Type 2 diabetes often have hypertension as well. Current recommendations for sodium intake range from 2,400 to 3,000 mg per day. With mild to moderate

Table 17.4
Cholesterol, total fat, and saturated fat content of selected meat, fish and poultry per 100 g portion.

Food item	Cholesterol (mg)	Total fat (g)	Saturated fat (g)
Beef, choice round tip, roasted lean	81	6.4	2.2
Beef, lean ground, broiled well done	101	17.6	6.9
Beef, regular ground, broiled well done	101	19.5	7.7
Beef liver, braised	389	4.9	1.9
Beef kidney, simmered	387	3.4	1.1
Lamb, choice loin, roasted	93	21.0	9.1
Pork, tenderloin, roasted lean	79	4.8	1.7
Pork, loin chop, broiled	82	15.8	5.8
Chicken, without skin, roasted			
Light meat	75	4.1	1.1
Dark meat	93	9.7	2.7
Salmon, Atlantic (cooked by dry heat)	71	8.1	1.3
Perch (cooked by dry heat)	115	1.2	0.2
Scallops, sea (raw)	33	0.7	0.1
Shrimp (cooked by moist heat)	195	1.1	0.3

Source: USDA, Nutrient Data Base for Standard Reference, Release 12 (March 1998).[73]

Table 17.5
Cholesterol, total fat, and saturated fat content of selected dairy products and eggs.

Food item	Portion size	Cholesterol (mg)	Total fat (g)	Saturated fat (g)
Whole milk (3.3% fat)	240 ml	33	8.1	5.1
Skimmed milk (non-fat)	240 ml	4	0.4	0.3
Cheddar cheese	28 g	30	9.4	6.0
Mozzarella cheese, part-skimmed milk	28 g	16	4.5	2.9
Cottage cheese, creamed	113 g	17	5.1	3.2
Cottage cheese, low fat (1%)	113 g	5	1.1	0.75
*Ice cream, vanilla (10% butterfat)	66 g	29	7.3	4.5
Egg, large whole	50 g	213	5.0	1.6

Source: Pennington JT, Bowes & Church's Food Values of Portions Commonly Used, 17th edn, 1998.[74]
* Premium ice creams contain 16% butterfat.

hypertension, ≤2,400 mg/day of sodium is recommended. The recommendation for patients with hypertension and diabetic nephropathy is ≤2,000 mg/day of sodium.[76]

Dietary fiber

The recommended level of dietary fiber intake is 20–35 g per day.[1] Dietary fiber can be classified as water-soluble or water-insoluble. Insoluble fibres, such as cellulose, lignin, and hemicellulose, increase stool volume and shorten intestinal transit time, but do not reduce serum cholesterol. Soluble fibers such as pectin, gums, mucilages, and some hemicelluloses, lower serum cholesterol; however, they do so only slightly more (5% reduction) than a diet low in saturated fat and cholesterol.[77–79] Whether high-fiber diets improve glycemic control in patients with Type 2 diabetes remains controversial.[10,80] Although increasing dietary soluble fiber intake (to 20 g/day or more) may be difficult to achieve by consuming natural food items, we still prefer to use that approach instead of using fiber supplements[1] (*Table 17.6*).[81]

Alcohol

Patients with Type 2 diabetes should avoid alcohol consumption. In addition to concerns about alcohol consumption for the general public, alcohol may be particularly detrimental to people with Type 2 diabetes. Alcohol intake increases serum triglyceride levels and induces insulin resistance, which may adversely affect glycemic control and raise blood pressure.[82,83] Alcohol consumption increases the potential for hypoglycemia in patients taking oral hypoglycemic agents or using insulin. This is especially true if no food is eaten at the time of the alcohol ingestion, or if binge drinking occurs. Alcohol provides 7 kcal (30 kJ) per gram, and the energy derived from alcohol can interfere with weight-loss efforts and may contribute to truncal adiposity.

Vitamins and minerals

In patients eating a variety of food and consuming adequate energy to maintain body-weight, there is no need for vitamin or mineral supplementation.[84] The diets of patients on reduced-energy diets for weight loss should be evaluated and any nutrient found to be low should be supplemented. Vitamin and mineral needs are increased during pregnancy and in times of illness or stress. Supplementation may be needed in those situations. Antioxidant vitamins, such as vitamin C and vitamin E, are of interest due to the hypothesis that they may protect LDL particles from oxidation or modification, and thus may prevent atherosclerosis.[85,86] Clinical trials to support this hypothesis are, however, lacking, therefore routine supplementation of these antioxidant vitamins in patients with Type 2 diabetes is not recommended.[52] Chromium supplementation in people with diabetes has not resulted in improved glycemic control unless the diet is deficient in chromium.[87–90] One recent study conducted in China reported a dose–response improvement in glycemic control and serum lipids with chromium supplementation; however, neither the dietary chromium intake nor the chromium status of the subjects was determined.[91] Patients with poor glycemic control or who use diuretics may need supplementation of magnesium.[2]

Phytochemicals

An area of growing interest and research is beginning to provide evidence that some substances in plants may play a beneficial role in disease prevention and treatment. One such example is sitostanol, a dietary plant sterol incorporated into a margarine, which lowers

Table 17.6
Soluble and insoluble fiber content of selected foods.

Food	Amount	Weight (g)	Insoluble (g)	Soluble (g)	Total (g)
Nuts					
Peanuts	1/2 cup	72.0	4.0	2.3	6.3
Filberts, hazelnuts	1/2 cup	67.5	2.6	1.7	4.3
Walnuts	1/2 cup	50.0	1.4	1.0	2.4
Almonds	1/2 cup	71.0	7.2	0.8	8.0
Fruit, fresh					
Orange	1 medium	131.0	1.2	1.9	3.1
Mango	1 medium	207.0	2.2	1.9	4.1
Cantaloupe	1/3 medium	307.0	1.0	1.5	2.5
Plums	2 medium	132.0	0.7	1.3	2.0
Strawberries	1 cup	149.0	2.8	1.0	3.9
Apple with skin	1 medium	138.0	1.8	1.0	2.8
Banana	1 medium	114.0	1.6	0.6	2.2
Grapes	1 cup	160.0	0.8	0.3	1.1
Vegetables, cooked or canned					
Squash, winter	1/2 cup	122.0	1.4	2.0	3.4
Broccoli	1/2 cup	92.0	1.4	1.2	2.6
Carrots	1/2 cup	78.0	1.5	0.9	2.4
Potato with skin	1/2 cup	78.0	0.8	0.7	2.0
Cabbage	1/2 cup	75.0	1.0	0.6	1.5
Turnips	1/2 cup	78.0	1.0	0.6	1.6
Green beans	1/2 cup	67.0	1.5	0.5	2.0
Peas, green	1/2 cup	80.0	3.0	0.5	3.4
Tomatoes	1/2 cup	78.0	0.8	0.3	1.0
Legumes dry, cooked, or canned					
Beans, lima	1 cup	188	6.2	7.4	13.6
Chick peas	1 cup	164	5.7	3.8	9.5
Beans, kidney	1 cup	177	8.2	2.8	11.0
Lentils	1 cup	198	9.2	1.1	10.3
Soybean curd, tofu	–	100	0.5	0.7	1.2
Breads					
Bread, wholewheat	1 slice	28.6	1.7	0.4	2.1
Bread, rye	1 slice	28.7	1.5	0.4	1.9
Tortilla, corn	1 piece	21.3	0.7	0.4	1.1
Bread, white	1 slice	25	0.3	0.2	0.5
Tortilla, flour	1 piece	24	0.5	0.2	0.7
Cereals					
Oatbran, cooked	1 cup	219.0	2.7	2.6	5.3
Oatmeal, cooked	1 cup	234.0	1.8	1.8	3.6
Oat cereal, ready to eat	1 cup	22.7	1.0	1.0	2.0
Couscous, cooked	1 cup	179.0	1.5	0.6	2.1
Rice, brown, cooked	1 cup	195.0	3.1	0.2	3.3
Rice, white, cooked	1 cup	205.0	0.8	0.2	1.0
Cream of wheat, cooked	1 cup	251.0	0.5	0.2	0.7
Cornflakes	1 cup	28.4	0.4	0.1	0.5

Adapted from Schakel SF, Sievert YA, Buzzard IM, in *CRC Handbook of Dietary Fiber in Human Nutrition*, 2nd edn, 1993.[81]

serum cholesterol by 10% and LDL-cholesterol by about 15% in mildly hypercholesterolemic subjects.[92] Cholesterol absorption efficiency is reduced, as indicated by reductions in total, VLDL-, and LDL-cholesterol levels, with an increase in HDL-cholesterol in mildly hyper-cholesterolemic men with Type 2 diabetes.[93,94] Other substances from plants, such as flavonoids, lutein, lycopene, lignans, and saponins, may eventually play a role in providing new ways to enhance diet and health. Until further research has been done, consumption of a wide variety of fruits, vegetables, and grains is the best way to obtain potentially beneficial phytochemicals with fewer risks of unknown adverse consequences.

Practical approach

Reduction of body fat is the cornerstone for management of Type 2 diabetes; however, long-term weight management remains a challenge for patients and health-care professionals. Implementation of an optimal diet is a complex process encompassing the elements of diet composition but extending into lifestyle changes necessary to overcome barriers to dietary compliance. Owing to its complicated nature, this challenge requires many different tools and techniques to meet the individual patient's needs.

Weight management

The patient and health-care professional should determine a realistic goal weight that can be achieved and maintained. The determinants of success in achieving weight-loss goals may vary. If the patient has continued to gain weight over a period of time, then slowing of weight gain or stabilization of weight may indicate success. Energy restriction alone can

have beneficial effects on glycemic control; thus an improvement in metabolic parameters is positive reinforcement for continued dietary change, even when actual weight loss is limited.[95,96] Gradual weight loss should be the goal for the overweight patient whose weight has been stable.[97] For the non-obese patient with Type 2 diabetes, a modest reduction in weight to lean levels (a BMI of 19 for women and 20 for men) is beneficial.

Determining current intake and then reducing energy by 250–500 kcal (1,050–2,100 kJ) per day will promote gradual weight loss of 0.25–0.5 kg per week if weight has been stable.[1] A thorough dietary history usually reveals one or more candidate foods or eating habits to target for change. Modifying food choices to reduce fat and/or carbohydrate intake may be an acceptable approach for some, while others prefer gradual reduction in portion size as a means to decrease overall intake. Change in food preference has been found to occur over a period of time.[98–101] Setting improved metabolic goals, such as improving glycosylated hemoglobin values or lowering serum triglyceride levels, often proves more productive and motivating than focusing on weight loss *per se* when using the modest energy-reduction approach for long-term weight management.

Weight loss can often be achieved in the short term, but long-term maintenance of reduced weight is more difficult.[102] Continued self-monitoring (keeping food records and weighing on a regular basis) is reported by individuals who have successfully maintained reduced weight, but increased physical activity seems to be the key to maintaining weight loss.[103–113] People tend to feel more confident in their overall weight management efforts when physical activity is included. The challenge is to find an activity the person likes and will continue to do. The patient's ability to increase physical activity determines how much decrease in food intake is required to facilitate weight loss. Finding a suitable energy-expending activity for older individuals with chronic illnesses is difficult. Osteoarthritis of hip or knee joints makes even walking difficult. Long-term complications of diabetes or peripheral vascular disease may lead to foot problems or even lower-extremity amputations, further decreasing physical activity. Cardiovascular disease may limit activity as well.

Medications can also adversely affect weight-loss efforts. Some, such as tricyclic antidepressants and antihistamines, may increase appetite.[114] Nonsteroidal anti-inflammatory drugs must be taken with food to avoid stomach irritation, thus increasing overall energy intake if care is not taken. Beta-blockers decrease metabolic rate, adding to the burden of energy imbalance.[115] When these factors are added to busy lifestyles with little time to devote to meal preparation and planning, making significant changes to dietary habits is a daunting challenge.

Barriers to dietary compliance

Patients with diabetes cite numerous obstacles to dietary compliance, including a sense of isolation, time pressures and competing priorities, lack of support from friends and family, social events, negative emotions, and feelings of deprivation.[116] Additional barriers identified by dietitians are: (a) denial, or a perception that diabetes is not serious, (b) poor understanding of the diet and its relationship to the disease, and (c) misinformation from unreliable sources.[117] Because dietary change is difficult and crucial to the achievement of the goals of dietary management, physician referral for dietary counselling is important. For approximately half of the patients with Type 2 diabetes in one study, lack of physician referral was the reason reported for not consulting a dieti-

tian.[118] Infrequent referral was deemed to be as ineffective in facilitating dietary changes as no referral for nutrition counselling[119] (*Table 17.7*).

Meal frequency and timing

Patients with Type 2 diabetes may benefit from a meal plan that includes 3–5 small meals per day. The meal plan needs to be flexible enough to encourage adherence, but consistency may help patients with hectic lifestyles and unstructured eating habits to limit overall energy intake. Eating breakfast, in particular, seems to reduce fat intake and minimize impulsive snacking.[120] The frequency of feeding does not appear to have an effect on rate of weight loss when energy intake is held constant; however, less fluctuation in satiety level occurs with more frequent feeding.[121,122] Increased frequency of eating could lead to weight gain, but advantages to eating smaller, more frequent meals have been noted.[123,124] Consuming multiple small meals lowers serum lipid and lipoprotein, insulin, and post-prandial glucose levels compared with a reduced number of meals, keeping energy content and food composition constant.[125–127] The temporal pattern of food intake had only a modest effect on overall blood glucose control.[128]

Diet composition

Carbohydrate

The amount of carbohydrate in the meal plan should be individualized and can be determined from food records kept over a period of several days.[129] Patients with Type 2 diabetes taking oral hypoglycemic agents or insulin need to maintain day-to-day consistency and meal-to-meal consistency in the amount of carbohydrate consumed, in order to avoid hypoglycemia. Emphasis should be placed on

Table 17.7
Barriers to successful weight loss in Type 2 diabetes mellitus.

Physical inactivity
    Physical limitations secondary to illness or injury
    Sedentary occupation and leisure-time activities
Medications
    Stimulate appetite and/or lead to increased food intake
    Decrease metabolic rate
Education
    Poor understanding of diet/disease relationship
    Misinformation
    Lack of referral for dietary counseling/follow-up
Psychological factors
    Sense of isolation
    Feelings of deprivation
    Negative emotions
    Denial of condition
Lifestyle/environment
    Time pressures/competing priorities
    Lack of support from family/friends
    Social events

inclusion of complex carbohydrates and simple sugars that occur naturally in foods such as fruit and milk.[130]

Nutritive sweeteners such as honey or fructose have been shown to have no advantage or disadvantage over sucrose.[1,2] Sucrose and other refined sugars can be substituted for other carbohydrate in the diet, but foods that contain them, such as pastries, cakes, and candy, are often high in fat. The high energy content of these foods, even in small amounts, can quickly sabotage weight-loss efforts. Fructose from fruit is not of concern as long as the total amount of carbohydrate is controlled. Intake of foods and beverages with high fructose corn syrup should be limited because of possible adverse effects on serum lipids.[22,131]

Sugar alcohols, such as sorbitol, vary in energy content, but provide approximately 2–3 kcal (8–12 kJ) per gram.[131] Hydrogenated starch hydrolysates (HSHs) are added to candies. Sugar alcohols and HSH can cause significant gastrointestinal distress (cramping and diarrhoea) if consumed in large amounts. As they induce a lower glycemic response than does sucrose, sugar alcohols and HSH should not be used to treat hypoglycemia.[1] Non-nutritive sweeteners can help to lower total carbohydrate and energy intake, especially if an individual drinks large quantities of sweetened beverages. Trying different sweeteners should be encouraged, to accommodate individual taste preferences. Non-nutritive sweeteners include saccharin, aspartame, and acesulfame K. Both saccharin and acesulfame K are non-caloric and are excreted unchanged from the body. Aspartame contains 4 kcal (17 kJ) per gram, but is used in such small quantities that energy contribution is negligible. Aspartame is not heat stable, cannot be used in cooking, and should not be used by people with phenylke-tonuria. Sucralose (trichlorogalactosucrose) has recently been approved for use in the US and provides no energy. Because it is heat stable, sucralose can be used in desserts and confections, as well as in beverages. Alitame and cyclamate are approved for use in some countries, but not in the US.[131]

Protein

Meat, poultry, fish, and dairy products are good sources of animal protein; however, these foods tend to be high in saturated and total fat unless low-fat selections are made. Dietary cholesterol intake also increases with increasing consumption of animal products. Consuming the recommended amount of 140–170 g of meat, poultry, or fish, along with two servings of milk per day provides approximately 20% of energy from protein. In addition to providing protein, low-fat dairy products are excellent sources of calcium, and red meats are good sources of iron and zinc.

An increasing number of people are following vegetarian diets. Such people tend to consume less total fat, saturated fat, and cholesterol than omnivores. In addition they consume more fiber, antioxidant-containing foods, and phytochemicals . Lacto-ovo vegetarians consume approximately 12–14% of their energy in the form of protein, while vegans obtain only about 10–12% of their energy from protein.[132] Legumes, such as soy beans, kidney beans, chick peas, other pulses, and nuts, are alternative sources of protein. As nuts are high in fat and energy, caution is required when energy restrictions are indicated for weight loss. Grain products and vegetables also provide substantial amounts of protein in the diet. When animal products are eliminated from the diet, it is important to ensure adequate intake of nutrients such as calcium, iron, zinc, and vitamin B_{12}.

Dietary fat

The total amount of fat in the diet should be individualized and determined by serum lipid and body-weight goals, with consideration of current eating habits. Some patients may do well on a diet obtaining 20% of energy from fat, while for others used to consuming high-fat foods, even limiting fat to 35–40% of their energy intake may be difficult. Fats and oils, red meat, poultry, fish, and dairy products account for approximately 90% of total fat intake in the US. Thus, intake of these foods must be reduced to lower total fat intake.[133] Two-thirds of the saturated fat in the American diet comes from animal fats, further emphasizing the need to limit the quantity of animal products eaten[45] (*Tables 17.4 and 17.5*).[73,74] Care must be used to evaluate invisible or hidden fats and oils in prepared foods, as these are often overlooked. Limiting the amount and type of fat added to the diet can also reduce total fat and saturated fat.

Trans fatty acids are found primarily in margarines and baked goods prepared with partially hydrogenated vegetable oils. Limiting these products will reduce the intake of *trans* fatty acids. It is estimated that approximately 3% of the total daily energy intake is provided by *trans* fatty acids in the US.

Small amounts of vegetable oils such as safflower, corn, or soybean oil, will provide sufficient amounts of essential fatty acids (*Table 17.8*).[73] Incorporating fish into the diet is the recommended way to obtain the n-3 polyunsaturated fatty acids for people with Type 2 diabetes (*Table 17.2*).[44]

Cis-monounsaturated fatty acids can be used to replace other types of fat in the diet without adverse effects on serum lipids or glycemic control.[61] This approach may enhance compliance for individuals with a high-fat intake. Because of the higher energy density of fat, attention to portion control

Table 17.8
Foods rich in cis-*monounsaturated and polyunsaturated fatty acids.*

Food	Saturated	Fatty acids (% of total fat)	
		Monounsaturated	Polyunsaturated
Oils			
Canola	7.1	58.9	29.6
Corn	12.7	24.2	58.7
Olive	13.5	73.7	8.4
Peanut	16.9	46.2	32.0
Safflower, high oleic	6.1	75.3	14.2
Safflower, high linoleic	9.1	12.1	74.5
Soybean	14.4	23.3	57.9
Sunflower, high oleic	9.7	83.6	3.8
Sunflower oil, high linoleic	10.3	19.5	65.7
Nuts and seeds			
Almonds	9.5	64.9	21.0
Cashew nuts	19.8	58.9	16.9
Filberts or hazelnuts	7.3	78.4	9.6
Macadamia nuts	15.0	78.9	1.7
Pecans	8.0	62.3	24.8
Pistachio nuts	12.7	67.5	15.1
Sesame seeds	14.0	37.8	43.8
Walnuts, English or Persian	9.0	22.9	63.2
Other			
Avocados	15.9	62.7	12.8
Olives, ripe	13.2	73.9	8.5

Source: USDA, Nutrient Data Base for Standard Reference, Release 12 (March 1998).[73]

and overall energy intake is critical to the achievement of weight-loss goals. Canola, olive, and peanut oil are good sources of monounsaturates. Highly monounsaturated varieties of sunflower and safflower oils are also available. Avocados, olives, and some nuts are other good sources of monounsaturates (*Table 17.8*).[73]

Fat substitutes: A number of fat substitutes that are carbohydrate-, protein-, or fat-based are now available. Gums, gels, and maltodextrins are examples of carbohydrate-based fat replacements adding creaminess and texture to items such as salad dressings. Protein-based replacements consist of microparticulated egg-white or milk protein, and are used in cheeses, salad dressings, and some bakery products. Most protein-based replacements will coagulate and lose the desired functional effect if subjected to high temperatures. Protein-based fat substitutes add 1–4 kcal (4–16 kJ) per gram.[133] Fat-based substitutes vary in energy value and are classified as either synthetic or modified fats. Olestra, a sucrose polyester, is an example of a synthetic fat that is not digested or absorbed by the body, thus contributing no energy. Olestra has been approved for use in snack chips, but it can cause gastrointestinal distress if consumed in large amounts. Because olestra may reduce absorption of fat-soluble vitamins, foods containing it must have additional quantitites of these vitamins.[134] Two examples of the modified fat substitute category are Caprenin and Salatrim. Caprenin contains caprylic (C8:0), capric (C10:0), and behenic (C22:0) acids. Salatrim is a modified triglyceride containing acetic, propionic, and stearic acids. Salatrim and Caprenin provide 5 kcal (20 kJ) per gram due to decreased absorption.[133,135] While reduced-fat products mimic the taste and feel in the mouth of higher-fat foods, they are of questionable benefit for weight control. Larger portions may be consumed, because of decreased satiety or because of the illusion that they contain less energy.[136–138] In fact, many fat-free products are only slightly lower in energy than the regular products they are designed to replace. Some foods containing carbohydrate-based fat substitutes contribute a significant amount of carbohydrate to the diet, and this must be taken into account by patients with diabetes when making food choices.

Cholesterol

Limiting lean meat, poultry, and fish to 140–170 g per day and choosing 2–3 servings of non-fat or low-fat dairy products will meet the recommended guidelines for cholesterol intake. Because of their high cholesterol content, certain other foods must also be limited. For example, egg yolks should be limited to 2–4 per week, including those used in cooking. Egg-whites or commercial egg substitutes can be used in place of whole eggs. Organ meats, such as liver and kidney, are very high in cholesterol and should be used sparingly. Some shellfish, such as shrimp, have a higher cholesterol content than other meats or fish, but may be eaten in moderation because they are lower in total fat and saturated fat[45] (*Tables 17.4 and 17.5*).[73,74]

Sodium

Intake of sodium tends to increase with increasing consumption of processed and convenience food items. A diet with no added table salt and limited processed foods can achieve the current recommendations. Sodium occurs naturally in meats and dairy products, but the amounts previously discussed can be included in the diet. Fruits and vegetables tend to be low in sodium. While manufacturers have begun to provide greater choices in reduced sodium products, the move toward reduced-fat foods has often lead to increased sodium content to enhance flavor in the lower-fat product.

Dietary fiber

Fruits, vegetables, and whole-grain products are primary sources of dietary fiber. The recommended amount of fiber is 20–35 g per day, much more than the usual intake of 10–13 g per day in the US.[1,2] Food sources of soluble fiber include legumes, barley, oats, and fruits. Vegetables, wheat, and other grains contain mainly insoluble fiber. Nuts and seeds also provide dietary fiber. (*Table 17.6*).[81] Guar gum and psyllium are sometimes used as supplements to increase fiber intake. Benefits of fiber in the diet include earlier satiety, possible promotion of weight loss, and modest reductions in blood cholesterol and glucose levels.[139] The most common side-effects of increased fiber intake are gastrointestinal discomfort and flatulence, which can be moderated by making gradual increases in fiber intake.

Tools and techniques

Determining effective ways of overcoming barriers to compliance with dietary guidelines is critical. Practice guidelines have been developed in the US to provide a systematic approach for provision of medical nutrition therapy for patients with Type 2 diabetes.[140] The major components of medical nutrition therapy are assessment, intervention, and evaluation. Intervention includes the nutrition prescription, education, and goal setting. To plan and implement an effective, individualized meal plan, the patient must be an active participant in this process.[141] Effectiveness of the medical nutrition therapy approach has been demonstrated by improved outcome measures, including fasting plasma glucose, glycosylated hemoglobin, serum lipids, and body-weight. Improved compliance and dietary intake were also reported in a study from Australia that focused on treatment of longer duration, greater simplicity, repetition, and cognitive motivational techniques.[142] Patients most likely to benefit from intensive nutrition therapy and additional appointments with a dietitian are those with diabetes of long duration, with poor metabolic control, and who have major obstacles to lifestyle changes.[143]

The importance of following a meal plan for improved glycemic control in Type 1 diabetes was recognized in the Diabetes Control and Complications Trial (DCCT).[144,145] Because changing dietary habits is essential to achieving long-term weight loss, and weight loss can bring about improvements in glycemic control, an effective meal plan that is followed should also be beneficial to patients with Type 2 diabetes.

A number of tools, ranging from simple to very complex, are available to facilitate meal planning for patients with diabetes.[129,146] Which meal-planning approach to use depends upon assessment of the individual patient's needs. *The Exchange Lists for Meal Planning* have long been used to help patients select appropriate foods and portion sizes. A simplified version of the exchange system was found to be an effective tool by many dietitians in the DCCT.[144] The carbohydrate-counting method has become a popular approach to meal planning because it can be used with varying degrees of complexity and allows greater flexibility.[147] Another tool is the glycemic index, a ranking of foods based on post-prandial blood glucose compared with a reference food.[148,149] However, the glycemic index is not used extensively in the US.

Conclusions

The goals of dietary management for Type 2 diabetes mellitus can be achieved using either a high-carbohydrate or a high-monounsaturated-fat diet as long as intake of dietary cholesterol and cholesterol-raising fat is limited. Emphasis should be on the total amount of carbohydrate, within the context of a healthy diet, rather than the type of carbohydrate. Reduction of total energy intake is essential to promote reduction of body fat, decrease insulin resistance, and improve glycemic control. Guidelines similar to those for the general public to ensure adequate intake of protein, dietary fiber, vitamins, minerals, and fluids are appropriate. Increased physical activity consistent with the patient's capabilities should be encouraged to help with weight management. Because of the difficulty associated with dietary change, patients should be referred to a qualified dietitian for counseling so that a realistic, individualized meal plan can be developed. Changing eating habits is a long-term process that requires continued attention by the patient and frequent follow-up with the dietitian.

References

1. American Diabetes Association. Nutrition recommendations and principles for people with diabetes mellitus. *Diabetes Care* 1994; **17**: 519–522.
2. Franz MJ, Horton ES, Bantle JP *et al.* Nutrition principles for the management of diabetes and related complications. *Diabetes Care* 1994; **17**: 490–518.
3. Abate N, Garg A, Peshock RM *et al.* Relationship of generalized and regional adiposity to insulin sensitivity in men with NIDDM. *Diabetes* 1996; **45**: 1684–1693.
4. Abate N, Garg A, Peshock RM *et al.* Relationships of generalized and regional adiposity to insulin sensitivity. *J Clin Invest* 1995; **96**: 88–98.
5. Chandalia M, Abate N, Garg A *et al.* Regional adiposity and insulin resistance in Asian Indian migrant men to the United States. *J Invest Med* 1995; **43 (Suppl 2)**: 303A.
6. Abate N, Garg A. Heterogeneity in adipose tissue metabolism: causes, implications and management of regional adiposity. *Prog Lipid Res* 1995; **34**: 53–70.
7. Markovic TP, Jenkins AB, Campbell LV *et al.* The determinants of glycemic responses to diet restriction and weight loss in obesity and NIDDM. *Diabetes Care* 1998; **21**: 687–694.
8. Bosello O, Armellini F, Zamboni M, Fitchet M. The benefits of modest weight loss in type II diabetes. *Int J Obes* 1997; **21 (Suppl 1)**: S10–S13.
9. Van Gaal LF, Wauters MA, De Leeuw IH. The beneficial effects of modest weight loss on cardiovascular risk factors. *Int J Obes* 1997; **21 (Suppl 1)**: S5–S9.
10. National Institutes of Health. Consensus development conference on diet and exercise in non-insulin-dependent diabetes mellitus. *Diabetes Care* 1987; **10**: 639–644.
11. Wing RR, Koeske R, Epstein LH *et al.* Long-term effects of modest weight loss in type II diabetic patients. *Arch Int Med* 1987; **147**: 1749–1753.
12. Liu GC, Coulston AM, Lardinois CK *et al.* Moderate weight loss and sulfonylurea treatment of non-insulin-dependent diabetes mellitus. *Arch Int Med* 1985; **145**: 665–669.
13. Hughes TA, Gwynne JT, Switzer BR *et al.* Effects of caloric restriction and weight loss on glycemic control, insulin release and resistance, and atherosclerotic risk in obese patients with type II diabetes mellitus. *Am J Med* 1984; **77**: 7–17.
14. Wolf RN, Grundy SM. Influence of weight reduction on plasma lipoproteins in obese patients. *Arteriosclerosis* 1983; **3**: 160–169.
15. Kennedy L, Walshe K, Hadden DR *et al.* The effect of intensive dietary therapy on serum high density lipoprotein cholesterol in patients with Type 2 (non-insulin-dependent) diabetes mellitus: a prospective study. *Diabetologia* 1982; **23**: 24–27.
16. Weisweiler P, Drosner M, Schwandt P. Dietary effects of very-low-density lipoproteins in Type 2 (non-insulin-dependent) diabetes mellitus. *Diabetologia* 1982; **23**: 101–103.
17. Shah M, Garg A. High-fat and high-carbohydrate diets and energy balance. *Diabetes Care* 1996; **19**: 1142–1152.
18. National Task Force on Prevention and Treatment of Obesity. Very low-calorie diets. *JAMA* 1993; **270**: 967–974.
19. Telch CF, Agras WS. The effects of a very low calorie diet on binge eating. *Behav Ther* 1993; **24**: 177–193.
20. Hollenbeck CB, Coulston A, Donner CC *et al.* The effects of variations in percent of naturally occurring complex and simple carbohydrates on plasma glucose and insulin response in individuals with non-insulin-dependent diabetes mellitus. *Diabetes* 1985; **34**: 151–155.
21. Jeppesen J, Chen Y-D I, Zhou M-Y *et al.* Effect of variations in oral fat and carbohydrate load on postprandial lipemia. *Am J Clin Nutr* 1995; **62**: 1201–1205.
22. Jeppesen J, Chen Y-D I, Zhou M-Y *et al.* Postprandial triglyceride and retinyl ester

responses to oral fat: effects of fructose. *Am J Clin Nutr* 1994; **61**: 787–791.

23. Grant KI, Marais MP, Dhansay MA. Sucrose in a lipid-rich meal amplifies the postprandial excursion of serum and lipoprotein triglyceride and cholesterol concentrations by decreasing triglyceride clearance. *Am J Clin Nutr* 1994; **59**: 853–860.

24. Peters AL, Davidson MB, Eisenberg K. Effect of isocaloric substitution of chocolate cake for potato in type I diabetic patients. *Diabetes Care* 1990; **13**: 888–892.

25. Forlani G, Galuppi V, Santacroce G *et al.* Hyperglycemic effect of sucrose ingestion in IDDM patients controlled by artificial pancreas. *Diabetes Care* 1989; **12**: 296–298.

26. Bornet F, Haardt MJ, Costagliola D *et al.* Sucrose or honey at breakfast have no additional acute hyperglycaemic effect over an isoglucidic amount of bread in type II diabetic patients. *Diabetologia* 1985; **28**: 213–217.

27. Coulston AM, Hollenbeck CB, Donner CC *et al.* Metabolic effects of added dietary sucrose in individuals with non-insulin-dependent diabetes mellitus (NIDDM). *Metabolism* 1985; **34**: 962–966.

28. Slama G, Haardt MJ, Jean-Joseph P *et al.* Sucrose taken during mixed meal has no additional hyperglycemic action over isocaloric amounts of starch in well-controlled diabetics. *Lancet* 1984; **2**: 122–125.

29. Bantle JP, Laine DC, Castle GW *et al.* Postprandial glucose and insulin responses to meals containing different carbohydrates in normal and diabetic subjects. *N Engl J Med* 1983; **309**: 7–12.

30. Malerbi DA, Paiva ESA, Duarte Al, Wajchenberg BL. Metabolic effects of dietary sucrose and fructose in type II diabetic subjects. *Diabetes Care* 1996; **19**: 1249–1256.

31. Bantle JP, Swanson JE, Thomas W, Laine DC. Metabolic effects of dietary sucrose in type II diabetic subjects. *Diabetes Care* 1993; **16**: 1301–1305.

32. Abraira C, Derler J. Large variations of sucrose in constant carbohydrate diets in type II diabetes. *Am J Med* 1988; **84**: 193–200.

33. Bantle JP, Swanson JE, Thomas W, Laine DC. Metabolic effects of dietary fructose in diabetic subjects. *Diabetes Care* 1992; **15**: 1468–1476.

34. Bantle JP, Laine DC, Thomas JW. Metabolic effects of dietary fructose and sucrose in types I and II diabetic subjects. *JAMA* 1986; **256**: 3241–3246.

35. Crapo PA, Kolterman OG, Henry RR. Metabolic consequence of two-week fructose feeding in diabetic subjects. *Diabetes Care* 1986; **9**: 111–119.

36. Bantle JP. Current recommendations regarding the dietary treatment of diabetes mellitus. *Endocrinologist* 1994; **4**: 189–195.

37. National Research Council. *Recommended Dietary Allowances*, 10th edn. Washington DC: National Academy; 1989.

38. Brodsky IG, Robbins DC, Hiser E *et al.* Effects of low-protein diets on protein metabolism in insulin-dependent diabetes mellitus patients with early nephropathy. *J Clin Endocrinol Metab* 1992; **75**: 351–357.

39. Zeller KR. Low-protein diets in renal disease. *Diabetes Care* 1991; **14**: 856–866.

40. Brenner BM, Meyer TW, Hostetter TH. Dietary protein intake and the progressive nature of kidney disease: the role of hemodynamically mediated glomerular injury in the pathogenesis of progressive glomerular sclerosis in aging, renal ablation and intrinsic renal disease. *N Engl J Med* 1982; **307**: 652–659.

41. Nakamura H, Ito S, Ebe N, Shibata A. Renal effects of different types of protein in healthy volunteer subjects and diabetic patients. *Diabetes Care* 1993; **16**: 1071–1075.

42. Jibani MM, Bloodworth LL, Foden E *et al.* Predominantly vegetarian diet in patients with incipient and early clinical diabetic nephropathy: effects on albumin excretion rate and nutritional status. *Diabetic Med* 1991; **8**: 949–953.

43. Kontessis P, Jones S, Dodds R *et al.* Renal, metabolic and hormonal responses to ingestion of animal and vegetable proteins. *Kidney Int* 1990; **38**: 136–144.

44. Padley FB, Gunstone FD, Harwood JL. Occurrence and characteristics of oils and fats. In: Gunstone FD, Harwood JL, Padley FB, eds. *The Lipid Handbook*, 2nd edn. London: Chapman & Hall; 1994: 49–183.

45. National Cholesterol Education Program.

Second Report of the Expert Panel on Detection, Evaluation, and Treatment of High Blood Cholesterol in Adults. Washington DC: National Institutes of Health, 1993.

46. Cater NB, Garg A. Serum low-density lipoprotein cholesterol response to modification of saturated fat intake: recent insights. *Curr Opin Lipidol* 1997; **8**: 332–336.

47. Kris-Etherton PM, Yu S. Individual fatty acid effects on plasma lipids and lipoproteins: human studies. *Am J Clin Nutr* 1997; **65** (Suppl): 1628S-1644S.

48. Bonanome A, Grundy SM. Effect of dietary stearic acid on plasma cholesterol and lipoprotein levels. *N Engl J Med* 1988; **318**: 1244–1248.

49. Cater NB, Heller HJ, Denke MA. Comparison of the effects of medium-chain triacylglycerols, palm oil, and high oleic acid sunflower oil on plasma triacylglycerol fatty acids and lipid and lipoprotein concentrations in humans. *Am J Clin Nutr* 1997; **65**: 41–45.

50. Cater NB, Denke MA. Comparison of effects of behenate oil, high oleic acid sunflower oil, and palm oil on lipids and lipoproteins in humans (abstr). *Circulation* 1996; **94**: I-97.

51. Prince MJ, Deeg MA. Do n-3 fatty acids improve glucose tolerance and lipemia in diabetics? *Curr Opin Lipidol* 1997; **8**: 7–11.

52. Garg A. Optimum dietary therapy for patients with non-insulin-dependent diabetes mellitus. *Endocrinologist* 1996; **6**: 30–36.

53. Mensink RP, Katan MB. Effects of dietary fatty acids on serum lipids and lipoproteins: a meta-analysis of 27 trials. *Arterioscler Thromb* 1992; **12**: 911–919.

54. Valsta LM, Jauhiainen M, Aro A *et al.* Effects of a monounsaturated rapeseed oil and a polyunsaturated sunflower oil diet on lipoprotein levels in humans. *Arterioscler Thromb* 1992; **12**: 50–57.

55. Berry EM, Eisenberg S, Haratz D *et al.* Effects of diets rich in monounsaturated fatty acids on plasma lipoproteins – the Jerusalem Nutrition Study: high MUFAs vs high PUFAs. *Am J Clin Nutr* 1991; **53**: 899–907.

56. Dreon DM, Vranizan KM, Krauss RM *et al.* The effects of polyunsaturated fat vs. monounsaturated fat on plasma lipoproteins. *JAMA* 1990; **263**: 2462–2466.

57. McDonald BE, Gerrard JM, Bruce VM, Corner EJ. Comparison of the effect of canola oil and sunflower oil on plasma lipids and lipoproteins and on *in vivo* thromboxane A$_2$ and prostacyclin production in healthy young men. *Am J Clin Nutr* 1989; **50**: 1382–1388.

58. Mensink RP, Katan MB. Effect of a diet enriched with monounsaturated or polyunsaturated fatty acids on levels of low-density and high-density lipoprotein cholesterol in healthy women and men. *N Engl J Med* 1989; **321**: 436–441.

59. Mattson FH, Grundy SM. Comparison of effects of dietary saturated, monounsaturated, and polyunsaturated fatty acids on plasma lipids and lipoproteins in man. *J Lipid Res* 1985; **26**: 194–202.

60. Grande FY, Matsumoto Y, Anderson JT, Keys A. Effect of dietary rapeseed oil on man's serum lipids. *Circulation* 1962; **26**: 653–654.

61. Garg A, Bonanome A, Grundy SM *et al.* Comparison of a high-carbohydrate diet with a high-monounsaturated-fat diet in patients with non-insulin-dependent diabetes mellitus. *N Engl J Med* 1988; **319**: 829–834.

62. Garg A. High-monounsaturated-fat diets for patients with diabetes mellitus: a meta-analysis. *Am J Clin Nutr* 1998; **67** (Suppl): 577S-582S.

63. Parillo M, Giacco R, Ciardulo AV *et al.* Does a high-carbohydrate diet have different effects in NIDDM patients treated with diet alone or hypoglycemic drugs? *Diabetes Care* 1996; **19**: 498–500.

64. Garg A, Bantle JP, Henry RR *et al.* Effects of varying carbohydrate content of diet in patients with non-insulin-dependent diabetes mellitus. *JAMA* 1994; **271**: 1421–1428.

65. Lerman-Garber I, Ichazo-Cerro S, Zamora-Gonzalez J *et al.* Effect of a high-monounsaturated fat diet enriched with avocado in NIDDM patients. *Diabetes Care* 1994; **17**: 311–315.

66. Campbell LV, Marmot PE, Dyer JA *et al.* The high-monounsaturated fat diet as a practical alternative for NIDDM. *Diabetes Care* 1994; **17**: 177–182.

67. Rasmussen OW, Thomsen C, Hansen KW *et al.* Effects on blood pressure, glucose, and lipid levels of a high-monounsaturated fat diet compared with a high-carbohydrate diet in

NIDDM subjects. *Diabetes Care* 1993; **16:** 1565–1571.

68. Parillo M, Rivellese AA, Ciardullo AV *et al.* A high-monounsaturated fat/low-carbohydrate diet improves peripheral insulin sensitivity in non-insulin dependent diabetic patients. *Metabolism* 1992; **41:** 1373–1378.

69. Garg A, Grundy SM, Unger RH. Comparison of effects of high and low carbohydrate diets on plasma lipoproteins and insulin sensitivity in patients with mild NIDDM. *Diabetes* 1992; **41:** 1278–1285.

70. Rivellese AA, Giacco R, Genovese S *et al.* Effects of changing amount of carbohydrate in diet on plasma lipoproteins and apolipoproteins in type II diabetic patients. *Diabetes Care* 1990; **13:** 446–448.

71. Nestel P, Noakes M, Belling B *et al.* Plasma lipoprotein lipid and Lp[a] changes with substitution of elaidic acid for oleic acid in the diet. *J Lipid Res* 1992; **33:** 1029–1036.

72. Mensink RP, Katan MB. Effect of dietary *trans* fatty acids on high-density and low-density lipoprotein cholesterol levels in healthy subjects. *N Engl J Med* 1990; **323:** 439–445.

73. US Department of Agriculture, Agriculture Research Service. USDA Nutrient Data Base for Standard Reference Release 12, (March 1998), Nutrient Data Home Page, http://www.nal.usda.gov/fnic/foodcomp.

74. Pennington JT. *Bowes & Church's Food Values of Portions Commonly Used*, 17th edn. Philadelphia: Lippincott; 1998.

75. American Diabetes Association. Treatment of hypertension in diabetes (consensus statement). *Diabetes Care* 1993; **16:** 1394–1401.

76. American Diabetes Association. Nutrition recommendations and principles for people with diabetes mellitus. *Diabetes Care* 1998; **21 (Suppl 1):** S32–S35.

77. Lalor BC, Bhatnagar D, Winocour PH *et al.* Placebo-controlled trial of the effects of guar gum and metformin on fasting blood glucose and serum lipids in obese, type II diabetic patients. *Diabetic Med* 1990; **7:** 242–245.

78. Uusitupa M, Siitonen O, Savolainen K *et al.* Metabolic and nutritional effects of long-term use of guar gum in the treatment of non-insulin-dependent diabetes of poor metabolic control. *Am J Clin Nutr* 1989; **49:** 345–351.

79. Aro A, Uusitupa M, Voutilainen E *et al.* Improved diabetic control and hypocholesterolaemic effect induced by long-term dietary supplementation with guar gum in type II (insulin-dependent) diabetes. *Diabetologia* 1981; **21:** 29–33.

80. Nuttall FQ. Dietary fiber in the management of diabetes. *Diabetes* 1993; **42:** 503–508.

81. Shakel SF, Sievert YA, Buzzard IM. In: Appendix I, Table 1, Dietary Fiber Values for Common Foods. In: Spiller GA, ed. *CRC Handbook of Dietary Fiber in Human Nutrition*, 2nd edn. Boca Raton: CRC Press, Inc.; 1993: 567–593.

82. Ben G, Gnudi L, Maran A *et al.* Effects of chronic alcohol intake on carbohydrate and lipid metabolism in subjects with type II (non-insulin-dependent) diabetes. *Am J Med* 1991; **90:** 70–76.

83. Yki-Jarvinen H, Koivisto VA, Ylikahri R, Taskinen M-R. Acute effects of ethanol and acetate on glucose kinetics in normal subjects. *Am J Physiol* 1988; **254:** E175–E180.

84. Mooradian AD, Failla M, Hoogwerf B *et al.* Selected vitamins and minerals in diabetes. *Diabetes Care* 1994; **17:** 464–479.

85. Jialal I, Grundy SM. Effect of combined supplementation with α-tocopherol, ascorbate, and β-carotene on low-density lipoprotein oxidation. *Circulation* 1993; **88:** 2780–2786.

86. Steinberg D, Parthasarathy S, Carew TE *et al.* Beyond cholesterol: Modifications of low-density lipoproteins that increase its atherogenicity. *N Engl J Med* 1989; **320:** 915–924.

87. Abraham AS, Brooks BA, Eylate U. The effects of chromium supplementation on serum glucose and lipids in patients with and without non-insulin-dependent diabetes. *Metabolism* 1992; **41:** 768–771.

88. Anderson RA, Polansky MM, Bryden NA, Canary JJ. Supplemental-chromium effects on glucose, insulin, glucagon, and urinary chromium losses in subjects consuming controlled low-chromium diets. *Am J Clin Nutr* 1991; **54:** 909–916.

89. Rabinowitz MB, Gonick HC, Levin SR, Davidson MB. Effect of chromium and yeast supplements on carbohydrate and lipid metabolism in diabetic men. *Diabetes Care* 1983; **6:** 319–327.

90. Rabinowitz MB, Levin SR, Gonick HC. Comparison of chromium status in diabetic and normal men. *Metabolism* 1980; **29**: 355–364.

91. Anderson RA, Cheng N, Bryden NA *et al.* Elevated intakes of supplemental chromium improve glucose and insulin variables in individuals with Type 2 diabetes. *Diabetes* 1997; **46**: 1786–1791.

92. Miettinen TA, Puska P, Gylling H *et al.* Reduction of serum cholesterol with sitostanol ester margarine in a mildly hypercholes-terolemic population. *N Engl J Med* 1995; **333**: 1308–1312.

93. Gylling H, Miettinen TA. Cholesterol absorp-tion, synthesis and LDL metabolism in NIDDM. *Diabetes Care* 1997; **20**: 90–95.

94. Gylling H, Miettinen TA. Serum cholesterol and cholesterol and lipoprotein metabolism in hypercholesterolaemic NIDDM patients before and during sitostanol ester-margarine treatment. *Diabetologia* 1994; **37**: 773–780.

95. Markovic TP, Campbell LV, Balasubramanian S *et al.* Beneficial effect on average lipid levels from energy restriction and fat loss in obese individuals with or without Type 2 diabetes. *Diabetes Care* 1998; **21**: 695–700.

96. Wing RR, Blair EH, Bononi P *et al.* Caloric restriction *per se* is a significant factor in improvements in glycemic control and insulin sensitivity during weight loss in obese NIDDM patients. *Diabetes Care* 1994; **17**: 30–36.

97. Food and Nutrition Board, Institute of Medicine, Thomas PR, ed. *Weighing the Options: Criteria for Evaluating Weight Management Programs. Committee to develop criteria for evaluating the outcomes of approaches to prevent and treat obesity.* Washington DC: National Academy Press; 1995.

98. Mattes RD. Fat preference and adherence to a reduced-fat diet. *Am J Clin Nutr* 1993; **57**: 373–381.

99. Mattes RD. Discretionary salt and compliance with reduced sodium diet. *Nutr Res* 1990; **10**: 1337–1352.

100. Bertino M, Beauchamp GK. Increasing dietary salt alters salt taste preference. *Physiol Behav* 1986; **38**: 203–213.

101. Bertino M, Beauchamp GK, Engelman K. Long term reduction in dietary sodium alters the taste of salt. *Am J Clin Nutr* 1982; **36**: 1134–1144.

102. National Institutes of Health Technology Assessment Conference Panel, Methods for voluntary weight loss and control: Technology assessment conference statement. *Ann Intern Med* 1993; **119**: 764–770.

103. Shick SM, Wing RR, Klem ML *et al.* Persons successful at long-term weight loss and maintenance continue to consume a low-energy, low-fat diet. *J Am Diet Assoc* 1998; **98**: 408–413.

104. French SA, Jeffery RW. Current dieting, weight loss history, and weight suppression: behavioral correlates of three dimensions of dieting. *Addict Behav* 1997; **22**: 31–44.

105. Klem ML, Wing RR, McGuire MT *et al.* A descriptive study of individuals successful at long-term maintenance of substantial weight loss. *Am J Clin Nutr* 1997; **66**: 239–246.

106. Harris JK, French SA, Jeffery RW *et al.* Dietary and physical activity correlates of long-term weight loss. *Obesity Res* 1994; **2**: 307–313.

107. Pronk NP, Wing RR. Physical activity and long-term maintenance of weight loss. *Obesity Res* 1994; **2**: 587–599.

108. Kayman S, Bruvold W, Stern JS. Maintenance and relapse after weight loss in women: behavioral aspects. *Am J Clin Nutr* 1990; **52**: 800–807.

109. Perri MG, McAllister DA, Gange JJ *et al.* Effects of four maintenance programs on the long-term management of obesity. *J Cons Clin Psychol* 1988; **56**: 529–534.

110. Perri MG, McAdoo WG, McAllister DA *et al.* Enhancing the efficacy of behavior therapy for obesity: Effects of aerobic exercise and a multicomponent maintenance program. *J Cons Clin Psychol* 1986; **54**: 670–675.

111. Jeffery RW, Bjornson-Benson WM, Rosenthal BS *et al.* Correlates of weight loss and its maintenance over two years of follow-up among middle-aged men. *Prev Med* 1984; **13**: 155–168.

112. Marston AR, Criss J. Maintenance of success-ful weight loss: Incidence and prediction. *J Int Obes* 1984; **8**: 435–439.

113. Colvin RH, Olson SB. A descriptive analysis of men and women who have lost significant

weight and are highly successful at maintaining the loss. *Addict Behav* 1983; **8**: 287–295.

114. Bray GA. Classification and evaluation of the obesities. *Med Clin N Am* 1989; **73**: 161–184.

115. Lamont LS. Beta-blockers and their effects on protein metabolism and resting energy expenditure. *J Cardpulm Rehabil* 1995; **15**: 183–185.

116. Schlundt DG, Rea MR, Kline SS, Pichert JW. Situational obstacles to dietary adherence for adults with diabetes. *J Am Diet Assoc* 1994; **94**: 874–876, 879.

117. Brown SL, Pope JF, Hunt AE, Tolman NM. Motivational strategies used by dietitians to counsel individuals with diabetes. *Diabetes Educ* 1998; **24**: 313–318.

118. Arnold MS, Stepien CJ, Hess GE, Hiss RG. Guidelines vs practice in the delivery of diabetes nutrition care. *J Am Diet Assoc* 1993; **93**: 34–39.

119. Close EJ, Wiles PG, Lockton JA *et al.* The degree of day-to-day variation in food intake in diabetic patients. *Diab Med* 1993; **10**: 514–520.

120. Schlundt DG, Hill JO, Sbrocco T *et al.* The role of breakfast in the treatment of obesity: a randomized clinical trial. *Am J Clin Nutr* 1992; **55**: 645–651.

121. Verboeket-van den Venne WPHG, Westerterp KR. Frequency of feeding, weight reduction and energy metabolism. *Int J Obes* 1993; **17**: 31–36.

122. Jenkins DJA, Ocana A, Jenkins AL *et al.* Metabolic advantages of spreading the nutrient load: effects of increased meal frequency in non-insulin-dependent diabetes. *Am J Clin Nutr* 1992; **55**: 461–467.

123. Nutrition Subcommittee of the British Diabetic Association's Professional Advisory Committee. Dietary recommendations for people with diabetes: An update for the 1990's. *Diab Med* 1992; **9**: 189–202.

124. Special Report Committee of the Canadian Diabetes Association. 1980 guidelines for the nutritional management of diabetes mellitus: a special report from the Canadian Diabetes Association. *J Can Diet Assoc* 1981; **42**: 110–118.

125. Bertelsen J, Christiansen C, Thomsen C *et al.* Effect of meal frequency on blood glucose,

insulin, and free fatty acids in NIDDM subjects. *Diabetes Care* 1993; **16**: 4–7.

126. Jenkins DJA, Ocana A, Jenkins AL *et al.* Metabolic advantages of spreading the nutrient load: effects of increased meal frequency in non-insulin-dependent diabetes. *Am J Clin Nutr* 1992; **55**: 461–467.

127. Jenkins DJA, Wolever TMS, Vuksan V *et al.* Nibbling versus gorging: Metabolic advantages of increased meal frequency. *N Engl J Med* 1989; **321**: 929–934.

128. Beebe CA, Cauter EV, Shapiro ET *et al.* Effect of temporal distribution of calories on diurnal patterns of glucose levels and insulin secretion in NIDDM. *Diabetes Care* 1990; **13**: 748–755.

129. Holler HJ, Pastors JG. *Diabetes Medical Nutrition Therapy: A professional guide to management and nutrition education resources.* Chicago, Alexandria: The American Dietetic Association, 1997.

130. Stephen AM, Sieber GM, Gerster YA, Morgan DR. Intake of carbohydrate and its components – international comparisons, trends over time, and effects of changing to low-fat diets. *Am J Clin Nutr* 1995; **62**: 851S–867S.

131. Position of The American Dietetic Association. Use of nutritive and nonnutritive sweeteners. *J Am Diet Assoc* 1998; **98**: 580–587.

132. Messina M, Messina V. *The Dietitian's Guide to Vegetarian Diets: Issues and Applications.* Gaithersburg, MD; Aspen Publishers, Inc., 1996.

133. Position of The American Dietetic Association. Fat replacers. *J Am Diet Assoc* 1998; **98**: 463–468.

134. Prince DM, Welschenbach MA. Olestra: a new food additive. *J Am Diet Assoc* 1998; **98**: 565–569.

135. Hahn NI. Replacing fat with food technology – a brief review of new fat replacement ingredients. *J Am Diet Assoc* 1997; **97**: 15–16.

136. Caputo FA, Mattes RD. Human dietary responses to perceived fat content of a midday meal. *Int J Obes* 1993; **17**: 237–240.

137. Lyle BJ, McMahon KE, Kruetler PA. Assessing the potential dietary impact of replacing dietary fat with other macronutrients. *J Nutr* 1992; **122**: 211–216.

138. Rolls B, Shide D, Hoeymans N *et al.* Information about the fat content of preloads, influences energy intake in women. *Appetite* 1992; **19**: 213.

139. Tinker LF, Wheeler ML. Fiber metabolism and use in diabetes therapy. In: Powers MA, ed. *Handbook of Diabetes Medical Nutrition Therapy.* Gaithersburg, MD: Aspen Publishers, Inc., 1996: 397–414.

140. Monk A, Barry B, McClain K *et al.* Practice guidelines for medical nutrition therapy provided by dietitians for persons with non-insulin-dependent diabetes mellitus. *J Am Diet Assoc* 1995; **95**: 999–1006.

141. Warshaw HS. Nutrition management of diabetes must be individualized. *Diabetes Care* 1993; **16**: 843–844.

142. Campbell LV, Barth R, Gosper JK *et al.* Impact of intensive educational approach to dietary change in NIDDM. *Diabetes Care* 1990; **13**: 841–847.

143. Franz MJ, Monk A, Barry B *et al.* Effectiveness of medical nutrition therapy provided by dietitians in the management of non-insulin-dependent diabetes mellitus: A randomized, controlled clinical trial. *J Am Diet Assoc* 1995; **95**: 1009–1017.

144. The DCCT Research Group. Nutrition interventions for intensive therapy in the diabetes control and complications trial. *J Am Diet Assoc* 1993; **93**: 768–772.

145. Delahanty LM, Halford BN. The role of diet behaviors in achieving improved glycemic control in intensively treated patients in the diabetes control and complications trial. *Diabetes Care* 1993; **16**: 1453–1458.

146. Diabetes Care and Education Dietetic Practice Group. *Meal Planning Approaches for Diabetes Management*, 2nd edn. Chicago: The American Dietetic Association, 1994.

147. Gillespie SJ, Kulkarni KD, Daly AE. Using carbohydrate counting in diabetes clinical practice. *J Am Diet Assoc* 1998; **98**: 897–905.

148. Foster-Powell K, Miller JB. International tables of glycemic index. *Am J Clin Nutr* 1995; **62**: 871S-893S.

149. Jenkins DJA, Wolever TMS, Taylor RH *et al.* Glycemic index of foods: a physiological basis for carbohydrate exchange. *Am J Clin Nutr* 1981; **34**: 362–366.

18

Patient self-empowerment: the route to improved clinical outcome and patient satisfaction

John Day

'The empowerment philosophy is based on the premise that human beings have the capacity to make choices and are responsible for the consequences of their choices. Empowerment is defined as an educational process designed to help patients develop the knowledge, skills, attitudes, and degree of self-awareness necessary to effectively assume responsibility for their health-related decisions.'[1]

Introduction

The idea that patients should undertake the principal role in the management of their diabetes is not new. Indeed, following the introduction of insulin in 1922, Joslin and colleagues in the USA and Lawrence in the UK each enshrined this in their systems of care.

However, in the 1930s and 1940s the excitement that followed the introduction of insulin and the success in preventing ketoacidosis were blunted by the realization that many patients still developed the late complications of diabetes. Major pharmacological efforts were undertaken to find different formulations of insulin and oral preparations which might provide patients with good overall control of their diabetes, preventing hypoglycaemia and hyperglycaemia alike. As a consequence of availability of different insulins and oral agents and the very large numbers of people with diabetes, systems of care were developed based on large centralized clinics. There was an overriding philosophy underpinning the systems of care, of the potential success of prescription, with neglect of the importance of patients' self-management.

In the 1960s and 1970s, the burden of the complications of diabetes became increasingly apparent, and frustration with the pharmacological tools available prompted moves to examine more closely the educational component of care. This was given considerable stimulus by the pioneering work of Leona Miller, which showed that an improved educational approach could have a dramatic effect on outcome.[2] Much of the original thrusts, of the education programmes which were developed, were knowledge- or information-transfer-based. The educational process was in many instances divorced from the clinical setting. Not only were many patients still admitted to hospital, for the institution of insulin treatment, especially children, but also large numbers of the big diabetes care centres provided special in-patient units for 'education'. The philosophy of 'treatment' either with the drugs available or with the provision of education was therefore maintained.

However, much more sophisticated scrutiny of educational processes was undertaken by such groups as the Diabetes Education Study Group of the European Association of Diabetes and the American Association of Diabetes Educators. There was a growing awareness that

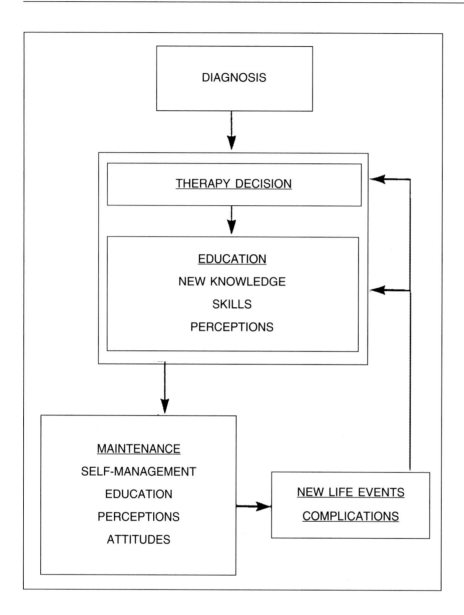

Fig. 18.1
Diabetes Care Cycle.

information transfer was just the first stepping stone to enable people to self-manage their condition and that psychological factors governing self-behaviour were much more important. Coincidentally, it was recognized that if success is to be achieved then the care systems must be changed to enable the process of what is now called 'self-empowerment' to be acquired.

Recent major clinical studies, the Diabetes Control and Complications Trial (DCCT) Study in insulin-treated diabetes, and the United Kingdom Prospective Diabetes Study (UKPDS) in non-insulin-treated diabetes, have delivered important messages in this regard. With regard to the DCCT Study, despite an enormous investment of professional time and money and the highly successful demonstration of the contribution of more-intensified treatment to the reduction of complications, less than 10% of subjects actually achieved and maintained the glycaemic targets which were set for them.[3] This would confirm most clinical experience, that despite our understanding and use of insulin and more intensive regimens, many people do not succeed in maintaining their blood sugars within a range which is likely to leave them free of the risk of long-term problems. On the positive side, however, if we examine the run-in period of the UKPDS, the most notable achievement was a considerable reduction in weight and improvement in blood sugar control achieved by dietary modification.[4] This was something that the patients achieved for themselves. Another striking recent study from Scotland revealed that many young people with diabetes failed to take significant amounts of the insulin prescribed for them, and that there was a clear-cut relationship not only between their lack of use of insulin and episodes of ketoacidosis, but also their glycosylated haemaglobin.[5] These studies emphasize the importance of self-management.

If we consider the life with diabetes, it can be summarized as a cycle (*Fig. 18.1*). Commencing with a diagnosis and a therapy decision, this is immediately followed by the requirement of some change in behaviour of the patient concerned. These changes demand the active participation of the subject, and we call this 'education', better defined as 'learning new behaviour'. Subsequently, these behaviours have to be maintained throughout the life of the individual. New life events, pregnancy, change in job, adoption of new social activities, etc., may require modification not only of therapy but also the adoption of new behaviours, e.g. frequency of injection, etc. Unfortunately, many subjects will develop complications and again require the learning of new activities (e.g. special foot care or adaptation of lifestyle) accompanied by further therapy changes.

The critical role of patient behaviour throughout this life cycle is such that unless the care process enables or empowers the patient to make these behavioural changes, they will not be adopted. There is now substantial evidence that processes of care which achieve this are associated with more successful outcomes, not only in diabetes but in other chronic disease such as hypertension and asthma.[6,7]

This chapter, therefore, examines the reasons why patients have difficulty in adopting and maintaining behaviours that are recommended to them, the recognition that shifting control of the illness from a medical team to the patient is a significant factor in helping people achieve these changes, and systems of care which enable this process of self-empowerment most likely to be more successful.

Factors governing effective self-care

Basic knowledge

Whilst new information is an essential part of the process of learning new behaviour, there is good evidence not only that IQ and behaviour are largely unrelated, but also that improvement in basic knowledge and metabolic control or other behaviours such as foot self-care are seldom correlated.[8] Many factors may be responsible for determining whether new information is used to adjust self-care behaviour. This seems to be determined largely by attitudes, perceptions and beliefs.

Targets

Clear recognition of the targets desired is critical. When patients are formally asked to indicate whether they believe themselves to be very well, moderately well, or poorly controlled, studies show that there is considerable discrepancy between belief and reality. Many subjects will recognize the ideal target to be aimed for but may have reset the target to meet their own needs, for example to avoid hypoglycaemia. The targets that are set by professionals may be perceived as unobtainable. A good example for this is the study by Frost in provision of dietary weight-reducing advice to people with non-insulin-dependent diabetes. They were divided into two groups, one of whom was provided with an average of 1,600 calories based on a formula which takes into account body mass index (BMI) and amount of exercise. The second group's calorie requirement was based on dietary history, with a subtraction of 500 calories giving a mean target of 1,200 calories. The latter failed to lose weight or improve their HbA_1, whereas the former despite a higher and hence more achievable target, improved significantly on both counts.[9] As indicated above in the DCCT Study, it was clear that the majority of patients could not achieve the targets that were set for them. Subsequently, it has been recognized that these targets were probably too tight and could only be achieved at the expense of considerable hypoglycaemia.

With regard to the matching of professional and patient targets, it is worth considering the fundamental processes of adult learning. Coles[10] has emphasized the need for patients to have an accurate 'picture' of the implications of the illness and the consequential behaviours required. Rather than the 'pot-filling' approach to education, where there is a multiple in-put of new information from which the individual is often expected to deduce the behaviours desired, the process should involve clear-cut demonstration of the picture from which are derived whatever new information, skills or attitudes are needed to create it. Almost all individuals have some image of the disease at diagnosis. This is often not recognized by professionals, and hence myths or false ideas may perpetuate inappropriate behaviour (for example, that on the one hand 'all people will develop complications' or alternatively 'people they know with diabetes never have any problems with it').

It is encumbent on the professionals, therefore, to ensure not only that the individuals have clear-cut targets to aim for, but also that these should be perceived as achievable, and if necessary negotiated. Continuous feedback must be provided as to the level of their achievement.

Health beliefs

Studies of health beliefs and their relationship to management of chronic disease reveal their importance. In making decisions about self-management, individuals undoubtedly[11] make decisions based on perceived benefits of, or barriers to, the adoption of new behaviours (although they may be unaware of this). Whereas professionals generally rate the medical benefits as outweighing the barriers, the judgement of the patient may be quite contrary. Whereas most individuals recognize the potential severity of the complications of diabetes, they may not appreciate their own vulnerability. The elegant studies of Bradley *et al.* in insulin-treated subjects showed that on a high to low rating scale, cancer and heart disease were followed by the complications of diabetes as potentially severe health problems, with hypoglycaemia rated as of least importance.[12] However, the same individuals when asked to consider their vulnerability to these problems reversed the order. Any one individual may have no 'belief' that they are at risk. Denial is well known to occur in up to 20% of the population. Amongst adolescents this may be the norm. Given such a belief set, there is no reason why an individual should adopt a more stringent approach to their self-management. The second important component of belief about health is whether the individual considers that they are personally responsible for the outcome of their illness. It has been traditional to consider that the medical/nursing team is responsible. This is clearly accurate in respect of severe acute illnesses, especially when surgery is required, but quite inappropriate to the management of chronic disease when active participation by the patient is vital. Three views about 'locus of control' may be held: that the responsibility lies primarily with the individual with the disease ('internal'), that it is the responsibility of the medical team ('external'), or thirdly, that it is a matter of pure chance as to what outcome may occur. Indeed, attitudes are also very variable in different cultural circumstances. Religious influences may be predominant or alternative medicine be more acceptable than traditional.

Many aberrant behaviours may be belief dependent. For example, falsification of blood sugar test results may be due to the failure of the individual to perceive tests as providing information to them as opposed to the doctor, to learned hopelessness that provision of tests makes no difference to the advice given and is not accompanied by useful interventions, or just perceived as socially useful in maintaining good relationships with the medical team. Ineffective choices of treatment, for example use of pumps or other devices, selected by patients may be based on false expectations that external control may solve their problem.[13] Fortunately, however, experience of measure-

ment of a patient's 'satisfaction with treatment' reveals that a switch from reliance on others to self-control or self-empowerment greatly enhances this.

Emotional adjustment

Mood and behaviour may be closely related. On the one hand, excessive anxiety, or on the other depression and despair, are major barriers to self-action. Studies do demonstrate higher rates either of anxiety or depression in people with diabetes, and in a significant number of individuals these may be critical features which influence self-management. In contrast, those with no anxiety about the illness are unlikely to adopt the difficult measures that are required to achieve the standards that are recommended. Coping skills, therefore, are undoubtedly mood related.[14,15]

Social environment

One of the major criticisms of clinical and educational approaches to diabetes has been that they have focused on the medical outcomes of the illness. However, for those with the diagnosis, the impact on their daily life may quite justifiably be perceived as far more important than the physical consequences. Furthermore, those important others, close family and friends, will also have views which may be supportive but can be unhelpful. On the one hand, their advice may be adopted by the sufferer more readily than those of the professional team and, on the other, constant 'good' advice from partners or parents may be construed as interference and thus rejected. In the process of developing effective self-empowerment, the importance of these influences cannot be overestimated. Subjects need to be able to recognize these themselves, and the supporting role of the health-care team is likely to be inappropriate if there is a failure to recognize when lifestyle objectives are overriding medical ones.

An integrated model of factors governing behaviour

Since there is such a wide range of influences that may be operating in any one individual, it is worth considering how these can be integrated for analytical purposes. The model of Ajzen and Fishbein is useful in this respect

(*Fig. 18.2*).[16] This is based on the well-accepted assumption that to change behaviour the individual must first want to do so. The various influences on this can be summarized as basic demographic variables such as age, sex, basic knowledge, and important social and attitudinal effects.[16] This model has been tested in a large diabetic population in The Netherlands, and significant relationships have been described between evidence of these influences and behaviour such as self-testing.[17] One of the most striking negative correlations was between

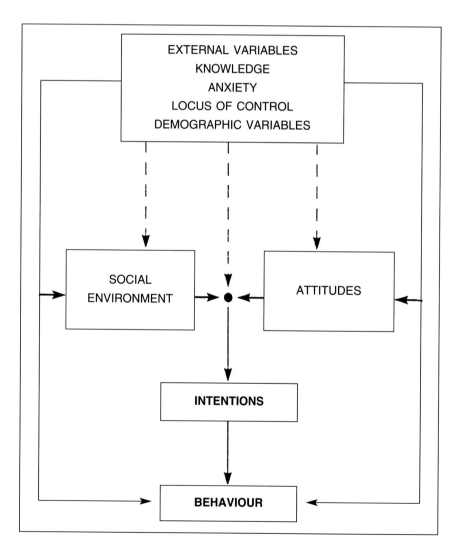

Fig. 18.2
Model of factors determining change in behaviour. Adapted from Ajzen I, Fishbein M. Understanding Attitudes and Predicting Social Behaviour, 1980.[16]

external locus of control or powerful others, i.e. behaviour. The Prochaska model of cycle of change behaviour amplifies this; starting with the pre-contemplative state, moving hopefully to contemplative (or intention to change) action and maintenance to avoid relapse.[18]

Identification of self-management or empowerment status of individuals

In order to ensure successful patient empowerment, it is necessary to determine which of the features described above (summarized in *Table 18.1*) in any one individual may be operative in promoting or preventing effective self-care behaviour. Unlike personality, beliefs and perceptions can be altered, but if professionals involved in clinical care are to facilitate the process, they need to take active steps to determine these. In the traditional medical model of care, these elements are frequently omitted.

In recent years a large number of the studies have been undertaken to determine whether quantitative assessment of these can be performed using specifically designed questionnaires. However, if care is not taken, the validity and reliability of these questionnaires may

Table 18.1
Factors governing self-management behaviour.

Knowledge
Self-management skills
Perception of desired targets
Perception of standards achieved
Perceived benefits/barriers
Locus of control
Role of important others
Effects in lifestyle
General emotional adjustment

be questionable. This is discussed in detail in Professor Bradley's *Handbook of Psychology and Diabetes*.[19] This contains examples of well-designed reliable and robust instruments. However, most of these are specific to only one of the factors. They are, therefore, cumbersome to use if a comprehensive picture of the individual is to be obtained. Recent work with questionnaires from the Ipswich group designed to incorporate these factors in single instruments for insulin-treated and non-insulin treated subjects, respectively, is very promising. Factor analysis of the insulin questionnaire identified nine discrete factors (*Table 18.2*),

Factor	No. of quests	Eigen value	Cronbach's alpha
Lifestyle	4	5.81	0.76
Perceived self-efficacy	7	3.21	0.71
Weight concerns	3	2.63	0.76
Perceived goals	2	1.87	0.83
Cost–benefit analysis	6	1.70	0.71
Outside support	2	1.53	0.45
Practical skills	3	1.50	0.65
Diet barriers	2	1.39	0.63
Emotional adjustment	5	1.19	0.75

Table 18.2
Factors identified by self-management questionnaire in 284 insulin-treated subjects.

Table 18.3

Relationship between factors identified and glycaemic control. Multiple regression – dependent variable HbA$_1$: predictor variables which explain 21% of variance in HbA$_1$ (r = 0.46)

	r	p
Practical self-management skills	−0.29	0.001
Emotional adjustment	0.27	0.002
Perceived goals	−0.23	0.01
Perceived self-efficacy	−0.26	0.003
Cost–benefit analysis	0.23	0.01

and these largely matched those that are discussed above, with the addition of two factors, one specifically related to perceived dietary barriers and one to weight concerns. Of the nine factor scores, five of them could be related to glycaemic control (*Table 18.3*). The remaining four were quite unrelated. The former were largely concerned with the medical self-management of the individual, and the latter to achieving a successful life with diabetes.[20] Similar factors were identified in the questionnaire for non-insulin-dependent patients. Both were discriminant in providing significantly different factor scores for subjects with different demographic characteristics, i.e. age, sex, duration of diabetes, and, in the case of non-insulin-dependent subjects, between those treated with diet alone and those treated also with tablets. These studies all validate the importance of the elements hypothesized above.

In day-to-day clinical practice, assessment of an individual is most likely to be based on a one-to-one interview. Studies of this process suggest that the agenda is usually medically based and more concerned with clinical outcomes than the attitudes, beliefs, and perceptions of the subject. However, the latter are so critical in determining the management which ultimately governs the clinical outcome that they need to be comprehensively addressed. A personal study by the author of sequential interviews performed by different personnel, including nurse educators, doctors, and dietitians, revealed that it was possible for reasonable reliability between interviewers to be achieved. However, all those involved in this study acknowledged that they had to adjust the agenda of their interviews and their style in order to achieve this. It is recommended that in our clinical assessment of those with diabetes we should not just itemize the clinical outcomes such as glycaemia control, weight, presence of complications, etc., but also complete a systematic list from time to time of their attitudinal status.

Facilitating or inhibiting self-empowerment?

Studies of educational and care processes have underlined the necessity of close examination of the attitudes and roles of the professional care team, the organization of care and methods of education, and identification of those which most effectively enable effective self-care and empowerment.

Role of professional advisers

Studies of interviews reveal that to a large extent the professional partner is the dominant one, does most of the talking, and controls the agenda. The excellent studies by Kaplan *et al.*[21] using audio recordings demonstrated that such behaviour has a negative outcome on self-management behaviour and indeed glycaemic control. In contrast, their intervention studies, in which they trained individuals with diabetes to take control of the interviews themselves, revealed a highly significant improvement in glycaemic outcome. Knowledge acquisition actually improved, presumably because the patients were asking questions which they perceived as relevant, and hence they 'learned' the answers. Outcomes were improved following interviews in which more emotion was expressed, whether by the subject with diabetes or the professional. It seems evident that if the barriers to self-empowerment are to be identified and adequate negotiation to take place, to eliminate such barriers a listening/counselling approach must be adopted. This may often require acquisition of new skills.

Attitudes of professionals

Despite frequent protests to the contrary, professionals like patients may find it difficult to change their behaviours. Those entering the caring professions very often do so with a desire to 'cure' or 'treat'. During training programmes largely based on the management of acute medical problems, these attitudes may become entrenched. Many may not wish to relinquish control to the patients, distrusting their ability to manage themselves. Similar inhibitions to those observed in patients apply to professional's change of behaviour, including social environment, peer pressures, and the individual's self-confidence. The presence or absence of desire to adopt new behaviours which may encourage self-empowerment are deep rooted and not necessarily profession related. Examination of many of the training curricula, whether for doctors or nurses, suggest that they tend to encourage a more prescriptive approach than that required for this purpose. Finally, all those involved need to perceive a benefit, not only for the patients but also for themselves. The importance of more successful medical outcomes as a consequence

of these approaches has therefore to be emphasized. It must be remembered, however, that there is nothing intrinsically wrong with the professional's agenda for a more successful medical outcome. The process of achieving self-empowerment should not take place at the expense of the requirement for appropriate medical supervision and treatment. Indeed, there have been some observations that when a system of care is developed to encourage improvement in quality of life but which does not take into account the medical aspects, glycaemic control may worsen. All those involved therefore have to recognize the dual roles that they serve and be able to switch from one to the other when appropriate.

Role perception

One of the major features for successful self-management is likely to be a change in perception or redefinition of roles. As indicated above, the professionals may find this difficult, but likewise the patients may be irritated and indeed resentful that they should be asked to take an active part in their management. Early after diagnosis it is necessary for the professionals to establish their roles and use all their persuasion to ensure that those with diabetes appreciate that it is an advisory one, and that success is only likely to be achieved if the role of self-doctoring is undertaken. Individuals may seek a whole range of manoeuvres to avoid this, and very often the professionals get drawn into the same process. For example, when poor glycaemic control is manifest there will be frequent requests for a change in insulin type or delivery system. The studies of Bradley[19] demonstrated that those seeking use of subcutaneous insulin infusion pumps very often did so in the desire to acquire a black box to control the illness for them.[13] It is very often more comfortable for the professional to respond to these cues and join the game of looking for an 'external' control system. Facing these issues may be very difficult and indeed create anger between the professional and patient partners, but failure to do so will result in ever-increasing fruitless consultation and lack of success.

Environment and organization of care

The encouragement of the self-empowerment process may be very dependent on the ways in which care is organized and the environment in which it takes place. For example, if the first response after establishing the diagnosis of insulin-dependent diabetes is admission to hospital for institution of insulin therapy, the major message is that this cannot be achieved by the patient themselves but is dependent on the armamentaria of the full medical team. The failure to discharge patients until 'perfect' metabolic control is achieved by such a team also cues the patient to believe that they might not achieve this themselves. Similarly, approaches to education may have the same implications if self-learning is substituted for by a formal hospital-based 'programme', especially when this also requires admission. Strict demands for adherence to particular testing or injection behaviours have the same effects. This may explain why many of the patients in the DCCT Study in the intensively treated group did not achieve the targets that were set for them, possibly because the regimen for injections, frequent testing, and frequent attendance was so rigid as to actually restrict self-adjustment.

It is recommended, therefore, that in the initial learning process, freedom is given to the patients to find out things for themselves. It is not desirable to achieve good glycaemic control in the first instance. It is probably better for

the initial prescription of insulin, for example, to be suboptimal, to allow the individual to observe high blood sugars and draw deductions for the reasons. This may then lead to their returning to the professional with questions such as, 'Shouldn't my insulin last longer?', 'Don't I need a larger dose?'. The consequence will be improved confidence of their own capabilities. The traditional hierarchy within hospital and clinic structures of doctors overseeing nurses or dietitians or other professionals may also be a barrier. Since the nurse educators are likely to play the most important role in the education counselling process, they must be perceived as having equivalent status. It is important therefore that their skills are made overt to the patient and not undermined by the way that clinics are organized (e.g. 'see the doctor first, then the nurse, and then the dietitian').

Continuity is also important. Short episodes with different professional personnel are likely to be least helpful. However, the long-term gains of patients achieving adequate self-empowerment in reducing clinic attendance and frequency of appointment, and ultimately shortening of consultation time, balance the initial time outlay. Finally, behaviours within clinics have to be discussed and agreed by all members of the team, and commitment of the principles of self-empowerment adopted. All too commonly, members of the staff may be observed reinforcing traditional institutional behaviour, e.g. remarks such as 'Have you brought your testing book' or alternatively reaching for the same book clutched by the patient before opening the conversation. Technological advances may also inhibit this process, e.g. a computer screen between the patient and the professional, with little eye-to-eye contact or, alternatively, the use of electronic transfer of data from a patient's meter into a doctor's office for him or her to remain the decision-maker. Finally, many clinics, involving as they do very large numbers of patients and staff, create an environment where activity and hurry are the most obvious features and are alien to effective communication. Not only do these processes need to be undertaken in a more comfortable environment but also one over which the patients themselves might feel some ownership.

'Patients' as teachers

Many studies indicate that patients may learn best from one another. Balint's emphasis on psychological processes, interpersonal relationships, and use of patient-centred discussion groups has had a major influence on the development of professional–patient relationships.[22] The work of Groen and Pelser several years ago elegantly demonstrated the use of group learning. Even when such groups were facilitated by non-professionals, they were highly effective in helping patients to manage their own illnesses.[23] The group process itself has a very positive motivating effect. Fears are sometimes expressed that inappropriate behaviours and attitudes may be developed, but with adequate facilitation this can be avoided. General experience is that it is usually the most positive attitudes that are likely to acquire consensus rather than the negative. Groups, however, are often difficult to set up and maintain. The rules of group processes have to be observed with careful timetabling and avoidance of newcomers dropping in and out.

However, as an alternative, individual patients may be invited or may offer to act as mentors on a one-to-one basis. In the programme of care, all should be offered the possibility of access to discuss their problems, whether in a group or on a one-to-one basis with fellow sufferers.

New technology

A large amount of written audio and visual material has been provided for patient education in attempts to empower them to look after themselves. Although much of this is exemplary in content, it is professionally produced and very often the professional voice is self-evident, whether it be in script, audio, or visual form. Improvements have taken place with videotapes in which the patients' voice can be better presented. However, new technology using multimedia allows a much more patient-oriented approach. As this material can be computer based and menu driven, it allows ease of access and choice of the material to be studied in a way which is not possible with written material and cumbersome with traditional video material. It places the learning process much more in the patient's hands. With programmes such as 'Learning Diabetes', this process is taken even further by the use of multiple video slips, enabling the user to obtain access to the attitudes, beliefs, and strategies adopted by a very wide range of subjects.[24] In the development of the latter programme it was notable that if the spoken voice was used to provide factual material, this was less successful than by neutral written script. Presumably this was because the former was perceived by the listener as professionals talking.

The role of lay associations

These can be extremely helpful in raising the profile of patient self-care and empowerment. A powerful group of those with diabetes is likely to include those who are most self-empowered and will help promote the principles. This works best where the lay and professional associations with responsibilities for the care of diabetes work closely in tandem, as, for example, in the British and Finnish

Diabetes Associations. Where there are separate bodies, professional- and patient-vested interests may become polarized and provide barriers to progress.

Professional training

As alluded to above, there may be significant failures in training of professionals of all groups in the appropriate communication skills and understanding of the psychological features of diabetes if they are to facilitate self-empowerment. Much medical and nursing training, based as it is on the acute care model, overlooks the demands of managing chronic diseases. This is not isolated to the management of diabetes: it can equally be applied to the management of those with respiratory, cardiovascular, neurological and musculo-skeletal chronic disorders. Self-empowerment has been shown to be equally successful in the management of hypertension. It must be recognized that every discussion with a patient, however brief, may have a learning element, whether intended or unintended. If the professional participant is unaware and untrained, then such communication may have a negative rather than a positive effect on the learning process and that of empowerment. It is now recognized that much more detailed training than is available in the traditional undergraduate or immediate postgraduate curriculum is necessary. All participants within a diabetes care team must be included in such training.

In the development of these training programmes it is strongly recommended not only that they should be multidisciplinary, involving all members of a team, but also that they should encourage active participation of the patients. The Diabetes Education Study Group (DESG) has long recognized this and has shown that, in the Workshop format, the involvement of those with diabetes as equal participants rapidly results in promotion of awareness of the needs for self-empowerment and the factors which may facilitate or hinder this process.

Summary

Self-empowerment not only improves clinical outcome, but also patient satisfaction with treatment and quality of life. It is possible to identify factors which hinder or help this process. These include:

- development of communication skills amongst all diabetes care personnel;
- provision of a system of regular assessment of factors likely to inhibit self-empowerment;
- examination of systems of care and implementation of changes to avoid processes which act as barriers;
- promotion of the role of patients as teachers;
- the use of educational materials based on patient's needs and wants;
- involvement of patients in the educational process; and
- strengthening the roles of patient association.

References

1. Feste C, Anderson RM. *Empowerment: from Philosophy to Practice*. Amsterdam: Elsevier Science BV, 1995: 139–144.
2. Miller LV, Goldstein G. More efficient care of diabetic patients in a county-hospital setting. *N Eng J Med* 1972; **286**: 1388–1391.
3. DCCT Research Group. The effect of intensive treatment of diabetes on development and progression of long term complications in insulin dependent diabetes. *N Engl J Med* 1993; **329**: 977–986.

4. UK Prospective Study of Therapies of Maturity-onset Diabetes. 1. Effect of diet, sulphonylurea, insulin or biguanide therapy on fasting plasma glucose and body weight over one year. *Diabetologia* 1983; **24**: 404–411.

5. Morris AD, Boyle DI, McMahon AD *et al.* Adherence to insulin treatment, glycaemic control, and ketoacidosis in insulin-dependent diabetes mellitus. *Lancet* 1997; **350** (9090): 1505–1510.

6. Partridge MR. *Asthma: Lessons from Patient Education.* Amsterdam: Elsevier Science BV, 1995: 81–85.

7. Cantor JC, Morisky DE, Green LW *et al.* Cost-effectiveness of educational interventions to improve patient outcomes in blood pressure control. *Prev Med* 1985; **14**: 782–800.

8. Dunn SM, Beeney LJ, Hoskins PL, Turtle JR. Knowledge and attitude change as predictors of metabolic improvement in diabetes education. *Soc Sci Med* 1990; **31**: 1135–1141.

9. Frost G. Comparison of two methods of energy prescription for obese non-insulin dependent diabetics. *Pract Diabetes* 1989; **6**: 273–275.

10. Coles C. Psychology in diabetes care. *Pract Diabetes* 1996; **13**: 55–57.

11. Rosenstock IM, Strecher VJ, Becker MH. Social learning theory and the health belief model. *Health Educ Q* 1988; **15**: 175–183.

12. Bradley C, Gamsu DS, Knight G *et al.* The use of diabetes specific perceived control and health belief measures to predict treatment choice and efficacy in a feasibility study of continuous subcutaneous insulin infusion pumps. *Psychol Health* 1987; **1**: 133–146.

13. Bradley C, Brewin CR, Gamsu DS, Moses JL. Development of scales to measure perceived control of diabetes mellitus and diabetes-related health beliefs. *Diabetic Med* 1984; **1**: 213–218.

14. Dunn SM. Reactions to educational techniques: coping strategies for diabetes and learning. *Diabetic Med* 1986; **3**: 419–429.

15. Bott U, Jorgens V, Grusser M *et al.* Predictors of glycaemic control in Type 1 diabetic patients after participation in an intensified treatment and teaching programme. *Diabetic Med* 1994; **11**: 362–371.

16. Ajzen I, Fishbein M. *Understanding Attitudes and Predicting Social Behaviour.* Englewood Cliffs NJ: Prentice Hall, 1980.

17. De Weerdt I, Visser AP, Kok G, Van Der Veen EA. Determinants of active self care behaviour of insulin treated patients with diabetes: implications of diabetes education. *Soc Sci Med* 1990; **30**: 605–615.

18. Prochaska JO, DiClemente CC. *Toward a Comprehensive Model of Change. Treating Addictive Behaviours.* New York: Plenum Press, 1986.

19. Bradley C. *Handbook of Psychology and Diabetes.* Chur, Switzerland: Harwood Academic Publishers, 1994.

20. Day JL, Bodmer CW, Dunn OM. Development of a questionnaire identifying factors responsible for successful self-management of insulin-treated diabetes. *Diabetic Med* 1996; **13**: 564–573.

21. Kaplan RM, Chadwick MW, Schimmel LE. Social learning intervention to promote metabolic control in type 1 diabetes mellitus: pilot experiment results. *Diabetes Care* 1985; **8**: 152–155.

22. Balint M. *The Doctor, his Patient and the Illness.* London: Pitman, 1957.

23. Groen JJ, Pelser HE. Newer concepts of teaching, learning and education and their application to the patient–doctor cooperation in the treatment of diabetes mellitus. *Ped Adolesc Endocrinol* 1982; **10**: 168–177.

24. Day JL, Rayman G, Hall L, Davies P. 'Learning Diabetes' – a multi-media learning package for patients, carers and professionals to improve chronic disease management. *Med Inform* 1997; **22**: 91–104.

Index

ABCD (Appropriate Blood pressure
    Control in Diabetes) 170
acarbose 305, 306
ACE genotype and diabetic
    nephropathy 170
ACE inhibitors 155–7, 166, 169–71,
    215, 303
acute coronary syndromes 209–22
adenosine diphosphate (ADP) receptor
    antagonists 214
adenosine triphosphate (ATP) 112
adipocyte 112–13
advanced glycation end-products see
    AGEs
AGE-LDL 79
AGE-receptor complex 71
AGEs 53–5, 153–4, 166
    anti-AGE strategies 82–3
    biochemistry of 68–9
    degradative mechanisms for removal
        of modified molecules 76–7
    endogenous 73–7
    exogenous 77
    formation with relevance to
        biological systems 73–7
    immunoreactivity 78, 81
        in glomerular podocyte cell 80
        in vitreous specimens 75
    impact on diabetic complications
        67–92
    in diabetic vascular complications
        77–82
    in macroangiopathy 77–9
    in microangiopathy 79–80
        in vitro evidence 81–2
        in vivo evidence 79–81
    long-lived molecules 74–5
    molecular structures 70
    receptor systems 70–3
    short-lived molecules 73
alanine aminotransferase (ALT) 287
albumin
    acylated insulin analogues binding
        to 251–3
    excretion rate (AER) 173
albumin/creatinine ratio 165
alcohol consumption 325

aldose reductase inhibitors (ARIs) 183
American Diabetes Association (ADA)
    7, 288, 317
angiotensin II 156, 166, 170
    receptor antagonists 171–2
angiotensin-converting enzyme (ACE)
    inhibition 166
angiotensin-converting enzyme
    inhibitors see ACE inhibitors
ankle brachial pressure index (ABPI)
    184
annual review 309–10
anti-CD3/CD4 monoclonal antibodies
    43
antigen-induced peripheral tolerance 44
antigen presenting cell (APC)-T cell
    interaction 34
antigen-specific immunotherapy 45–6
antigenic tolerance, immune deviation
    by 44
antihypertensive agents 298–300
    in normotension 172–3
antiplatelet agents 213–14
Antiplatelet Trialists' Collaboration
    214
antithrombin III 212
anti-TNF-α MoAb 44
apolipoprotein B 301
apoprotein B (ApoB) 73
applantation tonometry 148
L-arginine 155
L-arginine/NO pathway 142–3
arterial stiffness and endothelial
    function 146–8
Asp^{B28}-human insulin analogue see
    insulin aspart
aspirin 298–300, 302
atherosclerosis 143, 183, 209
autonomic neuropathy 181–2
    clinical features 182

Bacillus Calmette-Guerin (BCG)
    vaccination 39–40
beta-blockers 214
β-cell dysfunction 296
Bezafibrate Infarction Prevention (BIP)
    Study Group 214

blood glucose 305–7
blood pressure 281–2
blood pressure-lowering agents 302–3
body mass index (BMI) 117, 344
body-weight 282–3
brown adipose tissue (BAT) 114, 115,
    117
burden of diabetes 1, 6–9
Bypass Angioplasty Revascularization
    Investigation (BARI) trial 216

calcium channel blockers (CCBs) in
    diabetic nephropathy 171–2
callus formation 185
capsaicin 183
captopril in overt nephropathy 172
Captopril and Thrombolysis Study
    (CATS) trial 215
carbamazepine 183
carbohydrates 318, 328–30
cardiovascular disease (CVD) 131–4,
    146, 209, 296
cardiovascular risk
    assessment 297–304
    factors 295
    reduction in relation to therapeutic
        agents 170
    stratification 297–302
care
    cycle 342
    implementation 310–11
    organization 308–11
        in patient self-empowerment
            350–1
    requirements 308–9
CD4+ T cell subsets 42
Charcot arthropathy 188–90
Charcot foot 185
Charcot neuroarthropathy 183
cholesterol 322–3, 333
    intake 332
    levels 129
Cholesterol and Recurrent Events
    (CARE) study 134, 216, 301
cholesterol ester transfer protein
    (CETP) 126, 130
cigarette smoking 305

ciglitazone 269
clamp-derived insulin sensitivity index 279
Class II-peptide interaction 43
continuous subcutaneous insulin infusion (CSII) 241
coronary artery bypass grafting (CABG) 216
coronary artery disease 132
coronary circulation 144–5
coronary heart disease (CHD) 209–22, 298, 303
    management 213–18
cost of diabetes 1, 2
    to society 9–10
Coxsackievirus B (CBV) 36
cyclosporin A in prevention of Type 1 diabetes 37–8

diabetes
    animal models 144
    background 1
    burden of 1, 6–9
    education 307
    indirect costs to society 9–10
    terminology 1
    types 1
    see also Type 1 diabetes; Type 2 diabetes
Diabetes Control and Complications Trial (DCCT) 173–4, 217, 223, 224, 238, 342–3
diabetic dyslipidaemia 125–39
    epidemiology 131–4
    lipid lowering 133–4
    metabolism 125–31
    risk 132–3
diabetic embryopathy, DNA-AGE interactions as basis for 75–6
diabetic foot see foot problems
diabetic nephropathy 165–78
    and ACE genotype 170
    calcium channel blockers (CCBs) in 171–2
    ethnicity 168
    hypertension 168–9
    sodium restriction in 170–1
diabetic neuropathy (DN) 180–3
    clinical classification 180–1
    glycaemic control in 183
    treatment 183
diet 317–40
    compliance 328
    composition 318–33
    guidelines, barriers to compliance 333
    management goals 333
    meal frequency and timing 328
    practical approach 327–33
    scientific rationale 317–27
    total energy intake 317–18
    very low-calorie (VLCD) 318

diet-induced thermogenesis (DIT) 102
dietary fats 319–23, 330
dietary fibre 325, 332–3
    content of selected foods 326
DIGAMI study 217
dihydropyridine 171
diphethia toxin interleukin-2 recombinant fusion protein (DAB486 IL-2) 43
distal sensorimotor polyneuropathy, clinical and electrophysiological assessment 180
diurnal rhythm in hypertension 169
DNA-AGE interactions as basis for diabetic embryopathy 75–6
DNA chip technology 27
docosahexaenoic acid (DHA) 321
DPT-1 46
dyslipidaemia 281, 295

eicosapentaenoic acid (EPA) 321
end-stage renal disease (ESRD) 166
ENDIT 46
endothelial dysfunction 141–64
    and diabetes mellitus 143–4
    animal models 144
    clinical studies 144
    mechanisms 152–4
    therapeutic interventions 154–7
endothelial function 272, 282
    and arterial stiffness 146–8
endothelium, role of 149–52
endothelium-derived relaxing factor (EDRF) 141
erectile dysfunction 197–208
    aetiology 197–8
    history pro forma 200
    investigations 199–202
    management 202–4
    penile implants 205–7
    presentation 199
    psychological factors 199
    surgery 205–7
    vacuum devices 204–5
EUCLID study 172
euglycaemic insulin clamp 97, 275–7, 279
European Nicotinamide Diabetes Intervention Trial (ENDIT) 39
experimental allergic encephalitis (EAE) 44

FACET (Fosinopril vs Amlodipine Cardiovascular Events randomized Trial) 170
factors VII, IX, X and XII 212
fasting state 103
fat substitutes 331–2
fatty acids 330
financial costs 2, 4–6
fish oil 150–1, 155
flow-mediated dilatation (FMD) 146

foot-care education 191
foot problems 179–96
foot ulceration 179
    and amputation 182, 190
    biomechanical aspects 185
    classification 186–8
    footwear in 185
    grade 0 foot 186
    grade 1 ulcers 186–7
    grade 2 ulcers 187
    grade 3 ulcers 187–8
    grade 4 lesions 188
    management 186–8
    pathogenesis 180–6
    prevention 190–2
    risk factors 186
    screening 190–2
free fatty acids (FFAs) 112, 113, 118, 119, 125, 126

gangrene 188
    grade 5 lesions 188
genetic analysis 13–15
genetic heterogeneity, Type 2 diabetes 13, 21–7
genetic susceptibility, Type 1 diabetes 15, 35
genetics 13–32
gestational diabetes mellitus (GDM) 243
GISSI-2 213, 215
GISSI-3 215
glitazones 267, 271, 277
    combination with sulphonylureas or insulin 287
    contraindications 288
    monotherapy 287
    side-effects 287
Global Utilization of Streptokinase and Tissue Plasminogen Activator for Occluded Coronary Arteries (GUSTO-I) trial 212–13, 215
glomerular filtration rate (GFR) 165
glucokinase gene (GCK) 20
glucose clamp studies 97, 275–7, 279
glucose control 234
glucose disposition in peripheral target tissue 100
glucose metabolism, insulin actions on 99–102
glucose synthesis, intracellular routes in liver 102
glucose tolerance 295
    tests 278
glucose transporters 271
glucose uptake
    insulin-mediated 104
    insulin resistance of 108
glucotoxicity 53–66
    mediating 53
    PKC in 53–4
GLUT1 118, 270

GLUT2 102
GLUT4 99, 101, 217, 270
glutamate decarboxylase (GAD) 34, 36
glyburide 285
glycaemic control 224, 232, 237, 241,
    242, 245, 246, 305, 348
    diabetic neuropathy (DN) 183
    Type 1 diabetes 173–4
    Type 2 diabetes 174
glyceryl trinitrate (GTN) 150, 156
glycogen phosphorylase (GP) 102
glycogen synthase (GS) 99, 102, 270
glycogen synthetase 23
glycoprotein IIb/IIIa receptor 214
gradient gel electrophoresis 128
Gruppo Italiano per lo studio della
    Stretochinasi nell'Infarto
    miocardico 2 (GISSI-2) trial 213
GUSTO-1 212–13, 215

HDL 105, 111, 126, 211
    modified 126–9
HDL-cholesterol 105, 132, 167, 216,
    272, 281, 321, 322, 327
hepatic glucose production rates 273
hepatocyte nuclear transcription factor
    1α (HNF1α) 25
hexokinase II (HKII) 99
high-density lipoprotein see HDL
HLA-genes and Type 1 diabetes
    15–17
hormone dose–response curve 96
hormone-sensitive lipase (HSL) 101,
    105, 112
human insulin analogues 227
    see also specific analogues
human soluble insulin 226, 228
hydrogenated starch hydrolysates
    (HSHs) 329
hypercholesterolaemia 216
hyperglycaemia 295
    treatment 304
hyperinsulinaemic euglycaemic clamp
    procedure 97, 275–7, 279
hypertension 281–2, 295, 302–3
    clinical implications in diabetes
        168–9
    definition 168
    diabetic nephropathy 168–9
    diurnal rhythm in 169
    therapeutic options 169–70
Hypertension Optimal Treatment
    (HOT) study 302–3
hypertriglyceridaemia 125–6, 216, 301
hypoglycaemia, insulin therapy 237
hypoglycaemic agents 305–7

125I-labelled human soluble insulin 227
IDDM 151, 153
    see also Type 1 diabetes
IDDM1 17
IDDM2 17–18, 35

IDDM3 18
IDDM4 18
IDDM5 18–19
IDDM6 19
IDDM7 19
IDDM8 19
IDDM9 19
IDDM10 19
IDDM11 19
IDDM12 19–20
IDDM13 20
IDDM15 19
IDL 105
IGT 111–24, 277, 278, 280, 281, 282
    and obesity 118–20
immunointervention
    antigen identified for 45
    new approaches to 42–6
impact, of diabetes 1
impaired glucose tolerance see IGT
impotence
    investigation of 199
    presentation 199
insulin
    actions 106–7
    actions on glucose metabolism
        99–102
    dissociation process and subsequent
        absorption 226
    in prevention of Type 1 diabetes 38
    lipid metabolism 238
    primary structure 225
insulin analogues
    acylated, binding to albumin 251–3
    fast-acting 231–8
    increased isoelectric pH 249–51
    long-acting 248–53
    pre-mixed formulations 238–40
    rapid-acting 224–8
insulin aspart 229–31, 250
    in Type 1 diabetes 235–7
insulin-dependent diabetes see IDDM;
    Type 1 diabetes
insulin-like growth-factor 1 (IGF-1)
    82, 229
insulin Lispro 229, 230, 232–4
    clinical situations 244
    elderly diabetic patients 243
    external pump systems 241–2
    meal consumption and snacks
        240–1
    optimization strategies 244–6
    pregnancy 243–4
    safety 247–8
    serum insulin concentrations
        following bolus subcutaneous
        administration 239
    Type 1 diabetes 237
    Type 2 diabetes 235, 237
    young patients 242–3
insulin-mediated glucose disposal 100
insulin-mediated glucose uptake 104

insulin promoter factor (IPF-1) 25
insulin-receptor substrate-1 (IRS-1)
    gene 23
insulin receptors, IRS1 and IRS2 104
insulin resistance 93–110, 244, 272,
    296
    adaptation to 105–6
    before and after administration of
        troglitazone or placebo 279
    conditions associated with 107
    of glucose uptake 108
    pathophysiological features 102–5
    peripheral 274
    pre-diabetic conditions 277–81
    relevance to diabetes 108
    syndrome 95
    Type 2 diabetes 22, 274–7
insulin sensitivity 94, 107–8
    and plasma NEFA concentrations 101
    measurement in vivo 96–9
insulin sensitizers
    clinical studies 272–3
    mechanism of action 270–1
    pre-clinical studies 271
    safety 287
    Type 2 diabetes 267–93
    see also specific agents
insulin system 95
insulin therapy 223–65
    hypoglycaemia 237
    pharmacokinetic and
        pharmacodynamic studies
        228–31
    physical exercise 240
    preparation milestones 223
    primary 304
    quality of life issues 246–7
    secondary 307
    Type 2 diabetes 234–5
interferon-gamma (IFN-γ) 33, 42
interleukin 1 (IL-1) 211
interleukin 2 (IL-2) 42, 43
interleukin 4 (IL-4) 35, 42
interleukin 5 (IL-5) 42
interleukin 10 (IL-10) 42
intimal and medial thickness (IMT)
    282
intra-urethral prostaglandin 204
intravenous glucose tolerance test
    (IVGTT) 98, 274, 275, 277, 279,
    280
islet cell antibodies (ICAs) 33, 35
isolated systolic hypertension 173
isophane insuline 307

late autoimmune diabetes of the adult
    (LADA) 26
latent autoimmune diabetes in adults
    (LADA) 304
LDL 73, 77, 78, 105, 126, 153, 210,
    281
    modified 126–9

LDL-cholesterol 281, 303, 321, 323, 327
leptin 113–18, 283
 in animal models of obesity 114–16
 in human obesity 116–18
lifestyle adjustments 304–5
lignocaine 183
linkage analysis 13–14
lipids 174, 281
 abnormalities 152–3
 metabolism, insulin 238
 oxidation 281
lipohypertrophy 244
lipoprotein lipase (LPL) 105, 113
lipoproteins 211, 272, 295
 metabolism abnormalities 127
L-NMMA 142, 145, 146, 150
low-density lipoprotein see LDL

macrovascular complications 295
major histocompatibility complex (MHC) 35
maturity onset diabetes of the young (MODY) 24
Melbourne Diabetic Nephropathy Study (MDNS) 171
metformin 273, 274, 277, 285, 286, 288, 305, 306, 311
mexilitine 183
Michaelis–Menten approximation 96
microalbuminuria 165
 Type 1 diabetes 172
 Type 2 diabetes 172
microvascular disease 143
MIDAS (Multicentre Isradipine Diuretic Atherosclerosis Study) 170
minerals 325
MODY1 25
MODY2 24, 25
MODY3 25
MODYX 26
monoclonal antibodies, anti-CD3/CD4 43
monounsaturated fat 31
monounsaturated fatty acids 320, 330, 331
Multicenter Investigation of the Limitation of Infarct Size (MILIS) 213
MUSE 204
myocardial hypertrophy 272
myocardial infarction 299, 301

neuropeptide Y (NPY) 114
NHP insulin 224
nicotinamide, in prevention of Type 1 diabetes 38
NIDDM 151–3
 see also Type 2 diabetes
NIDDM1 25
nitric oxide (NO) 141, 156

nocturnal penile tumescence (NPT) monitoring 197–8
 traces 201–2
non-enzymatic glycation (NEG) reactions 68
non-esterified fatty acids (NEFA) 93, 94, 98, 101–5
non-HLA genes, and Type 1 diabetes 17, 20–1
non-insulin-dependent diabetes (NIDDM) see NIDDM; Type 2 diabetes
normoalbuminuria 172–3
normotension, antihypertensive agents in 172–3
NPH insulin 228, 231, 232, 234–6, 238, 239, 245–6, 249, 250, 253, 307
NPL insulin 238, 239

obesity 111–24, 295
 and IGT 118–20
 and Type 2 diabetes 118–20
 human, leptin in 116–18
 leptin in animal models 114–16
oral glucose tolerance test (OGTT) 117, 119
oxidative stress 152–3

pancreatic β-cell destruction 34
pancreatic insulin secretion 271, 281
patient self-empowerment 341–53
 attitudes of professionals 349
 care organization in 350–1
 emotional adjustment 345
 factors governing 343–52
 failures in professional training 352
 health beliefs 344–5
 identification of status of individuals 347–8
 new technology 351
 role of lay associations 351–2
 role of patients as teachers 351
 role of professional advisers 348–9
 role perception 349–50
 social environment 345–6
 targets 344
peripheral angiography 184
peripheral neuropathy, drug therapy 183
peripheral tolerance
 antigen-induced 44
 mechanisms of 41
peripheral vascular disease (PVD) 183–5
 clinical features 184
 treatment 185
peripheral vascular sympathetic denervation 183
peroxisome proliferator-activated receptor (PPAR) 270
peroxisome proliferator-activated receptor-γ (PPAR-γ) 23–4, 311

phenytoin 183
phosphoenolpyruvate carboxykinase (PEPCK) 102
phosphofructokinase (PFK) 99
phospholipid transfer protein (PLTP) 129
physical exercise, insulin therapy 240
phytochemicals 325–7
pioglitazone 53, 269, 271, 275, 276, 288
PKC
 activation in diabetes 54–5
 in glucotoxicity 53–4
 in TGF-β overexpression 56–8
 in vascular dysfunction 55–6
 potential mechanisms underlying development of chronic diabetic complications 55–60
 role in enhancing vascular permeability and stimulating neovascularization 59–60
plasma total cholesterol 321, 323
plasminogen activator inhibitor-1 (PAI-1) 106, 212, 280, 282, 295, 301
platelet-derived growth factor (PDGF) 211
platelet function 272
polycystic ovarian syndrome (PCOS) 280–2, 288
polyunsaturated fat 321
polyunsaturated fatty acids 320, 331
post-prandial dyslipidaemia 129–31
pramlintide 311
pregnancy, insulin Lispro in 243–4
protein intake 318–19, 330
protein kinase C see PKC
protein kinase C (PKC), activation 53–66
protein restriction 174
psychosexual counselling 203
psychosocial effects
 on patient 2–4
 on relatives 4
pulse wave velocity (PWV) 148–9
pulse waved analysis (PWA) 148–9, 151, 152
pyruvate dehydrogenase complex (PDH) 99

quality monitoring 310
quality of life issues in insulin therapy 246–7

renal disease, pathophysiology 165–6
renal function, assessing 165
renin–angiotensin system 170
repaglinide 311–12
retinoid X receptor (RXR) 269
rosiglitazone 269, 271, 284, 288, 311

St Vincent's declaration 190
saturated fatty acids 319–21

Second International Study of Infarct Survival (ISIS-2) trial 214
Semmes–Weinstein nylon monofilaments 190
smoking 305
social effects 2
sodium intake 323–5, 332
sodium restriction in diabetic nephropathy 170–1
statins 297–302
stroke 300
sulphonylureas 217, 273, 284–6, 288, 305, 311
Symptom Check List SCL-90 4
Syndrome X 131, 167

T cell reactivity in peripheral circulation 41
T cell repertoire 40–1
Th1 responses, inhibition of 43–5
Th1/Th2 cytokine balance 43, 46
Th1/Th2 paradigm 41–2, 43
thiazolidinedione 268
thiazolidine-2,4-dione 269
thiazolidinediones 269, 272, 283, 289, 311
    clinical indications 288
    effects on liver 273–4
Thrombolysis and Angioplasty in Myocardial Infarction Study Group (TAMI) 212
Thrombolysis in Myocardial Infarction II (TIMI-II) trial 213
thrombolytic therapy 215
thymus, role of 40–1
tissue-plasminogen activator (t-PA) 212
transaminases 287
transforming growth factor-β (TGF-β) 81, 166
    PKC in overexpression 56–8
triacylglycerol 322
tricyclics 183
triglyceride levels 128
troglitazone 269, 271–82, 287, 311
    adverse effects 287
    combination therapy 287, 288

with insulin 285–6
with metformin 285
with sulphonylurea and metformin 286
with sulphonylureas 284–5
drug interations 288
large-scale trials 283
monotherapy 283–4, 288
tumour necrosis factor alpha (TNF-α) 23, 33, 270, 271
Type 1 diabetes 1
    and HLA-genes 15–17
    and non-HLA genes 17, 20–1
    autoimmunity 40
    early environmental events 35
    genetic heterogeneity 13
    genetic susceptibility 15, 35
    glycaemic control 173–4
    insulin aspart 235–7
    insulin Lispro 237
    loci other than HLA (IDDM1) so far identified as being associated with 16
    microalbuminuria 172
    natural immune tolerance 40
    nephropathy 166–7
    pathogenesis 33–5
    prediction by genetic studies 26
    prevention 33–52
        strategies 35–6
    primary intervention 35–6
    randomized clinical intervention trials 37
    role of immunoregulation 35
    secondary prevention strategies 36
    specific immunotherapy 40
    tertiary prevention strategies 36
    see also IDDM
Type 2 diabetes 1
    and obesity 118–20
    candidate genes 22–4
    development 111
    dietary approach see diet
    genes identified by genome-wide searches 24–6
    genetic heterogeneity 13, 21–7
    glycaemic control 174

insulin Lispro 235, 237
insulin resistance 22, 274–7
insulin sensitizers 267–93
insulin therapy 234–5
metabolic abnormalities 268
microalbuminuria 172
monogenic 22–4
nephropathy 167
optimal control 295–315
polygenic 22–4
prediction by genetic studies 26
single genes identified and possible functional interaction 22–6
stepwise therapy 268, 289
treatment goals and benefits 303–4
treatment objectives 296–7
see also NIDDM
Type 3 diabetes 1
Type 4 diabetes 1

ultrasonic assessment of flow-mediated dilatation 146
United Kingdom Prospective Diabetes Study (UKPDS) 217, 223, 269, 296, 342–3

vascular endothelial growth factor (VEGF) 81–2
vascular endothelium 141
    functions 142
vascular smooth muscle 271–2
VEGF/VPF 53, 59–60
venous acclusion plethysmography 145–6
very-low-density lipoprotein see VLDL
vibration perception threshold (VPT) 181
vitamin C 154–5
vitamin E 154
vitamins 325
VLDL 105, 126, 129, 211, 272, 281
VLDL-cholesterol 321, 327
von Willebrand factor 295, 301

weight loss 306
weight management 327–8
white adipose tissue (WAT) 115